Clinics in
ORAL AND
MAXILLOFACIAL
SURGERY

Clinics in ORAL AND MAXILLOFACIAL SURGERY

SM Sharma MDS

Professor and Head
Department of Oral and Maxillofacial Surgery
AB Shetty Memorial Institute of Dental Sciences
Nitte University
Mangalore, Karnataka, India

Foreword
Rajendra Prasad

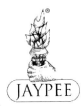

JAYPEE BROTHERS MEDICAL PUBLISHERS (P) LTD

New Delhi • Panama City • London • Philadelphia

Jaypee Brothers Medical Publishers (P) Ltd

Headquarters

Jaypee Brothers Medical Publishers (P) Ltd
4838/24, Ansari Road, Daryaganj
New Delhi 110 002, India
Phone: +91-11-43574357
Fax: +91-11-43574314
Email: jaypee@jaypeebrothers.com

Overseas Offices

J.P. Medical Ltd
83 Victoria Street, London
SW1H 0HW (UK)
Phone: +44-2031708910
Fax: +02-03-0086180
Email: info@jpmedpub.com

Jaypee Medical Inc.
The Bourse
111 South Independence Mall East
Suite 835, Philadelphia, PA 19106, USA
Phone: + 267-519-9789
Email: joe.rusko@jaypeebrothers.com

Jaypee Brothers Medical Publishers (P) Ltd
Shorakhute, Kathmandu
Nepal
Phone: +00977-9841528578
Email: jaypee.nepal@gmail.com

Jaypee-Highlights Medical Publishers Inc.
City of Knowledge, Bld. 237, Clayton
Panama City, Panama
Phone: + 507-301-0496
Fax: + 507-301-0499
Email: cservice@jphmedical.com

Jaypee Brothers Medical Publishers (P) Ltd
17/1-B Babar Road, Block-B, Shaymali
Mohammadpur, Dhaka-1207
Bangladesh
Mobile: +08801912003485
Email: jaypeedhaka@gmail.com

Website: www.jaypeebrothers.com
Website: www.jaypeedigital.com

Inquiries for bulk sales may be solicited at: jaypee@jaypeebrothers.com

This book has been published in good faith that the contents provided by the author(s) contained herein are original, and is intended for educational purposes only. While every effort is made to ensure an accuracy of information, the publisher and the author(s) specifically disclaim any damage, liability, or loss incurred, directly or indirectly, from the use or application of any of the contents of this work. If not specifically stated, all figures and tables are courtesy of the author(s). Where appropriate, the readers should consult with a specialist or contact the manufacturer of the drug or device.

Clinics in Oral and Maxillofacial Surgery

First Edition: **2013**

ISBN 978-93-5090-615-6

Printed at: S. Narayan & Sons

Dedicated to

Past, Present
and
Future Postgraduates

Foreword

Dental and oral organs are the part of digestive system of human body. Since they are exposed to various insults of environment and also exhibit their signs about systemic conditions, the science of dentistry has developed into various specialties.

Oral and maxillofacial surgery has many facets of ailment pertaining to these organs. As surgery is an important component and is most appealing as well as challenging for the dental students, the book *Clinics in Oral and Maxillofacial Surgery* has been authored by Dr SM Sharma. It is very apt that the practice of this science and controversies in modality of treatment and complications encountered are discussed in detail with suitable illustrations.

The completion, reasoning, and also suitable relevant description make the students/practitioners to understand and adopt this in their clinical works. The goal of any treatment is immediate relief from agony and, secondly, conservation of tissue as much possible, with careful, clear-cut dissection, controlling perioperative events, and promoting wound healing.

The contribution from basic medical sciences is defining anatomy, physiology, pathogenesis, and microbiological implication on oral tissues. The diagonosis and treatment planning is complex process of factual and reasonable judgment. The author has pointed out simple clues to arrive at diagnosis.

The postgraduate students can refer to this voulme for their applied knowledge in this specialty.

I hereby congratulate Dr SM Sharma for his contribution and wish him good success in his endeavor and also wish more work of this kind is produced by him in future.

Rajendra Prasad
Principal
AB Shetty Memorial Institute of Dental Sciences
Nitte University
Mangalore, Karnataka, India

Message

Professor Sharma has taken great efforts over several years to collect a very comprehensive volume of case studies illustrating the entire gamut of maxillofacial surgery. It is highly commendable that he has now decided to place this wealth of information at the disposal of postgraduates and faculty as a means of enhancing interest and understanding of clinical methodology.

Today, we have an overwhelming amount of books, specialized journals, and scholarly papers providing information about every facet of oral and maxillofacial surgery. Without knowledge and understanding, there can be no pursuit of clinical excellence, and the value of books and Internet searches cannot be underestimated. Nevertheless, only direct encounter with clinical situations and visualization of clinical problems awaken the mind to relate what is stored in memory to reality. As the process of logical decision making and adaptation of algorithms enable us to make choices with regard to optimal management of disease, and as we acquire the skills needed to implement therapies, our gradual transformation into maturity as clinicians takes place. Indeed, if we are sensitive enough, possess discipline to constantly improve our innate talents and remain humble, our clinical practice can truly have a transforming impact on our patients and also us.

The book *Clinics in Oral and Maxillofacial Surgery* places on record the considerable experience of Professor Sharma as a teacher and the lessons learnt in oral and maxillofacial surgery practice over several decades in the form of clinical cases. I am sure this book will be of immense value.

Paul C Salins
Vice-President/Medical Director
Chief, Craniofacial Surgery
Narayana Hrudayalaya Hospitals
Bengaluru, Karnataka, India

Preface

For quite sometime, I was thinking of writing a book, but a question remained that when there are so many books in the market, current trends, issues, contemporaries or advances, then what is the need of another book. During many years of my clinical experience and as an examiner, I felt that postgraduates should be thorough with the recent updates so that they can present and prepare themselves for the clinical examination. They should know a good clinical case presentation method with relevant questions normally an examiner asks and also specific examination cases, discussion, instruments, etc. I feel that there is a need of the book *Clinics of Oral and Maxillofacial Surgery* that will help students in the preparation for examination. The book will also be of immense value for students preparing for national board examination and even the faculty.

We are living in an era of explosion of knowledge. Definitely, new things and new cases are coming each day, and it is not the last word written here. Of course, postgraduates should also refer other specific books for detailed theory knowledge. Ultimately, goal is to provide the best knowledge and, thereby, a good care for our patients.

Listening to patient is more difficult and important rather just talking to him. Lord Platinom, one of the greatest teachers at the University College of Medicine in London, was of the firm opinion that if you listen to your patient long enough, he/she will fully guide you what is wrong with him/her.

Clinicians can learn many things from the patients either at bedside or chairside. Each patient is like a book. No two patients are alike even with the same disease, as every disease presents itself through the personality of the patient. The habit of learning books by heart does not work here. Books are necessary to keep in touch with the basics of clinical practice. I assure *Clinics in Oral and Maxillofacial Surgery* will bring vital information to enhance the knowledge of clinical aspects of the subject.

SM Sharma

Contents

Section 3: Carcinomas of Oral Cavity

Section

1

Basic Surgical Principles and Perioperative Management

Clinical Approach to Oral and Maxillofacial Surgical Patients

1

INTRODUCTION

Every patient is unique in the contemporary oral and maxillofacial surgery. The skills we bring to bear in daily clinical work-up are so diverse that positive impact we have on our profession and the health of our patient makes us proud to be known as Oral and Maxillofacial Surgeons.

Oral and maxillofacial surgery provide an extensive surgical services including management of traumatic injuries of maxillofacial structure, pathology and eventual reconstruction, minor oral surgery, placement of implant, orthognathic reconstruction of the facial deformity and distraction osteogenesis. Thus, the specialty is recognized for excellent ability and adapt to changes in public need for prosperous health, setting the highest goals.

Oral and maxillofacial surgery is a unique specialty that deals with the gentle structures of the facial skeleton, oral cavity and the neck and that covers a broad spectrum extending from oral malignancies, facial injuries, facial deformities and facial reconstruction to impacted 3rd molars, dental implants and generally minor oral surgery. This legacy of greatness must pass on to the next generation of oral and maxillofacial surgeons.

As an oral and maxillofacial surgeon, we are responsible for the diagnosis and treatment of traumatic, congenital, developmental and iatrogenic lesions in maxillofacial complex. Risk management in oral and maxillofacial surgery should begin with the golden rule. Treat patients the way you would treat your parents, spouse or children. The patients should receive the highest quality of care and for this listening to symptoms and concerns of the patients and appropriate evaluation through complete examination and diagnostic tests are the priorities.

Consider treatment options by joint clinics or clinicopathological discussions so that the best possible treatment is chosen. This will help to understand the risks, benefits and possible complications of the various treatment options including in some cases no treatment. The whole exercise should be legibly documented in records and explained to the patient and the family.

The management of oral and maxillofacial disorders besides the application of technical skills also requires training in basic sciences for diagnosis and treatment and a genuine sympathy and love for the patient.

Maxillofacial surgeon must also maintain good cordial behavior to his/ her fellow colleagues and subordinates.

This chapter addresses the rationale and method for gathering relevant medical and dental information (including the examination of the patient) and the use of this information for treatment. This process can be divided into the following four parts:

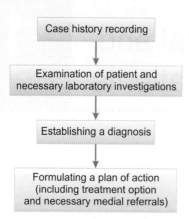

When did this problem start?

What did you notice first?

Did you have any problems or symptoms related to this?

What makes the problem worse or better?

Have the symptoms gotten better or worse at any time?

Have any tests been performed to diagnose this complaint?

Have you consulted other, oral and maxillofacial surgeons, or anyone else related to this problem?

What have you done to treat these symptoms?

CASE HISTORY

A detailed and concise compilation of all physical, dental, and social, factors relative and essential to diagnosis, prognosis, and treatment.

CHIEF COMPLAINT

The chief complaint is established by asking the patient to describe the problem for which he or she is seeking help or treatment.

- The chief complaint is recorded in the patient's own words as much as possible.

HISTORY OF THE PRESENT ILLNESS

The history of present illness is the course of the patient's chief complaint: when and how it began; direct and specific questions are used to elicit this information.

MEDICAL HISTORY

- Obtaining a medical history is an information gathering process for assessing a patient's health status. The medical history comprises a systematic review of the patient's chief or primary complaint, a detailed history related to this complaint, information about past and present medical conditions, pertinent social and family histories, and a review of symptoms by organ system

- An appropriate interpretation of the information collected through a medical history achieves three important objectives:
  - It enables the monitoring of medical conditions and the evaluation of underlying systemic conditions of which the patient may or may not be aware
  - It provides a basis for determining whether dental treatment might affect the systemic health of the patient, and
  - It provides an initial starting point for assessing the possible influence of the patient's systemic health on the patient's oral health and/or dental treatment.
- The components of a medical history may vary slightly, but most medical histories contain specific information under specific headings
- Information on the health of the patient can be arbitrarily divided into objective and subjective information
- The objective information consists of an account of the patient's past medical history, as well as information gained by physical and supplementary examination procedures (i.e. signs)
- The subjective information (i.e. symptoms) is a report of the patient's own sensory experience but can also be second hand, as in the case of children or others unable to communicate for

themselves. This second hand information is often used to confirm and supplement a patient's description of his or her complaint

- The past medical history is usually organized into the following subdivisions:

Serious or significant illnesses
Hospitalizations
Transfusions
Allergies
Medications
Pregnancy

Serious or Significant Illnesses

- The patient is asked to enumerate illnesses that required (or require) the attention of a physician, that necessitated staying in bed for longer than 3 days, or for which the patient was (or is being) routinely medicated
- Specific questions are asked about any history of heart, liver, kidney, or lung diseases; congenital conditions; infectious diseases; immunologic disorders; diabetes or hormonal problems; radiation or cancer chemotherapy; blood dyscrasias or treatment.

Hospitalizations

- A record of hospital admissions complements the information collected on serious illnesses and may reveal significant events such as surgeries that were not previously reported
- A history of blood transfusions, including the date of each transfusion and the number of transfused blood units, may indicate a previous serious medical or surgical problem that can be important in the evaluation of the patient's medical status.

Allergies

The patient's record should document any history of classic allergic reactions, such as urticaria, hay fever, asthma, or eczema, as well as any untoward

or adverse drug reaction to medications, local anesthetic agents, foods, or diagnostic procedures.

Medications

- An essential component of a medication history is a record of all the medications a patient is taking
- Identification of medications helps in the recognition of drug induced (iatrogenic) disease and oral disorders associated with different medications and in the avoidance of untoward drug interactions
- The types of medications, as well as changes in dosages over time, often give an indication of the status of underlying conditions and diseases.

Pregnancy

Knowing whether or not a woman of childbearing age is pregnant is particularly important when deciding to administer or prescribe any medication.

SOCIAL HISTORY

Different social parameters should be recorded; occupation; tobacco use when obtaining the social history, the clinician should take into account the patient's chief complaint and past medical history in order to gather specific information pertinent to the patient's oral and maxillofacial surgical management.

FAMILY HISTORY

Serious medical problems in immediate family members (including parents, siblings, spouse, and children) should be listed.

Disorders known to have a genetic or environmental basis (such as certain forms of cancer, cardiovascular disease including hypertension, allergies, asthma, renal disease, stomach ulcers, diabetes mellitus, bleeding disorders, and sickle cell anemia) should be addressed. Also noted are whether parents, siblings, or offspring are alive or dead; if dead, the age at death and cause of death are recorded. This type of information will alert the clinician to the patient's predisposition to develop serious medical conditions.

REVIEW OF SYSTEMS

The review of systems is a comprehensive and systematic review of subjective symptoms affecting different bodily systems. It includes the following categories:

- General
- Head, eyes, ears, nose, and throat
- Cardiovascular
- Respiratory
- Dermatologic
- Hematologic-lymphatic
- Neuropsychiatric.

EXAMINATION OF THE PATIENT— GENERAL PROCEDURE

A thorough and systematic inspection of the oral cavity and adnexal tissues minimizes the possibility of overlooking previously undiscovered pathologies. The examination is most conveniently carried out with the patient seated in a dental chair, with the head supported or examination table. Before seating the patient, the clinician should observe the patient's general appearance and gait and should note any physical deformities or handicaps.

The routine oral examination should be carried out. Laboratory studies and additional special examination of other organ systems may be required for the evaluation of patients with orofacial pain or signs and symptoms suggestive of salivary gland disorders or pathologies suggestive of a systemic etiology.

Examination carried out in oral and maxillofacial surgery clinic is restricted to that of the superficial tissues of the oral cavity, head, and neck and the exposed parts of the extremities. On occasion, evaluation of an oral lesion logically leads to an inquiry about similar lesions on other skin or mucosal surfaces or about the enlargement of other regional groups of lymph nodes. Although these enquiries can usually be satisfied directly by questioning the patient, the surgeon may also quite appropriately request permission from the patient to examine axillary nodes or other skin surfaces, provided the examination is carried out competently.

Evaluation Protocol

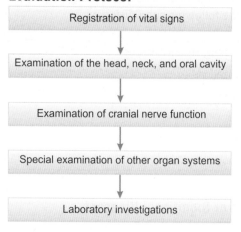

VITAL SIGNS

Vital signs (respiratory rate, temperature, pulse, and blood pressure) are routinely recorded as part of the examination.

In addition to being useful as an indicator of systemic disease, this information is essential as a standard of reference should syncope or other untoward medical complications arise during patient treatment.

Respiratory Rate

Normal respiratory rate during rest is 14–20 breaths per minute. Any more rapid breathing is called tachypnea and may be associated with underlying disease and/or elevated temperature.

Temperature

The normal oral (sublingual) temperature is 37°C (98.6°F), but oral temperatures <37.8°C (100°F) are not usually considered to be significant. Studies of sublingual, axillary, auditory canal and rectal temperatures in elderly patients indicate that these traditionally accepted values differ somewhat from statistically determined values. Recent drinking of hot or cold liquids or mouth breathing in very warm or cold air may alter the oral temperature. Also, severe oral infection may alter the local temperature in the mouth without causing fever.

Pulse Rate and Rhythm

The normal resting pulse rate is between 60 and 100 beats per minute (bpm). A patient with a pulse rate >100 bpm (tachycardia), even considering the stress of a surgery, should be allowed to rest quietly to allow the pulse to return to normal before the start of treatment. If the patient's pulse rate remains persistently high, medical evaluation of the tachycardia is appropriate because severe coronary artery disease or myocardial disease may be present. Note that the pulse rate normally rises about 5–10 bpm with each degree of fever.

Rates that are consistently < 60 bpm (bradycardia) warrant medical evaluation although sinus bradycardia, a common condition, can be normal.

Although a healthy person may have occasional irregularities or premature beats (especially when under stress) a grossly irregular pulse can indicate severe myocardial disease (arrhythmia or dysrhythmia), justifying further cardiac evaluation. Cardiac consultation is necessary for the accurate interpretation of most pulse rate abnormalities. Pulse rate abnormalities may be regular or irregular. Irregular rate abnormalities may be divided further into regularly irregular and irregularly irregular abnormalities.

Blood Pressure

Blood pressure should be measured with appropriate equipment and in a standardized fashion. Although sphygmomanometers are the most accurate devices, validated electronic devices or aneroid sphygmomanometers with appropriately sized cuffs are sufficient for blood pressure screening. Electronic devices are usually accurate to within 3 percent of a manual sphygmomanometer. Their ease of use in comparison with manual sphygmomanometers is a great advantage and encourages increased use. Both blood pressure and pulse are recorded, but irregular rhythms cannot be detected. To detect potential deviations, electronic devices should occasionally be calibrated against a manual sphygmomanometer.

If the cuff is applied too loosely, if it is not completely deflated before applying, or if it is too small for the patient's arm, the pressure readings obtained will be erroneously high and will not represent the pressure in the artery at the time of measurement.

CRANIOFACIAL REGION EXAMINATION

The ability to perform thorough physical examination of superficial structures of head, neck and oral cavity is essential. To perform this examination procedure successfully oral and maxillofacial surgeon should have knowledge of:

- Anatomy of craniofacial region
- He should know the technique for displaying mucosal surfaces and skin of craniofacial region with minimum discomfort to the patient
- He should have the knowledge of pathology of oral and maxillofacial region
- He should have ability to record both normal and abnormal findings
- He should know the general appearance of the patient and general nutritional status
- He should study the character of skin and the presence of petechiae and eruption
- He should be able to determine the reaction of pupil to light and accommodation especially when neurological disorders are being investigated
- Superficial and deep lymph nodes of the neck are examined from behind the patient when patient head is inclined forward
- Inner surfaces of lips mucosa of the cheek maxillary and mandibular mucobuccal fold the palate tongue sublingual space gingival and supporting structures
- Examine tonsillar and pharyngeal areas
- Examine the tongue, sublingual space, oropharynx
- Examine the occlusion.

FACIAL STRUCTURES

Observe the patient's skin for color, blemishes, moles, and other pigmentation abnormalities; vascular anomalies such as angiomas, telangiectasias, nevi, and tortuous superficial vessels; and asymmetry, ulcers, pustules, nodules, and swellings.

Note the color of the conjunctivae. Palpate the jaws and superficial masticatory muscles for tenderness or deformity. Note any scars or keloid formation.

LIPS

Note lip color, texture, and any surface abnormalities as well as angular or vertical fissures, lip pits, cold sores and, ulcers.

CHEEKS

Note any changes in pigmentation of the mucosa, a pronounced linea alba, leukoedema, hyperkeratotic patches, intraoral swellings, ulcers, nodules, scars, other red or white patches, and Fordyce's granules. Observe openings of Stensen's ducts and establish their patency by first drying the mucosa with gauze and then observing the character and extent of salivary flow from duct openings, with and without milking of the gland. Palpate muscles of mastication.

MAXILLARY AND MANDIBULAR MUCOBUCCAL FOLDS

Observe color, texture, any swellings, and any fistulae. Palpate for swellings and tenderness over the roots of the teeth and for tenderness of the buccinator insertion by pressing laterally with a finger inserted over the roots of the upper molar teeth.

HARD PALATE AND SOFT PALATE

Illuminate the palate and inspect for discoloration, swellings, fistulae, papillary hyperplasia, tori, ulcers, recent burns, leukoplakia, and asymmetry of structure or function.

Examine the orifices of minor salivary glands. Palpate the palate for swellings and tenderness.

TONGUE

Inspect the dorsum of the tongue (while it is at rest) for any swelling, ulcers, coating, or variation in size, color, and texture.

Observe the margins of the tongue and note the distribution of various papillae. Note the frenal attachment and any deviations as the patient pushes out the tongue and attempts to move it to the right and left up down to see ankyloglossia?

Wrap a piece of gauze around the tip of the protruding tongue to steady it, and lightly press a warm mirror against the uvula to observe the base of the tongue and vallate papillae; note any ulcers or significant swellings. Holding the tongue with the gauze, gently guide the tongue to the right and retract the left cheek to observe the foliate papillae and the entire lateral border of the tongue for ulcers, keratotic areas, and red patches. Repeat for the opposite side, and then have the patient touch the tip of the tongue to the palate to display the ventral surface of the tongue and floor of the mouth; note any varicosities, tight frenal attachments, stones in Wharton's ducts, ulcers, swellings, and red or white patches. Gently palpate the muscles of the tongue for nodules and tumors, extending the finger onto the base of the tongue and pressing forward if this has been poorly visualized or if any ulcers or masses are suspected. Note tongue thrust on swallowing.

FLOOR OF THE MOUTH

With the tongue still elevated, observe the openings of Wharton's ducts, the salivary pool, the character and extent of right and left secretions, and any swellings, ulcers, or red or white patches.

Gently explore and display the extent of the lateral sublingual space, again noting ulcers and red or white patches.

GINGIVAE

Observe color, texture, contour, and frenal attachments. Note any ulcers, marginal inflammation, resorption, festooning, Stillman's clefts, hyperplasia, nodules, swellings, and fistulae.

TEETH AND PERIODONTIUM

Note missing or supernumerary teeth, mobile or painful teeth, caries, defective restorations, dental arch irregularities, orthodontic anomalies, abnormal jaw relationships, occlusal interferences, the extent of plaque and calculus deposits, dental hypoplasia, and discolored teeth.

TONSILS AND OROPHARYNX

Note the color, size, and any surface abnormalities of tonsils and ulcers, tonsilloliths, and inspissated secretion in tonsillar crypts. Palpate the tonsils for discharge or tenderness, and note restriction of the oropharyngeal airway. Examine the faucial pillars for bilateral symmetry, nodules, red and white patches, lymphoid aggregates, and deformities. Examine the postpharyngeal wall for swellings, nodular lymphoid hyperplasia, hyperplastic adenoids, postnasal discharge, mucus secretions.

SALIVARY GLANDS

Note any external swelling that may represent enlargement of a major salivary gland. A significantly enlarged parotid gland will alter the facial contour and may lift the ear lobe; an enlarged submandibular salivary gland (or lymph node) may distend the skin over the submandibular triangle. With minimal manipulation of the patient's lips, tongue, and cheeks, note the presence of any salivary pool, and note whether the mucosa is moist, covered with scanty frothy saliva, or dry. To evaluate parotid gland function, dry the cheek mucosa around the orifice of each parotid duct, and massage or "milk" the gland and duct externally, observing the amount and character of any excreted material. With a normal gland, clear and freely flowing saliva will be readily apparent.

When salivary flow is reduced, there may be a brief flow of viscous or cloudy saliva, followed by a small amount of apparently normal saliva; this emphasizes the need for careful observation of the initial flow. Psychic stimuli (such as asking the patient to think of a cold refreshing lemon drink on a hot day) may also be used to increase the flow of parotid saliva during the examination. Palpate any suspected parotid swelling externally at this time, recording texture and any tenderness or nodularity; distinguish parotid enlargement from hypertrophy and spasm of the masseter muscle.

For the submandibular and sublingual glands, use bimanual palpation (insert the gloved index finger beside the tongue in the floor of the mouth and locate the two salivary glands and any enlarged submandibular lymph nodes, using a second finger placed externally over the gland); note the location, texture, and size of each gland and any tenderness or nodules. Dry the orifices of both Wharton's ducts and note the amount and character of the excreted saliva as one and then the other submandibular glands and ducts are "milked." Palpate Wharton's duct on each side for any salivary calculi. When either the parotid or the submandibular/sublingual salivary flow appears minimal, flow may often be stimulated by either gustatory stimuli (such as lemon juice swabbed on the tongue dorsum) or painful stimuli (e.g. pricking the gingiva with an explorer). With stimulation of the salivary flow, minor salivary gland function can be demonstrated by the appearance of multiple small beads of saliva on the dried upper- and lower-lip mucosa.

Temporomandibular Joint

Mandibular deviation while opening and closing the jaw
Range of vertical and lateral movements
Palpate the joints, and listen for clicking and crepitus during opening and closing of the jaw
Note any tenderness over the joint or masticatory muscles
Explore the anterior wall of external auditory meatus for tenderness

NECK AND LYMPH NODES

Examination of the neck includes examination of the submandibular and cervical lymph nodes, the midline structures (hyoid bone, cricoids and thyroid cartilages, trachea, and thyroid gland), and carotid arteries and neck veins.

With the patient's neck extended, note the clavicle and the sternomastoid and trapezius muscles, which define the anterior and posterior triangles of the neck. Palpate the hyoid bone, the thyroid and cricoid cartilages, and the trachea, noting any displacement or tenderness.

Palpate around the lower half of the sternomastoid muscle, and identify and palpate the isthmus and wings of the thyroid gland below and lateral to the thyroid cartilage, checking for any nodularity, masses, or tenderness. If local or generalized thyroid enlargement is suspected, check to ascertain whether the mass moves up and down with the trachea when the patient swallows. Observe the external jugular vein as it crosses the sternomastoid muscle, and with the patient at an angle of approximately 45° to the horizontal, note any distension and/or pulsation in the vein. Distension more than 2 cm above the sternal notch is abnormal; in severe right-sided heart failure, distension as far as the angle of the mandible may be seen. Place the diaphragm of the stethoscope over the point of the carotid pulse, and listen for bruits or other disturbances of rhythm that may indicate partial occlusion of the carotid artery.

Palpate for lymph nodes in the neck commencing with the most superior nodes and working down to the clavicle. Palpate anterior to the tragus of the ear for preauricular nodes; at the mastoid and base of the skull for posterior auricular and occipital nodes; under the chin for the submental nodes; and further posterior for submandibular and lingual-notch nodes. The superficial cervical nodes lie above the sternomastoid muscle; the deep cervical nodes lie between the sternomastoid muscle and cervical fascia. To examine the latter, ask the patient to sit erect and to turn his or her head to one side to relax the sternomastoid; use thumb and fingers to palpate under the anterior and posterior borders of the relaxed muscle, and repeat the procedure on the opposite side. Next, palpate the posterior cervical nodes in the posterior triangle close to the anterior border of the trapezius muscle. Finally, check for supraclavicular nodes just above the clavicle, lateral to the attachment of the sternomastoid muscle.

Normal lymph nodes may be difficult to palpate; enlarged lymph nodes (whether due to current infection, scarring from past inflammatory processes, or neoplastic involvement) are usually readily located. Many patients have isolated enlarged and freely movable submandibular and cervical nodes from past oral or pharyngeal infection. Nodes draining areas of active infection are usually tender; the overlying skin may be warm and red, and there may be a history of recent enlargement.

Nodes enlarged as the result of metastatic spread of a malignant tumor have no characteristic clinical appearance and may be small and asymptomatic or grossly enlarged. Classically, nodes enlarged due to cancer are described as "fixed to underlying tissue" (implying that the tumor cells have broken through the capsule of the lymph node or that necrosis and inflammation have produced perinodular scarring and adhesions), but this feature will usually be absent except with the most aggressive or advanced tumors.

Gradually enlarging groups of nodes in the absence of local infection and inflammation are a significant finding that suggests either systemic disease [e.g. infectious mononucleosis or generalized lymphadenopathy associated with human immunodeficiency virus (HIV) infection] or a lymphoid neoplasm (lymphoma or Hodgkin's disease); such a finding justifies examination for (or inquiry about) lymphoid enlargement at distant sites, such as the axilla, inguinal region, and spleen, to confirm the generalized nature of the process. A successful outcome to cancer treatment is dependent on early detection and treatment, and hence the need for rapid follow up investigation whenever unexplained lymph node enlargement is detected during examination of the neck.

Enlargement of supraclavicular and cervical nodes may occur from lymphatic spread of tumor from the thorax, breast, and arm as well as from tumors of the oral cavity and nasopharynx. Conditions to be considered in a patient with cervical lymph node enlargement include acute bacterial, viral, and rickettsial infections of the head and neck (e.g. acute abscesses, infectious mononucleosis, cat-scratch disease, and mucocutaneous lymph node syndrome); chronic bacterial infections, such as syphilis and tuberculosis; leukemia, lymphoma, metastatic carcinoma, collagen disease, and allergic reactions and sarcoidosis.

Preoperative Care and Evaluation

2

INTRODUCTION

Preoperative care and evaluation of oral and maxillofacial patient is the preparation and management of a patient prior to surgery. It includes both physical and psychological preparation. Although importance of a thorough history and physical examination remains key element in the preoperative evaluation of all patients.

Preoperative patient management period, maxillofacial pathology, defects and injuries are assessed and accurate decision is made for a surgical intervention. Patient is appropriately apprised of the problems, procedure and the need for surgery as well as options available and necessary preoperative evaluation and preparation is completed.

DEFINITION

The patient management period during which oral and maxillofacial pathology, defects and injury are assessed and diagnosed, an accurate decision is made for a surgical intervention; the patient and family are appropriately appraised of the condition; problem and need for surgery as well as options available.

PREOPERATIVE EVALUATION

Preoperative evaluation of a patient before surgery for the purpose of detecting factors that could affect surgical outcome and may include in addition to a thorough examination, laboratory testing, echo study, imaging procedures, and neurosurgical consultation. Preoperative patient conditions are significant predictors of postoperative complications.

Aim

- Patients who are physically and psychologically prepared for surgery tend to have better surgical outcomes
- Preoperative teaching meets the patient's need for information regarding the surgical experience, which in turn may alleviate most of patients fears. Patients who are more knowledgeable about what to expect after surgery, and who have an opportunity to express their goals and opinions, often cope better with postoperative pain and decreased mobility
- Preoperative care is extremely important prior to any invasive procedure, regardless of whether the procedure is minimally invasive or a form of major surgery
- Preoperative teaching must be individualized for each patient. Some people want as much information as possible, while others prefer only minimal information because too much knowledge may increase their anxiety
- Patients have different abilities to comprehend medical procedures; It is important for the patient to ask questions during preoperative teaching sessions.

Table 2.1: Modified American Society of Anesthesiologists (ASA) physical status may be more practical in recent use for preoperative risk assessment

A normal healthy patient
A patient with mild systemic disease
A patient with severe systemic disease that limits activity but is not incapacitating
A patient with severe systemic disease that is a constant threat to life
A moribund patient who is not expected to survive 24 hours without the operation

Description Assessment (Table 2.1)

- Preoperative care involves many components, and may be done the day before surgery in the hospital, or during the weeks before surgery on an outpatient basis
- Many surgical procedures are now performed in a day surgery setting.

Physical Preparation

- Physical preparation may consist of a complete medical history and the patient's surgical and anesthesia background
- The patient should inform the physician and hospital staff if he or she has ever had an adverse reaction to anesthesia (such as anaphylactic shock), or if there is a family history of malignant hyperthermia
- Laboratory tests may include complete blood count, electrolytes, prothrombin time, activated partial thromboplastin time, and urinalysis
- The patient will most likely have an electrocardiogram (ECG) if he or she has a history of cardiac disease, or is over 50 years of age
- A chest X-ray is done if the patient has a history of respiratory disease
- Part of the preparation includes assessment for risk factors that might impair healing, such as nutritional deficiencies, steroid use, radiation or chemotherapy, drug or alcohol abuse, or metabolic diseases such as diabetes
- The patient should also provide a list of all medications, vitamins, and herbal or food supplements that he or she uses
- Latex allergy has become a public health concern. Latex is found in most sterile surgical gloves, and is a common component in other medical supplies including general anesthesia masks, tubing, and multi-dose medication vials
- The night before surgery, skin preparation is often ordered, which can take the form of scrubbing with a special soap or possibly scalp or facial hair removal from the surgical area
- Shaving hair is no longer recommended because studies show that this practice may increase the chance of infection
- Instead, adhesive barrier drapes can contain hair growth on the skin around the incision.

Psychological Preparation

- Patients are often fearful or anxious about having surgery. It is often helpful for them to express their concerns to health care workers. This can be especially beneficial for patients who are critically ill, or who are having a high-risk procedure
- The family needs to be included in psychological preoperative care
- If the patient has a fear of dying during surgery, this concern should be expressed, and the surgeon notified. In some cases, the procedure may be postponed until the patient feels more secure
- Children may be especially fearful. They should be allowed to have a parent with them as much as possible, as long as the parent is not demonstrably fearful and contributing to the child's apprehension. Children should be encouraged to bring a favorite toy or blanket to the hospital on the day of surgery
- Patients and families who are prepared psychologically tend to cope better with the patient's postoperative course. Preparation

leads to superior outcomes since the goals of recovery are known ahead of time, and the patient is able to manage postoperative pain more effectively.

SYSTEMIC ASSESSMENT

Cardiovascular System

- A variety of problems—ischemic heart disease (IHD), congestive cardiac failure (CCF), cardiac arrhythmias, valvular heart disease, cardiomyopathies, hypertension
- Cardinal symptoms—exercise intolerance and chest pain.

To assess the cardiovascular status
- Pulse (rate, rhythm, character)
- BP
- Cardiac murmers, added heart sounds.

Other signs like
- Hepatomegaly
- Ankle edema
- Basal crepitations in lung
- Neck vein distension.

General Examination

- Clubbing—associated with congenital heart disease or subacute endocarditis
- Cyanosis—seen when capillary oxygen saturation is less than 85 percent
  - Central cyanosis—seen in tongue and lips, due to desaturation of central arterial blood as in right to left heart shunt
  - Peripheral cyanosis—noticed in hand and feet, may be due to circulatory shock, CCF, abnormalities of peripheral circulation, or exposure to cold.

Pulse
- Rate—physiological variation
- Pulse chart is valuable
- Rhythm—irregularities are seen due to premature beats, intermittent heart block, ectopic

- Carotid pulse (Corrigan's sign) associated with large volume pulse as in anemia, thyrotoxicosis, or fever.

Jugular Venous Pressure
- Is an indicator of the pressure in the right atrium
- Maybe elevated in heart failure, constrictive pericarditis, cardiac tamponade, etc.
- Heart sounds and murmers
- S1 and S2 normal physiological heart sounds
- S3—abnormal if >40 years
- S4—abnormal in young,indicative of ventricular stiffness
- Murmers are caused by turbulent flow
- High velocity murmers—mitral or aortic regurgitation
- Low velocity murmers—mitral stenosis.

Cardiac Investigations
- Chest X-ray
  - Assess cardiomegaly
  - Atrial or ventricular hypertrophy
  - Calcifications
    - Pericardial
    - Valvular
    - Myocardial or coronary artery
    - Lung field
- ECG—to record the electrical activity of heart
- ECHO—involves use of ultrasound with contrast agent to assess cardiac structure and function, useful to determine
  - Valve stenosis and regurgitation
  - Vegetations >2 mm
  - Aortic aneurysms and dissections
  - Cardiomyopathies, pericardial effusion.

Other Investigations
- Nuclear imaging (SPECT)
- Radionuclide angiography (MUGA)
- Positron emission tomography (PET)
- Cardiac catheterization

- Digital subtraction angiography
- Cardiovascular magnetic resonance (CMR).

Risk of surgery in patients with cardiac problems as described by Lee et al.

High-risk Surgery

- History of IHD
- CCF
- Previous stroke
- Diabetes mellitus
- Renal failure
- Cardiovascular system.

Management

Ischemic Heart Disease

- Patient maybe already on medications like β-blockers, diuretics or nitrates and are continued up to the time of premedication
- Those with history of angina at rest transdermal or IV nitrates are given preoperatively.

Hypertension

WHO defines hypertension as:
- Systolic BP >160 mm Hg
- Diastolic BP >95 mm Hg

Accordingly 4 groups of patients:
- Diastolic BP 95–110 mm Hg
- Diastolic BP 110–120 mm Hg
- Diastolic BP >120 mm Hg
- Elevated systolic BP 200–250 mm Hg
  - Assess end organ disease

If treatment is required, then surgery can be postponed for 4–6 weeks to allow optimization of therapy.

Congestive Cardiac Failure

GA can cause cardiac muscle depression and hypokalemia, ionotropic agents like dopamine or dobutamine.

Valvular Heart Disease

Appropriate antibiotic prophylaxis against endocarditis.

Arrhythmias

Ventricular tachycardia and ectopic should be treated preoperatively.

Respiratory System

Physical Examination

- Observe for pattern of breathing and degree of chest expansion
- Cyanosis and clubbing
- Dyspnea, cough, hemoptysis, wheeze, chest pain.

Asthma

- In well controlled asthmatics, salbutamol inhalation or nebulization is done prior to anesthesia to prevent bronchospasm and laryngospasm
- Elective surgery is undertaken if PEFR is 250 – 300 L/min
- In severe asthma a short course steroid, prednisone 40–80 mg/day can be used
- Other drugs that are used are antileukotrienes and theophylline
- Atelectasis and increased risk of pneumonia are seen in asthmatics postoperatively
- Histamine releasing drugs like
- d-tubocurarine, morphine, atracurium are avoided.

Chronic Obstructive Pulmonary Disease

- Chronic bronchitis
- Emphysema
- Smoking is the most common cause.

Management

- Hydration to mobilize mucus secretion
- Inhaled *b* agonists or inhaled ipratropium
- Oral and parenteral steroids used if wheezing is detected preoperatively
- Production of mucopurulent sputum may indicate need for antibiotics
- Nitrous oxide and narcotics are avoided in anesthesia.

Table 2.2: Management of difficult airway
Recognition of difficult airway
Preparation for difficult airway positioning of patient for airway manipulation
Awake intubation technique
Technique for anesthetized patient with difficult airway
Technique for patient who cannot be ventilated or intubated
Confirming the position of endotrachel tube
Extubation or tube exchange for a patient with known difficult airway

Upper airway, examination is carried out for intubation (Table 2.2)

Mallampati Classification (Figs 2.1 to 2.4)

Depending on structures visible

Class I: Hard palate, soft palate, uvula and faucillapillors (Fig. 2.1)

Class II: Hard palate, soft palate and uvula (Fig. 2.2)

Class III: Hard palate and soft palate (Fig. 2.3)

Class IV: Hard palate only (Fig. 2.4).

Liver Diseases

Important Functions of Liver

1. Metabolism of glucose, amino acids, fatty acids and cholesterol
2. Production of bile
3. Detoxification of drugs and waste products
4. Synthesis (albumin, coagulation factors)
   - Each of these factors will influence the safe conduct of anesthesia
   - While assessing liver disorders history of jaundice is recorded (indicates hepatitis, cholecystitis or gallstones)
   - Assess evidence of clotting disorders.

Investigations

- Blood tests
- Liver function tests
  - Serum albumin
  - Prothrombin time
- Liver biochemistry
  - Serum aspartate and alanine amino-transferases-reflects hepatocellular damage
  - Serum alkaline phosphatase-reflects cholestasis
  - Total protein
- Viral markers
- Additional blood, immunological (AMA, ANCA), genetic investigations
- Urine tests for bilirubin and urobilinogen
- Imaging techniques for defining gross anatomy
- Liver biopsy for histology
- Liver diseases and anesthesia
- Serum albumin is a valuable guide to assess severity of chronic liver disease
- Prothrombin time is a sensitive indicator of both acute and chronic liver disease.

Liver Enzymes

- Aspartate aminotransferase (a mitochondrial enzyme), also present in heart, muscle, kidney and brain. High levels in hepatic necrosis, MI, muscle disease and CCF
- Alanine aminotranferase (cytosol enzyme)—specific for liver diseases
- International normalized ratio INR is the ratio PT (patient)/PT (control sample)
  Normal value—0.8–1.2
  For patients on anticoagulants—2–3
  INR of 5—bleeding tendencies
  < 0.5—high chances of having a clot.

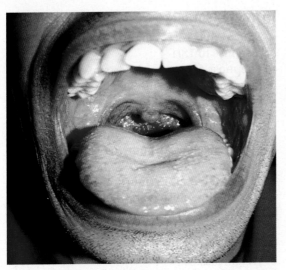

Fig. 2.1 Class I: Visualized intraoral anatomy: Soft palate, fauces, uvula, anterior and posterior pillars
Implications: Generally associated with an easy intubation

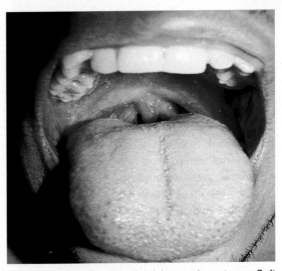

Fig. 2.2 Class II: Visualized intraoral anatomy: Soft palate, fauces, uvula
Implications: Generally associated with an easy intubation

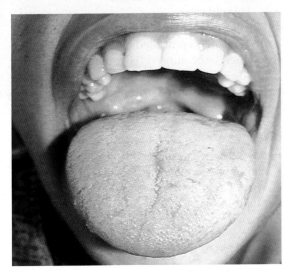

Fig. 2.3 Class III: Visualized intraoral anatomy: Only soft plate, base of uvula
Implications: Potential for intubation difficulty

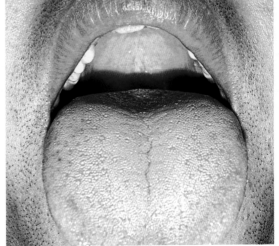

Fig. 2.4 Class IV: Visualized intraoral anatomy: The hard palate but not the soft palate
Implications: Potential for intubation difficulty

Imaging Techniques
- Ultrasound examination
  - Splenomegaly/hepatomegaly
  - Focal liver disease
  - Parenchymal liver disease
  - Lymph node enlargement

- CT
  - Assess size, shape, density of liver and can determine focal diseases
- MRI
- MRCP (MR Cholangiopancreatography)
- Radionucleide imaging

- PTC (percutaneous transhepatic cholangiography).

Preparation

- During premedication, IM drugs are avoided due to preexisting bleeding tendency
- Opiates are avoided, benzodiazepenes are given
- Vitamin K is administered when necessary to the jaundiced patient
- Central venous monitoring is advisable for patients with cirrhosis
- In obstructive jaundice, oral bile salts are administered to avoid postoperative renal failure and endotoxemia
- If factors II, VII, IX, and X are reduced they may respond to vitamin K
- In case factor V and X are reduced then infusion of fresh frozen plasma is given.

Surgery in Diabetic Patients

A diagnosis of diabetes is made if:

- Fasting venous blood glucose level >140 mg/dL (7.8 mmol/L)
- An abnormal glucose tolerance test
- Glucose concentration in excess of 200 mg/dL after ingestion of 75 g of glucose.

Preoperative Management

- Patients with diet controlled diabetes mellitus can be safely maintained without food or glucose infusion before surgery
- Patients on oral hypoglycemics should discontinue them the evening before surgery. In case of long acting agents like chlorpropamide, they are discontinued 2 or 3 days prior to surgery
- Patients on insulin require glucose and insulin preoperatively
- In patients undergoing major surgical procedures one half of the morning dose of insulin with 5 percent dextrose at 100–125 mL/hr subsequent insulin admin is guided by frequent (4–6 hr) blood glucose determinations.

Thyroid Disorders

- The normal T3:T4 ratio is 15:1,are released in response to TSH
- The most common lab tests to assess thyroid function are measurement of total thyroid hormone levels by RIA,
  - Normal levels—5012 pg/dL
  - Higher value—hyperthyroidism
  - Lower value—hypothyroidism
- T3 resin uptake

Higher values of T3 resin uptake are associated with hypothyroidism and lower values with hyperthyroidism.

Hyperthyroidism

- Weight loss
  - Palpitations
  - Restlessness
- Surgical risk—cardiac failure
  - Thyroid crisis
- Elective surgery is deferred until hyperthyroidism is controlled
- If emergency surgery is required-IV sodium iodide is used to block hormone from the gland
- *b* antagonists used to control the effects of thyroid hormones.

Hypothyroidism

- Poses a lesser surgical and anesthetic risk when compared to hyperthyroidism
- Weight gain
- Muscle weakness
- Bradycardia.

Surgical Risk

- Pretoperative heart failure
- Mental confusion postoperatively
- Delayed wound healing.

Chronic Renal Failure

Impaired renal function will show:

- Acid base and electrolyte imbalance
- Anemia

- Hypertension and IHD
- Coagulation disorders
- Delayed gastric emptying, gastric reflux, etc.

Preoperative Management

- Routine hemofilteration or dialysis is done for surgical patients
- All intercurrent therapy should be continued up to the day of surgery
- Opioid premedication is avoided (bleeding tendencies)
- Doses of analgesics are titrated against effect
- Enfluorane is avoided.

Laboratory Investigations

- The single most useful measure of renal health is GFR (normally, 100-125 mL/min/1.73 sqm of body surface area in an adult)
- Mild-to-moderate renal insufficiency—25-50 mL
- Severe renal deficiency—10-25 mL
- Frank renal failure — >10 mL
- GFR is measured clinically by determining the clearance of endogenous creatinine
- Other indicators of renal problems are proteinuria, hematuria, pyuria, all detectable by urine analysis.

Drug Therapy

Patients on Anticoagulant Therapy

- Warfarin (coumadin)
- Heparin.

Indications

- Deep venous thrombosis (DVT)
- Pulmonary embolism
- Unstable angina
- Acute MI.
  Oral anticoagulation therapy does not need to be changed for minor oral surgical procedures and exodontia if patients INR range is 2-3.

Heparin Window

- Describes the time before and after a surgical procedure when the patient's warfarin therapy is replaced with low molecular weight heparin.
- The standard protocol is to
  - Discontinue warfarin 4 or 5 days before the scheduled procedure,
  - Initiate unfractionated IV heparin or low molecular weight heparin
- After the International normalized ratio (INR) falls below the therapeutic range, and then discontinue heparin before surgery (4–5 hours before surgery when using unfractionated IV heparin and 12–24 hours before surgery when using LMWH)
- After surgery, when the risk of bleeding is minimized, both heparin and warfarin are restarted. Once the INR is within the therapeutic range, heparin therapy is stopped, while oral anticoagulation using warfarin continues.

Corticosteroid Therapy

- Normal secretion—25-30 mg/day
- At the time of trauma or surgery—300-500 mg/day
- In patients on steroid therapy, ACTH production is supressed.

Management

Adrenal cortical function is assessed using synthetic ACTH.

Regimen

- 100 mg IV at the time of induction followed by 100 mg IV every 6 hours for 3 days
- 25 mg at induction followed by 25 mg q6h for 24 hours for intermediate surgery
- 25 mg q6h for 48 hours for major surgeries.

Oral Contraceptives

- Oral contraceptives + surgery will reduce the action of antithrombin III

- Before elective surgery, combined pill should be stopped 4 weeks prior
- If surgery is an emergency, then prophylactic heparin should be considered.

Antiepileptic Therapy

- Patients on chronic antiepileptic therapy have hepatic microsomal enzyme induction
- Higher than normal doses of hypnotics and analgesics will be required for anesthesia and pain relief.

Antihypertensives

Are maintained up to the time of surgery, which will maintain normal BP and blood volume.

Surgery in the Special Patient

Pediatric Patients

The normal physiology of these patients makes them differ from adults in their response to drugs and anesthesia

Children have
- Large tongue
- Small nasal airway
- Small mandible
- Short neck
- All these makes airway very easily compromised
- Children have relatively large surface areas that can allow excessive heat loss when they are left uncovered in operating room
- Dosing of drugs is usually best decided based on manufacturer's recommendations.

Pregnant and Lactating Patients

- Are relative contraindications for elective oral and maxillofacial surgical procedures
- If surgery cannot be deferred then patient's obstetrician is consulted with
- When feasible surgery should be conducted under LA
- Drugs like aspirin, diazepam, steroids, promethazine, and tetracycline are best avoided in pregnancy

- Medications for lactating mothers include paracetamol, cephalexin, erythromycin, lignocaine, pentazocine, antihistamines.

NPO Status

For all patients, abstain from any oral intake except for medications with sips of water for 8 hours before elective surgery.

Aspiration Prophylaxis Regimen

- For patients who are not considered at increased risk for aspiration of gastric contents
  - Solid food permitted until 6 hours before surgery
  - Clear liquids (not milk or juices containing pulp) until 2 hours before surgery
- Obese, diabetic or patients on narcotic therapy (delayed or incomplete gastric emptying)
  - Require longer fasting periods
  - Additional pretreatment with metoclopromide, H_2 antagonists
  - Maintenance IV fluid should be started.

NPO Status and Antibiotic Prophylaxis

Antibiotic prophylaxis depends on:
- Type of pathogens encountered during surgery
- The type of operative wound
- Class I wound—no antibiotic prophylaxis
- Class II wound—single dose of appropriate antibiotic prior to skin incision
- Class III wound—parenteral antibiotic with aerobic and anerobic activity
- Class IV wound—same as with Class III wound but should be continued postoperatively.

Medicolegal Aspects

- Documented Informed consent which is legally valid
- Patient awareness of various drugs used and the procedure
- Perioperative complications and deaths.

Informed Consent

- The patient's or guardian's written consent for the surgery is a vital portion of preoperative care

- By law, the physician who will perform the procedure must explain the risks and benefits of the surgery, along with other treatment options
- However, the nurse is often the person who actually witnesses the patient's signature on the consent form. It is important that the patient understands everything he or she has been told. Sometimes, patients are asked to explain what they were told so that the health care professionals can determine how much is understood
- Patients who are mentally impaired, heavily sedated, or critically ill are not considered legally able to give consent. In this situation, the next of kin (spouse, adult child, adult sibling, or person with medical power of attorney) may act as a surrogate and sign the consent form
- Children under age 18 must have a parent or guardian sign.

Preoperative Teaching
- Preoperative teaching includes instruction about the preoperative period, the surgery itself, and the postoperative period
- Instruction about the preoperative period deals primarily with the arrival time, where the patient should go on the day of surgery, and how to prepare for surgery. For example, patients should be told how long they should be NPO (nothing by mouth), which medications to take prior to surgery, and the medications that should be brought with them
- Instruction about the surgery itself includes informing the patient about what will be done during the surgery, and how long the procedure is expected to take. The patient should be told where the incision will be
- It is also important for family members (or other concerned parties) to know where to wait during surgery, when they can expect progress

information, and how long it will be before they can see the patient
- Knowledge about what to expect during the postoperative period is one of the best ways to improve the patient's outcome. Instruction about expected activities can also increase compliance and help prevent complications
- Additionally, the patient should be informed about intermaxillary ligation, early ambulation (getting out of bed). The patient should also be taught that the respiratory interventions decrease the occurrence of pneumonia, and that early leg exercises and ambulation decrease the risk of blood clots
- Patients hospitalized postoperatively should be informed about the tubes and equipment that they will have. These may include multiple intravenous lines, drainage tubes, dressings, and monitoring devices
- Pain management is the primary concern for many patients having surgery. Preoperative instruction should include information about the pain management method that they will utilize postoperatively. Patients should be encouraged to ask for or take pain medication before the pain becomes unbearable, and should be taught how to rate their discomfort on a pain scale. This instruction allows the patients, and others who may be assessing them, to evaluate the pain consistently. If they will be using a patient-controlled analgesia pump, instruction should take place during the preoperative period.

Normal Results
- The anticipated outcome of preoperative care is a patient who is informed about the surgical course, and copes with it successfully
- The goal is to decrease complications and promote recovery.

Principles of
Postoperative Care

3

INTRODUCTION

Postoperative care of maxillofacial surgical patient like orthognathic, trauma or cancer patients are quite as important as their preoperative preparation; deficient care in *either area may produce an unsatisfactory* outcome, irrespective of standard of surgery.

POSTOPERATIVE CARE

- Provides physiological support when patient is temporarily incapacitated
- Gives adequate pain relief
- Anticipates and takes early action on complications
- Maintains good team communication
- Regularly reviews the treatment plan.

Definition

Postoperative care covers the period of time, the surgery ends to the time patient regains consciousness. Care includes correct positioning of the patient relative to surgery performed and application of minimum pressure and strain on operative site, maintenance of open airway, body temperature, fluid balance and monitoring sign of developing shock.

Aim

It is to enable the patient to return to pain-free and independent life quickly.

Main points in the postoperative treatment plan includes:
- Prophylaxis
- Monitoring problems contingency planning for adverse events makes them easy to manage.

Recovery from Major Surgery

The recovery from major surgery can be divided into 3 phases:
1. An immediate or postanesthetic phase
2. An intermediate phase
3. A convalescent phase
   - During the first two phases, care is principally directed at maintenance of homeostasis, treatment of pain and prevention and early detection of complications
   - The convalescent phase is a transition period from the time of hospital discharge to full recovery.

Immediate Postoperative Period

- Major causes of early complications and death following major surgery are acute pulmonary, cardiovascular and fluid derangements
- The patient can be discharged from the recovery room to postoperative ward when cardiovascular, pulmonary and neurologic functions have returned to baseline
- *Operating room to recovery room:* The attending surgeon and responsible assistant should

accompany the patient to recovery room with recovery room note and postoperative orders.

"Many of the physiological disorders which are easily recognized in fully awake, nonmedicated patients are modified, abated or entirely eliminated by residual anesthesia. In recovery room, this presents major difficulties in recognizing problems such as hypoxia, hypoventilation and hypovolumia."

- Patients who require continuing ventilator or circulatory support or who have other conditions that require frequent monitoring are transferred to an ICU
- Postoperative orders must be advised of the nature of the operation and patient's condition. It should cover.

Monitoring

Vital signs: Blood pressure, pulse and respiration should be recorded until stable. When an arterial catheter is in place, blood pressure and pulse should be monitored continuously.

Central venous pressure: Indicated when operation has caused large blood losses/fluid shifts.

Fluid balance: Aids in hydration and helps to guide intravenous fluid replacements. A bladder catheter can be placed for frequent measurement of urine output. In the absence of bladder catheter, the surgeon should be notified if the patient is unable to void within 6–8 hours after operation.

Respiratory care: Patient may require mechanical ventilation, supplemental oxygen by mask or nasal prongs. For intubated patients, tracheal suctioning or other forms of respiratory therapy must be specified. For extubated patients, deep breathing exercises frequently to avoid atelectasis.

Position in Bed and Mobilization

- Patient should be turned from side-to-side every 30 minutes until conscious and then hourly for the first 8–12 hours to minimize atelectasis
- Early ambulation to reduce venous stasis
- Upright position to increase diaphragmatic excursions

- Venous stasis may be minimized by intermittent compression of the calf by pneumatic stockings.

Diet Orders

Wright estimated that 50 percent of persons in surgical wards of private, public hospitals are at various stages of starvation.

Orders should include
- Time to start clear fluids
- Aim of nutrition therapy is to achieve positive nitrogen balance and to provide adequate calories
- *Nitrogen requirement*: Nitrogen loss (urine urea × 0.028 + 2) approx = 3-6 g/d
- Energy requirements = 50 percent glucose + 30 percent fat
- Electrolytes + vitamins added to feeds.

Administration of Fluids and Electrolytes

Based on maintenance needs and replacement of gastrointestinal losses from drains, fistulas or stomas.

Drainage Tubes

- Drain care—character and quantity
- Suctin—type and pressure
- Irrigation fluids.

Medications

- Antibiotics
- Analgesics
- Gastric acid suppressants
- Deep vein thrombosis prophylaxis
- Corticosteroids
- Antipyretics
- Laxatives
- Stool softeners.

Laboratory Examinations and Imaging

- Daily chest radiograph
- Blood counts
- Serum electrolytes
- Liver function test, if needed
- Renal function test, if needed.

Routine Daily Checks for all Surgery Patients

Subjective

- Greeting with general questions to assess his mental state
- Postoperative patient who is hungry is usually a patient who is doing well.

Objective

- Look for pain reaction on face, pallor, cyanosis
- Take patients hand for peripheral perfusion
- Look for temperature chart:
  - Fever is common usually after major surgery
  - If temperature persists, source of infection may be: chest, urine, surgical wound (in order of occurrence)

Cardiovascular Status

- Check for BP, pulse, RR, oxygen saturation
- "Blue jumpers and warm trousers"
  Urine output
  Pressure areas
  Wound.

Intermediate Postoperative Period

- Starts with complete recovery from anesthesia and lasts for the rest of hospital stay
- In this period, patient recovers most basic functions and become self-sufficient and able to continue convalescence at home.

Wound Care

- Bulky dressings are not usually used for incised wounds
- Area can be inspected daily for signs of infection
- Skin sutures left in place until wound healed soundly
- Removal of the dressing and handling of the wound during first 24 hours should be done with aseptic technique
- If wound becomes infected one or two sutures removed prematurely to allow egress of infected material
- Wounds of head and neck sutures can be removed in 4–6 days checking apposition, swelling, gaping of wound edges.

Fluid and Electrolytes

- Maintenance calculations
- Calculate ongoing losses
  - Blood loss
  - Other parameters
- From practical standpoint most losses or gains of body fluids are from ECF
- Improper fluid balance:
  - Preoperative: Causes prompt hypotension with induction of anesthesia
  - Intraoperative: complete replacement of blood loss + 45 mL/hr of RL up to total of 300 mL

Postoperative Fluid Management

- Based on vitals (blood loss + urine output)
- Replacement includes loss + maintenance
- In postoperative period 1 lts of fluid is given to replace urine volume necessary to handle excretion work load (900 mL urine + 600 mL insensible loss)
- IV fluid of choice 5 percent dextrose in normal saline @ 100 mL/hr
- Next day add 40 mEq of K^+.

Monitoring of Fluid Replacement

- Pulse
- BP
- Urine output
- CVP.

Complications of Fluid Balance

- Hypotension and tachycardia earliest postoperative sign of circulatory instability
- Minimum urine output of 30–50 mL/hr to be maintained.

Clinical Features of Fluid Overload

- Weight gain
- Heavy eyelids
- Dyspnea.

Mathematics of Fluids

Distribution of body fluids: "rule of thirds"
- Colloid stays in vascular compartment
- Saline stays in extracellular compartment
- Dextrose eventually goes to all compartment.

Flowchart 3.1: pH control in body

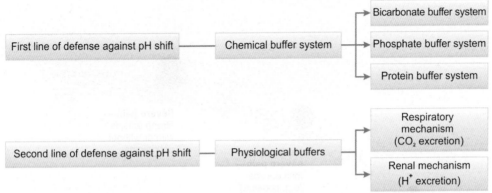

Acid-base Balance

This occurs from altered excretion of CO_2, impaired excretion of H^+ ions from kidney or productions of lactic acid (Flowchart 3.1).

Respiratory acidosis
Causes
- Atelectasis
- Pneumonia
- Airway obstruction

treated by underlying cause, assist ventilation.

Respiratory alkalosis
Causes
- Hyperventilation (apprehension, pain, brain injury)

treated by reducing ventilatory rates.

Metabolic acidosis
Causes
- Acute circulatory failure or renal damage
- Chloride excess
- Loss of GI fluids
- Administration of unbalanced salt solutions

treated by sodium bicarbonate

Metabolic alkalosis
Causes
- Loss of acids,
- Retention of bases
- Hypokalemia.

treated by rehydration.K^+, Cl^-

Opioids for Severe Pain (Fig. 3.1)
- *Morphine-like agonists*: Morphine, hydrocodone
- Oxycodone, codeine
- *Mixed agonist/antagonists*: Butorphanol nalbuphine
- Dezocine
- *Partial agonist*: Buprenorphine.

Multimodal Pain Control

Patient controlled IV analgesia by morphine. If patient experiences pain, patient activates device, bolus dose of morphine is delivered.

Postoperative Edema
- Edema of face and neck may be alarming in its appearance after maxillofacial surgeries
- However only edema causing respiratory arrest is of significance to the patient
- If this is anticipated then tracheostomy has to be performed specially in case of IMF.

Management
- Head up position
- Hydrostatic pressure amounts to 2 mm Hg for every 2.5 cm of vertical height above heart and gravity must be allowed to act for the patient and not against him
- Oxygen to be administered in case of stridor.

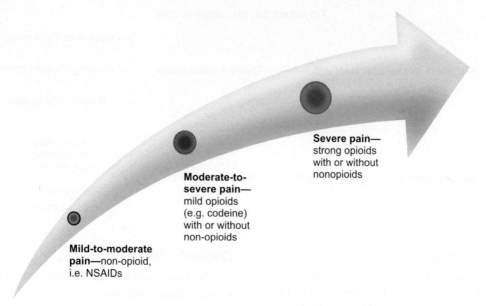

Fig. 3.1: WHO pain relief ladder

Pulmonary Care

- Postoperative pulmonary complications can be prevented by early mobilization
- Proper meticulous NPO status
- Frequent changes in position
- Encouragement to cough
- Incentive spirometer
- Chest physiotherapy

Cardiovascular System Care

- Hemodynamic stability
- Control of heart rate with digitalis, beta-blockers
- Treatment of hypokalemia if any
- Ventricular dysarythmias prevented by oxygen, analgesia, electrolyte balance.

Gastrointestinal Prophylaxis

- Maxillofacial trauma patients more prone to stress ulcers
- Superficial erosions due to reduced blood flow and not due to gastric acidity
- Prevention is by early enteric feedings, sucralfate, proton pump inhibitors.

Care of Drain and Catheter

- Observance of aseptic methods during cannulation
- Frequent change of tubings, rotation of insertion sites
- Use of sialistic catheters
- Drain is usually removed once it has stopped draining, or minimal drainage.

Postoperative Complications and Management

4

INTRODUCTION

Postoperative period is crucial because consciousness and reflex may still be impaired. It is critical since the first 24–48 hours is most important to monitor basic physiological parameters, such as CVS, respiratory, renal, and laboratory tests to optimize and sustain recovery.

DEFINITION

- Any expected or unexpected problem that arise during postoperative period which includes time the surgery ends to the time patient regains consciousness.

Aspiration
Reduced consciousness
Neurologic deficits
Mechanical disruption of normal anatomy
Local pharyngeal anesthesia
Recumbent position

Risk factors
Age
Type of anesthesia
Type of surgery
Recent meal
Delayed gastric emptying
Decreased lower esophageal sphincter tone
Obesity
Neuromuscular disorders

- The most frequent are bleeding, infection, change in position of occlusion or protracted pain.

Precautions

- Avoid heavy preanesthetic sedation
- Adequate preoperative starvation
- Nasogastric tube to remove liquid from stomach
- Metoclopramide 10 mg prokinetic to hasten gastric emptying
- H_2 antagonists to inhibit secretion of gastric acid.

Symptoms

- Restlessness
- Tachycardia
- Occasionally cyanosis.

Signs: Auscultation of breath sounds, chest X-ray

Investigations: Chest X-ray, sputum examination, blood routine (Fig. 4.1).

Treatment

- Removal of foreign body
- Use of steroids
- Broad-spectrum antibiotics.

Sore Throat

Throat pack—First postoperative concern in OMFS.

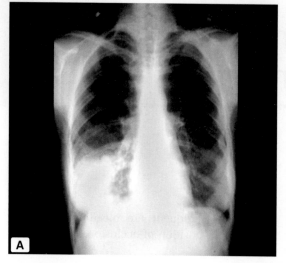 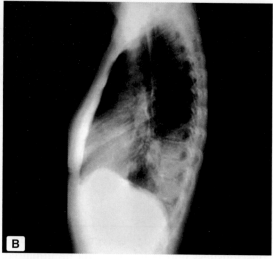

Fig. 4.1: Chest X-rays

Etiology

- Trauma during intubation
- Irritation of larynx
- Trauma to pharynx.

Management

- Tongue should be cleaned of blood
- Lozenges
- Salt water gargling
- Cup of tea.

Nausea and Vomiting

- Dehydration, electrolyte imbalance, aspiration of vomitus raises intracranial pressure
- Emergency bedside tray consisting wire cutter, wire twister should be kept ready in case of intermaxillary wire removal or arch bar adjustment or removal.

Etiology

- Patient factors
  - Age
  - Weight
  - Anxiety
  - Sex
  - Past medical history

- Surgical factors
  - Duration
  - Type of surgery
- Anesthetic factors
  - Drugs used
  - Hypoxia
  - Poor airway management.

Management

- Stop all oral fluids until bowel sounds are present
- Phenothiazines
- Gastric suction in case of protracted nausea and vomiting
- Antihistamines
- Dopamine antagonists
- Anticholinergic drugs
- Seratonin antagonists
- Dexamethasone 2–8 mg IV.

Regurgitation

- Passive movement of gastric contents into the pharynx under the force of gravity
- Anesthesia reduces the barrier pressure
- Head down position

- Increased gastric pressure, pregnancy, full stomach, high intra-abdominal pressure, gas from face-mask ventilation
- Incompetence of cardiac sphincter.

Urinary Retention

- Voluntary effort 8–12 hours postoperatively
- Secondary to anesthesia, drugs and recumbency
- Prerenal
  - Decreased cardiac output
  - Volume depletion
- Renal
  - Acute tubular necrosis
- Postrenal
  - Obstructive uropathies
  - Bladder atony secondary to medications
- Urinary tract infections.

Treatment

- Suprapubic hot packs
- Assisted ambulation
- 10–12 hours straight catheter. No more than 500–700 ml should be removed or else bladder spasm and syncope could result
- Correct volume depletion
- Fluid bolus
- Diuretics.

Polyuria

- Excessive volume administration
- Pharmacologic diuresis
- Osmotic diuresis.

Edema

Etiology

- Physical trauma
- Infections
- Increased venous pressure
- Decreased lymphatic flow
- Excessive sodium retention
- Cardiac failure, immobility.

Management

- Position site of surgery above the level of heart

- Good hemostasis
- Judicious use of steroids
- Compression of area of surgery.

Stress Gastritis

Seen in 25–40 percent of ICU patients, clinically significant bleeding in 2–10 percent of patients.

Risk Factors

- Mechanical ventilation for >48 hours
- Coagulopathy
- Significant burns
- Head injury.

Treatment

- Antacids
- Proton pump inhibitors
- Sucralfate.

Hyperthermia

Temperature >100°F for more than 6 hours warrant further investigations.

Immediate Fever

- Medications
- Blood products
- Trauma from surgery
- Hypersensitivity reactions
- Altered thermoregulatory mechanisms
- Idiosyncratic reactions.

Acute Fever

- 24–72 hours
- Atelectasis
- Aspiration pnuemonia.

Subacute Fever

- Pulmonary embolism
- Urinary tract infections
- Surgical site infections
- Intravascular catheters.

Management

Care of IV line and catheter.

Hypotension

McLean defines it as inadequate blood flow to vital organs or failure of cells of vital organs to utilize oxygen.

Etiology

- Hypoxia
- Hypercarbia
- Coronary insufficiency
- Arrhythmias
- Electrolyte imbalance
- Endotoxic shock
- Pulmonary embolism
- Transfusion reactions
- Fat embolism.

Diagnosis

- Healthy patient tolerates well
- Renal failure in prolonged hypotension
- Hematocrit
- Orthostatic vital signs supine then sitting or standing taken within 30 sec or 1 minute increase in heart rate of 20 or a decrease in systolic pressure of 20 indicates significant volume depletion.

Management

- 300 ml of normal saline or ringer lactate IV over 10 minutes
- Trendelenburg position
- Ephidrine 10 mg IV or phenylephrine drip
- Myocardial ischemia
- Myocardial ischemia is an imbalance between myocardial oxygen supply and demand.

Hypertension

It causes wound hematomas and disruption of suture lines.

Common Causes

- Compliance
- Pain
- Bladder distension
- Drugs

- Fluid gains and loses
- Confusion
- Hypercapnia.

Rare Causes

- Renovascular hypertension
- Cushing's disease
- Hyperaldosteronism
- Hyperthyroidism
- Pheochromocytoma
- Increased intracranial pressure.

Diagnosis

Signs

- Vital signs
- Anxious patient
- Flushed skin
- Respiratory distress
- Epistaxis
- Full bladder.

Symptoms

- Pain at operated site
- Headache
- Nausea
- Vomiting
- Visual changes.

Management

- Antihypertensive regimen
- Control of pain
- Assess renal status.

Hypertensive Emergencies

- Diazoxide—300 mg IV or 150 mg followed by 50 mg increments
- Hydralazine-propranolol 10 mg hydralazine in 10 ml normal saline with 1 mg propranolol given in 2 ml aliquots
- Frusemide 10 mg IV if the patient is in positive fluid balance
- Morphine, if pain is the cause; 5 mg IV and 2 mg increments are added.

Myocardial Ichemia

- Symptoms may be masked
- History and elevated cardiac specific blood enzyme levels
- ST segment depression on ECG.

Management

- Increased FiO_2
- Nitroglycerin infusion.

Cardiac Arrhythmias

- Ischemia
- Ectopy
- Acid–base imbalances
- Drugs
- Preexisting cardiac problems
- Hypercapnea
- Pain
- Fluid overload.

Management

- Correct hypoxia
- Adequate pain control
- Correct fluid and electrolyte imbalances.

Pulse

Sinus Tachycardia

- Unrelieved pain
- Hypoxia
- Hypercapnea
- Hypovolemia

Sinus Bradycardia

- Hypoxia
- Vagal stimulation

Needs treatment only if it is causing symptoms.

PULMONARY COMPLICATIONS

- Exacerbation of COPD or asthma
- Hypoxemia
- Aspiration
- Upper airway obstruction
- Postobstructive pulmonary edema
- Pneumonia

- Pleural effusion
- Tracheal lacerations or rupture
- Bronchospasm.

Risk Factors

Patient-related

- Smoking
- Lung conditions
- General health status
- Age
- Obesity.

Procedure-related

- Site of surgery
- Type of surgery
- Duration of surgery
- Type of anesthesia.

Pathophysiology

- Lack of normal pattern of spontaneous breaths
- Spontaneous deep breaths to maximal lung inflation are eliminated from the pattern of breathing
- Alveolar collapse begins to produce transpulmonary shunting.
- Recumbent position
- Superior lobes of lungs ventilated
- Perfusion is preferential to dependent lobes
- Shunting of blood
- Lower lobe alveoli begin to collapse.

Pulmonary Interstitium

- Hydrostatic pressure increases
- Oncotic pressure decreases
- Capillary permeability increases
- Impaired mucociliary transport
- Normal cough reflex suppressed
- Ventilatory response to hypercapnea and hypoxemia decreases.

Hypoxemia

- PaO_2 <90 percent
- Anesthesia induced hypoventilation
- Loss of upper airway muscle tone
- Volume overload

- Inability to clear secretions
- Upper airway edema
- Aspiration
- Pulmonary embolism
- Exacerbation of COPD and asthma.

Treatment

- Supplemental oxygen
- Noninvasive positive pressure ventilation.

Upper Airway Obstruction

- Lack of adequate air movement
- Intercoastal and suprasternal retractions
- Discoordinate abdominal and chest wall movements
- Complete obstruction is silent.

Etiology

- Incomplete recovery
- Laryngospasm, precipitated by irritation of glottis by secretions of blood or a foreign body.
- Airway edema
- Children are more susceptible to upper airway edema because of small diameter of their upper airway
- Tonsillar or adenoid hypertrophy.

Management

- Warmed and humidified 100 percent oxygen by mask
- Chin lift jaw thrust to relieve obstruction
- Head elevation and fluid restriction
- Dexamethasone
- Reintubation.

Laryngeal Edema

- Postnasal or oral intubation
- Usually in infants and children due to narrow anatomy of glottis.
- Can be prevented by use of glucocorticoids, ultrasonic nebulizers, tracheostomy.

Respiratory Failure

1. Early postoperative failure:
   - <48 hours, failure develops over minutes

   - Mechanical etiology
   - Life threatening
   - Occurs in patients with severe trauma and preexisting lung disease
2. Late postoperative failure:
   - >48 hours
   - Triggered by pulmonary embolism, opioid overdose.

Clinical Features

- Tachypnea of 25–30 breaths/min
- Tidal volume < 4 mL/kg.

Treatment

- Emergency intubation
- Adequate ventilation
- Treat underlying cause.

Pneumothorax

- Autogenous rib grafts
- Subclavian central venous lines
- Neck dissections
- Flaps.

Signs

- Tachypnea
- Tachycardia
- Cyanosis
- Hyperresonance
- Absent breath sounds.

Management

- Intermittent needle aspiration
- Chest tube placement.

Aspiration Pneumonitis

- General anesthesia that tend to obtund reflexes
- Drug overdose with resultant CNS depression
- Seizure disorders
- Previous history of CVAs
- Tracheostomy
- Esophageal motility disorders
- Bowel obstruction.

Pathophysiology

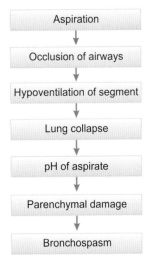

Diagnostic Findings

- Dyspnea
- Cough
- Wheezing
- Fever
- Tachycardia
- Hypotension
- Shock
- Cyanosis
- Unilateral radiodense infiltrates, most commonly seen in the right upper lung if the patient is supine at aspiration, or possibly bilateral diffuse infiltrates.

Management

- Trendelenburg position
- Pharyngeal and endotracheal suction should be started immediately
- Bronchoscopy for the removal of particulate matter from the airway
- Bronchodilators (aminophylline)
- Hydrocortisone.

Prevention

- This includes identification and appreciation of patients who are at particular risk

- Cimetidine or an antacid in an effort to decrease the acidity and amount of gastric secretions
- Rapid-sequence intubation is recommended in these patients
- Extubated in an alert and fully awake condition
- A suction source should be readily available at the bedside at all times.

Bronchospasm

- Reflex stimulation of airways
- Hyperreactive airway (COPD, asthama, smokers).

Management

- Beta2 sympathomimetic bronchodilators
- Steroids.

Pulmonary Edema

Pathophysiology

- Disruption of pulmonary basement membrane by large negative intrapleural pressure
- Fulminant life-threatening pulmonary edema within minutes
- Signs of respiratory obstruction, desaturation, distress
- Cardiac involvement leads to life-threatening dysrhythmias.

Management

- 100 percent O_2
- Lasix 1 mg/kg
- IPPV
- Morphine-venodialator.

Management of postoperative pulmonary complications:

- Lung expansion maneuvers
- Adequate pain control.

Delayed Awakening

- Persistent effects of drugs
- Decreased cerebral perfusion
- Septicemia
- Hemorrhage

- Fat embolism
- Air embolism
- Metabolic causes
- Electrolyte and acid-base imbalances
- Hypothermia
- Hypoglycemia.

Neurologic Damage

Signs and Symptoms

- Slurred speech
- Visual changes
- Agitation
- Confusion
- Numbness
- Muscular weakness
- Paralysis.

Etiology

- Fat emboli
- Uncontrolled hypertension
- Coagulopathies.

Emergence Delirium

- Hypoxemia
- Acidemia
- Hyponatremia
- Hypoglycemia
- Sepsis
- Pain
- Alcohol withdrawal
- Drugs used preoperatively may precipitate delirium.

Management

- Oxygen
- Fluid and electrolyte replacement
- Adequate analgesia
- Diazepam 2.5–5 mg IV, if severe.

Awareness and Recall

Etiology

- Pharmacodynamic variability
- Faulty equipment
- Light anesthetic techniques.

Long-term Effects

- Anxiety
- Post-traumatic stress disorder.

Convulsions

Etiology

- Hyperthermia
- Anoxia
- Hypocalcemic tetany
- Toxemia.

Treatment

IV diazepam.

Jaundice

- Halothane hepatitis
- Hepatotoxic effects of drugs
- Incompatible transfusions
- Large hematomas
- Viral hepatitis.

Hemorrhage

- If large volumes of blood have been transfused, then hemorrhage may be exacerbated by consumption coagulopathy
- May also be due to preoperative anticoagulants or unrecognized bleeding diathesis.

Thromboembolism

- Changes in composition of blood
- Damage to blood vessel walls
- Decreased blood flow.

Risk Factors

- Extensive trauma
- Infection
- Heart failure
- Blood dyscrasias
- Malignancy
- Metabolic disorders.

Investigations

- Venography
- Radioactive fibrinogen uptake

- Ultrasonography
- Impedance plethysmography.

Management

- Elimination of stasis
- Mechanical methods
  - Graded compression stockings
  - Intermittent pneumatic compression
- Pharmacological management.

Wound Dehiscence

- Poor blood supply
- Excess suture tension
- Long-term steroids
- Immunosuppressive therapy
- Radiotherapy.

OPHTHALMOLOGICAL COMPLICATIONS

- Loss of protective reflexes
- Tear production, tear film stability reduced
- Chemical injuries
- Direct trauma to eyes.

Management

Occlusive dressings, viscous ointments or gels.

Wound Hematoma

- Neck wound hematomas cause pain pressure, dysphagia, respiratory distress
- Should be treated by emergency re-exploration and evacuation
- Vocal cord paralysis
- Result of manipulation of recurrent laryngeal nerve
- Primary concern is aspiration
- Bilateral vocal cord paralysis is a serious complication.

Postoperative Parotitis

It is a staphylococcal infection of parotid gland limited to elderly, poor oral hygiene usually seen

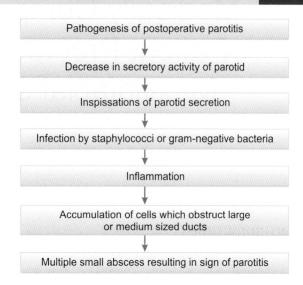

after 2nd postoperative week associated with prolonged nasogastric intubation, dehydration, etc. pathology consist decrease secretion of parotid gland which gets infected by staphylococci or gram-negative bacteria from the oral cavity resulting in inflammation, accumulation of cells that obstruct the duct eventually resulting in formation of small abscess.

Clinical Feature

- First appears as pain or tenderness at the angle of the jaw progressing with high temperature
- Swelling and redness in the parotid area
- Parotid feels firm
- In laboratory investigation leukocytosis may be seen.

Management

- Adequate fluid intake
- Avoid anticholinergics
- Minimize trauma
- Improve oral hygine (mouthwash, irrigation, moisturizing measures, etc).

Medically Compromised Patient Preparation for Maxillofacial Surgery

5

INTRODUCTION

- Maxillofacial surgeon may come across various medical and systemic conditions that are challenging for various surgical procedures. Hence, thorough knowledge is a prerequisite before planning for surgical intervention. Proper planning will help in minimizing chances of adverse event; thus, protecting patients from anxiety, injury, sleepless night heartache or litigation
- The initial contact with any new patient should be carefully orchestrated to achieve specific goals:
  - Assessment of patients surgical needs
  - Identification of potential management problems
  - Formulation of a treatment plan in light of the patients oral and medical status
  - Preparation of the patient for indicated procedures.
- The disorders discussed are:
  - Cardiac dysfunction
  - Pulmonary dysfunction
  - Hypertension
  - Renal dysfunction
  - Hepatic dysfunction
  - Endocrine dysfunction
  - Thyroid dysfunction
  - Adrenal dysfunction and patients taking steroids
  - Dysfunction of the immune system
- An arbitrary guideline for the patient selection for treatment may be based on the classification of physical status of the American Society of Anesthesiology (ASA) (Table 5.1).

CARDIOVASCULAR SYSTEM

Examination

Symptoms
- Dyspnea
- Wheezing
- Syncope
- Angina

Table 5.1: The American Society of Anesthesiologists classification of physical status				
ASA I	ASA II	ASA III	ASA IV	ASA V
Definition				
A patient without any systemic disease	Patient with mild systemic disease	Patient with severe systemic disease limiting activity	Patient with incapacitating disease that is constant threat to life	A moribund patient not expected to survive 24 hours with or without surgery

- Orthopnea
- Pedal edema
- Palpitations.

Signs
- Cyanosis
- Jugular venous distention
- Clubbing of the finger nails
- Carotid bruits
- Alteration in pulses and abnormal cardiac rhythms
- Pedal edema
- Presence of third or fourth heart sound
- Cardiac murmurs.

Routine Preoperative Tests
- Chest radiographs—PA and Lateral views
- Electrocardiography
- Exercise stress test
- Echocardiography
- Nuclear stress tests
- Radionuclide ventriculography
- Ambulatory echocardiography.

Cardiac Abnormalities
- Ischemic heart disease
- Angina pectoris
- Myocardial ischemia
- Congestive heart failure
- Cardiac valve abnormalities:
  - Aortic stenosis
  - Mitral stenosis
  - Aortic regurgitation
  - Mitral valve regurgitation
  - Mitral valve prolapse
  - Prosthetic heart valves.

Endocarditis Prophylaxis Recommended

High Risk
- Prosthetic heart valves
- Prior bacterial endocarditis
- Cyanotic congenital heart disease
- Surgically constructed shunts.

Moderate Risk
- Acquired valvular dysfunction
- Hypertrophic cardiomyopathy
- Mitral valve prolapse with regurgitations.

Endocarditis Prophylaxis Not Recommended
- Isolated atrial septal defect
- Surgical repair of ASD, VSD
- Prior coronary artery bypass graft
- Mitral valve prolapse without regurgitation
- Previous rheumatic fever
- Cardiac pacemaker.

Standard regimens for antibiotic prophylaxis to minimize risk of bacterial endocarditis due to oral surgical procedures is described in Table 5.2.

Hypertensive Patient
- Hypertension is the presence of elevated pressure that places patients at increased risk of organ damage
- Degree of hypertension
  - Emergencies
  - Urgencies
  - Mild uncomplicated
  - Transient.

Primary Agents for Use in Hypertensive Emergencies
- Sodium nitroprusside 0.25–10 µg/kg/m IV infusion
- Labetalol 10-80 µg IV bolus every 10 min
- Intravenous nitroglycerin 5–100 g/min IV infusion.

Management of Hypertensive Urgencies
- Sublingual nifedipine 5–10 mg
- Oral clonidine 0.2 mg initial then 0.1 mg/hr.

Preoperative Management of Hypertensive Patient
- Patients ideally should undergo elective surgery only when in normotensive state
- Elective surgical procedures on patients with sustained preoperative diastolic blood pressure

Table 5.2: Antibiotic prophylactic regimens			
Adults, not allergic to penicillin	Adults, allergic to penicillin	Children, not allergic to penicillin	Children, allergic to penicillin
2 g amoxicillin 1 hour before procedure	600 mg clindamycin 1 hour before procedure or	50 mg/kg amoxicillin 1 hour before procedure or	20 mg/kg clindamycin 1 hour before procedure or
2 g ampicillin IM or IV within 30 minutes before procedure	600 mg clindamycin IV within 30 minutes before procedure or	50 mg/kg ampicillin IM or IV within 30 minutes before procedure	20 mg/kg IV clindamycin within 30 minutes prior to procedure or
	2 g cephalexin 1 hour before procedure or		50 mg/kg cephalexin or cefadroxil 1 hour before procedure or
	1 g cefazolin IM or IV within 30 minutes before procedure or		25 mg/kg IM or IV cefazolin 30 minutes before procedure or
	500 mg azithromycin or clarithromycin 1 hour before procedure		15 mg/kg azithromycin or clarithromycin 1 hour before procedure

higher than 110 mm Hg especially in persons with end organ damage should be delayed until blood pressure is better controlled over a course of several days

- Mild-to-moderate hypertension often resolves after administration of anxiolytic agents such as midazolam.

Choice of Anesthetic Agents

- Ketamine is contraindicated
- Barbiturates, benzodiazepines, opioids, propofol are equally safe in inducing anesthesia in most hypertensive patients

Postoperative Management

- Hypertension in the postoperative is often multifactorial and can be due to the volume overload, pain, bladder distension
- If acute treatment is necessary IV nicardipine or sublingual nifedipine.

DIABETES MELLITUS

- Patients with diabetes mellitus (DM) have 50 percent chance of undergoing surgery in their lifetime

- The morbidity and mortality of these procedures are enhanced greatly by the physiologic effects of hyperglycemic microangiopathies
- Insulin-dependent diabetes mellitus (IDDM) applies to all forms of diabetes in which exogenous insulin is required to prevent diabetic ketoacidosis (Type 1 DM)
- Noninsulin-dependent diabetes mellitus (NIDDM) is used to denote any condition in which some endogenous insulin is present to prevent ketoacidosis
- Management of any patient begins with the initial assessment that includes age of onset, manifestation, requires exogenous insulin, susceptibility to ketoacidosis, blood glucose concentration.

Drug History

- Exogenous insulin is used for patients who have no function of beta cells of the pancreas and require an exogenous source of insulin to prevent ketoacidosis.

Preoperative Assessment

Cardiovascular

- History (hypertension, angina, infarction)

- Blood pressure
- ECG.

Neurologic
- Peripheral neuropathy
- Autonomic examination.

Renal
- Proteinuria
- Serum creatinine levels
- Urinalysis.

Metabolic
- Home glucose control
- Glycosylated Hb
- Electrolytes.

Preparation

Patients with IDDM
- Stop administration of long-acting insulin
- Substitute intermediate acting insulin.

Patients with NIDDM
- Stop administration of long-acting sulfonyl-ureas, stop administration of metformin, and reinforce dietary advice
- Minor surgical procedures, such as routine extractions, biopsies and procedures that are minimally stressful can be performed without altering the patient's usual regimen
- Patient should have the usual morning meal and oral medication
- Patient should be treated early in the day and have the capillary blood glucose level evaluated.
- Moderate surgical procedure that induces a certain amount of surgical stress, such as removal of impacted tooth, administration of general anesthesia (GA)
- Medications stopped evening before surgery
- Should be scheduled in the morning and not be subjected to prolonged fasting
- Patients with IDDM should hold their dose of regular insulin and alter the dose of intermediate-acting insulin

- Traditionally the dose is one-fourth or one-half of the actual dose
- One of the protocols for control of the IDDM during the perioperative period is the split dose technique
- All long-acting preparation is changed to short acting. A glucose infusion is begun and subcutaneous (SC) insulin is given according to need demonstrated by hourly capillary glucose evaluations
- Mix 50 U of regular insulin in 500 ml of normal saline (1U/h = 10 ml/hr)
- Initiate IV infusion at 0.5–1U/hour
- Measure blood glucose concentration every hour and adjust infusion rates accordingly.

Postoperative Care

- Continue the glucose infusion
- Check the serum glucose and acetone levels
- After the patient has voided completely, start checking urine fractional samples for glucose and acetone
- Write orders on a sliding; scale the amount of insulin to be given for specific urine glucose levels

Units of CZI	Urine sugar
10–20	4
10–15	3
5–10	2
0–5	1

HEMOPHILIA, ANTICOAGULATION

- One of the most important factors in successful surgery lies in the control of bleeding
- Bleeding disorders may be either (Table 5.3):
  - *Intrinsic*: Results from congenitally deficient or dysfunctional components of the hemostatic system
  - *Acquired*: because of an underlying condition or disease

Laboratory Screening Tests

- Bleeding time
- Platelet count
- Partial thromboplastin time (PTT)
- Prothrombin time (PT)

Table 5.3: Intrinsic and acquired bleeding disorder	
Intrinsic bleeding disorder	Acquired bleeding disorder
Hemophilia A	Thrombocytopenia
Hemophilia B	Decresed production of platelets
von Willebrand's disease	Increased destruction of platelets
	Patients on anticoagulants
	Liver disease

Bleeding Time

- Von Willebrand's disease
- Thrombocytopenia caused by drug
- Autoimmune thrombocytopenia
- Pregnancy
- Hypersplenism
- Cirrhosis
- Drugs such as warfarin
- Vessel abnormality.

Platelet Count

- *Normal:*190000–400000 per microliter
- Thrombocytopenia ranges from 50000-100000
- However, the minor surgical procedures, such as tooth extraction and biopsy are usually tolerated
- Placing Gelfoam or microfibrillar collagen in the socket accelerates the formation of platelet plug.

Partial Thromboplastin Time

- *Normal*: 22–36 seconds
- Tests the factors involved in the intrinsic coagulation pathway, viz VIII, IX, XI, XII
- Hemophilia A
- Hemophilia B.

Prothrombin Time

- The normal range is 11–14 seconds
- Examines the efficiency of the extrinsic and common coagulation pathways, viz II, V, VII, X
- Increase in PT could be due to vitamin K deficiency, fat malabsorbtion, Coumadin

therapy, liver disease and disseminated intravascular coagulation (DIC)

$$International\ normalized\ ratio\ (INR) = \frac{Patient\ PT^C}{Control\ PT}$$

Management of Bleeding

- In case in which immediate anticoagulation is required the use of fresh frozen plasma is management of choice
- When bleeding is not severe the best therapeutic approach is to stop warfarin and follow the patient with a frequent PT/INR measurements until the desired level is reached
- For simple tooth extractions in a patient with an INR level 2.5 or lower, the use of local antifibrinolytic agents should be adequate
- *Tranexamic acid*: 10 ml of 4.8 percent aqueous solution can be used
- Direct pressure at the extraction sites
- Full liquid diet followed by soft diet for 5 days
- No aspirin postoperatively.

Management of Hemophilia

- Disorder is a sex-linked recessive trait
- The successful management is the adequate maintenance of the antihemophilic globulin (AHG)
- The normal AHG is 50–100 percent.
- Factor VIII replacement can be provided through blood, plasma, fresh frozen plasma and cryoprecipitate.

THYROID DISORDERS

Patients having thyroid disorders can be classified broadly into.
- Hypothyroid
- Euthyroid
- Hyperthyroid.

Investigations

Blood TSH, T_3 and T_4.

Imaging

- Ultrasonography (USG) (cysts)
- Radioisotope scans—gland uptake.

Cytopathology
- Fine needle aspirate (FNA)/biopsy (FNB)
- Hyperthyroidism leads to hypermetabolic state in the body resulting in catabolic state with tachycardia, diarrhea and heat tolerance
- If the patient is subjected to stress, thyroid storm occurs.

Management
- Monitor the hormone levels intra- and postoperatively
- Continuous monitoring of the vital parameters
- Check for signs
- If the patient is in a thyroid storm treat by cooling the patient, intravenous infusion of glucose and IV fluids.

ADRENAL DISEASES

Common adrenal disorders that have to be dealt with during surgical procedure are:

Cushing's Syndrome

Signs
- Centripetal obesity
- Moon face
- Buffalo hump
- Hypertension
- Thin skin and purpura
- Muscle weakness
- Osteoporotic changes and fractures.

Addison's Disease

Signs
- Postural hypotension
- Salt and water depletion
- Weight loss and lethargy
- Hyperpigmentation
- Scars, mouth and skin creases due to pigmentation effect of increased adrenocorticotropic hormone secretion
- Vitiligo
- During surgery attention must be paid in maintaining optimum levels of carbohydrates in the body, sodium and potassium ion levels and the blood pressure
- Patients with adrenal insufficiency should be supplemented with adequate exogenous steroids prior to procedure to help the patient combat with stress.

Intra- and Postoperative Management
- Continuous monitoring of the vital signs
- Adequate intravenous corticosteroid supplements to prevent adrenal crisis
- Maintain fluid and electrolyte balance.

RENAL DISEASE

Renal Failure and Acute Glomerulonephritis
- Disturbances in the renal function leads to changes in the acid-base balance, serum calcium, and phosphorous levels
- Postoperative infection
- Associated hypertension secondary to fluid retention and edema.

Preoperative Investigations
- Renal profile
- Urinalysis
- Electrolytes
- USG of kidneys

Management
- Monitoring of acid-base balance and electrolyte
- Renal profile-tests intra- and postoperatively
- Potassium overload during fluid replacement is to be avoided
- Patients should be covered with broad spectrum antibiotics.

HEPATIC DISEASE
- A history of chronic alcohol intake, substance abuse, repeated blood transfusions and viral hepatitis is indicative of probable silent liver disease
- The liver is the site for various drugs and anesthetic gases biotransformation and synthesis of vitamin K

- A patient with viral hepatitis should be handled with care to avoid inadvertent transmission of the disease

Preoperative Investigations
- *Liver enzymes*: SGOT, SGPT
- *Total bilirubin*: Direct and indirect
- Serum albumin
- Serum alkaline phosphatase
- Bleeding time and clotting time
- Prothrombin time
- USG liver.

Management
- Avoid anesthetic gases that are metabolized in the liver
- Correction of coagulation deficiency by IV vitamin K, fresh frozen plasma transfusions
- Careful intra- and postoperative management of blood volume, urine volume
- Appropriate precautions and sterilization techniques to prevent transmission of disease in carrier of viral hepatitis.

RESPIRATORY DISEASE
- *Cough*: What?
- Dry sputum (color?), blood
- *Wheeze*: Expiratory noise
- *Stridor*: Inspiratory noise
- *Dyspnea*: Distress on effort

- *Pain*: General/inspiratory
- *Infections*: Pneumonia
- Airflow obstruction
  - Asthma
  - Chronic obstructive pulmonary disease
  - Restrictive pulmonary change
- Gas exchange failure
  - Reduced surface area, fibrosis, fluid
- Tumors.

Preoperative Investigations
- Routine chest radiographs
- Pulmonary function test
- Blood investigations like arterial blood gases
- Sputum AFB culture
- Bronchoscopy if required.

  The patient should be on bronchodilators pre-intra- and post- operatively.

  Carry inhaler for use in case of emergency

IMMUNOCOMPROMISED PATIENT

Common Causes of Immunosupression
- Advanced age
- Malignancy
- Malnutrition
- Acquired/congenital immunodeficiency
- Trauma
- Burns
- Radiation.

Section

2

Examination of Maxillofacial Trauma Patient

Initial Assessment and Emergency Care of Maxillofacial Trauma Patient

6

INITIAL ASSESSMENT

Trauma is the leading cause of death in the first four decades of life. Trauma team can play a major role in reducing the incidence of death in such patients.

Advanced trauma life support protocol
- Primary survey and resuscitation
- Secondary survey
- Continued postresuscitation monitoring & re-evaluation
- Definitive treatment

Trimodal Death Distribution

Trimodal death distribution is described in Figure 6.1.

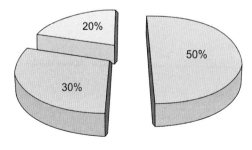

- Immediate: Trauma to first one hour
- Early: First four hours
- Late: 2–5 weeks

Fig. 6.1: Trimodal death distribution

- *First peak*: Nonsalvageable within minutes
- *Second peak*: Salvageable within minutes to hours
  - Hemopneumothorax
  - Fractures, abdominal organ injuries, pelvic fractures, etc.

The concept of 'Golden hour' emphasizes upon the urgency necessary for successful management. It refers to a time period lasting from a few minutes to first few hours following traumatic injury being sustained by a casualty, during which there is the highest likelihood that prompt medical treatment will prevent death

The first 10 minutes of prehospital care given to patients at the site of injury is Platinum 10 minutes

- *Third peak:* Days to weeks.

  Patient dies because of sepsis during this period.

PREPARATION

- Prehospital
  - Stabilization of airway
  - Control of external bleeding
  - Immobilization and transport
- Inhospital
  - Triaging the casualties
  - Identification of life-threatening injuries
  - Resuscitation and stabilization
  - Any other injury
  - Definitive care.

TRIAGE

- Triage is a protocol for immediate classification of the seriousness of the accident (Fig. 6.2)
- The term comes from the French word *trier*, meaning to 'sort out or cull out' wool into various categories depending upon the quality, a term used by Napoleon's surgeon
- It has been defined as 'doing the greatest good for the greatest number'

- A process of prioritizing patients based on the severity of their condition
- This protocol must be uniform, understandable and universally accepted. The aim of prehospital triage is the rapid and accurate on site identification of high-risk patients based on (Fig. 6.3):
1. Severity of the injury and its physiological effect—injury anatomy.

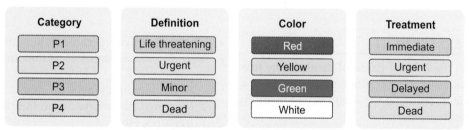

Fig. 6.2: Triage categories

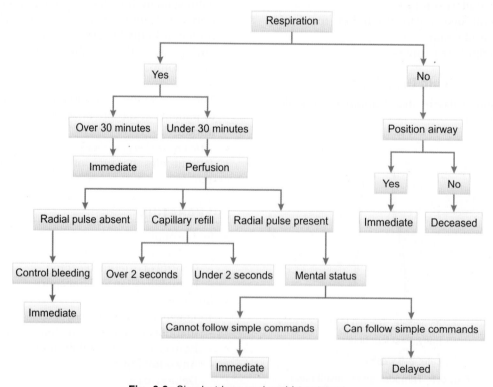

Fig. 6.3: Simple triage and rapid treatment

Table 6.1: Injury severity score

Region	Injury description	AIS	Square top three
Head and neck	Cerebral contusion	3	9
Face	No injury	0	0
Chest	Flail chest	4	16
Abdomen	Complex rupture spleen	5	25
Extremity	Fractured femur	3	0
External	No injury	0	0
	Injury severity score		50

Table 6.2: Revised trauma score

Coded value	Respiratory rate	Systolic BP	Glasgow coma score
4	10–29	>89	13–15
3	>20	76–89	9–12
2	6–9	50–75	6–8
1	1–5	1–49	4–5

predicting death. It is scored from the first set of data obtained on the patient, and consists of Glasgow coma scale, systolic blood pressure and respiratory rate.

$RTS = 0.9368\ GCS + 0.7326\ SBP + 0.2908\ RR$

- Values for the RTS are in the range 0 to 7.8408. The RTS is heavily weighted towards the Glasgow coma scale to compensate for major head injury without multisystem injury or major physiological changes. A threshold of RTS <4 has been proposed to identify those patients who should be treated in a trauma center, although this value may be somewhat low (Table 6.2).

PRIMARY SURVEY

A = Airway and cervical spine
B = Breathing
C = Circulation and hemorrhage control
D = Dysfunction of the central nervous system
E = Exposure.

Airway Maintenance

Recognize Airway Obstruction

The conditions associated with airway obstruction in the acutely injured and stabilized trauma victim must be recognized by using following algorithm.

Look	Listen	Feel
Signs of obvious airway obstructions	Any abnormal sounds during respiration	Any asymmetry on inspiration and expiration

Assess the Patency

- Signs of respiratory distress
  - i. Stridor
  - ii. Cyanosis
  - iii. Anxiety
  - iv. Tachypnea rate >25/min
  - v. Intercostals retraction
  - vi. Use of accessory muscles.

Causes of upper airway obstruction in trauma patient

- Tongue position
- Aspiration of foreign bodies
- Regurgitation of stomach contents
- Facial/tracheal/laryngeal fractures.

Conditions that influence airway management

1. **Syndromes:**
   i. Treacher Collins syndrome
   ii. Crouzon and Apert syndrome
   iii. Pierre Robin syndrome
   iv. Hemifacial microsomia
   v. Down syndrome
   vi. Goldenhar syndrome
2. **Infections:** Epiglottitis, bronchitis, pneumonia, abscess (submandibular, retropharyngeal, Ludwig's angina), papillomatosis, tetanus.
3. **Trauma:** Foreign body, cervical spine injury, fractures, soft tissue edema.
4. **Neoplastic:** Upper and lower airway tumors, radiation therapy.
5. **Inflammatory:** Rheumatoid arthritis, ankylosing spondylitis, (TMJ) syndrome, scleroderma, sarcoidosis, angioedema.
6. **Endocrine/metabolic:** Acromegaly, diabetes mellitus, myxedema, goiter, obesity.

Clear the Airway and Reposition the Patient

Allow the patient to maintain an existing airway through self posturing than to jeopardize the airway by forcing him or her to assume another position.

Airway Maneuvers and Adjuncts

- Chinlift/jaw thrust maneuver
- Oral and nasopharyngeal airways
- Bag-valve mask ventilation.
- Perform endotracheal intubation (Fig. 6.6) or surgical airway if unable to intubate.

Airway Maintenance Techniques

1. Chin lift
2. Jaw thrust
3. Oropharyngeal airway
4. Nasopharyngeal airway

The triple maneuver, head tilt/chin lift, jaw thrust and open mouth done together is the most reliable method to maintain a patent upper airway.

Definitive Airway

Indications

- Unconscious
- Severe maxillofacial fracture

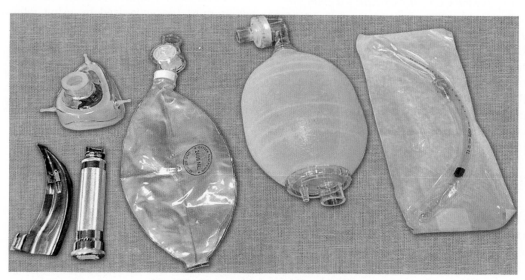

Fig. 6.6: Endotracheal intubation equipment

- *Risk for aspiration*: Bleeding/vomiting
- Risk for obstruction
- Neck hematoma/laryngeal, tracheal injury, stridor
- Inadequate respiratory effort
- Tachypnea/hypoxia/hypercapnia/cyanosis
- *Severe head injury*: Need for hyperventilation.

Laryngoscopy
- *Direct*: Through a laryngoscope
- *Indirect*: Through a laryngeal mirror
- One can inspect the base of tongue, valleculae, epiglottis, aryepiglottic folds, piriform fossa, vestibular and vocal fold

Anatomy of the visualization of the vocal cords with a laryngoscope:
- Alignment of 3 axes.
- Curved blade is inserted into the vallecula.
- Straight blade is inserted directly into esophagus.
- Visualization of cord may be facilitated by BURP maneuver.

Airway adjuncts
- Guedel
- Laryngeal mask airway (LMA) (Fig. 6.7)
- ETC/Combitube.

Invasive airway access—surgical airway
- Cricothyroidotomy
  - Needle cricothyrotomy
  - Percutaneous cricothyrotomy
- Tracheostomy.

Needle cricothyrotomy and transtracheal jet insufflations
- First described by Sanders in 1969
- Indications
  - When edema of the glottis
  - Fracture of the larynx
  - Severe oropharyngeal hemorrhage obstructs the airway and an endotracheal tube cannot be placed into the trachea
- Jet insufflation can provide up to 45 minutes of extratime before a definitive airway is established
- It is performed by a large bore cannula 12–14 gauge through the cricothyroid membrane into the trachea
- Cannula is connected to an oxygen source with a Y connector or side hole
- Intermittent sufflation 1 second on and 4 seconds off is accomplished by occluding the Y connector.

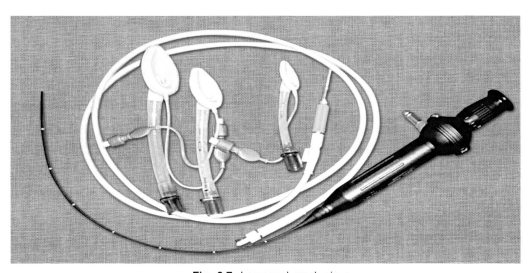

Fig. 6.7: Laryngeal mask airway

Cricothyroidotomy

Indications

  i. Maxillofacial trauma
 ii. Oropharyngeal obstruction
iii. Condition in which oral and nasal intubation is contraindicated
 iv. Spinal cord injury.

Contraindications

- Age; in children under the age of 10–12 years
- Crush injury to the larynx
- Pre-existing laryngeal or tracheal pathological condition; obstruction secondary to tumor or subglottic stenosis.

Procedure

- The space between thyroid and cricoid cartilage, i.e. cricothyroid membrane is the site of the cricothyrotomy
- Usual width 2.7–3.2 cm and height 0.5–1.2 cm
- Once the anatomy is identified and marked, local or general anesthesia is administered
- The head and neck is placed in a slightly extended position
- Unless contraindicated a horizontal incision is made through skin and subcutaneous tissue
- The incision is made superior to the cricoid cartilage
- A Trousseau dilator is inserted and spread vertically, to enlarge the opening of the membrane.

Advantages

- More rapid
- Less complications
- Improved cosmetic result
- Less soft tissue thickness to pass through Contraindicated in children, laryngeal infection.

Tracheostomy

- Tracheotomy is a surgical procedure in which an opening is made in the anterior wall of the trachea to establish airway
- In contrast, tracheostomy is the surgical creation of and opening into the trachea through the neck, with the tracheal mucosa being contact with the skin.

Indications

- Major laryngeal trauma.
- Inability to intubate or perform needle cricothyrotomy.
- Laryngeal foreign body or pathology.
- Prolonged ventilation.
- Facilitation of management of cervical spine injuries or oncological resections of the head and neck.

Contraindications

- When a cricothyrotomy may be performed more safely
- Expanding hematoma in the neck.

Procedure

- *Incisions*: Both vertical and horizontal are advocated. In the emergency situation, the vertical incision has been advocated. The incision is made from the inferior to the cricoid cartilage to the suprasternal notch
- For improved cosmetic results in an elective tracheostomy horizontal incision is advocated
- Retraction and dissection exposes the pre tracheal fascia and the thyroid isthmus
- Two principles must be adhered
  - Cricoid cartilage and the 1st tracheal ring must not be cut or injured
  - The incision into the trachea must not be extended below the 4th tracheal ring
- A tracheostomy hook is placed between the 1st and 2nd tracheal ring
- Various entrance incision into the trachea is advocated such as U incision-inverted U-T incision and cruciform
- The inverted incision advocated by Bjork and Dukes is preferred.

Complications

- Tracheal stenosis, bleeding, obstruction of tube, mucosal ulceration, cartilaginous necrosis
- Hemorrhage, hypoxia, pneumothorax, sub cutaneous emphysema, tracheesophageal fistula, damage to recurrent laryngeal nerves
- Hemorrhage, infection, aspiration.

Cervical spine injury
- Multisystem trauma, altered consciousness or blunt trauma above the level of clavicle
- Hyperextension to be avoided
- Neutral position by means of, spine board and bolstering device
- Semirigid cervical collar to be avoided—stabilize only 50 percent of movements.

Breathing and Ventilation
- Expose patient's chest for chest wall excursions
- Inspection of wounds
- Palpation without spinal movement
- Detect injuries to chest wall
- Percussion for presence of air or blood
- Auscultation to assure gas flow to lungs.

Identify
- Pnuemothorax
  - Open
  - Closed
  - Tension
- Massive hemothorax
- Flail chest with contusion.

Circulation
- Hemorrhage is the most common cause of early post-injury death.
- Ominous signs:
  - Altered level of consciousness
  - Pale skin
  - Rapid thready central pulse.

Shock
- Abnormality of the circulatory system that results in inadequate organ perfusion and tissue oxygenation. Any patient who is cold and tachycardic is in shock until proven otherwise
- Shock in trauma patient is hypovolemic until proven otherwise
- Systolic BP maintained till 30 percent of loss
- Tachycardia occurs before drop in systolic BP
- Tachycardia is present if rate is greater than 160 in an infant, 140 in preschool child, 120 from 5 years to puberty and 100 in adult

Table 6.3: Effect of blood loss			
Blood loss	*<15%*	*15–30%*	*>40%*
Heart rate	<100	>120	>140
SBP	N	N	Highly low
Cap refill	N	Delayed	-do-
RR	14–20	20–30	>35
CNS	Anxious	++	Lethargic

Abbreviations: SBP, systolic blood pressure; RR, respiratory rate; CNS, central nervous system

- Changes in vital signs with percentage blood volume lost (Table 6.3).

Fluid Resuscitation
- Crystalloid, colloid or blood.
- Crystalloid in the ratio of 3 ml of crystalloid to 1 ml blood.
- *Colloids*:
  - Albumin 5%
  - Gelatin
  - Hydroxyethyl starches
  - Dextran.

blood product replacement
- Class III and IV hemorrhage—packed red blood cells
- Thrombocytopenia (platelets <50,000)—platelets
- PT/PTT >1.5 normal—fresh frozen plasma
- Hemophilia A, von Willebrand's disease, factor XIII deficiency, microvascular bleeding in transfused patients with fibrinogen concentrations <80–100 mg/dl—cryoprecipitate.

Acid-base balance
- Early hypovolemic shock → tachypnea → respiratory alkalosis → mild metabolic acidosis...does not require treatment
- Longstanding or severe shock → tissue ↑ perfusion → ↑ anaerobic metabolism → severe metabolic acidosis → treat with fluids
- If pH <7.2 → sodium bicarbonate.

Therapeutic decisions
Rapid response to initial ↑ fluid administration: Patient has lost <20 percent of blood volume. No

further transfusion required but cross matched blood should be kept available.

Transient response
Respond to fluid but once slowed perfusion indices will deteriorate. Have lost 20–40 percent of blood volume or still bleeding. Continue fluid administration and initiate blood transfusion

Minimal or no response
- Usually require surgical intervention to control exsanguinating hemorrhage
- Rarely due to pump failure secondary to cardiac contusion or tamponade. CVP monitoring helps to differentiate between two.

Evaluation of response to treatment
- Return of normal BP, pulse pressure and pulse rate, are signs that circulation is stabilizing
- Improved skin circulation and CNS status do show enhanced perfusion
- Urinary output can be easily measured and is one of prime monitors
- CVP monitoring can be useful in complicated cases
- Urine output reflects renal blood flow
- Adequate volume replacement should produce approximately
  - 50 ml/hr in adult
  - 1 ml/kg/hr in children
  - 2 ml/kg/hr in babies; 1yr.

Disability: Brief Neurological Examination
- Detail neurological examination at the end of primary survey
- Establishes level of consciousness, pupillary size and reaction
  - A: Alert
  - V: Response to vocal stimuli
  - P: Responds to pain
  - U: Unresponsive
- Changes in neurological examination may indicate intracranial pathology or reflect hypovolemia or decreased oxygenation of CNS.

Indications for CT
- Patients with seizure activity
- Unconsciousness lasting longer than a few minutes
- Abnormal mental status
- Abnormal neurological evaluation
- Clinical evidence of skull fracture
- Also suggested for patients with blunt trauma and who have experienced loss of consciousness or mild amnesia.

Exposure
- Patient should be completely undressed to facilitate thorough examination and assessment
- Patient should be kept warm during this stage

Adjuncts to Primary Survey and Resuscitation
- ECG :
  - *Dysrhythmias*: Blunt cardiac injury
  - PEA: Tamponade, pneumothorax, hypovolemia
  - Bradycardia, VPCs: Hypoxia.
- *Urinary catheter*: Volume status, renal perfusion
- *Gastric catheter*: Decompress stomach, reduce risk of aspiration
- *Monitoring*: BP, pulse oximeter, arterial blood gas level, RR
- *X-rays and diagnostic studies*:
  - Chest, CS, pelvis
  - Diagnostic peritoneal lavage
  - USG abdomen.

Neurological Consequences Associated with Maxillofacial Injury

7

INTRODUCTION

Maxillofacial region has all special structures and centers for breathing, speech, vision, hearing, mastication, and diglution and is highly vulnerable to wide variety of injuries. These injuries can often be dramatic and for the patients are frequently disfiguring leading to considerable psychological damage. This injuries often disrupt the appearance and ability to express emotion. Hence it is crucial to establish an early, clear understanding of the mechanism of injury.

Patient sustaining maxillofacial injuries are at a great risk of accompanying injuries. Localized injury to the face resulting in fractures may also involve brain and meninges. In many cases maxillofacial injuries distract attention from more critical often life-threatening injuries.

- Road traffic accidents accounts for 70 percent of brain injuries
- Brain injury is 10 times more common than spinal injury
- Twice more common in males than females
- Alcohol intoxication in at least 30–50 percent of head injuries
- Correlation exists between midfacial injuries and central nervous system (CNS) trauma
- Intracranial hemorrhage cannot be excluded in patients with maxillofacial fractures even when a GCS score of 15 and normal neurological findings. Hence, accurate and systematic assessment is essential
- Predictors such as nausea, vomiting, seizures, skull base injuries and closed head injuries enhance the likelihood of a intracranial hemorrhage and have to be considered.

PATHOPHYSIOLOGY

- Brain receives about 1/5th of total cardiac output
- $CPP = MAP - ICP$
- Intracranial pressure: 0–15 cm of H_2O.

1 liter per min at rest (cerebral blood flow) or 49 mL/100 gm of brain/min
• Normal
At 25-39 mL/100 gm/min
• Confusion and sometimes loss of consciousness
At 8 mL/100 gm/min
• Neuronal death

CLASSIFICATION OF HEAD INJURIES

1. According to duration since impact:

Primary: Inertial brain injury (Figs 7.1 to 7.3)
Contact brain injury
a. Cerebral contusions (Figs 7.1A and B)
b. Skull fractures (Figs 7.3A and B)
c. Concussions

Secondary: Hematoma formation
a. Extradural hematoma (Fig. 7.4)
b. Acute subdural hematoma (Figs 7.5A and B)
c. Chronic subdural hematoma
d. Intracerebral hematoma

Primary Brain Injury (Figs 7.1 to 7.3)

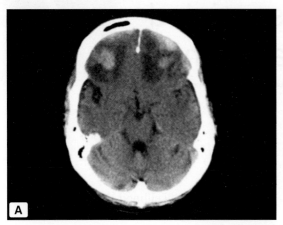 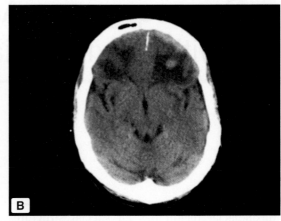

Figs 7.1A and B: Contusions

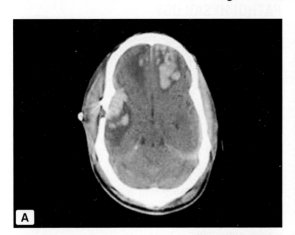 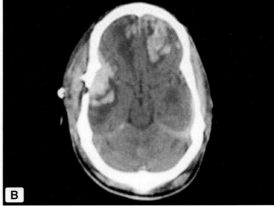

Figs 7.2A and B: Multiple contusions

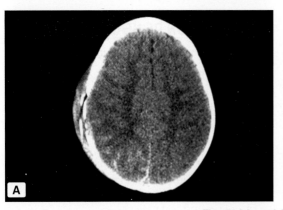 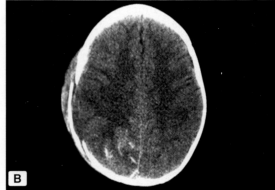

Figs 7.3A and B: Skull fracture

2. According to extent of involvement:
- Focal
- Diffuse

3. According to severity of injury:
- Mild
- Moderate
- Severe

4. According to site of impact:
- Coup injuries
- Counter-coup injuries.

PRIMARY ASSESSMENT

- Level of consciousness
- Pupil

Secondary Brain Injury (Figs 7.4 to 7.8)

- Motor power
- Glassgow comma scale.

Unilateral nonreactive pupillary dilatation in head trauma commonly heralds uncal herniation secondary to an expanding supratentorial mass lesion.

Alarming findings

Bradycardia and papillary dilatation

SECONDARY ASSESSMENT

"Three S's":

Simple

Systematic

Standardized

- It is a complete head to toe detailed examination of the patient

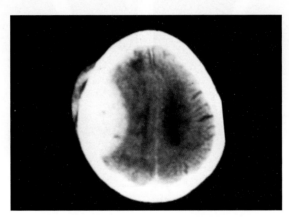

Fig 7.4: Extradural hematoma

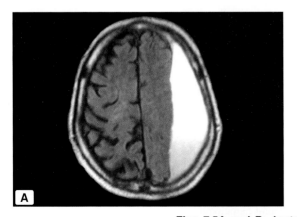
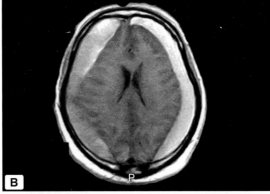

Figs 7.5A and B: Acute subdural hematoma

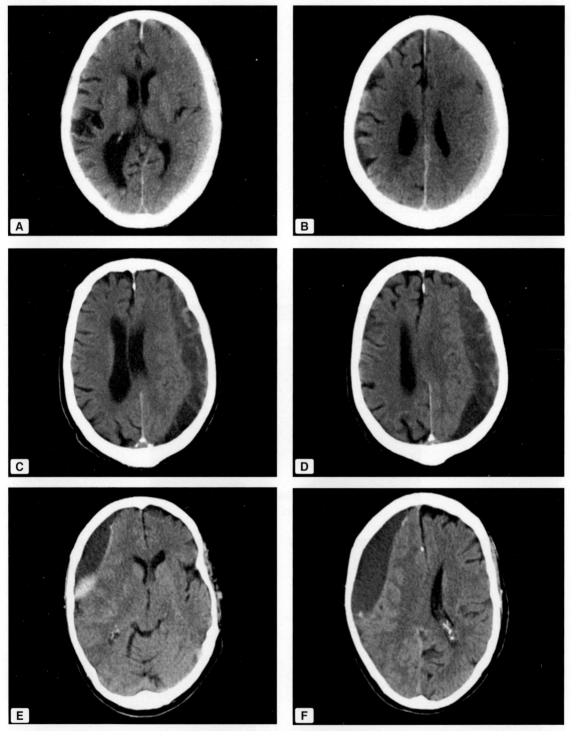

Figs 7.6A to F: Subdural hematoma

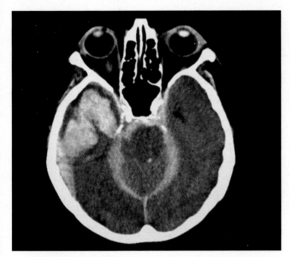

Fig 7.7: Multiple hemorrhages after trauma

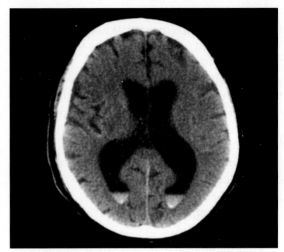

Fig 7.8: Intraventricular hemorrhage

- Full history and reassessment of vital signs
- Complete neurological examination including GCS
- Special investigations such as radiographs, lab investigations
- Facial grimace in response to pain above but not below the clavicles
- Hypotension without evidence of hemorrhage.

Associated Trauma

- Scalp
- Periauricular region
- Periorbital region
- Face
- Cervical spine.

NEUROLOGICAL EXAMINATION

The neurological examination consists of the following components:

1. Higher cognitive function as assessed by the mental status examination.
2. Cranial nerves.
3. Motor system.
4. Sensory systems.
5. Stance and gait.

CRANIAL NERVES EXAMINATION

CN I: Olfactory

- Usually not tested
- Rash, deformity of nose
- Test each nostril with essence bottles of coffee, vanilla, peppermint.

CN II: Optic

- With patient wearing glasses, test each eye separately on eye chart/card using an eye cover
- Examine visual fields by confrontation by wiggling fingers 1 foot from patient's ears, asking which they see move
- Keep examiner's head level with patient's head
- If poor visual acuity, map fields using fingers and a quadrant-covering card
- Look into fundi.

CN III, IV, VI: Oculomotor, Trochlear, Abducens

- *Look at pupils:* Shape, relative size, ptosis.
- Shine light in from the side to asses pupil's light reaction
- Assess both direct and consensual responses

- Assess afferent papillary defect by moving light in arc from pupil to pupil. While doing arc test, have patient block light so that light can only go into one eye at a time
- Follow finger with eyes without moving head: test the 6 cardinal points in an H pattern
- Look for failure of movement, nystagmus
- Convergence by moving finger towards bridge of patient's nose
- Test accommodation by patient looking into distance, then a hat pin 30 cm from nose.

CN V: Trigeminal

- *Corneal reflex*: Patient looks up and away
- Look for blink in both eyes, ask if can sense it
- *Facial sensation*: Sterile sharp item on forehead, cheek, jaw
- Repeat with dull object. Ask to report sharp or dull
- If abnormal, then temperature, light touch
- *Motor*: Patient opens mouth, clenches teeth. Palpate temporalis and masseter muscles as they clench.

CN VII: Facial

- Inspect facial droop or asymmetry
- *Facial expression muscles*: Patient looks up and wrinkles forehead
- Examine wrinkling loss
- Feel muscle strength by pushing down on each side
- Examine the facial expression.

CN VIII: Vestibulocochlear (Hearing, Vestibular Rarely)

Do specific tests like:
- Weber's test: Lateralization
- Rinne's test: Air vs Bone conduction

CN IX, X: Glossopharyngeal, Vagus

- *Voice*: Hoarse or nasal
- Patient swallows, coughs
- Examine palate for uvular displacement
- *Patient says "Ah"*: Symmetrical soft palate movement
- Gag reflex.

CN XI: Accessory

- From behind, examine for trapezius atrophy, asymmetry
- Patient shrugs shoulders
- *Patient turns head against resistance*: Watch, palpate SCM on opposite side.

CN XII: Hypoglossal

- Listen to articulation.
- Inspect tongue in mouth for wasting, fasciculations.
- *Protrude tongue*: Unilateral deviates to affected side.

EXAMINATION OF MOTOR SYSTEM

Components of the Motor Examination

- Abnormal involuntary movements
- Posture
- Muscle bulk
- Tone
- Power
- Coordination
- Deep tendon reflexes.

EXAMINATION OF SENSORY SYSTEM

Components of the Sensory Examination

- Light touch
- Pain and temperature
- Vibration sense
- Position sense
- 2 point discrimination
- Double simultaneous stimuli (extinction).

Investigations Require in Head Injury Patients

- Hemogram
- Blood chemistry
- Coagulation profile

- Blood grouping and cross matching
- Arterial blood gas analysis
- Wound swab.

IMAGING

- Plain skull X-ray
- CT scan
- MRI.

Indications

1. GCS <15 at 2 hours after injury
2. Vomiting >2 episodes
3. Age >65 years
4. Confusion
5. Loss of consciousness
6. Seizures
7. Deteriorating consciousness
8. Confusion persisting after initial assessment
9. Resuscitation
10. Progressive headache
11. Multiple trauma
12. Any sign of base of skull fracture, open skull fracture.

UNCONSCIOUS PATIENT

- Always pause and observe an unconscious or drowsy patient for a few moments before disturbing them
- Change in level of consciousness is the single most important information.

History (Specific Indicator Points)

- Subarachnoid hemorrhage: Coma of sudden onset
- Subdural hematoma: History of trauma with concussion, followed a few days later with fluctuating drowsiness and stupor
- Extradural hematoma: Concussion followed by a brief lucid interval before rapidly deepening coma
- A history of headache before coma frequently present with intracranial space occupying lesion of any cause.

Pattern of Breathing

- Cheyne–Stokes respiration—subdural hematoma
- Altered respiration pattern—Raised ICP.

CRITICAL CARE IN HEAD INJURY

The aim is prevent secondary injury to the damaged neuron

- Prevent hypoxia
- Prevent hypotension
- Control hyperglycemia
- Maintain normal serum Na^+ level.

CONTRIBUTION OF NEUROSURGEON IN TRAUMA TEAM

Treating associated head injury and spine injury, management of CSF leak, meningitis, and whenever access and repair of anterior cranial fossa—single stage repair is required.

Maxillofacial Trauma: First 24 Hours in Intensive Care Unit

8

INTRODUCTION

Airway management hemodynamic monitoring are the prime concern of acute phase of severe maxillofacial injuries. In addition to comprehensive physiological monitoring facial trauma with or without life-threatening complication may arise isolated injury or it may be associated with significant injury elsewhere. Assessment may be systematic or repeated in overall management.

Concept of Intensive Care

- In 1854, Florence Nightingale left for the Crimean War, where the necessity to separate seriously wounded soldiers from less-seriously wounded was observed
- Nightingale reduced mortality from 40 to 2 percent on the battlefield, creating the concept of intensive care.

INTENSIVE CARE UNIT

Major trauma victims often spend the first 24 hours in ICU or high dependancy units (Figs 8.1A to C):
ICU = Intensive Care Unit
- Serves as a place for monitoring and providing care of patients with potentially severe physiological instability requiring artificial support
- Level of care is greater than what is available in the ward

Major roles for ICU
Diagnosis of injuries and clearing spine
Oxygen support
Optimization of: • Hemodynamics   • Oxygenation   • Homeostasis   • Normalization of temperature   • Coagulation

- Treating underlying comorbidities
  Discussing the injuries and treatment plan with the family.

Criteria for ICU Admission

- Avoid patients with 'too well to benefit' and 'too sick to benefit'
- Thus ICU admission decision may be based on one of the following criteria:
  - Prioritization
  - Diagnosis
  - Objective.

PRIORITIZATION

- Assessed as priority 1–4
- This system defines those that will benefit most from the ICU (priority 1) to those that will not benefit at all (priority 4).

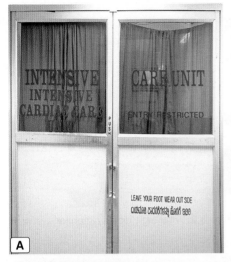
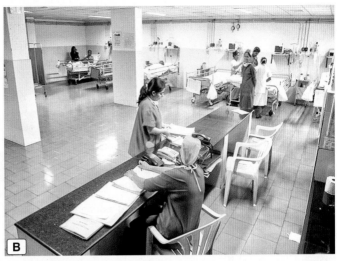
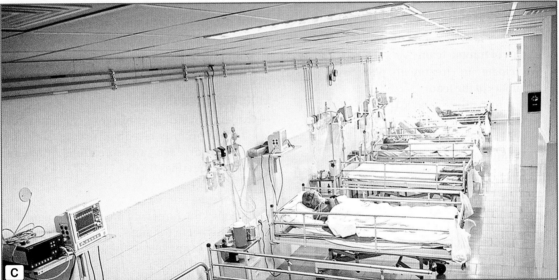

Figs 8.1A to C: Intensive care unit

Priority 1: Critically ill, unstable patients.

For example, postoperative acute respiratory failure, hemodynamic shock, trauma patients with GCS <8.

Priority 2: Patients requiring intensive monitoring and may need immediate intervention.

For example, Patients with chronic comorbid conditions

Priority 3: Unstable/critically ill patients with less chance of recovery.
For example, Patients with metastatic malignancy complicated by infection, cardiac tamponade, or airway obstruction.

Priority 4: These patients are generally not appropriate for ICU admission.

Facial injuries resulting in life-threatening conditions include
Facial injuries resulting in airway compromise (e.g. panfacial fractures with gross displacement, mobility, or swelling; comminuted fractures of the mandible; gunshot wounds; profuse bleeding; foreign bodies)
Anterior neck injuries, resulting in airway compromise (e.g. penetrating injuries, laryngeal or tracheal injuries)
Injuries resulting in profuse blood loss (e.g. penetrating neck, facial fractures, however rare)

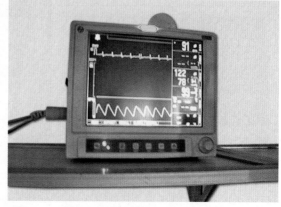

Fig. 8.2: Vital sign display monitor

Maxillofacial ICU Personnel Responsibility

- They may be involved in the initial trauma call as part of trauma team
- Participate in treatment plan with other members of the team
- Ability to institute good ICU care early
  - Keeping the patient warm
  - Well oxygenated
  - Ventilated
  - Early insertion of lines
  - Monitoring vital signs (Fig. 8.2)
- When patient reaches ICU it is important to discuss with all other teams:
  - What the injuries are?
  - What plan is for their area of interest?
    For example, neurosurgery, orthopedic, anesthesiology
- How the patient responded to:
  - IV Fluids
  - Anesthesia
- Rapidly assess airway, breathing, and circulation and ensure ongoing appropriate resuscitation
- Go through case sheet of information, about the patient ambulance, casualty notes, radiology, operating notes, anesthesiology or old prescriptions.

What are the Emergency Conditions?

- Systolic BP <90 (adult patient)
- Respiratory rate <9 or >30 (adult patient)
- Child (<12 years) heart rate > 130.

Emergency Intubation

- Evidence of airway or respiratory compromise (stridor, profuse bleeding, use of accessory muscles or "see-saw" breathing, impaired swallowing) (Figs 8.3 to 8.7).
- GCS <12
- Penetrating trauma
- Any open fractures with mechanism suggestive of multisystem trauma
- Evidence of spinal cord injury with neurologic deficit
- Any injury with uncontrolled bleeding
- Any child younger than 1 year of age
- Scalp degloving.

Sequel of Facial Injury

Obstruction of airway
↓
Asphyxia
↓
Cerebral hypoxia
↓
Brain damage/ death

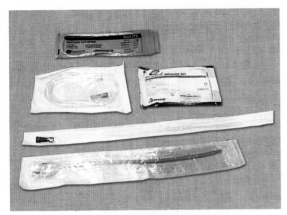

Fig. 8.3: RT tube, urinary catheter, ET tube, suction tube, etc.

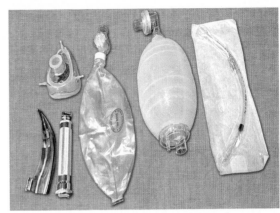

Fig. 8.4: Emergency intubation set

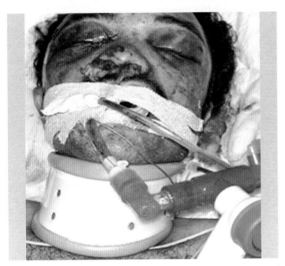

Fig. 8.5: Trauma patient with spinal collar and intubated

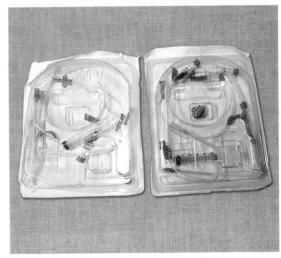

Fig. 8.6: Endotracheal tube

- Is the patient fully conscious? And able to maintain adequate airway?
- Semiconscious or unconscious patient rapidly suffocate because of inability to cough and adopt a posture that held tongue forward.

What is Emergency?

- Focus on clinical problem that requires
  - Resuscitation
  - Emergency
  - Urgent
  - Routine
- Immediate identification and management to preserve life

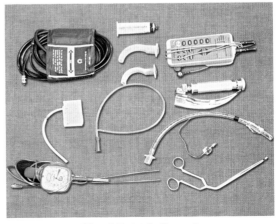

Fig. 8.7: Intubation set

- Hence focus on resuscitation but not on definitive treatment
- Many conditions may be considered clinically "urgent".

  For example, contaminated wounds, open fracture. But these can be left until the patient is fully stabilized with little or no increase in mortality or morbidity.

Emergency Care

1. Airway care
2. Control of profuse bleeding
3. Management of vision threatening injuries.

Trimodal Distribution of Death—3 Peaks

- Instantaneous or within seconds
- If untreated or within minutes or an hour after accident and this period is known as Golden hour
- Occurs in hospital after a week or more due to sepsis or multiorgan failure.

Principles

- To prevent further injury by inept and over enthusiastic treatment
- To save life of patient, to achieve pretreatment quality of life
- To restore function
- To prevent the 3rd peak from occurring.

Maxillofacial Injuries

- Maxillofacial trauma with or without life threatening complications, may arise following isolated injury or it may be associated with significant injuries elsewhere
- A large number of patients predominantly younger age die due to trauma and if prompt and proper management is instituted, many of them can be saved with an acceptable quality of life

- Maxillofacial trauma is a challenge as it compromises airway, vision, circulatory status and neurological centers
- Life saving role is an important one in the second peak and also in prevention of third peak in ICU
- Treatment divided into following phases:
  - Emergency or initial care
  - Early care
  - Definitive care
  - Secondary care or revision.

Emergency Care (Figs 8.8 to 8.11)

- C-spine stabilization
- Preserve the airway
- Control of hemorrhage
- Prevent or control shock
- Control of life-threatening injuries, head injuries, chest injuries, compound limb fractures, intra-abdominal bleeding.

Stabilization of Associated Injuries

C-spine injury suspected

- Avoid any movement of spinal column
- Establish and maintain proper immobilization until vertebral fractures or spinal cord injuries ruled out
  - Lateral C-spine radiographs
  - CT of C-spine
  - Neurologic examination
- Retropharyngeal hematoma secondary to cervical spine injury can also occasionally result in airway obstruction and its presence should alert the clinician to the possibility of cervical spine injury
- In each trauma patient, first priority is to assess the airway at the same time protecting the cervical spine
- In many cases initial assessment requires a verbal response from the patient
  - What happened?
  - How do you feel?

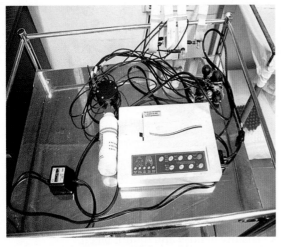

Fig. 8.8: ECG machine

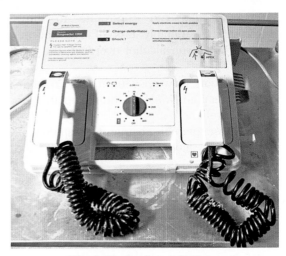

Fig. 8.10: Cardiac defibrillator

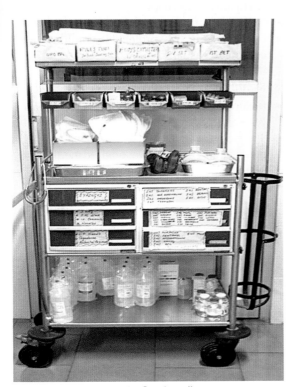

Fig. 8.9: Crash trolley

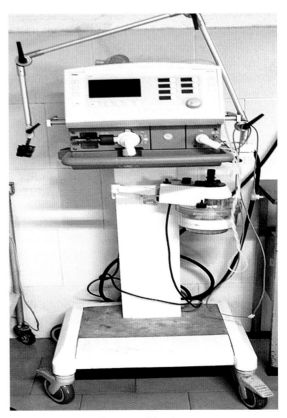

Fig. 8.11: Ventilator

- Many factors can contribute to airway compromise notably loss of consciousness (associated with alcohol overdose and brain injury)
- Obstruction may arise from foreign bodies (chewing gum, sweets, dentures, teeth, blood and secretions)
- The most common obstructing materials that threaten the airway in facial injuries are blood and vomit.
- Trauma to the front of neck can result in direct injury to upper airway and an expanding hematoma due to arterial bleeding
- Occasionally displaced midface fracture may cause airway obstruction
- The face can be regarded as 'crumple zone'.

Conclusion

- Fortunately life-threatening maxillofacial injuries are uncommon (Fig. 8.12)
- However they do occur in well-defined high-risk groups and as such, it is important that clinicians maintain high index of suspicion and treat these emergencies accordingly in 24 hours
- The best outcome for these traumatized patients is associated with treatment by a multi-disciplinary trauma team, which includes a maxillofacial surgeon who has the experience in these situations
- Important realization is the fact that the first 24 hours is crucial and that will determine the outcome of accident and it is during this period that maxillofacial trauma and proper management by the ICU team is important for increasing the salvage rate among these patients, leading to a good quality of life and better economics for the nation and community.

CASE PRESENTATION

- A 21 years female patient reported to casualty with chief complaint of injury on the face due to RTA

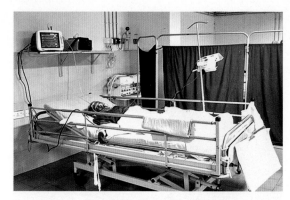

Fig. 8.12: Patient in ICU

- History of nose and mouth bleed
- History of anterograde amnesia
- No history of loss of consciousness
- No history of ear bleed
- No history of seizures
- No history of vomiting or nausea
- One episode of projectile vomiting after coming to casualty.

Past Medical History

- Recurrent episodes of giddiness from past 5 years
- 3 episodes of seizures (?) 5 years back, sought medical consultation, was advised medications. Medications were discontinued 2 years back
- History of breathlessness at night.

Personal History

- Mother reports – mild depression (following father's death due to electrocution)
- ↑ sleep, ↓ appetite
- History of bruxism present
- Mixed diet 3times/day
- Bowel/bladder habits regular.

Family History

Nothing contributory.

Drug History

No previous history of any drug allergy.

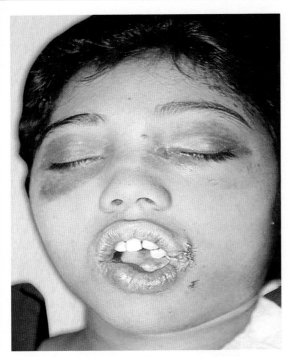

Fig. 8.13: Trauma patient with circumorbital ecchymosis

General Physical Examination

- Patient is moderately built and nourished
- Patient is conscious, oriented to place and person, confused conversation, drowsy but arousable, moving all limbs, eye opening on command, obeying simple orders (Fig. 8.13)
- GCS = E3 M6 V4 = 13/15
- Vitals
  Pulse: 98/min
  BP: 100/60 mm Hg
  RR: 20 b/min
  Temperature: Afebrile
  P° I° Cy° Cl° L° E°

Cardiovasular System

S1, S2 heart sounds heard.

Respiratory System

NVBS, bilateral air entry to lungs + crowing sound.

Pulmonary Artery

Soft, nontender, bowel sounds heard.

Central Nervous System

- B/L pupils reactive to light (direct and indirect reflexes present)
- Cranial nerves normal

Local Examination (Figs 8.14 to 8.16)

Inspection

- Severe facial edema
- Bilateral circumorbital edema and ecchymosis
- Active bleeding from nose/mouth
- Abrasion over left forehead and angle of mandible region
- Deep laceration over left commissure of mouth
- Inability to close and difficulty to open mouth
- Interincisal mouth opening 2.5 cm
- Flattening of malar region (more on left side).

Intraoral

- Displaced maxillary fracture between 21 and 22
- Displaced mandibular fracture between 42 and 43
- Hard and soft palatal tear present
- Ecchymosis present in lower lingual vestibule.

Palpation

- Step deformity and tenderness
  - Bilateral infraorbital rim, left zygomatic arch, left palate involving alveolus, right parasymphyseal region, left angle of mandible
- Crepitus
- Paresthesia present over bilateral cheek, upper lip, lateral aspect of nose and left half of lower lip.

Provisional Diagnosis

- Panfacial trauma involving
  - Le Fort II fracture

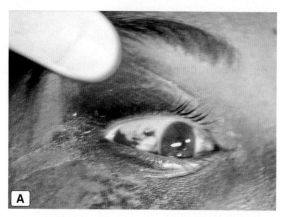
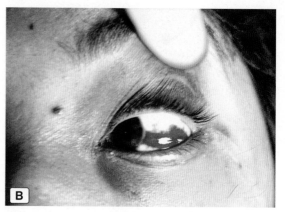

Figs 8.14A and B: Subconjuctival ecchymosis

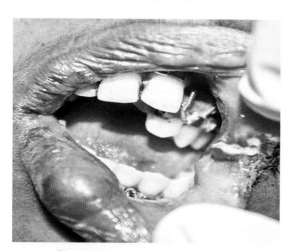

Fig. 8.15: Intraoral soft tissue injury

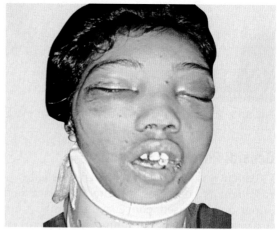

Fig. 8.16: ICU patient stabilized with cervical collar

- Left palatal fracture involving alveolus
- Bilateral infraorbital rim fracture
- Left zygomatic arch fracture
- Right parasymphyseal fracture
- Left angle of mandible fracture

Investigations (Figs 8.17 to 8.21)

CT Scan

Hematological investigations
- HIV: Negative
- HBsAg: Negative

- HCV: Negative
- Blood group: O⁺
- TLC: 14, 100/ mm³
- DLC: N-90%, L-5%, E-5%
- ESR: 0.5 mm/hour
- Serum creatinine: 0.9 mg/dL
- Blood urea: 13 mg/dL
- Na: 133.1 mmol/L
- K: 3.3 mmol/L
- Cl: 99 mmol/L
- BT: 2 min
- CT: 3 min 30 sec.

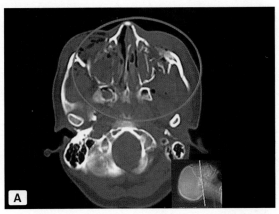
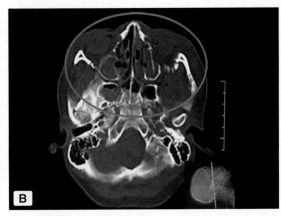

Figs 8.17A and B: CT showing fracture of orbital wall

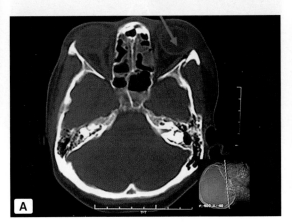
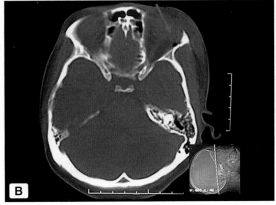

Figs 8.18A and B: CT showing fracture of lateral orbital wall

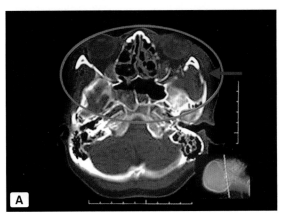
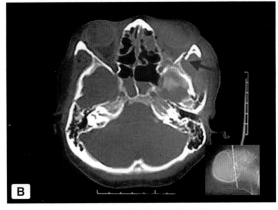

Figs 8.19A and B: CT showing fracture of zygomatic arch and orbital lateral wall

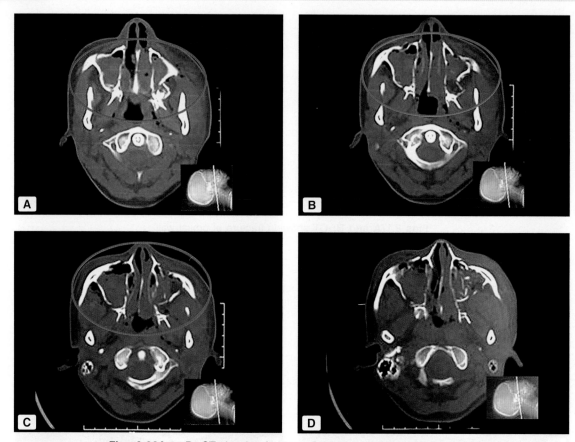

Figs 8.20A to D: CT showing fracture of anterior wall of maxillary sinus

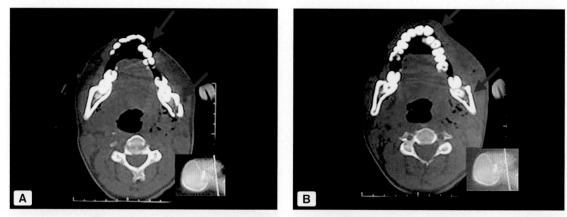

Figs 8.21A and B: CT showing fracture of mandible-symphysis and condyle

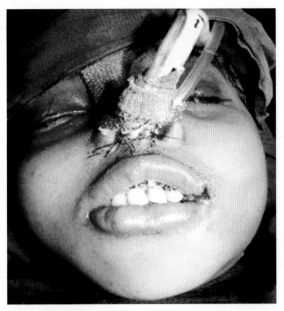

Fig. 8.22: Patient intubated

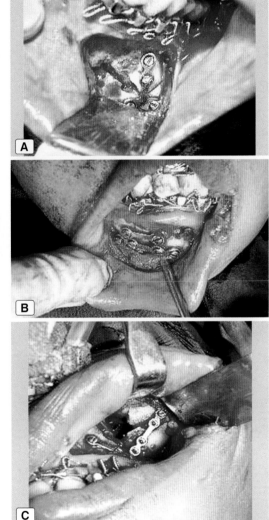

Figs 8.23A to C: Intraoperative bone plating

Management

Initial Management

Patient was shifted immediately to intensive care unit (Fig. 8.22)

- *Airway compromise*: Temporarily reduce the fractured facial bones encroaching on the airway

- *Severe hemorrhage*: Immediate surgery to ligate associated major vessels and to reduce the fracture segments

- *Large open wounds*: Debride and close in a layered fashion. Wounds that are to be used later for access to repair fractures may be closed in a temporary manner (Fig. 8.23 to 8.28).

- *Concomitant procedures*: Debriding and stabilizing maxillofacial inuries

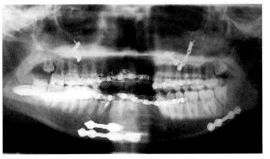

Fig. 8.24: Postoperative OPG showing bone plating

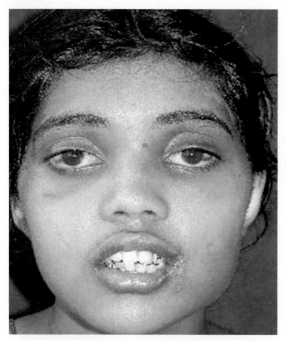

Fig. 8.25: Postoperative 20 days

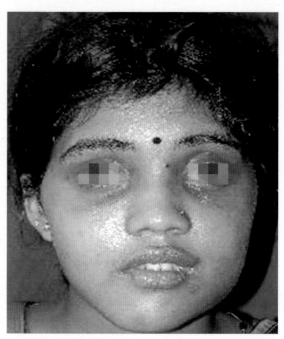

Fig. 8.26: Postoperative 3 months

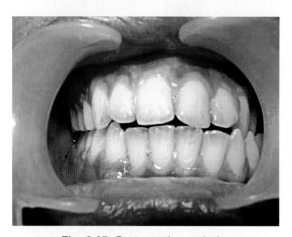

Fig. 8.27: Postoperative occlusion

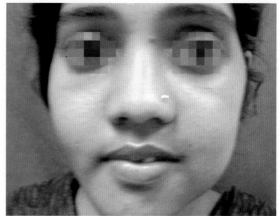

Fig. 8.28: Postoperative 6 months

Basic Principles for the Management of Maxillofacial Trauma

9

INTRODUCTION

- Primate evolution has made human face very vulnerable to frontal impacts. In other species, face is more protective. Most mammals like gorilla have prognathous jaws. In homo sapiens, the sense of smell has become less important and mastication less aggressive. Concurrently, the nose and jaws have receded (Fig. 9.1)
- Injury has become a major public health problem and education 1.2 million people die as a result of road traffic accidents each year. Average 3,242 persons die each day around the world from RTA. By 2020, RTA will become the 2nd leading cause of disability and the 3rd leading cause of death
- 60% of patients with severe facial trauma have multisystem trauma and the potential for airway compromise.
  - 20–50 percent concurrent brain injury.
  - 1–4 percent cervical spine injuries.
  - Blindness occurs in 0.5–3 percent
- 25 percent of women with facial trauma are victims of domestic violence
- 25 percent of patients with severe facial trauma will develop Post-traumatic stress disorder.

Etiology

1. Typical causes:
   i. Direct violence
   ii. Indirect violence
2. Crush injuries:
   i. Automobile accidents RTA
   ii. Aeroplane crash
   iii. Mining accidents.
3. High velocity missiles.
4. Predisposing causes like presence of cyst, tumors, osteomyelitis, presence of 3rd molars, etc.

Components of Trauma System

i. Prehospital care
ii. In hospital care
iii. Rehabilitation
iv. Prevention
v. Education
vi. Research.

APPROACH TO A SUSPECTED FRACTURE

1. History
2. Symptoms
3. Physical examination
4. Imaging.

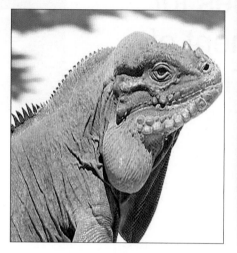 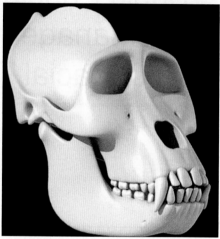

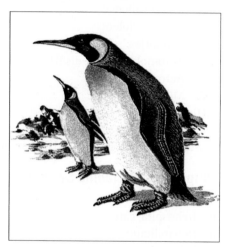 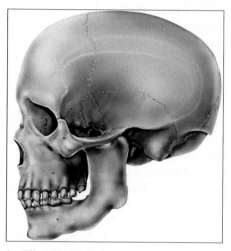

Fig. 9.1: Jaw pattern in different species

History

Ample history.

Specific Questions

1. Was there loss of consciousness? If so, how long?
2. How is your vision?
3. Hearing problems?
4. Is there pain with eye movement?
5. Are there areas of numbness or tingling on your face?
6. Is the patient able to bite down without any pain?
7. Is there pain with moving the jaw?

Obtain a history from the patient or witnesses about:

- Cause of fracture
- Degree of force
- Specific symptoms

- Time since injury
- Allergies
- Medications.

Physical Examination

1. Symmetry/deformity
2. Lacerations/abrasions/ecchymoses
3. Palpable step deformities
   a. Orbital rims
   b. Zygomatic arches
   c. Nose
   d. Frontal Bones
   e. Mandibular borders
4. Movement of dental arches
5. Fractured/avulsed/mobile teeth
6. Visual disturbances
   a. Diplopia
   b. Reflexes
   c. Extraocular muscle function
   d. Acuity
   e. Fields.
7. Intranasal Inspection
   a. Hematoma
   b. Airway obstruction
   c. CSF rhinorrhea.
8. Facial movement (including jaw excursions)
9. Facial sensation.

Clinical Examination

1. Inspection of the face for asymmetry.
2. Inspect open wounds for foreign bodies.
3. Palpate the entire face.
   a. Supraorbital and
   b. Infraorbital rim
   c. Zygomatico/frontal suture
   d. Zygomatic arches.
4. Inspect the nose for asymmetry, telecanthus, widening of the nasal bridge.
5. Inspect nasal septum for septal hematoma, cerebrospinal fluid or blood.
6. Palpate nose for crepitus, deformity and subcutaneous air.

7. Palpate the zygoma along its arch and its articulations with the maxilla, frontal and temporal bone.
8. Check facial stability.
9. Inspect the teeth for malocclusions, bleeding and step-off.
10. Intraoral examination.
11. Manipulation of each tooth.
12. Check for lacerations.
13. Stress the mandible.
14. Tongue blade test.
15. Palpate the mandible for tenderness, swelling and step-off.

Radiographic Examination (Table 9.1)

Basic Principles of Treatment of Severe Maxillofacial Injuries

1. Preservation of life.
2. Maintenance of function.
3. Restoration of appearance (esthetics).

Preservation of Life

ABC to be followed:

1. Airway management
2. Bleeding control
3. Conscious restoration, circulation maintenance.

Table 9.1: Structure and best view	
Mandible	
Condyle/coronoid	Lateral oblique
Ramus/body	Waters
Condyle and neck	Reverse Towne's
Symphysis	Occlusal
Symphysis/body/ ramus	Panoramic
Maxilla and zygoma	
Waters	
Lateral	
Submentovertex view (jug handle)	
Frontal and orbital floor	
Caldwell	
Waters	

Airway Management

i. Chin lift.
ii. Jaw thrust.
iii. Oropharyngeal suctioning.
iv. Manually, move the tongue forward.
v. Maintain cervical immobilization.
vi. Oro or nasopharyngeal airways.
vii. Endotracheal intubation.
viii. Be prepared for cricothyroidotomy.
ix. In extensive injuries, tracheostomy may be indicated.

Bleeding Control

i. Maxillofacial bleeding:
   a. Direct pressure.
   b. Avoid blind clamping in wounds.
ii. Nasal bleeding:
   a. Direct pressure.
   b. Anterior and posterior packing.
iii. Pharyngeal bleeding:
   a. Packing of the pharynx around endotracheal tube.

Principles of fracture management
Reduction—aligning of fragments to original anatomic position
Fixation for re-establishment of form, function and occlusion
Immobilization until bony union occurs
Control of infection
Rehabilitation

REDUCTION

Restoration of the fractured fragments to their original anatomic position. Can be brought about by
Close reduction (alignment without visualization of fracture line)
Open reduction (alignment with visualization of fracture line)

Close Reduction

Advantages

i. Conservative
ii. Inexpensive
iii. Convenient
iv. Short procedure, stable
v. Secondary bone healing
vi. No great operator skill needed
vii. No foreign object left in the body.

Disadvantages

i. Absolute stability not possible
ii. Long period of IMF, difficult nutrition
iii. Muscle atrophy and stiffness
iv. TMJ problems
v. Irreversible loss of bite force
vi. Weight loss
vii. Decrease range of motion of mandible.

Open Reduction

Advantages

i. Early return to normal jaw function
ii. Normal nutrition and oral hygiene
iii. Can get absolute stability
iv. Primary bone healing
v. Don not require patient's compliance
vi. Less myoatrophy
vii. Helpful in epileptics, early work, etc.

Disadvantages

i. Need for an open procedure
ii. Prolonged anesthesia
iii. Expensive hardware
iv. Some risk to neuromuscular structures
v. No manipulation is possible
vi. Need much operator skill
vii. Higher frequency malocclusion, facial nerve damage and scarring.

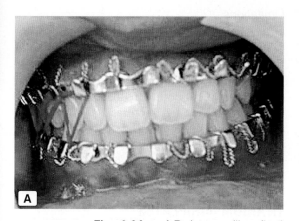

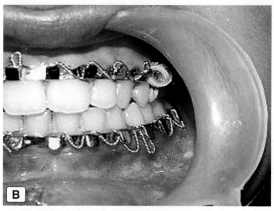

Figs 9.2A and B: Intermaxillary fixation with help of Eric arch bar and elastics

FIXATION

Fixation
Nonrigid fixation
Semirigid fixation
Rigid fixation

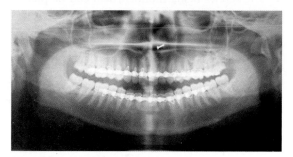

Fig. 9.3: OPG showing Eric arch bar in place (condylar fracture)

Nonrigid

Dental Wiring

- Direct wiring
- Essig's wiring
- Eyelet wiring
- Risdon's wiring
- Multiloop wiring.

Arch Bars

- Jelenko
- Erich pattern (Figs 9.2 and 9.3)
- German silver notched.

Gunning's splint

i. Edentulous patient
ii. Rigid fixation is not possible
iii. To establish the occlusion.

Cap splint

i. Used in adult patients with few firm teeth available
ii. Expensive and construction is also time consuming.

Rigid Fixation

- Intraosseous wiring (semirigid)
- Plates and screws
- Kirchener wire
- Lag screws.

Compression Plates (Fig. 9.4)

Noncompression osteosynthesis
Monocortical miniplate osteosynthesis
Michilet et al developed the concept of miniplate osteosynthesis in late 1960s.

Goals

- Perfect anatomical reduction
- Complete stable fixation
- Painless mobilization of injured region around its articulation.

Advantages

- Smaller incisions and less soft tissue dissection are necessary for their placement
- Because of smaller size and thinner profile of the plates, these are less palpable and reduces the necessity of plate removal. The smaller size of the miniplate may decrease the stress shielding seen following rigid fixation
- The screws being monocortical can be placed in areas of mandible adjacent to tooth roots with minimal risk of tooth injury (Figs 9.5 to 9.7).

Limitations

- Because of their smaller size, miniplates are not as rigid and this decreased rigidity may lead to torsional movements of the fracture segments under functional loading, resulting in infection or nonunion or both. This also precludes their use in comminuted fractures.
- Also because of reduced stability, reduced function is recommended after fracture fixation. A soft diet for 3–6 weeks and some surgeons also recommend 1–2 weeks of IMF.

TITANIUM MINIPLATES

Lag Screws

Indications

- It is ideal for wide sagittal fractures or lamellar fractures that have large area of interfrag-

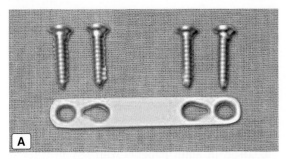
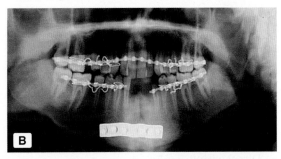

Fig. 9.4A and B: (A) Compression plate; (B) OPG showing compression plate *in situ*

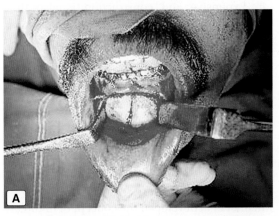
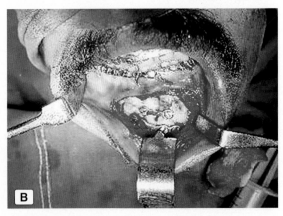

Figs 9.5A and B: (A) Showing symphysis fracture; (B) Showing intraoperative miniplate fixation

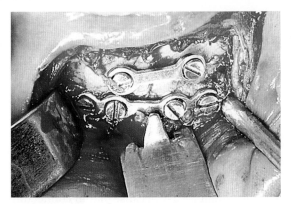

Fig. 9.6: Showing 2 hole and 4 hole miniplate *in situ*

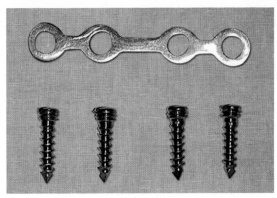

Fig. 9.7: Showing 4 hole plate and locking screw

mentary contact and friction between the lamellae
- Median fractures of the mandible with bicondylar neck fractures
- Comminuted fractures.

Types
- True lag screw
- Cortical lag screw.

Principle
- Length of the fracture should be at least equal to the height of the mandible and twice the height of the atrophic mandible.
- At least two lag screws for functionally stable fixation
- Insertion of lag screw along the bisector of the angle formed by perpendiculars to the bone surface and to the fracture line.

Advantages
- Minimal hardware requirement
- The need for few specialized instruement
- Possibility of application with miniplate system
- Direct central application of compression forces
- An even distribution of forces on fragment interface

- Rotational stabilization by close interdigitation of the fracture serration
- Interfragmentary mechanical rest and stability
- Best condition of primary fracture healing
- Easy removal of screws.

Technique
- A true lag screw has threads only on its terminal end. When used the threads engage the distal cortex and the head seats agginat the proximal cortex, resulting in compression and mechanical rest.
- The gliding hole is drilled first in the outer cortical plate. This is achieved with a 2.7 mm drill bit protected by a corresponding drill sleeve.

Reconstruction plates
- It is a load bearing plate.
- If the bone loss is severe or in a comminuted fracture, reconstruction plate will provide stability and support the fracture segments during healing.
- At least sscrews should be placed in each segment and if an osseous gap has to be bridged atleast 4 screws in each segment should be applied.

NEWER DEVELOPMENT IN OSTEOSYNTHESIS (FIGS 9.8 TO 9.16)

3-D Plates (Figs 9.8 and 9.9)

- Developed by Fermand M in 1995
- Differs from other miniplate system
- The basic concept of three dimensional mini plate fixation is geometrically closed quadrangular plate secured with screws creates create stability in three-dimensions (Fig. 9.14)
- The smallest component is a cube or square stone
- The stability is gained over a defined surface area
- The maintenance of quadrangular position of the arms of the plate to each other is essential to optimal stability

- The principle is further based on the idea that plate is not positioned along the trajectories but over the weak structure lines
- The fixation points remain in the vicinity of the fracture line
- The connecting arms should be positioned rectangle to the fracture line.

Advantages of 3-D Plates

- Stability is achieved by configuration not by thickness or length
- Adjustment is easy because of thin connecting arms of the plate
- Screws adapt to each part of the plate without any tension on the bone
- There is no need for the exact adaptation of plate to the bone
- Minimal dissection is required as compared to the other plating system, hence blood supply is not hampered.

Trapezoidal Condylar Plates (Figs 9.10 and 9.11)

C Meyer specifically developed for osteosynthesis of low subcondylar and high subcondylar fractures.

Advantages

- It respects the principle of functionally stable osteosynthesis of Champy (1976)

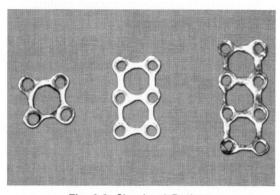

Fig. 9.8: Showing 3-D plates

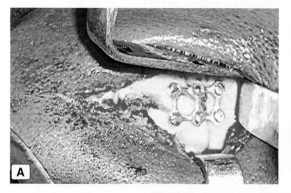

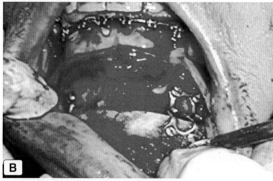

Fig. 9.9A and B: showing 3-D plates *in situ* intraoperative

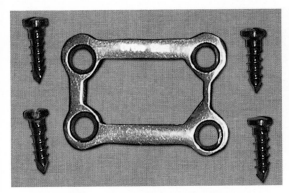

Fig. 9.10: Trapezoidal miniplate

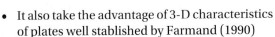

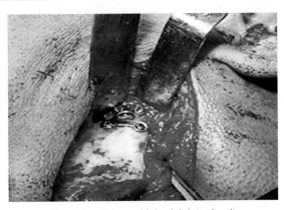

Fig. 9.11: Trapezoidal miniplate *in situ*

- It also take the advantage of 3-D characteristics of plates well stablished by Farmand (1990)
- Enhanced stability, less periosteal dissection and possible osteosynthesis of small fragments (Fig. 9.15)
- Plates are available in various sizes 4 and 9 holes with different bridges in order to allow anatomical variations.

LOCKING PLATES (FIG. 9.7 TO 9.12)

- These plates are designed with threaded hole through which the screws pass
- This provides two separate points of fixation for each screw, one into the bone and second in the threads of screw hole in the plate. The screw lock into the plate independent of the bone and therefore plates provide fracture stability without requiring direct contact with the bone (Fig. 9.16).

Advantages of Locking Plate Over Compression Plate

- Precise adaptation of the plate to the bone is not required as the screws lock into the plate independent of the bone
- Because the plate is not compressed against the bone more periosteum remains viable to aid in the fracture healing
- If a screw loosens in a compression plate, it is a mobile foriegn body that may become infected, exposed, or painful
- In the locking plate, if the screw become loose in the bone, it remain fixed to the plate.

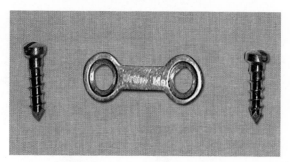

Fig. 9.12: Titanium locking plates

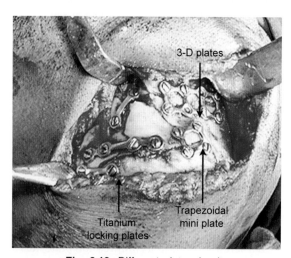

Fig. 9.13: Different plates *in situ*

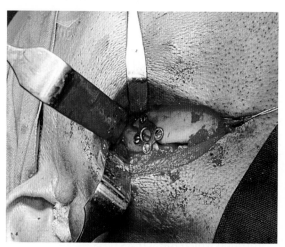

Fig. 9.14: Trapezoidal miniplate in use

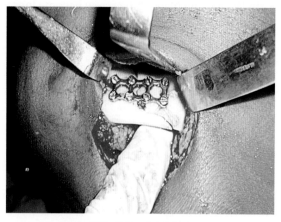

Fig. 9.15: 3 D miniplate in use

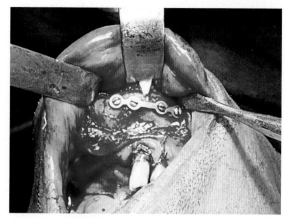

Fig. 9.16: Locking miniplate in use

10

Dentoalveolar Fractures

DEFINITION

Dentoalveolar fractures are those in which avulsion, subluxation or fracture of the teeth occurs in association with a fracture of the alveolus. Early recognition and management can improve tooth survival and functionality trauma to the teeth are not life-threatening however associated maxillofacial injuries can compromise the airway, mostly maxillary teeth are at higher risk than mandibular. Fractures of this types are more common in permanent teeth than deciduous teeth.

It may occur as an isolated clinical entity or in conjunction with any other soft tissue or facial bone fracture.

Isolated dentoalveolar fracture seen among children and adolescents and boys are three times at risk than girls.

ETIOLOGY

  i. RTA (minor accidents)
  ii. Collisions and falls
  iii. Cycling accidents
  iv. Epileptic seizures
  v. Iatrogenic damage during:
     – Extraction of teeth
     – Endoscopy procedure
     – Endotreacheal intubation.

Classification of Dentoalveolar Injuries (Andreasen and Andreasen 1994)

- *Dental hard tissue injury:* Crown infracture and fracture with or without root fracture.

- *Periodontal injury:* Concussion, subluxation, intrusion, extrusion, lateral luxation, avulsion.
- *Alveolar bone injury:* Intrusion of teeth with fracture of socket, alveolus or jaws.
- *Gingival injury:* Contusion, abrasion, laceration, degloving
- Combination of the above

Dental Hard Tissue Injury

- Occurs as a result of direct trauma or by forcible impaction against the opposing dentition
- Anterior teeth damaged by direct impact while posterior ones damaged by impaction between the two jaws (Fig. 10.1)
- Upper teeth intrusion is more frequent and impact against lower teeth may lead to vertical splitting
- Meticulous clinical and radiographical examination are very essential to determine the degree of dental damage and chest X-ray when missing or knocked out tooth is suspected
- Early treatment is imperative to relieve pain and preserve tooth.

Treatment objectives: Preservation of damaged teeth

Depends upon
- Complexity of maxillofacial injury
- Age of the patient
- General dental condition
- Site of injury
- Wishes of the patient.

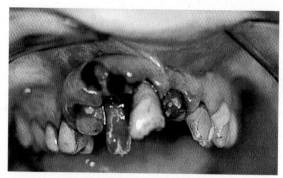

Fig. 10.1: Dentoalveolar fracture

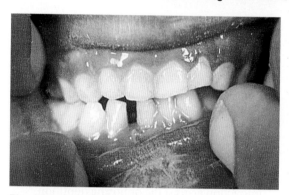

Fig. 10.2: Disturbed occlusion as the result of fracture

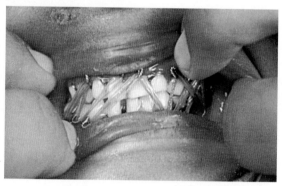

Fig. 10.3: Short-term IMF with elastics

Prognosis is influenced by
- Open root apices
- Intact gingival tissue
- Absence of root fracture
- Periodontal-bone support.

Injuries to the Primary Dentition

- 70% involve maxillary central incisors
- Intrusion, lateral luxation and avulsion are the commonest
- Intruded teeth are likely to normally erupt spontaneously
- Damage to developing permanent teeth by displaced tooth are recognizable problem

Management of Injuries to Primary Dentition

- Fractured, extruded or grossly displaced teeth are to be extracted

- Less displaced with no occlusal interference should be monitored since extraction carries risk to permanent one (Fig. 10.2).

Management of Injuries to Permanent Dentition (Fig. 10.3)

Crown fracture

- Dressing of exposed dentin, minimal pulpotomy or pulp extirpation and restoration of damaged part of the tooth

Root fracture
(Oblique, vertical or transverse)
- Inevitable extraction
- Saving the tooth by:
  a. Rigid splinting for a minimum of 8 weeks
  b. Devitlaiztion (RCT) with eventful apico surgery
  c. Orthodontic extrusion *or crown lengthening*

Injuries to periodontal tissues
- Force distributed over several teeth or impact cushioned by overlying soft tissue may result into:
  a. Concussion
  b. Subluxation
  c. Intrusion
  d. Displacement and avulsion
  e. Fracture of teeth structure
- Looseness and displacement of teeth carries a high risk of subsequent pulp necrosis
- As with root fracture, late complications can be resorption, canal obliteration, ankylosis and loss of alveolar bone

Management of injuries to the periodontal tissues
- Loosened, laterally luxated and extruded teeth should be repositioned and splinted for 1–3 weeks respectively by semi rigid splint: (Fig. 10.3).
  a. Acid-etch composite
  b. Arch bar
  c. Orthodontic wire
  d. Soft stainless-steel wire-loop
  e. Vacuum formed splint.
- Avulsed teeth necessities immediate replantation and semirigid splinting for 1-2 weeks and prognosis is influenced by:
  a. Stage of root development
  b. Length of exposure
  c. Medium storage
  d. Handling and splinting

Alveolar fracture
- Alveolar injury in mandible is associated with complete fracture of tooth-bearing area and in maxilla is often isolated injury
- Teeth damage might be no existed but the potential devitilzation should be expected
- Alveolar fractures are often seen as two distinct fragment containing teeth but comminuted fracture is possible
- Alveolar fracture in mandible my go along with mandible fracture and impacted fracture into the maxilla may appear to be immobile

- Midline split of palate with unilateral Le Fort I lead to large dentoalveolar fracture
- Fracture of tuberosity and fracture of antral floor is a recognized complication of upper molars extraction.

Management of injuries to the alveolar bone (Block or plate fracture)
- Finger manipulation
- Reduction (closed) and fixation
- Rigid wire and composite splint
- Elimination of premature contact and occlusal trauma
- Short inter-maxillary fixation.

Management of tuberosity fracture
- Removal of comminuted fracture of loss alveolar bone and teeth and repair of soft tissue
- Delay of extraction of teeth in case of tuberosity fracture for (6–8 weeks)
- Mandatory extraction of a tooth from a block fracture should be carried out surgically.
- Splinting of a tooth of fractured tuberosity in to other standing teeth for one month.

Injuries to the gingival and soft tissues
- Damage to the lip observed more with anterior dento-alveolar fracture
- Embedded of portion of a tooth or foreign bodies in soft tissues is very substantial
- Laceration of the gingiva is associated with dento-alveolar fracture
- Degloving of the mental region is a common injury to the lower anterior teeth.

Management of soft tissue injuries
- Inspection of a full thickness perforating wound
- Debridement and copious lavage with chlorhexidine solution
- Removal of denuded piece of bone
- Repair of soft tissue injury
- Application of external support strapping to help in tissue adaptation
- Antibiotic prescription.

Mid-facial Fractures

11

INTRODUCTION

Mid-face fractures rarely occur in isolation and are often a component of a panfacial or maxillary-mandibular fracture pattern. The evolution of open reduction and internal fixation techniques in the treatment of facial fractures over the past 2 decades has supplanted the need for prolonged periods of intermaxillary fixation and facilitated early functional rehabilitation.

Appropriate application of the general principles can minimize morbidity and ensure a return to premorbid facial appearance and occlusion. Improved diagnostic capabilities, use of open surgical techniques, advance rigid fixation devices, advances in techniques of resuscitation, and more focused surgical training have markedly improved the care of the facial trauma patient.

Mid-face fractures are defined as an area bounded superiorly by a line drawn across the skull from frontozygomatic suture across the fronto nasal and fronto maxillary sutures on the opposite side and inferiorly by the occlusal plane of the upper teeth.

- Causes:
  - Road traffic accidents
  - Altercation
  - Sport
  - Falls
- Commonest site:
  - Nasal 50%
  - Zygomatic 22%
  - Occular 12%

SURGICAL ANATOMY

- Physical characteristics of the mid-facial skeleton
- Articulation with the base of the skull
- Involvement of the brain and cranial nerves
- Involvement of the orbit
- Disturbance of the occlusion
- Paranasal sinuses
- Important blood vessels
- Articulation with the base of the skull
- Match box phenomenon
- Areas of weakness
- Buttress system
  - Vertical buttress
  - Horizontal buttress.

CLASSIFICATION (TABLE 11.1)

A. Lefort I, II, III, IV
B. As per the direction of fracture line (Erich):
  - Horizontal
  - Pyramidal
  - Transverse
C. Depending on the relation of fracture line to zygomatic bone:
  - Sub zygomatic
  - Supra zygomatic
D. Depending on the level of fracture:
  - Low level
  - Mid level
  - High level
E. Rowe and William's classification:

Table 11.1: Mid-face fracture

Lefort
- I
- II
- III
- IV

As per the direction of fracture line (Erich)
- Horizontal
- Pyramidal
- Transverse

Depending on the relation of fracture line to zygomatic bone
- Subzygomatic
- Suprazygomatic

Depending on the level of fracture
- Low level
- Mid level
- High level

Rowe and William's classification
- Fractures not involving the occlusion
- Fractures involving the occlusion

Modified Lefort classification
- Lefort I, Ia
- Lefort II, IIa, IIb
- Lefort III, IIIa, IIIb
- Lefort IV, IVa, IVb

a. fractures not involving the occlusion:
 1. Central region
    - Fractures of the nasal bones and/or nasal septum
      - Lateral nasal injuries
      - Anterior nasal injuries
    - Fractures of the frontal process of the maxilla
    - Fractures of types A and B which extend into the ethmoid bone
    - Fractures of types A, B and C which extend into the frontal bone.
 2. Lateral region
    Fractures involving the zygomatic bone, arch and maxilla excluding the dentoalveolar component.

b. Fractures involving the occlusion:
 1. Dentoalveolar fractures
 2. Subzygomatic
    - Lefort I (low level or Guerin)
    - Lefort II (pyramidal)
 3. Suprazygomatic
    Lefort III (high level or craniofacial dysjunction)
F. Modified Lefort classification:
  - Lefort I – Low maxillary fracture
    Ia – Low maxillary fracture/multiple segments
  - Lefort II – Pyramidal fracture
    IIa –Pyramidal fracture and nasal fracture
    IIb –Pyramidal fracture and NOE fracture
  - Lefort III –Craniofacial dysjunction
    IIIa – Craniofacial dysjunction and nasal fracture
    IIIb –Craniofacial dysjunction and NOE
  - Lefort IV – Lefort II or III and cranial base fracture
    IVa –Supraorbital rim fracture
    IVb –Anterior cranial fossa and orbital wall fracture

LeFort I (Low Level, Subzygomatic, Guerin's, Horizontal, Floating Fracture) (Fig. 11.1)

- Horizontal fracture line above the level of floor of the nose involving lower third of septum and the mobile fragment consists of the palate, the maxillary alveolar process and lower third of pterygoid plates and associated portion of palatine bone. May occur as single or in combination with II and III
- Allows motion of the maxilla while the nasal bridge remains stable.
 Radiographic findings:
 Fracture line which involves:
 - Nasal aperture
 - Inferior maxilla
 - Lateral wall of maxilla.

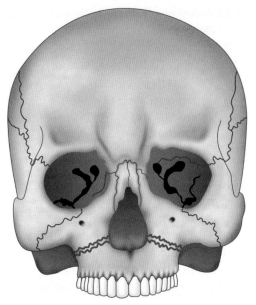

Fig. 11.1: LeFort I fracture line

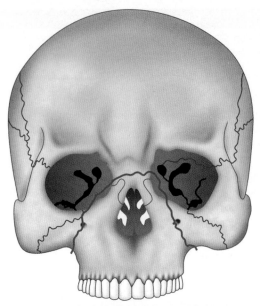

Fig. 11.3: LeFort II fracture line

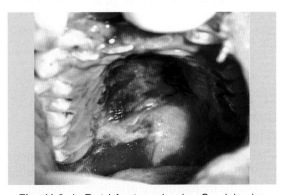

Fig. 11.2: LeFort I fracture showing Guerin's sign

LeFort II (Pyramidal/Subzygomatic Fracture) (Fig.11.3)

From the nasal bridge the fracture invariable enters the medial wall of the orbit, involving the lacrimal bone and then recrosses the orbital rim at the junction of the middle third and the lateral two third, medial to, or through infraorbital foramen. The fracture line runs beneath the zygomaticomaxillary suture, traversing the lateral wall of the antrum to extend backward horizontally through the pterygoid plate.

Clinical findings of LeFort (Fig. 11.2)
Facial edema
Ecchymosis in buccal, lingual and palatal (Guerin's sign)
Malocclusion of the teeth
Motion of the maxilla while the nasal bridge remains stable-grating sound
Cracked-pot sound and # of cusps
Mid palatal split

Clinical findings of LeFort II
Moon face
Bilateral circumorbital ecchymosis
Bilateral subconjunctival hemorrhage-medial half
Step deformity at infraorbital margin
Nasal flattening
Traumatic Telecanthus
Epistaxis or CSF rhinorrhea
Movement of the upper jaw and the nose

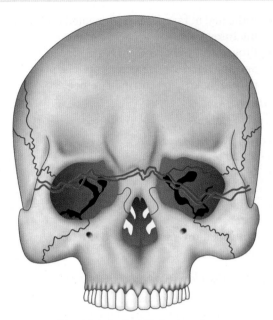

Fig. 11.4: LeFort III fracture line

Radiographic findings: Fracture line which involves:
- Nasal bones
- Medial orbit
- Maxillary sinus
- Frontal process of the maxilla.

LeFort III Fracture (Fig.11.4)

Fracture extends through the zygomaticofrontal suture and the nasofrontal suture and across the floor of the orbits to effects a complete separation of the mid-facial structures from the cranium.

Clinical findings of LeFort III
Gross edema of face-Panda facial within 24-48 hr
Bilateral circumorbital/periorbital ecchymosis and gross edema-Racoon eyes.
Tenderness and separation of frontozygomatic sutures
Dish faced deformity
Epistaxis and CSF rhinorrhea
Motion of the maxilla, nasal bones and zygoma
Severe airway obstruction

Radiographic imaging: Fracture through
- Zygomaticofrontal suture
- Zygoma
- Medial orbital wall
- Nasal bone.

MAXILLARY FRACTURE MANAGEMENT

General Considerations
- Restoration of occlusion is must for correct reduction
- Fixation is maintained by external/internal skeletal fixation until consolidation is achieved.
- Immobilization for 6–8 weeks to stable segments
- IMF for 3–4 weeks.

Methods of Reduction
1. Closed reduction.
2. Open reduction.

Manual/Closed Reduction
- Simple manipulation by hand
- By dental impression compound
- By rubber dam sheet/ ribbon gauze/rubber catheters
- By using special instruments-Disimpaction forceps.

Rowe's Maxillary Disimpaction Forceps and Hayton Williams Forceps-I Fracture

For II# -Asche`s/Walsham`s Septal Forceps.

Fixation of LeFort Fractures

External Fixation

Craniomandibular
- Box frame
- Halo frame
- Plaster of Paris head cap.

Craniomaxillary
- Supraorbital pins
- Zygomatic pins
- Halo frame

Suspension by cheek wires from Halo-frame or head cap.

Pin fixation (supraorbital pins)
- Simple method
- "Wooden screw "pattern pins
- Landmarks for pin placement
- Supraorbital pins linked with upper silver cap splint
- Great advantage – without IMF
- Important to check occlusion in postoperative day
- Occasionally a discrepancy.

Box Frame

Combined middle 3rd and mandibular fracture
- Fractured mandible is reduced first
- Middle 3rd fracture is mobilized and occlusion re-established
- Temporary IMF
- Supraorbital pins inserted and craniomaxillary fixation established
- IMF released.

Halo Frame

Plaster of Paris head cap and cheek wires

- Indicated in rare cases of elongated middle 3rd fractures
- Progressive tightening
- Special head cap attachments via plaster of paris of head caps and halo frame.

Disadvantage
Lack of stability.

Transfixation of maxilla
- Rapid form of fixation
- Useful in the rare situation- profuse leak of CSF and risk of aerocele
- Achieved by Steinmann pin or Stout Kirschner wire
- Transfixation pin is linked to head cap or haloframe.

Internal Fixation (Figs 11.5 to 11.11)

1. Direct osteosynthesis
   - Transosseous wiring at fracture sites
     - High level (frontozygomatic and frontonasal)
     - Mid level (orbital rim/zygomatic buttress)
     - Low level (alveolar /midpalatal)

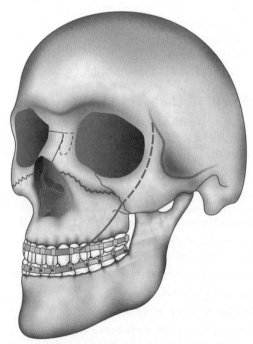

Fig. 11.5: Lateral wiring   **Fig. 11.6:** Frontozygomatic wiring

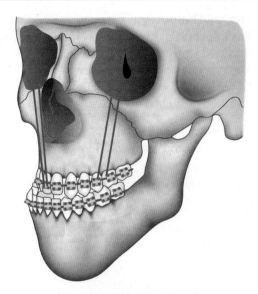

Fig. 11.7: Infraorbital rim wire

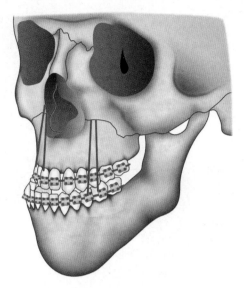

Fig. 11.8: Pyriform aperture wire

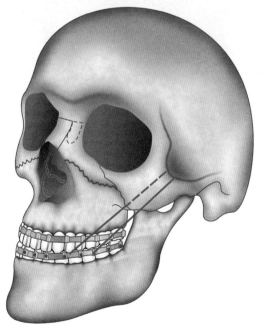

Fig. 11.9: Circumzygomatic wire

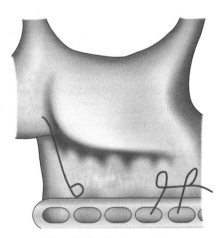

Fig. 11.10: Buttress wiring

– Miniplates
– Transfixation with Kirschner wire or Steinman pin:
  - Transfacial
  - Zygomatic–septal

Internal fixation
Suspension wires to mandible (Fig. 11.9)
• Frontal – Central or lateral
• Circumzygomatic
• Zygomatic

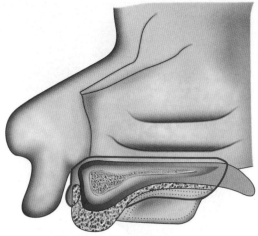

Fig. 11.11: Circumpalatal wire

- Infraorbital
- Pyriform aperture (Fig. 11.8).

Adam's Wiring (1942)

Disadvantages of Fixation by Wire Suspension:
- Lack of compensation of dislocating forces direction posteriorly
- Difficult to ensure a correct facial projection
- Tooth borne appliances offer only direct control the occlusal level of fractures
- Lack of 3 dimensional stability.

Complications of Fixation by Wire Suspension
- Mid-face shortening
- Widening and retrusion of paranasal areas.

Sequence of Internal Fixation
- Top to bottom – Merville (1974)
- Outer facial frame
- Bottom to top to middle—Manson and Kelly et al.

Open Reduction and Internal Fixation by Interosseous Wiring

Introduced by Adams 1942
Later refined by Manson et al
- Reconstruction of the sinus wall fragment between the 2 anterior pillars was omitted

- Pterygoid buttress was not operated
- Posterior height of mid-face –restore the ramus
- Mid-face projection – ORIF of the nasomaxillary and zygomaticomaxillary buttresses
- Upper mid-face – Open reduction of zygomatic and nasoethmoidal fracture was performed.

Open Reduction and Internal Fixation by Miniplates, Microplates, and Screws
- Champy et al 1976
- Harle and Duker in 1975
- Luhr in 1979.

Surgical approaches to maxillary fractures (Figs 11.12 to 11.17)

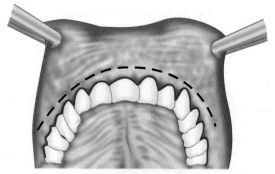

Fig. 11.12: Intraoral approach

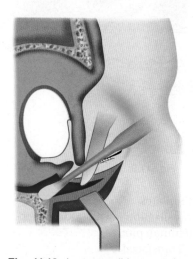

Fig. 11.13: Lower eyelid approach

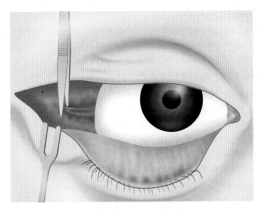

Fig. 11.14: Transconjunctival lateral canthotomy

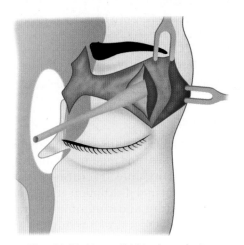

Fig. 11.15: Upper lid blepharoplasty

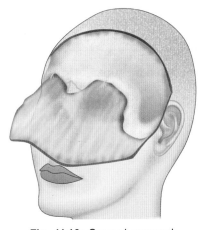

Fig. 11.16: Coronal approach

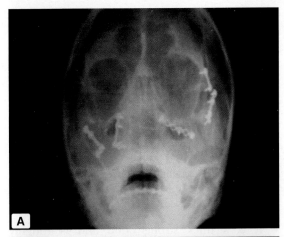

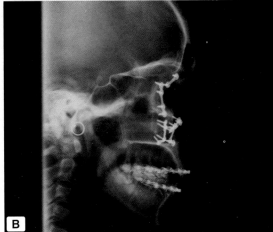

Figs 11.17A and B: Showing postoperative radiograph

ZYGOMATICOMAXILLARY COMPLEX FRACTURES (FIG. 11.18)

Introduction

- Zygomatic fractures are common facial injuries
- It is the most common facial fracture of the second in frequency after nasal fractures
- The high incidence of zygoma fractures probably relates to the zygoma's prominent position within the facial skeleton.

Anatomy

- It is the major buttress of facial skeleton and principal structure of the lateral mid-face

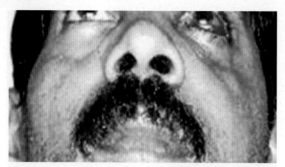

Fig. 11.18: Left zygomatic complex fracture involving orbit showing subconjuctival echymosis

- It is a thick strong bone and is roughly quadrilateral in shape with an outer convex surface and inner concave
- It has temporal, orbital, maxillary and frontal processes
- It articulates with four bones: the frontal, sphenoid, maxilla and temporal.

Terminology and Fracture Pattern

The malar bone represents a strong bone on fragile supports and it is for this reason that, though the body of the bone is rarely broken, the four processes fontal, maxillary and zygomatic are frequent sites of fracture.

HD Gillies, TP Kilner, D Stone, 1927

Zygomatic or malar fractures are the terms commonly used to describe fractures that involve the lateral one-third of the mid-face. Other names for this fracture are:

- Zygomaticomaxillary complex
- Zygomaticomaxillary compound
- Zygomatico-orbital
- Zygomatic complex
- Malar
- Trimalar
- Tripod.

Classification

Rowe and Killey (1968)
Type I: No significant displacement
Type II: Fracture fo the zygomatic arch
Type III: Rotation around vertical axis • Inward displacement of orbital rim • Outward displacement of orbital rim
Type IV: Rotation around longitudinal axis • Medial displacement of frontal process • Lateral displacement of frontal process
Type V: Displacement of the complex enbloc • Medial • Inferior • Lateral (Rare)
Type VI : Displacement of orbitoantral partition • Inferiorly • Superiorly
Type VII : Displacement of orbital rim segments
Type VIII : Complex comminuted fractures

Rowe (1985)

1. Group A: Stable fracture—showing minimal or no displacement and requires no intervention.
2. Group B: Unstable fracture—with great displacement and distruption at the frontozygomatic suture and comminuted fracture. Requires reduction as well as fixation.
3. Group C: Stable fracture—other types of zygomatic fractures, which requires reduction, but no fixation.

Fractures of the Zygomatic Arch Alone

1. Minimum or no displacement.
2. V type in fracture.
3. Comminuted fracture.

Diagnosis of ZMC Fracture (Figs 11.19 to 11.21)

In a typical case diagnosis may be made at sight once the characteristic appearance has been

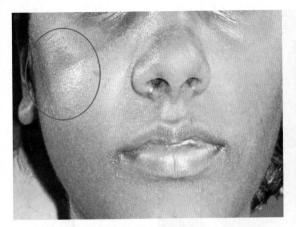

Fig. 11.19: Clinical presentation of right side zygomatic complex fracture

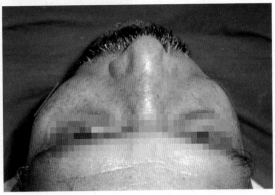

Fig. 11.20: Flattening on left side of face

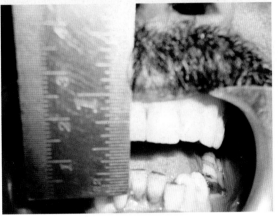

Fig. 11.21: Reduced mouth opening

Signs and Symptoms
Periorbital ecchymosis and edema
Flattening over the zygomatic arch
Ecchymosis of the maxillary buccal sulcus
Deformity of the zygomatic buttress of the maxilla
Trismus
Abnormal nerve sensibility
Epistaxis
Subconjuctival ecchymosis
Crepitation from air emphysema
Displacement of the palperbral fissure
Unequal pupillary level
Diplopia
Enophthalmos

fully recognized. A peculiar facies is present, due chiefly to a certain flatness of contour and absence of expression on the affected side.
HD Gillies, TP Kilner, D Stone, 1927

Inspection and Palpation

- It should be performed from the frontal, lateral, superior and inferior vantages
- Note symmetry, pupillary levels and presence of orbital edema and subconjuctival ecchymosis and anterior and lateral projection of zygomatic bodies

- The most useful method of evaluating the position of the body of the zygoma is from the superior view
- Intraoral examination to evaluate buccal ecchymosis in the superior buccal sulcus
- Palpation of the infraorbital rim, frontozygomatico suture, body of the zygoma and arch.

Radiological Evaluation (Figs 11.22 to 11.24)

- Plain film radiography
  - Water's view
  - Submentovertex
- CT scan.

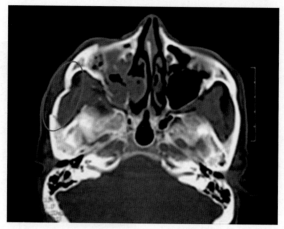

Fig. 11.22: Zygomatic arch fracture

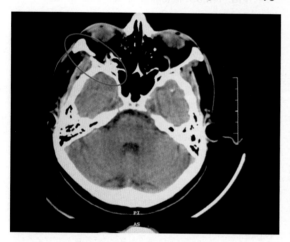

Fig. 11.23: Zygoma fracture

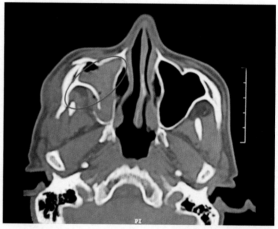

Fig. 11.24: Fracture of anterior wall of maxillary sinus

TREATMENT INDICATIONS FOR SURGERY

- Alteration in facial contour
- Globe displacement—enophthalmus/exophthalmus/ diplopia
- Muscle/fat/nerve entrapment
- Mechanical restriction of mandibular movement.

TIMING OF SURGERY

- Early: Surgery performed prior to significant swelling
- Late: After resolution of significant edema

- If possible surgery should be performed within 7–14 days before significant healing has begun
- Stable nondisplaced fractures may be observed weekly for proper healing.

SURGICAL APPROACHES

Temporal Approach (Gillies Approach)

- Isolated arch fractures/minimally displaced ZMC fractures—no direct visualization
- 2–3 cm incision in hairline below and parallel to anterior branch of temporal artery

- Through and through superficial temporalis fascia
- Rows zygomatic elevator passed medial to arch for elevation in a sweeping upward and outward direction.

Intraoral Keen Approach

- Incision in maxillary buccal suicus in region of canine sulcus, periosteum is elevated and elevator passed deep to arch superiorly
- Again no visual access for direct fixation.

OPEN REDUCTION TECHNIQUES

- Lateral brow incision
- Infracilliary (blepheroplasty) incision
- Infraorbital crease incision
- Supratarsal fold
- "Crows foot" incision
- Bicoronal/Hemicoronal flap.

FIXATION V/S NONFIXATION

- Nondisplaced fractures should be followed clinically without surgical intervention
- One or two point fixation may be adequate for stable, minimally displaced fractures
- Direct fixation at the site of fracture techniques for unstable, comminuted, and grossly displaced fractures.

DIRECT FIXATION TECHNIQUES

- Wiring—24–30 gauge stainless steel wire
- Mini bone plates
- Steinmann pins.

INDIRECT FIXATION

- Fixation away from the fracture site
- Steinmann pins / transfacial pin
- Temporary packing with penrose drains, gauze, gelfoam, silastic, antral balloon
- Attachment of external framework
- Extent of fixation obviously dictated by fracture—miniplate fixation is generally the most common stabilization technique.

Complications
Infraorbital nerve disordres
Persistent diplopia
Enophthalmos
Blindness
Infection
Maxillary sinusitis
Ankylosis of zygoma to coronoid process
Malunion of zygoma

NASOETHMOIDAL ORBITAL FRACTURE

Introduction

- Naso-orbital ethmoid fractures involves central mid-face nasal bone, frontal process of maxilla and ethmoid bone
- These have variously been described as fracture of the ethmoids, naso-orbital fractures, nasoethmoidal injuries and nasoethmoido-maxillofronto-orbital complex
- Although nasal fractures are the most common facial fracture, they often go unnoticed by both surgeons and patients. Patients with nasal fractures usually present with some combination of deformity, tenderness, hemorrhage, edema, ecchymosis, instability, and crepitation; however, these features may not be present or may be transient (Tremolet de Villers, 1975)
- To further complicate the matter, edema can mask underlying nasal deformity, crepitation, and instability; thus, many surgeons and patients fail to pursue further diagnosis and appropriate treatment. If untreated, nasal fractures can result both in unfavorable appearance and in unfavorable function, especially when the underlying structural integrity of bone and cartilage is lost.

Pathophysiology

The nasal bones and underlying cartilage are susceptible to fractures because the nose maintains a prominent position and central location on the face and because it has a low breaking strength. Patterns of fracture are known to vary with the momentum of the striking object and the density of the underlying bone (Murray, 1984). As with other facial bones, younger patients tend to have larger nasoseptal fracture segments, whereas older patients are more likely to present with more-comminuted fracture patterns (Cummings, 1998).

Causes

- Road traffic accidents
- Sports injuries
- Fights
- Work related accidents
- Falls are a more common cause of nasal injury in children.

Frequency

- Fracture of nasal bones is the most common site-specific bone injury of the facial skeleton. Nasal fractures account for 39–45 percent of all facial fractures (Hussain, 1994)
- Sex: The male-to-female ratio in nasal fractures is greater than 2:1
- Age: The incidence is increased in patients aged 15–30 years (Muraoka, 1991)
- A small but significant increase in the number of nasal fractures is noted in the elderly population because of a higher rate of falls
- Most nasal bone fractures in young adults are related more to altercations and sporting injuries and less to motor vehicle accidents; however, these rates vary according to the location of the conducted study and the association with alcohol (Muraoka, 1991; Hussain, 1994; Scherer, 1989; Logan, 1994).

Surgical Anatomy

- The skeletal foundation of nasoethmoidal complex consists of a strong triangular shaped frame (Fig. 11.25)
- On each side the frontal process of maxillary bone and the nasal process of the frontal bone are united above at glabella. The triangle is completed inferiorly by the premaxilla
- Behind the frame lies interorbital space situated between the medial walls of the orbit

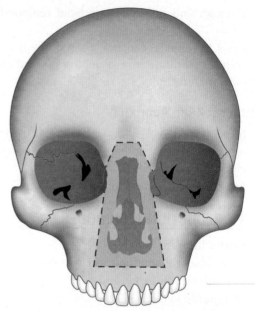

Fig. 11.25: Nasoethmoidal complex

each of which is formed by the thin lacrimal bone and the lamina papyracea (orbital plate) of the ethmoid which overlie the ethmoid sinuses
- This space contains the nasal septum, turbinates, ethmoid sinuses and is bridged above by the cribriform plate of the ethmoid.

Classification of the Nasoethmoidal Injuries

Rowe and Williams Classification

1. Isolated nasoethmoid and frontal region injuries without other fractures of the mid-face.
   - Bilateral
   - Unilateral
2. Combined nasoethmoidal and frontal region injury with other fractures of mid-face
   - Bilateral
   - Unilateral.

Markowitz Classification

Depending on the velocity and point of impact
- Type I: Nasal-orbital-ethmoid fracture: Involves only one portion of the medial orbital rim with

its attached medial canthal tendon, may occur unilateral or bilateral

- Type II: Nasal-orbital-ethmoid fracture: May occur in bilateral or unilateral form and may be large segments or comminuted. Most commonly the canthus remains attached to a large central segment

Clinical Features
Frontal depression
Nasal deformity
Traumatic telecanthus
CSF rhinorrhea
Diplopia
Hemorrhage (due to rupture of anterior and posteior branches of ethmoidal artery)

- Type III: Nasal-orbital-ethmoid fracture: This fracture includes comminution involving central fragment of bone where the medial canthal tendon attaches. The canthus is rarely avulsed completely but on occasions the fragments of bone are so small that the reconstruction is not possible, in these cases transnasal wiring of the canthus is required.

Diagnosis of Telecanthus
- An increased intercanthal distance may result from severance, avulsion or displacement laterally while still attached to the fragment of bone. Traumatic telecanthus should be differentiated from hypertelorism where in there is increased interpupillary distance
- The criteria for making diagnosis:
  - A high index of suspicion
  - Measurement: The intercanthal distance should be measured carefully with dividers and particular attention should be paid to the distance of the midpoint of the nose from each canthus to reveal the possibility of the unilateral displacement. The normal intercanthal distance is 33–34 mm
  - Palpebral fissure: This should be scrutinized carefully since characteristically it becomes narrowed and almond shaped. Medial

angle becomes blunt with obliteration of the caruncle and may be displaced downwards and laterally particularly when there is associated comminution and displacement of zygomatic complex
  - Eyelids: These become lax and epicanthal fold is more prominent. Flattening of the bottom of the naso-orbital valley is the earlier sign of traumatic disruption of the canthal region
  - Canthal ligament: Diminished tension of the canthal ligament
  - Eye: diplopia.

Imaging
- Plain films are of almost no use in diagnosing NOE fractures as most will be undetected
- CT is of greatest value and provides more insight into NOE injuries. Thin axial slices provide the basic detail of the extent of the injury. Coronal sections are essential to reveal the details of the fractures of the middle third of the orbit.

Treatment
Eight steps for the management of such injuries are presented:
  i. Surgical exposure
  ii. Identification of the medial canthal tendon/tendon-bearing bone fragment
  iii. Reduction/reconstruction of medial orbital rim
  iv. Reconstruction of medial orbital wall
  v. Transnasal canthopexy
  vi. Reduction of septal fractures
  vii. Nasal dorsum reconstruction/augmentation
  viii. Soft tissue adaptation.

Surgical exposure
Through Existing laceration
H-shaped incision
Vertical or horizontal nasal radix
Bilateral Z
Open sky approach (w incision)
Bicoronal plus lower lid incision

*Identification of the Medial Canthal Tendon/
Tendon-bearing Bone Fragment*

- The canthal tendon is almost never avulsed from bone, but it is usually attached to a bony fragment. The proper identification of this fragment and its reduction produces an esthetically acceptable result
- If the tendon is severed or avulsed one should tag the thicker anterior component with braided tendon wire or suture.

Reduction/Reconstruction of Medial Orbital Rim

- Transnasal reduction of the canthal bearing bone fragment is the most important step in preserving the intercanthal distance
- In simple fractures simple repositioning and fixation with a small bone plate or wire may be all that is necessary. In more comminuted injuries transnasal wiring has advantages over plates
- A hole is made through the unstable bone fragment as well as the bone on the contra lateral side. A double 30 gauge wire is then threaded through 2 holes transnasally with a awl and wire is tightened.

Reconstruction of Medial Orbital Wall

- Reconstruction of both bony orbital volume and shape is important to achieve normal eye position
- Materials used: Autogenous bone (calvarial bone).

Reduction of Septal Fractures

Most NOE fractures are associated with fracture of perpendicular plate of ethmoid bone. Simple intranasal manipulation of the septum with Asch forceps to place it in the midline is adequate using upward and anterior force with the forceps.

Nasal Dorsum Reconstruction/Augmentation

Nasal dorsum reconstruction with a cantilevered bone graft provides long lasting dorsal nasal support and prevents the characteristic saddling that occurs after NOE injuries. This procedure is mainly of esthetic importance.

Soft Tissue Adaptation

A thermoplastic nasal stent may be used early in the post surgical period to help to redrape the soft tissues deeply into the naso-orbital valley to prevent thickening of the soft tissue giving the appearance of an increased intercanthal distance

Conclusion

No other facial fracture is more challenging to repair than an NOE fracture. The complex anatomy of the region and difficulty with the access makes the surgeons' task more demanding. Fortunately, significant contributions made by a host of surgeons and new instrumentation and technology have culminated in a better understanding of NOE injuries and their treatment.

NASAL FRACTURES (FIGS 11.26 TO 11.29)

- Most common of all facial fractures
- Injuries may occur to other surrounding bony structures.
- They are 3 types
  - Depressed
  - Laterally displaced
  - Nondisplaced.

Clinical findings
Nasal deformity
Edema and tenderness
Epistaxis
Crepitus and mobility

Diagnosis

- History and physical examination
- Lateral or Waters view to confirm your diagnosis.

Treatment

- Control epistaxis
- Drain septal hematomas.

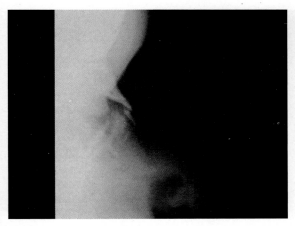

Fig. 11.26: Radiograph showing nasal fracture

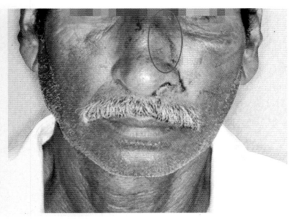

Fig. 11.27: Nasal bone fracture

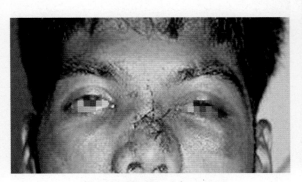

Fig. 11.28: Nasal fracture

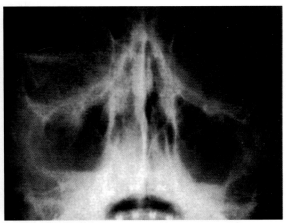

Fig. 11.29: Radiograph showing nasal fracture

ORBITAL BLOWOUT FRACTURES (FIGS 11.30 TO 11.32)

Orbital Trauma

Anatomy

- Bones of the orbit
- Fracture lines rupture of dura mater causes CSF to escape into orbit
- Medial wall, floor of the orbit.
- Muscles of the eye
- Common tendinous ring
- Eyelids.

Etiology and Epidemiology

- Males > females, 4:1.
- Orbitozygomatic fractures second in frequency of facial fractures.
- RTA, assaults, sport injuries.

Fracture Patterns

Type I: Nasal-orbital-ethmoid fractures
- Involves only one portion of medial wall with its attached medial canthal ligament.
- May be unilateral or bilateral

Type II: Nasal-orbital-ethmoid fractures
- Comminuted or large segments.

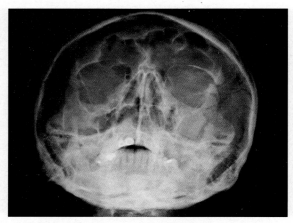

Fig. 11.30: PNS view shows lateral rim fracture

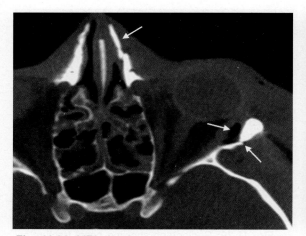

Fig. 11.31: MRI showing nasal and orbital lateral rim fracture

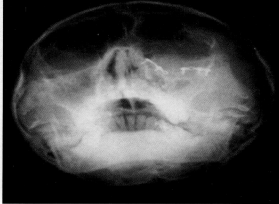

Fig. 11.32: PNS showing infraorbital rim fracture—postoperative

- Medial canthal ligament attached to the large central segment.
- Reduction is required.

Type III: Nasal-orbital-ethmoid fractures
Comminution involving the large central fragments where the medial canthal ligament attaches.

Clinical Features

The periorbital tissues
- Edema
- Circumorbital ecchymosis
- Subconjunctival hemorrhage

- Orbital emphysema.

The eyelids
- Abnormality of the palpebral fissure.
- Height, width, inclination.
- Mobility (ptosis, pseudoptosis)
- Integrity of the margins and tarsal plates.

The ligaments
- Alteration in the canthal level.
- Alteration in the ocular level
- Increased intercanthal distance (telecanthus)
- Alteration in the ocular level.

The eye
- Preservation of vision
- Limitation of the ocular movements
- Presence of diplopia
- Exopthalmos or enopthalmos
- Pupilary reflexes
- Ophthalmic injuries
- Increased interpupilary distance.

The lacrimal apparatus
- Wounds involving the puncta
- Epiphora
- Wounds involving the passages.

Neurological defecits
- Paraesthesia of the infraorbital, supraorbital or supratrochlear nerves.
- Paresis of extraocular muscles
- Paresis of facial nerve.

The orbit
- Pain on palpation and /or deformity at
  - The superior margin
  - The frontozygomatic suture
  - The inferior margin
  - The nasomaxillary and nasofrontal suture.
  - Zygomatic bone and/or arch.
  - The lateral antral wall.

The mandible
- Limited opening with deviation to the opposite side.
- Restricted lateral excursion to the same side.
- Limited opening with deviation to the opposite side.

Physical Examination
- Difficult in traumatized patient
- ABC's (ATLS)
- Palpation of superior, inferior, lateral, medial, zygoma, maxilla and mandible done in sequential order
- Ophthalmologic evaluation
- Visual acuities (subjective and objective)
  - Pupillary function
  - Ocular motility
  - Anterior chamber for hyphema
  - Fundoscopic examination
- Test for pupilary reflexes

- Intraorbital pressure
- Forced duction testing
- Jones test
- Hess chart
  - Pictorial record of ocular movement of each eye
  - Dissociation test which shows ocular movement of non fixing eye in all positions of gaze.

Imaging
- Plain radiography.
  - Waters view
  - Reverse waters view
  - AP skull and PA skull view
- Computed tomography.
- Radiographic interpretation
- PA skull view
- Computed tomography
- Coronal CT scan of orbits demonstrating loss of orbital floor on the left in contrast to the normal orbital floor on the right.
- Coronal view computed tomography scan of patient showing left orbital floor fracture with herniation of orbital contents
- Medial wall fracture
- Orbital roof fracture.

General Principles
Classification for the purpose of treatment.
a. No treatment
b. Indirect reduction with:
  - No fixation
  - Temporary support
  - Direct fixation
  - Indirect fixation
c. Direct reduction and fixation
d. Immediate reconstruction by grafting
e. Delayed reconstruction by osteotomy and /or grafting
f. Late restoration of contour by onlay grafts.

Optimum time for surgery
(NL Rowe and JLL Williams)

Factors to be considered:
1. Ophthalmic injuries
2. Progressive proptosis

3. Deterioration in visual acuity
4. The visual integrity on the unaffected side
5. The necessity for immediate operation for other facial or general injuries
6. General condition of the patient
   - Distinct advantage in not operating for 5–7 days as the edema would resolve facilitating ease of operation
   - 5–10 days critical period.
   - Early surgery necessary within 3 days in children with diplopia and mainly within 7 days in adults .

Order of repairs
- Work from stable to unstable
- Use occlusion as guide
- Generally stabilize mandible, zygoma and palate before mid-face or before orbit and NOE
- Skin incisions for orbital fractures
- Bicoronal incision (Tessiers)
- Used for the purpose of extensive orbital surgery especially when roof has to be visualized.
- Bicoronal incision
- Hemicoronal approach
- Multiple eyelid incisions
- Lateral brow incision
- Blepharoplasty incision
- Lynchs incision
- Subciliary incisions
- Transconjunctival incisions
- Lateral canthotomy
- Lateral brow incision.

Approaches to orbital rim
- Transconjunctival approach
- Tessier for correction of congenital orbital deformities
- Converse posttraumatic orbital deformities.
- Advantage: no external scar.

Blow-out fractures
Smith and Regan
- Pure and impure fracture.

Mechanism
- "Force necessary to fracture the orbital floor"
- Current theory on the pathophysiology of orbital wall fractures postulates either a "Hydraulic" or a "Buckling" mechanism

- Fracture of the orbital floor was consistently produced at and above a force of 2.08 J
- Orbital floor fractures can occur at low energies with direct ocular trauma only ("pure" hydraulic mechanism).

Two main theories
Hydraulic Theory
Buckling Theory

Diagnosis
- 2 mm thick section CT scan. 100% accuracy. (Hammerschalg et al)
- Forced duction test
- Infraorbital nerve paresthesia.
  Evaluation of ocular changes secondary to blowout fractures
- Assessment of diplopia
- Measurement of globe position.

Timing of surgery
- Management of blowout fractures involving the orbital floor has been controversial over the past several decades
- A 2-week waiting period has been found to be of little benefit and possibly harmful to their motility. Hence, it is advocated surgery within the first few days after injury as it may help to avoid permanent motility restriction.

Orbital floor materials
Titanium and Vitallium mesh
Gelatin film
Polydiaxone
Polyamide mesh
Polyglactin 910
Polyglactin 910
Polypropelene
Silicones
Bone-derived biomaterials • Fresh-frozen bone • Freeze-dried bone • Demineralized bone • Deproteinated bone
Non-bone substitutes • Hydroxyapatite • Tricalcium phosphate
Marlex mesh
Medpor

Complications of orbital trauma
- Hemorrhage
- Retrobulbar hemorrhage
- Superior orbital fissure syndrome
- Orbital apex syndrome
- Caroticocavernous fistula
- Canalicular injuries.

Retrobulbar Hemorrhage

- Hot angry eye
- This is a very rare condition that can result in loss of vision
- Where bleeding into the orbital space can result in compression of the optic nerve, leading to ischemia and eventually blindness
- It can follow both trauma and surgery to the orbital region
- Trauma
- Infraorbital
  - Zygomatic
  - Le Fort
- Postoperatively
  - Blepheroplasty
  - Zygomatic reduction
  - LeFort reduction.

Symptoms
- Orbital pain
- Decreased visual acuity or blindness
- Diplopia if vision preserved

Signs
- Proptosis with globe that is very hard on palpation
- Increased intraocular pressure on tonometry
- Marked subconjuctival edema and ecchymosis
- Opthalmoplegia.

Treatment
- Immediate action
- Remove any sutures in the area, for pressure relief
- Medication
  - Mannitol 1 g/kg as 20% infusion
    - Osmotic diuretic
    - Contraindicated in congestive cardiac failure.

- Acetazolamide 500 mg IV
- Dexamethasone 8 mg PO
- Papaverine 40 mg smooth muscle relaxant
- Dextran-40 500 ml IV improves perfusion.

Superior Orbital Fissure Syndrome
Instructive example of precise anatomical localization of a lesion by neurological signs.

Signs and symptoms
- Gross and persistent edema of the periorbital tissue
- Proptosis and subconjuntival hemorrhage
- Ophthalmoplegia and ptosis
- Dilatation of pupil
- Direct light reflex absent
- Consensual reflex preserved
- Corneal reflex lost
- Loss of sensation over forehead.

Endoscopic repair of orbital blow-out fractures
Fracture types can be evaluated and repaired endoscopically without the need for an eyelid incision.

It offers improved visualization, anatomic fracture repair, no risk of postoperative eyelid complications, and good clinical results.

Trigeminocardiac Reflex

- In the early 20th century, trigeminocardiac reflex (TCR) has gained much clinical attention, in the form of the oculocardiac reflex (OCR) which is the cardiac response (mainly bradycardia) associated with stimulation of the ophthalmic division of the trigeminal nerve during ocular surgeries
- Schaller, for the first time, demonstrated that a similar reflex occurs with stimulation of the intracranial portion of the trigeminal nerve.

Trigeminocardiac reflex
Defined as the sudden onset of parasympathetic dys-rhythmia, sympathetic hypotension, apnea or gastric hypermotility during stimulation of any of the sensory branches of the trigeminal nerve

Pathophysiology
(Central Neurogenic Reflex)

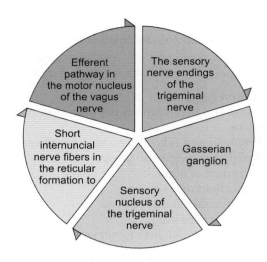

- Hypercapnia
- Hypoxemia
- Light general anesthesia
- Age (more pronounced in children)
- The nature of the provoking stimulus (stimulus strength and duration)
- Drugs

Drugs known to increase the trigeminocardiac reflex include:
- Potent narcotic agents (sufentanil and alfentanil)
- Beta-blockers, and
- Calcium channel blockers.

   Narcotics may augment vagal tone through their inhibitory action on the sympathetic nervous system. Beta-blockers reduce the sympathetic response of the heart and by so doing, augment the vagal cardiac response resulting in bradycardia. Calcium channel blockers result in peripheral arterial smooth muscle relaxation and vasodilatation causing reduction in blood pressure.

Clinical significance of the trigeminocardiac reflex and why it should be treated: Trigeminocardiac reflex is a transient response to the trigeminal nerve manipulation in its extra or intracranial course which subsides with cessation of the stimulus. But, in the most serious forms of severe bradycardia and asystole, administration of vagolytic agents is warranted in addition to cessation of the stimulus. The importance of the trigeminocardiac reflex which may range from mild bradycardia which responds to simple cessation of the stimulus to asystole and severe bradycardia requiring additional intervention with vagolytics. In some rare but serious cases, it may lead to death if not detected early and appropriate measures taken.

Management of the trigeminocardiac reflex: The most important "management option" for the trigeminocardiac reflex is to be aware of its potential danger and minimize any mechanical stimulation of the nerve.

Treatment

Cessation of the manipulation, and administration of vagolytic agents or adrenaline.

Clinically, the trigeminocardiac reflex has been reported to occur during craniofacial surgery, balloon-compression rhizolysis of the trigeminal ganglion, and tumor resection in the cerebellopontine angle. Apart from the few clinical reports, the physiological function of this brainstem reflex has not yet been fully explored. From experimental findings, it may be suggested that the trigeminocardiac reflex represents an expression of a central neurogenic reflex leading to rapid cerebro vascular vasodilatation generated from excitation of oxygen sensitive neurons in the rostral ventrolateral medulla oblongata. By this physiological response, the adjustments of the systemic and cerebral circulations are initiated to divert blood to the brain or to increase blood flow within it. As it is generally accepted that the diving reflex and ischemic tolerance appear to involve at least partially similar physiological mechanisms, the existence of such endogenous neuroprotective strategies may extend the actually known clinical appearance of the trigeminocardiac reflex and include the prevention of other potentially brain injury states as well.

CLINICAL CASES (FIGS 11.33 TO 11.44)

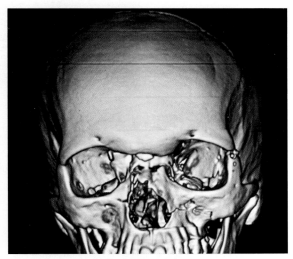

Fig. 11.33: 3D CT showing nasal fracture

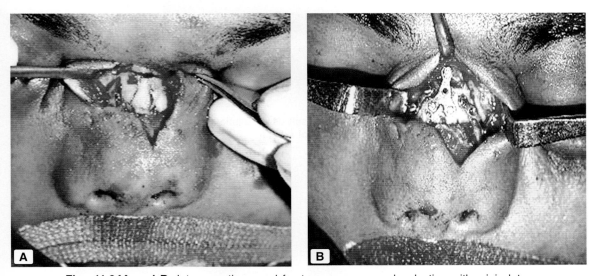

Figs 11.34A and B: Intraoperative nasal fracture exposure and reduction with mini plates

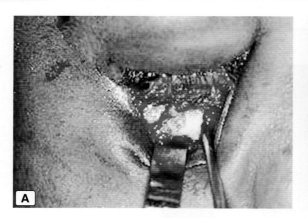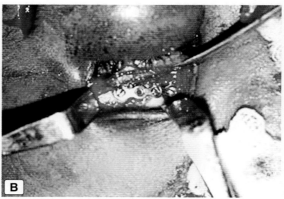

Figs 11.35A and B: Intraoperative infraorbital rim fracture exposure and reduction with mini plates

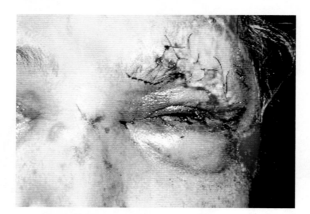

Fig. 11.36: Showing soft tissue injuries and periorbital edema

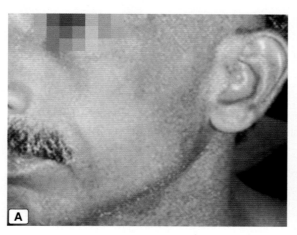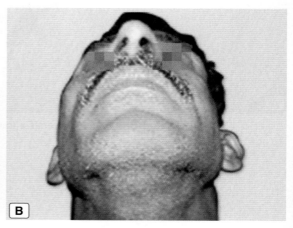

Figs 11.37A and B: Preoperative left zygomatic arch fracture

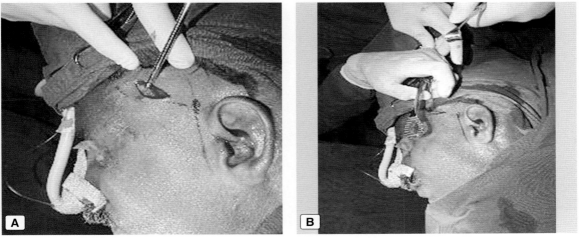

Figs 11.38A and B: Intraoperative left zygomatic arch fracture reduction by Gillies temporal approach

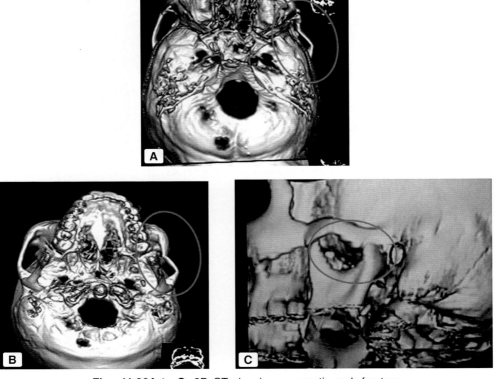

Figs 11.39A to C: 3D CT showing zygomatic arch fracture

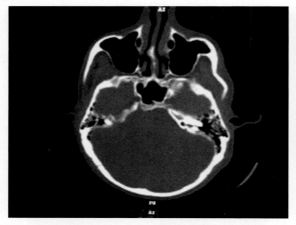

Fig. 11.40: CT showing zygomatic fracture

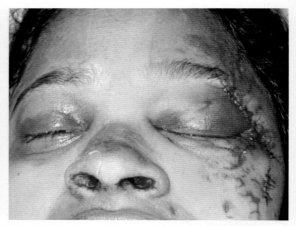

Fig. 11.41: Left frontozygomatic fracture

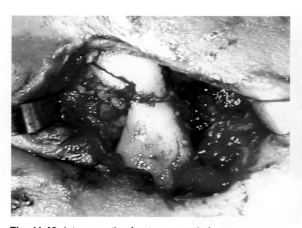

Fig. 11.42: Intraoperative frontozygomatic fracture exposure

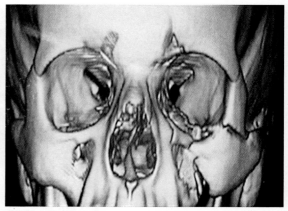

Fig. 11.43: 3D CT Intrafrontozygomatic fracture

ZYGOMATIC ARCH FRACTURE RIGHT SIDE (FIG. 11.44)

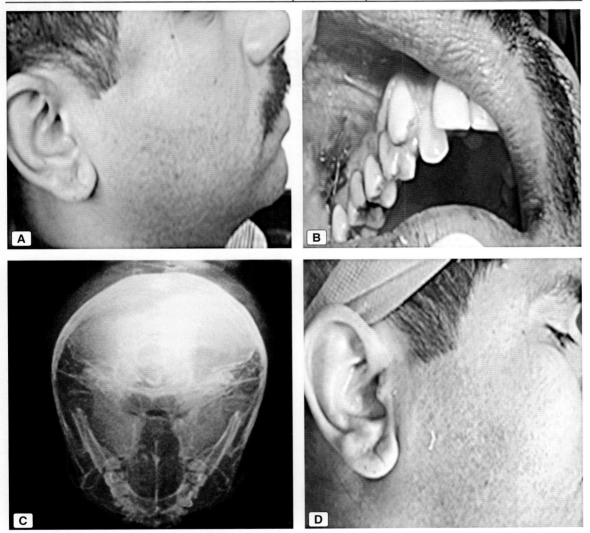

Figs 11.44A to D: Zygomatic arch fracture right side: (A) Preoperative clinical picture showing depression at preauricular region. (B) Intraoral suturing. (C) Jug handle view showing fractured zygomatic arch. (D) Postoperative clinical picture

Mandibular Fractures

12

INTRODUCTION

Mandibular fracture is more common than middle third fracture. It could be observed either alone or in combination with other facial fractures. Minor mandibular fracture may be associated with head injury owing to the cranio-mandibular articulation. Mandibular fracture may compromise the patency of the airway in particular with loss of consciousness. Mandible is more sensitive to lateral impact than frontal one. Fracture of condyle regarded as a safety mechanism to the patient.

- Frontal force of 800–900 lb (350–400 N) is required to cause symphyseal fracture
- Frontal impact is substantially cushioned by opening and retrusion of the jaw
- Long canine tooth and partially erupted 3rd, molar represent line of relative weakness.

Factors influencing site of fracture and displacement
Anatomy of the mandible and attached muscle (canine and wisdoms)
Weakening areas of mandible (resorption and pathology)
Direction of force of the blow
Age of the patient

ANATOMICAL CONSIDERATIONS

Attached Muscles

- Masseter
- Temporalis
- Medial and lateral pterygoid
- Mylohyoid
- Geniohyoid and genioglosus
- Anterior belly of digastric.

Effects of Muscles on Displacement

- Transverse midline fracture (symphysial) stabilizes by the action of mylohyoid and geniohyoid
- Oblique fracture (parasymphysial) tends to overlap under the influence of muscles action
- Bilateral parasymphysial fracture results in backward displacement associated with loss of tongue control when the level of consciousness is depressed.

Incidence of mandibular fractures	
Body fractures	33.6%
Subcondylar fracture	33.4%
Fractures at the angle	17.4%
Alveolar fractures	6.7%
Ramus fractures	5.4%
Midline fractures	2.9%
Fracture of coronoid process	1.3%

CLASSIFICATION

Kruger's General Classification

- Simple or closed
- Compound or open
- Comminuted

- Complicated or complex
- Impacted
- Greenstick
- Pathological.

Rowe and Killey's Anatomic Classification

I. Fractures not involving the basal bone
   - Dentoalveolar fractures
II. Fractures involving the basal bone
   - Single unilateral
   - Double unilateral
   - Bilateral
   - Multiple.

Factors influencing site of fracture and displacement
Anatomy of the mandible and attached muscle (canine and wisdoms)
Weakening areas of mandible (resorption and pathology)
Direction of force of the blow
Age of the patient

Favorable or Unfavorable

- Aimed towards angle fractures. The direction of fracture line is important for resisting the muscle pull
- They are influenced by the medial pterygoid-masseter "sling"
- They can be vertically or horizontally in direction
- Favorable fracture line makes the reduced fragment easier to stabilize
  - If the vertical direction of the fracture favours the unopposed action of medial pterygoid muscle, the posterior fragment will be pulled lingually
  - If the horizontal direction of the fracture favors the unopposed action of masseter and pterygoid muscles in upward direction, the posterior fragment will be pulled lingually.

Kazanjian and Converse Classification

Class I: When the teeth are present on both sides of the fracture line

- An adequate number of teeth of suitable shape and stability.
- An adequate number of teeth whose shape or stability is unsuitable.
- Lateral compression splint, arch bars or cast metal splints.

Class II: When the teeth are present only on one side of the fracture line
a. Short edentulous posterior fragment
   - If favorable – IMF
   - If unfavorable – ORIF
b. Long edentulous posterior fragment
   - If favorable – IMF
   - If unfavorable – ORIF

Class III: When both the fragments are edentulous
- Simple fractures without much displacement—gunning type splints
- Simple fractures which are unfavorable—ORIF
- Compound fractures—surgical intervention.

AO Classification

Relevant to Internal Fixation
   F : No. of fracture
   L : Location of the fracture
   O : Occlusion status
   S : Soft tissue involvemrnt
   A : Associated fractures of the facial skeleton

Fracture of the Angle and Body
- Pain, tenderness and trismus
- Extraoral swelling at the angle with obvious deformity
- Step deformity behind the molar teeth
- Movement and crepitus at the fracture site
- Derangement of occlusion
- Intraoral buccal and lingual hematoma
- Involvement of inferior alveolar nerve
- Gingival tear if fracture in tooth area
- Tooth involvement and possible longitudinal split fracture.

Midline Fracture
- The most common missed fracture
- Types—symphysial or parasymphysial

- Commonly associated with one or both condylar fracture.
- Unilateral fracture leads to over-riding of the fragments and bilateral may contribute in loss of voluntary tongue control.
- Long canine tooth represent a weak area and contributes to parasymphysial fracture.

CLINICAL ASSESSMENT AND DIAGNOSIS (FIGS 12.1 TO 12.13)

1. History of trauma
2. Clinical Examination
   - Extaroral
     - Inspection—assessment of asymmetry, swelling, ecchymosis, laceration and cut wounds
     - Palpation for tenderness, pain, step deformity and malfunction.
   - Intra- and paraoral
     - bleeding, hematoma, gingival tear, gagging of occlusion and step deformity and sensory and motor deficiency
3. Radiographs (Figs 12.3 to 12.5 and 12.7 to 12.10)
   - Plain radiograph
     - OPG

- Lateral oblique
- PA mandible
- AP mandible (Reverse Towne)
- Lower occlusal
– CT scan
– 3D CT imaging
– MRI.

Principles of Treatment

Similar to Elsewhere Fractures in the Body
- Reduction of fragments in good position
- Immobilization until bony union occurs

These are achieved by
- Close reduction and immobilization
- Open reduction and rigid fixation

Definitive Treatment

Objective
- Restoration of functional alignment of the bone fragments in anatomically precise position utilizing the present teeth for guidance.

Reduction and Fixation of the Jaw (Fig. 12.2)
- Close reduction and IMF (traditional method by means of manipulation).

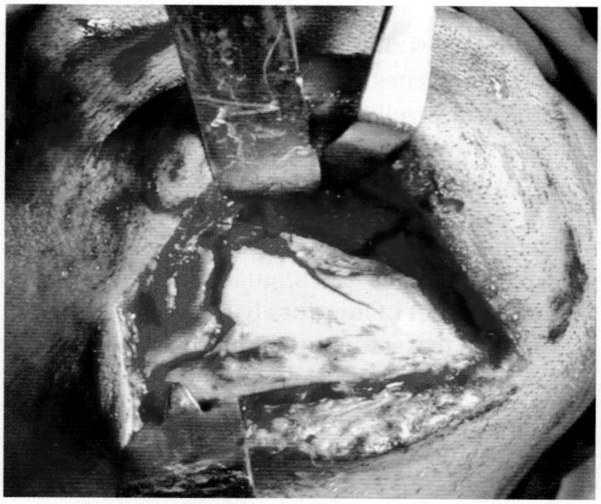

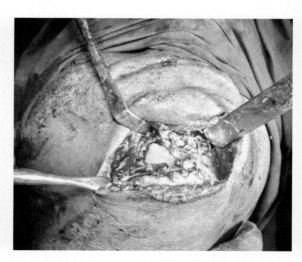

Fig. 12.1: Showing intraoperative symphysis fracture exposure

Fig. 12.2: Showing intraoperative symphysis fracture plating

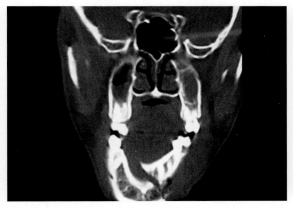

Fig. 12.3: Radiographic image of symphyseal fracture

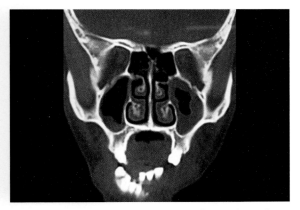

Fig. 12.4: Radiographic image of symphyseal fracture with lingually displaced fracture

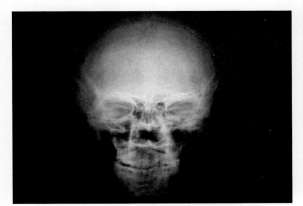

Fig. 12.5: PA skull showing bilateral parasymphyseal fracture

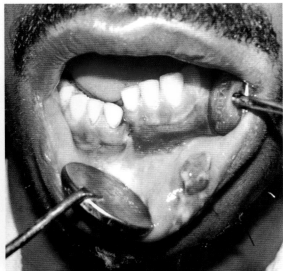

Fig. 12.6: Clinical appearance of displaced symphyseal fracture

- Open reduction and semi-rigid fixation (using interossous wirings).
- Open reduction and rigid fixation (using bone palates osteosynthesis).

Close Reduction

- Arch bars
  - Jelenko
  - Erich pattern
  - German silver notched

- Cap splints
- *IMF prior to rigid fixation*
- Bonded brackets
- IMF screws
- Dental wiring:
  - Direct wiring
  - Eyelet wiring
- Minimal displacement
- IMF for 6 weeks.

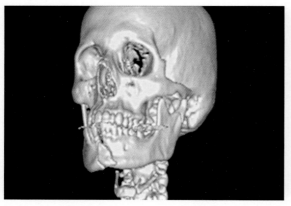

Fig. 12.7: 3D CT showing parasymphyseal fracture (oblique view)

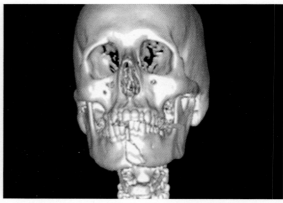

Fig. 12.8: 3D CT showing parasymphyseal fracture (frontal view)

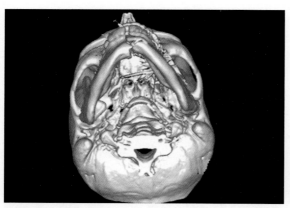

Fig. 12.9: 3D CT showing parasymphyseal fracture (basal view)

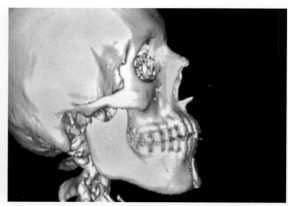

Fig. 12.10: 3D CT showing parasymphyseal fracture (lateral view)

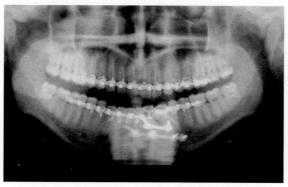

Fig. 12.11: OPG showing parasymphyseal fracture

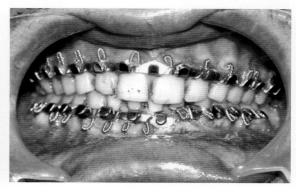

Fig. 12.12: Clinical photograph of closed eduction

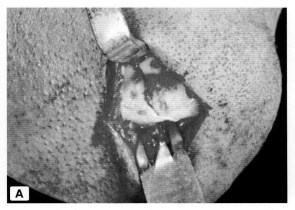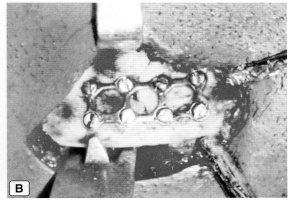

Figs 12.13A and B: intraoperative symphyseal fracture exposure and fixation with 3D plate

Open Reduction and Fixation

Surgical approaches to the mandible
- Intraoral approach
    a. Symphysis and parasymphysis region– degloving incision
    b. Body, angle, ramus region – transbuccal incision
- Extraoral approach
    - Submandibular Risdon's incision
    - Postramal Hind's incision
- Intraosseous or transosseous wiring
- Compression plates
- Mini plates
- Lag screws.

Teeth in the Fracture Line

- The fracture is compound into the mouth.
- The tooth may be damaged or lose its blood supply.
- The tooth may be affected by some preexisting pathology.

Absolute Indications

- Longitudinal fracture
- Dislocation or subluxation from socket
- Presence of periapical infection
- Infected fracture line
- Acute pericoronitis.

Relative Indications

- Functional tooth that would be removed
- Advanced caries or periodontal diseases
- Doubtful tooth which would be added to existing denture.
- Tooth in untreated fracture presenting more than 3 days after injury.

Management of Teeth Retained in Fracture Line

- Good quality intraoral periapical radiograph (Fig. 12.14)
- Insinuation of appropriate systemic antibiotic therapy
- Splinting of tooth if mobile
- Endodontic therapy if pulp is exposed
- Immediate extraction if fracture becomes infected
- Follow up for 1 year and endodontic therapy if there is a loss of vitality.

Edentulous Body Fracture

- Bucket handle type of fracture

Management of edentulous body fractures

Gunning splint
- Old modality
- Rigid fixation is not possible
- To establish the occlusion.

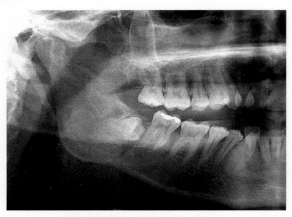

Fig. 12.14: Radiograph showing fracture line passing in the region of impacted tooth

Fracture Mandible in Children

- Conservative therapy
- Close reduction

- Open reduction and fixation is usually not necessary
- Plating at the inferior border
- Resorbable plates
- Cap splints:
  - Open cap splints
  - Close cap splints.

Complications of Open Reduction and Direct Fixation During Mandibular Fracture Management

During primary treatment:
- Infection
- Damage to inferior alveolar, mental and sometimes facial nerve.
- Gingival and periodontal complications.

Late complications
- Malunion
- Delayed union
- Nonunion.

Condylar Fractures

13

INTRODUCTION

Condylar injuries deserve special consideration apart from those of the rest of the mandible due to their anatomic differences, variations in clinical picture, unique management protocols and distinct healing potential. The management of mandibular condylar injuries is one of the most controversial areas in the treatment of facial trauma. Fractures involving the mandibular condyle are the only facial bone fractures which involve a synovial joint. Severe displcement of fractured condyle can cause malocclusion. abnormal mouth opening; and impaired function.

Condyle	29.1%
Angle	24.5%
Symphyseal and parasymphyseal	22%
Body	16%
Dentoalveolar	3.1%
Ramus	1.7%
Coronoid	1.3%

ETIOLOGY OF CONDYLAR INJURIES

- Facial injuries are most commonly associated with falls, motor vehicle accidents, sports-related trauma and interpersonal violence.
- Injury to the condyle may be caused by a variety of mechanisms, which also vary according to the characteristics of the group studied.

- In adults, motor vehicle accidents account for the majority of condylar fractures, while interpersonal violence, work-related incidents, sporting accidents and falls play significant but lesser roles.
- In children, falls and bicycle accidents are the major causes, with motor vehicle accidents also contributing significantly.
- Different still are in elderly, falls again constitute the primary etiologic factor, followed by assaults and automobile accidents.
- Other less obvious causes of injury to the temporomandibular joint (TMJ) include orotracheal intubation, whiplash injury, childbirth and weight lifting.

CLASSIFICATIONS

Wassmund (1934) described five types of condylar fractures:

Type I: Fracture of the neck of the condyle with relatively slight displacement of the head.

Type II: Fractures which produce an angle of 45 to 90 degree, resulting in tearing of the medial portion of the capsule.

Type III: The fragments are not in contact, and the head is displaced *mesially* and forward owing to traction of the lateral *pterygoid* muscle. The fragments confined to the glenoid fossa. The capsule is torn, and the head is outside the capsule.

Type IV: Fractures where the condylar head articulates in an anterior position to the articular eminence.

Type V: Vertical or oblique fractures through the head of the condyle.

MacLennan (1952) Classification

Type I: Nondisplaced fracture.

Type II: Fracture deviation, where there is simple angulation of the condylar process to the major fragment (e.g. greenstick fracture).

Type III: Fracture displacement, where there is simple overlap of the condylar process and major mandibular fragments.

Type IV: Fracture dislocation, where the head of the condyle is completely disrupted from the articular fossa.

Lindahl in 1977

Proposed a classification based on radiographic views in two planes at right angles to each other. He took into consideration three major aspects. They are the anatomic location of the fracture, relationship of condylar fragment to mandible and relationship of condylar head to the glenoid fossa.

- Anatomic location of the fracture
  - Condylar head
  - Condylar neck
  - Subcondylar
- Relationship of condylar fragment to mandible
  - Nondisplaced
  - Deviated
  - Displacement with medial or lateral overlap
  - Displacement with anterior or posterior overlap
  - No contact between fractured segments
- Relationship of condylar head to fossa
  - Nondisplaced
  - Displacement
  - Dislocation

Spiessl and Schroll (1972)

- Nondisplaced fracture
- Low-neck fracture with displacement, mostly with contact between fragments
- High-neck fracture with displacement, mostly without contact between fragments
- Low-neck fracture with dislocation
- High-neck fracture with dislocation
- Intracapsular fracture of condylar head.

Injuries of the TMJ other than fractures
Contusion
Effusion and Hemarthrosis
TMJ Sprain
Subluxation
Dislocation

DIAGNOSIS OF CONDYLAR INJURIES

Diagnosis is based on a suggestive history, determination of the direction of force, clinical signs and symptoms and radiographic visualization of the joint and subcondylar region.

CLINICAL FEATURES

An overall evaluation of the patient with traumatic injury should precede evaluation of the maxillofacial region. Numerous symptoms point generally to traumatic damage in the joint region. They include pain, tenderness and swelling in the joint region, limitation of mouth opening and malocclusion. Supplementing these suggestive symptoms, different fracture types provide characteristic symptoms.

- Unilateral malocclusion
  - Premature tooth contact
  - Contralateral open bite
  - Deviation of midline to side of injury
  - Swelling over the preauricular region
  - Restricted mouth opening
  - Bleeding from the ear
  - Mandibular mid line shifted to the affected side
  - Ecchymosis over the mastoid occasionally [Battle's sign].

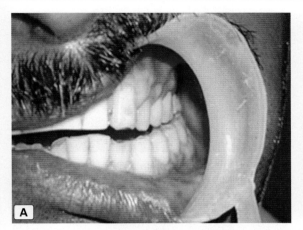
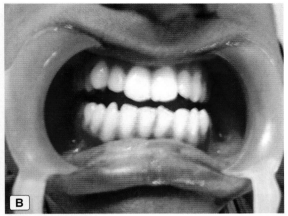

Figs 13.1A and B: Occlusion in unilateral condylar injuries

Unilateral condylar fracture (Fig. 13.1)
Deviation to the ipsilateral side
Gagging of occlusion on ipsilateral molar teeth
Painful limitation of protrusion and laterl excursion to the opposite side

Bilateral condylar fracture
Undisplaced and intracapsular fracture—occlusion not disturbed
Displaced fracture—anterior open bite
Pain and limitation of opening, protrusion and lateral excursion

Goals
Stable occlusion
Restoration of interincisal opening
Full range of mandibular excursive movements
Minimize deviation
Relief from pain
Avoid internal derangement of the TMJ
Avoid growth disturbance

RADIOGRAPHY (FIGS 13.2 TO 13.5)

- Conventional radiography
- Orthopantomogram (OPG)
- Lateral oblique view of mandible
- Posteroanterior (PA) view of mandible
- Reverse Towne's view
- Transcranial views for TMJ
- CT scan
- Magnetic resonance imaging (MRI).

MANAGEMENT GOALS

The objective of the maxillofacial surgeon treating condylar fractures is primarily directed towards functional rehabilitation.

CONSERVATIVE AND FUNCTIONAL MANAGEMENT

- Objective is either to allow bony union to occur where there is no significant displacement of the condyle or in the case of fracture dislocation, to produce an acceptable functional pseudoarthrosis by re-education of the neuromuscular pathways
- The aims of conservative and functional treatment are to encourage active movement of the jaw as early as possible provided that the patient can bring his or her teeth into normal occlusion. Excessive pain or persistent malocclusion will require periods of intermaxillary fixation. Such a period of fixation should not exceed 10 days if there is a risk of ankylosis. In the case of children one must be aware of the remarkable remodelling capacity of the condyle which may persist.

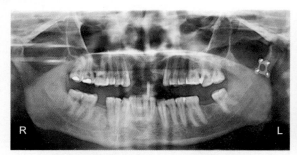

Fig. 13.2: Orthopantomogram (OPG) showing trapezoidal plate in place after condylar fracture fixation

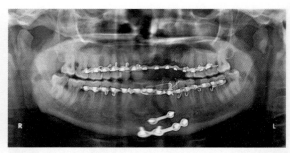

Fig. 13.3: Orthopantomogram (OPG) showing condylar and parasymphysial fracture (fixed with mini plates)

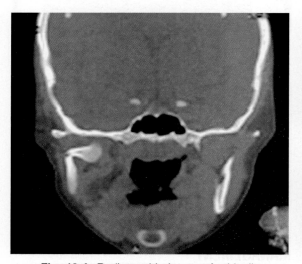

Fig. 13.4: Radiographic image of mideally displaced condyle

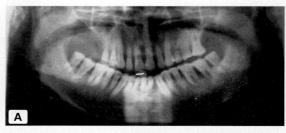

A

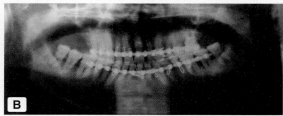

B

Figs 13.5A and B: Illustrating closed reduction treatment given for a case of right subcondylar fracture (A) Preoperative, (B) Postoperative

CLOSED REDUCTION (FIGS 13.5A AND B)

Placement of *archbars or splints*, immobilizing the jaws for 2–4 weeks has been the mainstay of therapy for many decades.

Displaced fractures of the neck of the condyle, the joint must be relieved of stress by opening the occlusion by 2–3 mm with an acrylic block in the distal molar region in the side of the fracture. This therapy is known as 'extension by means of a *fulcrum*'. The height of the fulcrum depends on the radiographically determined degree of ramus shortening. After 8 days, the fixation is removed and the patient is followed by functional movements with elastics applied in the anterior region.

OPEN REDUCTION (FIGS 13.6 TO 13.11)

- In open reduction, the objective is to perform a repositioning of the fractured condyle as near to its anatomical location as possible. This is achieved by exposing the condylar fragment, reducing it to a normal relationship with the mandibular fragment and then fixing it in that position

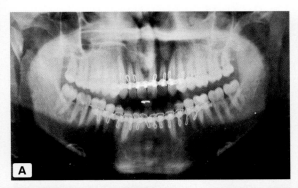

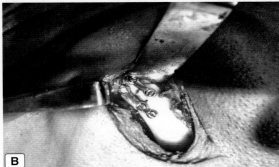

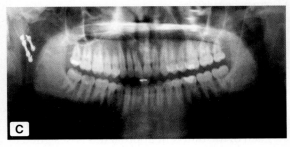

Figs 13.6A to C: Illustration of open reduction for a case of right subcondylar fracture. (A) Preoperative, (B) Intraoperative, (C) Postoperative

- Surgical access in cases of fracture dislocations tends to be difficult with a real risk to branches of 7th cranial nerve and the maxillary artery.

Indications

Zide and Kent (1983) divided indications for open reduction of a condylar fracture into absolute and relative.

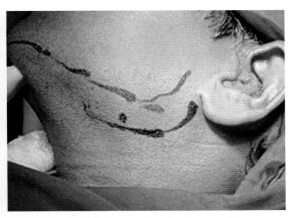

Fig. 13.7: Intraoperative incision marking

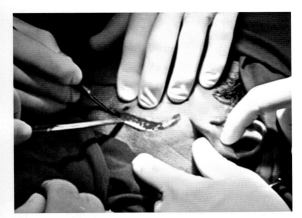

Fig. 13.8: Intraoperative incision

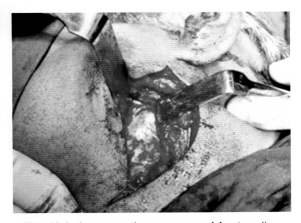

Fig. 13.9: Intraoperative exposure of fracture line

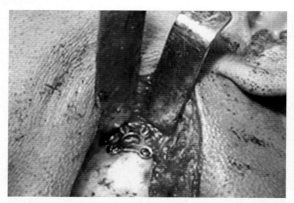

Fig. 13.10: Intraoperative fixation of fracture with traphezoidal plate

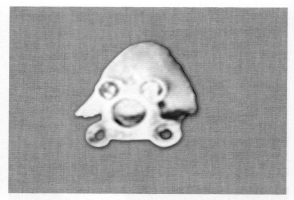

Fig. 13.11: Traphezoidal plate fixed to condylar stump

The absolute indications
Displacement of the condyle into the middle cranial fossa
Inability to achieve occlusion with a closed reduction
Lateral fracture-dislocation of the condyle and
Invasion of the joint space with a foreign body

Relative indications for open reduction
Bilateral condylar fractures where establishing vertical facial height is important
Associated injuries that dictate early immediate function
Associated medical conditions that indicate an open reduction is preferable to maxillomandibular fixation and
Conditions in which treatment has been delayed and early healing in a malaligned position has commenced

Surgical Approaches

- The selection of surgical approach for open reduction depends on a variety of factors, which include the level at which the fracture has occurred, the degree of displacement or dislocation and the planned method of fixation. Other factors are the quest for optimal access for visualization and instrumentation, esthetic factors like scarring, minimizing injury to vital structures like nerves, blood vessels and ducts of salivary glands

Various surgical approaches
Preauricular
Horizontal incision over the zygomatic arch
Endaural
Retroauricular
Submandibular
Retromandibular
Intraoral
Rhytidectomy
Endoscopy

- The advantages of all extraoral approaches are that a fracture is visualized and approached more directly than from an intraoral approach. Each of the different approaches is designed to prevent or minimize injury to the branches of the facial nerve. The major disadvantages of all extraoral approaches are visible scars and possible injury to the branches of the facial nerve
- It is claimed that the intraoral technique obviates the known complications of external open reduction such as the possibility of facial nerve injury, external scar, ischemic compromise to the proximal segment and undoubted technical facilities. The main disadvantage of this approach is that exposure of the condylar segment is limited.

Methods of Immobilization of the Condyle

Once the proximal segment is visualized and the fracture reduced, the fragments can be immobilised in a number of ways.

Methods of immobilization of the condyle
Simple soft tissue repair without fixation
Transosseous wiring
Bone pins
Glenoid fossa-condyle suture
Kirschner wire
Intramedullary screws
Bone plating

- Three useful plating techniques are described:
    i. Extraoral approach through the preauricular route
    ii. Intraoral approach
    iii. Osteotomy—Extracorporeal reduction technique through a submandibular incision.

Specific Treatment of Condylar Fractures

The following factors should be considered
The age of the patient whether under 10 years of age, 10–17 years of age, adults
Whether the fracture is intracapsular or extracapsular (low condylar neck or high condylar neck)
Site, whether unilateral or bilateral
Whether the occlusion is undisturbed or whether there is malocclusion

Children under 10 Years of Age

- This group has been shown to be more likely to develop growth disturbance or limitation of movement than other groups
- If malocclusion is present entirely as a result of condylar injury it should be disregarded because spontaneous correction will take place as the dentition develops
- Displaced condylar neck fractures will undergo functional restitution in most cases
- Unilateral and bilateral fractures are treated the same

- Treatment should be entirely functional where possible
- Indirect immobilization by intermaxillary fixation is indicated for control of pain and should be released after 7–10 days
- Where an intracapsular fracture has been diagnosed careful follow-up and monitoring of growth is required.

Adolescents

- Ten to seventeen years of age
- Malocclusion is an indication for intermaxillary fixation for 2–3 weeks. The dentition at this stage is suitable for application of simple eyelet wires.

Adults

Unilateral intracapsular fractures: The occlusion is usually undisturbed and the fracture should be treated conservatively without immobilization of the mandible.

Unilateral condylar neck fractures
- If the fracture is undisplaced the occlusion will generally be undisturbed and no active treatment is necessary
- A fracture dislocation will often induce significant malocclusion due to shortening of ramus height and premature contact of molar teeth on that side
- A low condylar neck fracture is probably best treated by open reduction in these circumstances
- In the case of a high condylar neck fracture with extensive displacement and malocclusion, intermaxillary fixation is applied and maintained until stable bony union has occurred, i.e. 3–4 weeks.

Bilateral intracapsular fractures: The occlusion is usually slightly damaged in these cases. The degree of displacement of the two condyles may not be the same and it is best to immobilize the mandible for the 3–4 weeks required for stable union.

Bilateral condylar neck fractures: These fractures present the major problem in treatment. There is usually considerable displacement of one side and/or the other. Even if displacement is not evident when first seen, the fractures are inherently unstable and functional treatment is contraindicated.

COMPLICATIONS

- Complications that occur concurrent with or early after treatment of condylar fractures include the following:

Early complications
Fracture of the tympanic plate and middle ear injury
Fracture of the glenoid fossa
Damage to cranial nerves
Vascular injury

- The late complications of condylar injury commonly include the following:

Late complications
Malocclusion
Growth alteration
Temporomandibular joint dysfunction (Internal derangement)
Ankylosis

CONCLUSION

- Fractures of the mandibular condyle constitute a significant portion of mandibular fractures. A number of clinical signs and symptoms are characteristic of injury to the condylar apparatus. The use of plain radiographs in multiple view, or CT scans discloses most condylar fractures and displacements, if any. A number of classification systems are available to help in treatment planning and record keeping.
- Nonsurgical treatment is adequate for a majority of condylar fractures. A period of immobilization

followed by active functional therapy is indicated for most cases. Surgical management has specific indications, and can be accomplished through a wide variety of techniques. In general, complications are not common following condylar trauma. Important among the possible complications are ankylosis, growth disturbances and internal derangement.

SOME MORE CASES (FIGS 13.12 TO 13.15)

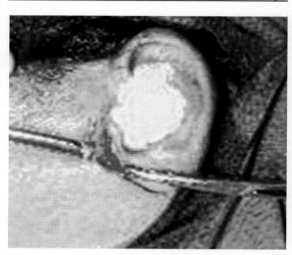

Fig. 13.12: Preauricular incision for condylar exposure

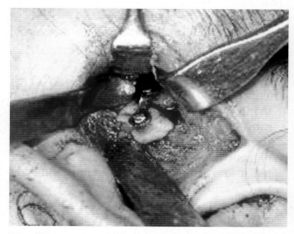

Fig. 13.13: Exposure and fixation of condyl with help of two hole miniplate

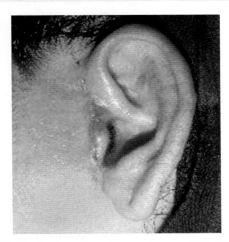

Fig. 13.14: Postopertive closure of preauricular incision

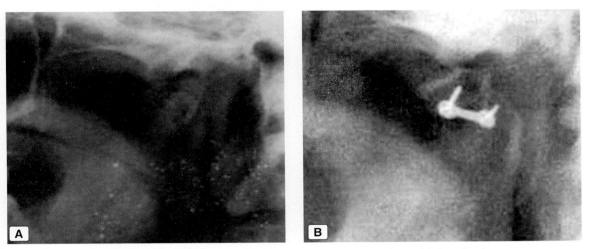

Figs 13.15A and B: Pre- and postoperative radiograph after miniplate fixation

Cerebrospinal Fluid Rhinorrhea

14

INTRODUCTION

Cerebrospinal fluid (CSF): "Third circulation"—Clear fluid bathing the cerebral hemispheres, cerebellum and layers of meninges that is produced on a daily basis in the ventriculocisternal portion of the nervous system, It is essentially an *ultrafiltrate of plasma*. It is 5–10% of intracranial volume. Approximate amount 50–160 mL, it forms at the rate of 20–22 mL/hr or 500 mL/day and renewed three times a day, mostly made in choroid plexus traverses, ventricles, convexities, uptaken by arachnoid villi, normal pressure between 50–180 mm H_2O, but pressure is maintain by relative balance between CSF secretion and CSF resorption, it surrounds and cushions brain, pathologic communication with outside world can lead to problem. The CSF circulates from ventricles through *foramina Luschka and Magendie to subarachnouid space*.

DEFINITION

Cerebrospinal fluid (CSF) rhinorrhea results from a direct communication between the CSF-containing subarachnoid space and the mucosalized space of the paranasal sinuses.
- *Main site of formation:* Choroid plexus around the lateral ventricles.

Functions
- Water Cushion
- Protection
- Buoyancy
- Nutrition
- Removal of metabolic wastes.

Historical Perspective
- First reported in the 17th century
- Dandy in 20th century, reported first successful repair utilizing a bifrontal craniotomy for placement of a fascia lata graft
- Extracranial approaches introduced mid-20th century
- Endoscopic approaches were introduced and popularized in the 1980s and early 1990s.

Objectives
- Understand the classification system for various causes of CSF rhinorrhea
- Understand the pathophysiology and diagnosis of CSF rhinorrhea
- Review diagnostic testing techniques (chemical markers and CSF tracers) as well as localization studies
- Review both medical and surgical strategies in treatment of CSF rhinorrhea.

CLASSIFICATION OF CSF RHINORRHEA

Based on established pathophysiology of CSF rhinorrhea
- This has important clinical implications for the selection of treatment strategies and patient counseling about prognosis
- Initial schemes–traumatic leaks and nontraumatic leaks

- Accidental trauma—Eighty percent of all CSF rhinorrhea
- Non-traumatic—Four percent of all CSF rhinorrhea
- Procedure-related—Sixteen percent of all CSF rhinorrhea.

Traumatic
- Accidental
  - Immediate
  - Delayed
- Surgical
  - Complication of neurosurgical procedures
    i. Transsphenoidal hypophysectomy
    ii. Frontal craniotomy
    iii. Other skull-base procedures
  - Complication of rhinologic procedures
    i. Sinus surgery
    ii. Septoplasty
    iii. Other combined skull base procedures.

Nontraumatic
- Elevated intracranial pressure
  - Intracranial neoplasm
  - Hydrocephalus
    i. Noncommunicating
    ii. Obstructive
  - Benign intracranial hypertension
- Normal intracranial pressure
  - Congenital anomaly
  - Skull-base neoplasm
    i. Nasopharyngeal carcinoma
    ii. Sinonasal malignancy
  - Skull-base erosive process
    i. Sinus mucocele and osteomyelitis
  - Idiopathic.

Pathophysiology
- CSF produced by choroid plexus (20 mL/hr)
- CSF circulates from ventricles through foramina Luschka and Magendie to subarachnoid space
- Total CSF volume is 140 mL = 20 mL (ventricles) + 50 mL (intracranial subarachnoid space) + 70 mL (paraspinal subarachnoid space)
- CSF pressure ranges 40 mm H_2O (infants) - 140 mm H_2O (adults)

- CSF pressure maintained by relative balance between CSF secretion (choroid plexus) and CSF resorption (arachnoid villi)
- CSF resorption rate plays major role in determining CSF pressure
- CSF rhinorrhea requires disruption of barriers that normally separate the contents of the subarachnoid space from the nose and paranasal sinuses
- Pressure gradient is also required to produce flow of CSF.

Conditions with elevated intracranial pressure and associated CSF rhinorrhea
- Nontraumatic CSF rhinorrhea
- Benign intracranial hypertension (BIH)
- Empty sella syndrome (ESS).

DIFFERENTIAL DIAGNOSIS
- CSF otorrhea presents as CSF rhinorrhea
- Sinonasal saline irrigations
- Seasonal and perennial allergic rhinitis
- Vasomotor rhinitis.

Clinical Presentation (Fig. 14.1)
- Unilateral watery nasal discharge
- Salty taste
- Positional variation
- History trauma or surgery
- Weight loss
- Presence of inflammatory paranasal sinus disease
- Headache
- History of single or multiple episodes bacterial meningitis.

Physical Examination (Fig. 14.2)
- Position testing
- Halo sign
- Glistening moist nasal mucosa on side of CSF leak
- Clear fluid stream
- Papilledema
- Abducens nerve palsy
- Traumatic CSF rhinorrhea and physical stigmata of recent or distant maxillofacial trauma.

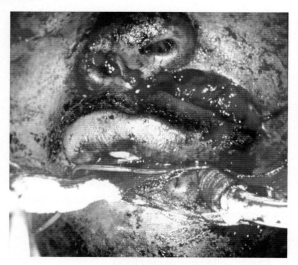

Fig. 14.1: CSF rhinorrhea in midfacial trauma case

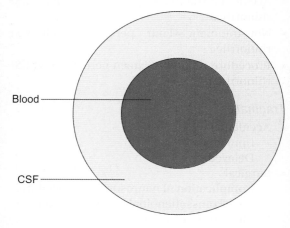

Fig. 14.2: Diagrammatic presentation of classical halo sign

Diagnostic Testing

Two types of testing
1. Identification substance serves as marker CSF.
2. Agent administration that documents communication (intradural and extradural space).

Chemical Markers

- Glucose—The CSF has glucose concentration equal to or greater than half the glucose concentration of the serum—58–90 mg/100 mL
- Beta-2 transferrin—A specific iron binding protein found only in CSF, aqueous humor and perilymph. It is a sensitive and specific method of detecting presence of CSF. It is not found in blood, mucus and tears, thus, making it specific marker of CSF at the time of maxillofacial injury where this materials are inhibitor to provide CSF leak diagnosis clinically. Beta 2 transferrin is an isolated form.

Method of testing-
- – Sample requirement – 0.5 mL of body fluid
- – Plain tubes – no additive
- – Transport at room temperature
- – If delayed more than 2 hours send at 4°C
- – An additonal 1 mL serum is recommended if patient is suspected of alcohol intoxication.

CSF Tracers

- Visible dyes (Intrathecal fluorescin).
- Radionuclide markers (Radioactive iodine (^{131}I) serum albumen (RISA), technetium (^{99}Tc)-labeled serum albumin and diethylene triamterine penta acetic acid (DTPA), and Indium (^{111}In)-labeled DTPA).
- Radiopaque dyes (metrizamide).

Chemical markers	CSF tracers
Glucose	Visible dyes
Beta-2 transferrin	Radionuclide markers
	Radiopaque dyes

Localization Studies

- Radionuclide cisternography
  - – Poor spatial resolution.
- MR cisternography
  - – Long scan acquisition times required that produce thick image slices that cannot identify small skull-base defects.
- CT cisternography (Metrizamide)
  - – Difficult to reliably interpret, even with slices of 1 mm.

All above studies assume presence active CSF flow (intermittent or very small leaks may not be identified)

- Nasal endoscopy after intrathecal fluorescin infusion.

MANAGEMENT

Multidisciplinary Approach

- Maxillofacial surgeon
- Otolaryngologist
- Neurosurgeon.

Conservative Treatment of CSF Rhinorrhea

- Subarachnoid drainage through a lumbar catheter
- Strict bed rest
- Head elevation
- Stool softeners
- Patient advised to avoid coughing, sneezing, nose blowing, and straining.

Transcranial Techniques

- After craniotomy, defect site identified, and tissue graft placed to close the defect.
- *Materials used:* Fascia lata grafts, muscle plugs, and pedicled galeal flaps may be used.
- A tissue sealant, such as fibrin glue, may be used to hold the grafts into position.
- Access to the cribriform plate region and roof of the ethmoid requires a frontal craniotomy.
- Extended craniotomy and skull-base techniques with even greater brain compression provide access to the sphenoid sinus defects.
- Potential morbidities include brain compression, hematoma, seizures, and anosmia.
- High failure rates (25%) despite direct access.

Extracranial Techniques

- Endoscopic repair of CSF rhinorrhea provides adequate visualization of defect.
- Intrathecal fluorescin facilitates defect identification.
- Prepare defect site for grafting.
- Mucosa within 5 mm of the margins of the skull-base defect must be removed to facilitate mucosal grafting.

- Graft material:
  - Temporalis fascia, fascia lata, muscle plugs, pedicled middle turbinate flaps (mucosa alone or mucosa and bone), autogenous fat, free cartilage grafts (from the nasal septum or the cartilaginous auricle), and free bone grafts (from the nasal septum or calvarium) Acellular dermal allograft
    Higher failure with pedicled intranasal grafts versus free grafts
  - Underlay technique
  - Larger defects require layered reconstruction less risk of delayed recurrence and meningoencephalocele formation
  - Never place mucosal grafts intracranially (intracranial mucocele after repair can occur)
  - Surgical sealant (fibrin glue) may be used to help hold the grafts in place
  - Absorbable nasal packing is placed adjacent to the grafts, and nonabsorbable packing used to support absorbable packing.

Pure endoscopic approaches provide excellent access to the ethmoid roof, cribriform plate, and most of the sphenoid sinus.

Lateral sphenoid leaks may require an extended approach, which incorporates endoscopic dissection of the medial pterygomaxillary space.

Osteoplastic flap or a simple trephine might be required for repair of defects through the posterior table of the frontal sinus.

Postoperative care includes:

- Strict bed rest for several days and antistaphylococcal antibiotics
- Observation in ICU for first 24 hours
- Continue lumbar drain for 4–5 days
- Nasal packing removed after several days
- Operative site may be checked through serial nasal endoscopy
- Patients advised to avoid strenuous activity, sneezing, coughing for 6 weeks after repair.
  Primary cases successful repair: 85–90%

Secondary endoscopic repair also has high likelihood of success.

Endoscopic techniques offer several advantages.

Excellent visualization afforded by nasal endoscopy facilitates identification of the defect and graft placement.

Endoscopic repair is also well-tolerated, especially compared with intracranial techniques.

Report outcomes are excellent for both primary and secondary endoscopic repairs.

Management Strategy

Indications
- Failed conservative management
- Intraoperative recognition of a leak (during sinus surgery, skull-base surgery, and craniotomy)
- Large defects/leaks (especially in association with pneumocephalus)
- Idiopathic leaks (spontaneous leaks)
- Open traumatic head wounds with CSF leakage.

Traumatic (Nonsurgical) Etiology
- Conservative measures (reduces ICP and promotes spontaneous closure)
- Persistent rhinorrhea-explore and repair
- Extracranial endoscopic techniques and open transcranial procedures (massive head injury requiring urgent operative exploration) might be warranted.

Intraoperative Injury with Immediate Recognition
- The CSF leaks noted intraoperatively should be repaired immediately during functional endoscopic sinus surgery (FESS)
- Intracranial and skull-base procedures include deliberate violations of the dura; provide a watertight seal at the end of the procedure.

Operative Injury with Delayed Recognition
- Conservative therapy for a few days warranted since some leaks will close
- Can pursue operative intervention for massive leaks early

- Significant delay between time of surgery and CSF leak diagnosis-conservative measures less successful, and early surgical intervention warranted.

Nontraumatic Leaks
- Usually require surgical repair
- Can attempt conservative measures
- Treat underlying etiology along with CSF rhinorrhea (neoplasm, hydrocephalus, etc.)
- Always consider unrecognized elevation of ICP (ESS or BIH) in cases of spontaneous CSF leaks
- Operative repair in ESS and BIH usually necessary.

CSF Fistula
- Fracture skull, dural, arachnoid tear
- Risk of meningitis and even the death
- Spontaneous cessation in 66% by 10th day
- High index of suspicion of rhinorrhea, otorrhea, pneumocephalus—X-ray skull, CT scan, MRI brain to rule out site of fistula.

Complications of CSF rhinorrhea:
- Meningitis
- Tension pneumocephalous

CONCLUSION

1. Categorize leaks
2. Beta-transferrin assay and several CSF tracer studies available, but have limitations
3. High-resolution CT provides detailed information about the bony skull-base anatomy
4. MRI assesses soft tissue issues, including unrecognized tumors and coincidental meningoencephaloceles
5. Many CSF leaks respond to conservative management (observation plus measures to minimize ICP)
6. Traumatic CSF rhinorrhea tends to resolve with conservative measures alone
7. Nontraumatic CSF rhinorrhea require operative repair
8. Extracranial techniques are first line for CSF rhinorrhea.

Maxillofacial Trauma: Case Presentation

15

CASE NUMBER 1

A 20-year-male patient complains of headache, inability to close his teeth and pain in front of ear on right side since 1 day.

History of Presenting Illness

- Gives history of fall from bike while driving yesterday near Someshwara and sustained injuries and contusion over lower jaw region
- Patient was conscious whole time and gives no history of any vomiting or ENT bleeding following accident
- Gives history of bleeding from chin laceration and mouth
- Patient was drowsy and was taken to nearby hospital where primary treatment was given. Patient had one episode of seizure and 3 episodes of vomiting following which CT scan of head was done which showed cerebral edema along with fracture of mandible at parasymphysis region on left side and condyle on right side
- Patient got discharge and came to hospital.

Past Medical History

No history of hypertension, diabetes mellitus, epilepsy, asthma.

Drug History

Patient not on any medication, and does not give history of allergy to any drug.

Personal History

- Sleep normal, bowel and bladder habits normal
- No history of substance abuse.

Clinical Examination

Systemic Examination

- Patient conscious, cooperative
- Pupils bilateral equal in size and reacting to light.

Vitals

- BP—132/82 mm Hg
- Pulse—74 b/min, regular
- RR—22 cycles/min.

CNS

- Cranial nerves—normal
- GCS—15/15; E4,M6,V5
- Pupils—bilateral equal and reactive
- No motor or neurosensory deficit noted
- No cerebellar signs noted

CVS—S1 and S2 heard
RS—bilateral equal air entry
Per abdomen—NAD.

Head and Neck Examination

Face

- Facial asymmetry noted, chin deviated to left side, and mild edema noted over right pre-auricular area
- A single laceration of about 2/0.5 cm size present over chin area not involving deep muscles (Fig. 15.1)

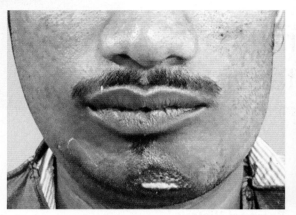

Fig. 15.1: Chin soft tissue injury

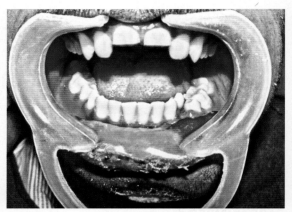

Fig. 15.2: Intraoral soft tissue injuries and disturbed occlusion

- On palpation lower border continuity present in left premolar region with a distinct step palpable
- Bony crepitus felt over right TMJ area, condyle could not be palpated on right side, tenderness present over right preauricular area.

Eyes

No abnormality detected.

Nose

No abnormality detected.

Ears

No abnormality detected.

Inspection

- Mouth opening restricted – 25 mm
- Deviation present on mouth opening towards right side.

Palpation

Tenderness severe in nature on right preauricular region.

Intraoral

- Deranged occlusion
- Arch form disrupted between 34 and 35 with displacement of anterior arch segment lingually (Fig. 15.2).

CASE NUMBER 2

A 24-year male patient with alleged RTA following which he sustained injury to the face:
- Patient was pillion rider and was under the influence of alcohol
- Ellis class 3 fracture of 11 and 21
- Overriding of fracture segments noted
- Ecchymosis present in left vestibule involving lower lip mucosa on left side (Fig. 15.3).

Radiographic Findings

- OPG suggestive of displaced condylar head fracture on right side and left body fracture (Fig. 15.4)
- No history of loss of consciousness
- History of giddiness for 2–4 minutes
- No history of vomiting/seizures
- History of bleeding from both ears
- Unable to open the jaw and bite properly
  Medical history: No relevant history.

General Examination

Conscious and oriented
    GCS – 15/15
    Vitals – BP – 140/100 mm Hg
          Pulse – 78/min
          Respiratory rate – 24/min
    CVS – NAD

CNS – NAD
RS – NAD

Local examination

Inspection
E/O
On examination facial asymmetry with swelling on right side of the face, bleeding from both ears (Fig. 15.5)

Difficulty in opening the mouth deviation of jaw to right side (Fig. 15.6)

I/O
- Deranged occlusion (Fig. 15.7)

- Posterior open bite present
- Sublingual ecchymosis present (Fig. 15.3).

Palpation
E/O: Depression present in right condylar fossa
   Bony crepitation present
      TMJ tenderness present
I/O: No dentoalveolar fracture
      No step deformity present

Investigations
PA Cephalometric (Open Mouth)
Medially displaced right condylar fracture (Fig. 15.8).

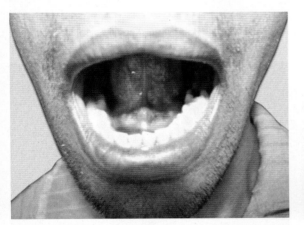

Fig. 15.3: Intraoral photograph showing mild sublingual ecchymosis

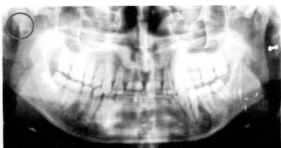

Fig. 15.4: OPG showing fracture: Right condyl and left parasymphysis

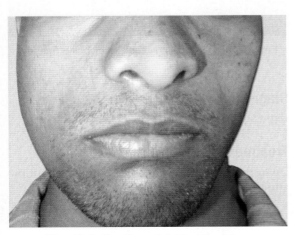

Fig. 15.5: Swelling of right side of face

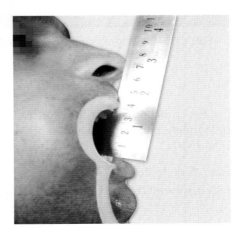

Fig. 15.6: Reduced mouth opening

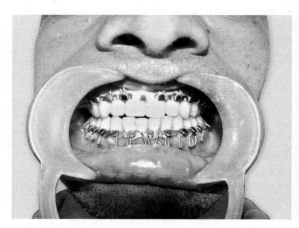

Fig. 15.7: Preoperative stabilization

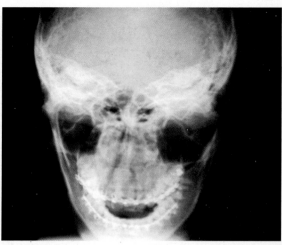

Fig. 15.8: PA skull showing medially displaced condyle

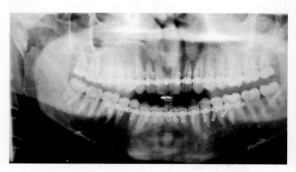

Fig. 15.9: OPG showing right parasymphysis and condylar fracture

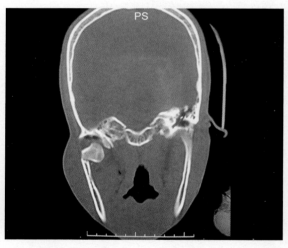

Fig. 15.10: CT showing medially displaced condyl

OPG

OPG shows subcondylar fracture on right side and incomplete parasymphysis fracture on right side (Fig. 15.9).

CT Scan (Fig. 15.10)

Medially displaced right subcondylar fracture.

Diagnosis

Right subcondylar fracture.

Treatment

Open reduction internal fixation through submandibular approach (Figs 15.11 and 15.12).

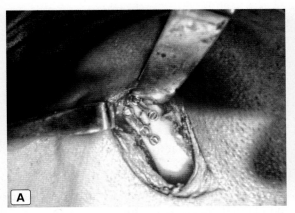

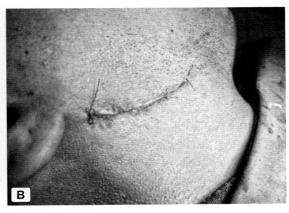

Figs 15.11A and B: (A) Intraoperative open reduction; (B) Intraoperative after closure

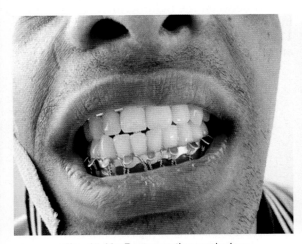

Fig. 15.12: Postoperative occlusion

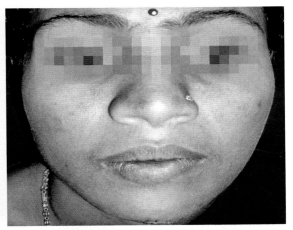

Fig. 15.13: Extraoral photograph

CASE NUMBER 3

A 20 years female patient complains of pain over the right side of the face while opening the mouth since 1 week.

- History of trauma to the symphysis region 1 week back-fall from the table
- Patient was unconsciousness for 15 minutes following the trauma
- History of giddiness for 2–4 minutes
- No history of vomiting/seizures
- History of bleeding from both ears
- Unable to open the jaw and bite properly.

Medical History

No relevant history.

Extraoral Examination (Fig. 15.13)

- Face—Asymmetry was noted due to the swelling on the right side of face
- Nose, eyes—Normal
- Lip—Competent and laceration was noted on the lower lip
- Lymph nodes—Bilateral submandibular lymph nodes were palpable.
  One in number

Nontender

Soft-in consistency

- Mouth opening was reduced.

Local Examination

Inspection

E/O: Facial asymmetry present

Swelling on right side of face

Trismus present

Deviation of jaw to right side

A 4 cm laceration which had been sutured was seen over skin.

I/O: Deranged occlusion (Fig. 15.14)

Posterior open bite present.

Palpation

E/O: Depression present in right condylar fossa.

Bony crepitation present.

TMJ tenderness present.

Muscles of mastication was tender on palpation.

I/O: Ellis class II facture of 11.

Ellis class I fracture of 21.

Ellis class III fracture of 22.

Radiographs

Diagnosis

Bilateral subcondylar fracture (Fig. 15.15).

Treatment Given

Erich arch bar placement for maxillary and mandibular arch (Fig. 15.16).

Small piece of impression compound was placed between the right occlusal surface of the molar and premolar, red elastics was placed. After 12 hours, the impression compound was removed and occlusion was achieved (Fig. 15.17).

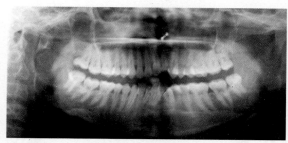

Fig. 15.15: OPG shows bilateral subcondylar fracture – Radiolucent line running through left subcondylar region and the fractured segment is displaced on the right side

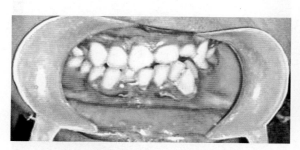

Fig. 15.14: Preoperative occlusion

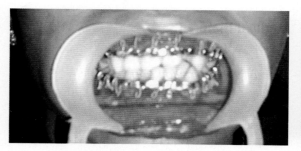

Fig. 15.16: Postoperative photograph

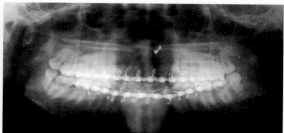

Fig. 15.17: Postoperative radiograph following conservative management

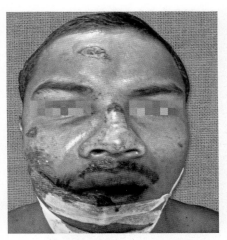

Fig. 15.18: Extraoral photographs

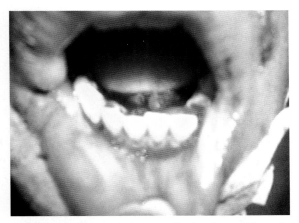

Fig. 15.19: Intraoral photograph showing sublingual ecchymosis

CASE NUMBER 4

A 25-year-male patient complains of laceration and abrasion of the face and inability to open the mouth and bleeding from the oral cavity (Fig. 15.18).

History of Presenting Illness

- Patient complains of alleged RTA and sustained injury to the face and the lower jaw
- No history of loss of consciousness, vomiting, seizures, bleed from the nose
- History of alcohol intoxication
- Patient was conscious, well-oriented to time place

Medical history—Nothing significant

Drug allergy—No history of drug allergy.

General Physical Examination

- GCS – 15/15
- VITALS
  - BP – 150/90 mm Hg
  - Pulse – 88/min
- CVS, CNS, RS – NAD
- Pupils bilaterally reacting to light
- Extraocular muscles – NAD

Extraoral Examination

Inspection

- Abrasion 2.5 cm × 2.5 cm present over the right forehead region, 2.5 cm × 1.5 cm over the bridge of the nose, 1.5 cm over the right philtrum region and over the skin of right zygomatic region (Fig 15.18)
- Laceration about 2.5 cm present at right side angle of the mouth on the lower lip (Fig. 15.19)
- A 3.5 cm laceration present over the skin over submental region with active bleeding
- Slight edema noticed over the lower half of the face.

Palpation

- Step deformity present bilaterally in the left and right parasymphysis region
- No palpable step noticed in the maxilla, zygomatic complex region.

Intraoral Examination

Inspection

- Trismus present
- Mouth opening decreased to 1½
- Tenderness while opening the mouth
- Occlusion was deranged
- Sublingual ecchymosis present
- Totally avulsed tooth interim restorative treatment (IRT) 33 and partially avulsed tooth IRT 43.

Palpation

Step deformity in the right and left parasymphysis region at the region of 33 and 43.

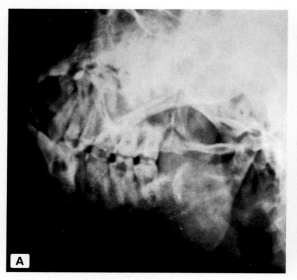

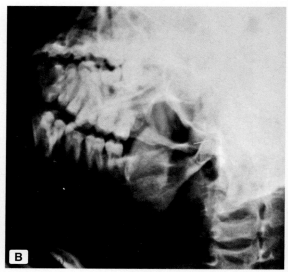

Figs 15.20A and B: Both the left and right lateral oblique views did not show any signs of condylar fracture

Provisional Diagnosis

- Bilateral fracture of parasymphysis region
- Bilateral subcondylar fracture—No (Figs 15.20A and B).

Investigations

Diagnosis

Bilateral parasymphysis fracture at the region of 23 and 32 (Fig. 15.21)

Treatment Plan

- Intermaxillary fixation using Erichs arch bar
- Open reduction and internal fixation.

Intraoperative (Figs 15.22 and 15.23)

- Skin prepared with povidone iodine
- Extraoral submandibular incision placed, incision extended over the lacerated wound
- Bilaterally fracture site identified and fracture site reduced after securing IMF intraorally
- Two 4 hole plate with gap placed over the lower border of mandible. 8 mm screw fixed bilaterally
- Two 2 hole with gap plate fixed above the 4 hole plate and fixed with 6 mm screws
- Muscle closed with 3-0 vicryl. Skin closed with 3-0 Ethilon, subcuticular suture

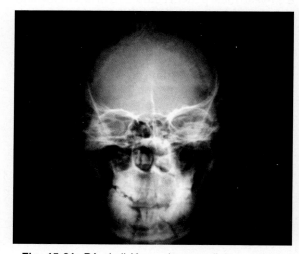

Fig. 15.21: PA skull X-ray shows radiolucent lines running bilaterally at the parasymphysis region

- Dynaplast pressure dressing placed.

CASE NUMBER 5 (FIGS 15.24 TO 15.27)

Diagnosis

Displaced fracture of condylar head fracture on right side and mandibular body on left side.

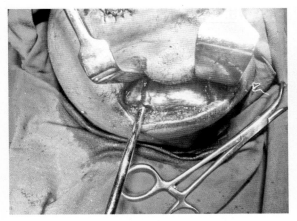

Fig. 15.22: Intraoperative fracture site exposure

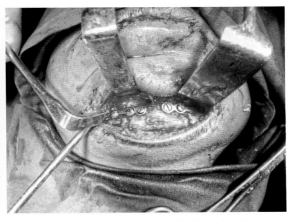

Fig. 15.23: Intraopertive miniplate fixation

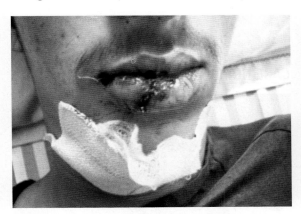

Fig. 15.24: Extraoral photograph

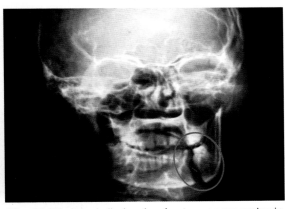

Fig. 15.25: PA skull showing fracture parasymphysis left side, and right condylar head fracture

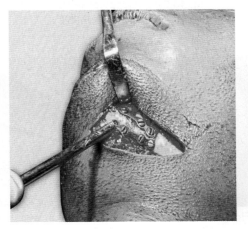

Fig. 15.26: Intraoperative miniplate fixation

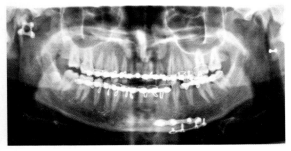

Fig. 15.27: Postoperative radiograph showing traphezoidal plate for condylar fracture

Treatment Plan

Open reduction and internal fixation of right condylar head fracture with titanium TCP plates and of left side body with conventional titanium miniplates.

CASE NUMBER 6 (FIGS 15.28 AND 15.29)

Diagnosis

Malunited coronoid fracture of left side.

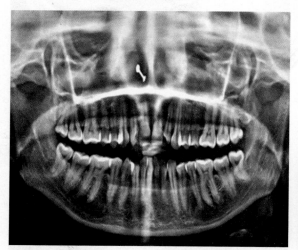

Fig. 15.28: OPG showing left coronoid fracture

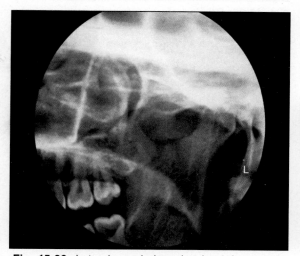

Fig. 15.29: Lateral ramal view showing left coronoid fracture (L)

CASE NUMBER 7 (FIG. 15.30)

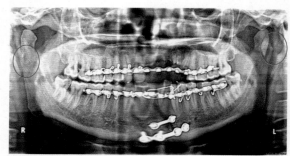

Fig. 15.30: OPG showing bicondylar with parasymphysis fracture

CASE NUMBER 8 (FIGS 15.31 AND 15.32)

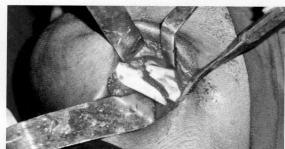

Fig. 15.31: Intraoperative fracture of parasymphysis region

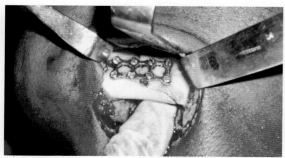

Fig. 15.32: Open reduction and fixation with locking plate and screw

CASE NUMBER 9 (FIGS 15.33 TO 15.35)

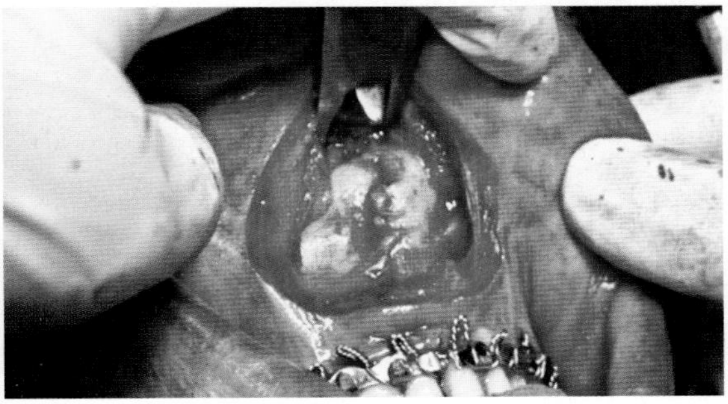

CASE NUMBER 10 (FIGS 15.36 TO 15.38)

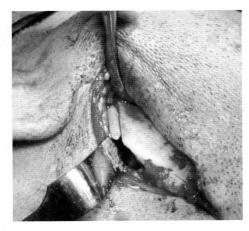

Fig. 15.33: Intraoperative fracture of symphysis

Fig. 15.36: Intraoperative showing mandibular angle fracture

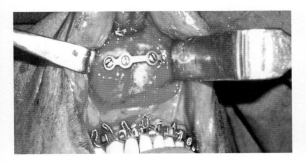

Fig. 15.34: Intraoperative 4 hole locking plate

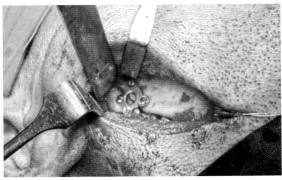

Fig. 15.37: Intraoperative showing angle fracture reduction and fixation with 3D mini plate (*Curtesy:* Dr Muralee)

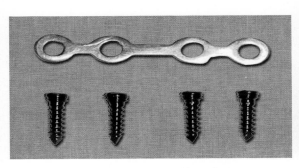

Fig. 15.35: 4 hole locking plate

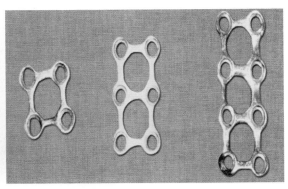

Fig. 15.38: 3D mini palte

CASE NUMBER 9 (FIGS 15.33 TO 15.35)

CASE NUMBER 10 (FIGS 15.36 TO 15.39)

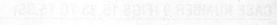

Fig. 15.32: Intraoperative fixation of symphysis

Fig. 15.36: Preoperative alveolar mandibular angle fracture

Fig. 15.34: Intraoperative of the occlusal plate

Fig. 15.37: Intraoperative showing angle fracture reduction and fixation with 2.0 mm plate (Champy's) (N Mathod)

Fig. 15.35: A lower 15.5 mm plate

Fig. 15.38: 2.0 mm plate

Section

3

Carcinomas of Oral Cavity

Examination of an Ulcer

16

INTRODUCTION

An ulcer is a localized defect in the continuity of an epithelial surface. It is usually associated with an inflamed base of granulation tissue with or without necrotic slough. The majority is chronically inflamed; the slough at their base represents inadequate drainage. Acutely inflamed ulcers may have an outer rim of cellulitis. Weak ulcers are those with low quality granulation tissue and hence delayed healing; they are usually due to ischemia or infections such as tuberculosis ulcers.

The incidence and prevalence varies across the world.

DEFINITION

An ulcer is a break in the continuity of the covering epithelium, either skin or mucous membrane due to molecular death of cells.

What causes oral ulcers? Oral ulcers may have a great many causes, Although in some no cause is identified oral ulcers (Fig. 16.1) are termed 'acute' if they persists for less than three weeks duration, and 'chronic' if they persists for longer than three weeks

PARTS OF AN ULCER

Margin

It may be described as area between the edge and the normal surrounding tissue.

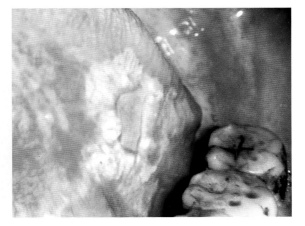

Fig. 16.1: Ulcer on lateral surface of tongue

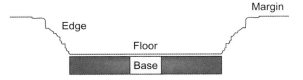

Edge

Lies between the floor and the margin.

Different Types of Edges

Sloping edge
- Seen in a healing ulcer
- Inner part is red due to granulation tissue
- Middle part is white due to scar/fibrous tissue

- Outer most part has a bluish tinge due to a thin layer of epithelial proliferation.

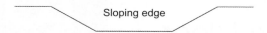

Sloping edge

Undermined edge
Characteristic of a tuberculous ulcer. Disease process advances in a deeper plane (in the subcutaneous tissue). Also seen in bedsore, carbuncle, meleney's ulcer, tropical ulcer.

Undermined edge

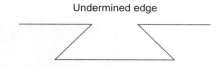

Punched out edges
Seen in gummatous, trophic ulcer, occurs due to end arteritis with rapid destruction of full thickness of the skin.

Punched out edge

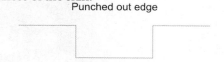

Raised and beaded edges (with a pearly white color)
- Is seen in a rodent ulcer (Basal cell carcinoma)
- Occurs due to a slow growth of tissue at the edge of the ulcer.

Raised and beaded

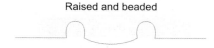

Everted Edges (Rolled out Edges)
Seen in carcinomatous ulcer due to excessive proliferation of malignant cells over the normal skin.

Floor

It is the one that is seen. Floor may contain discharge, granulation tissue.
- Wash-leather appearance is seen in syphilitic ulcers

- Bluish unhealthy granulation tissue seen in tuberculosis ulcers
- No granulation tissue is often present in ischemic ulcers—in this case structures such as tendons may lie bear in the base of the ulcer
- Solid brown or gray dead tissue suggests full-thickness skin death
- The redness of the granulation tissue is proportional to the underlying vascularity of the ulcer site (and therefore of the ulcer's ability to heal).

Base

Is the one on which the floor rests. It may be bone, or soft tissue.

Depth

Is defined height: in millimeters
Anatomically: which structures are visible.

Relations

It is important to define the relation of the ulcer with surrounding structures, especially those deep to it. The examiner must try to ascertain whether the ulcer is adherent to deep structures.

Local Lymph Nodes

Check for
- Enlargement
- Tenderness.

State of the local tissues to be assessed
Local blood supply
Local nerve supply
For evidence of previously healed ulcers

CLASSIFICATION

Clinical

- *Spreading ulcer*: Here the edge is inflamed and edematous
- *Healing ulcer*: Edge is sloping with healthy pink/red granulation tissue with serous discharge

- *Callous ulcer*: Floor contains pale, unhealthy granulation tissue.

Pathological

- Specific ulcers
- Malignant ulcer
- Nonspecific ulcer.

HISTORY

A detailed history is an essential component of the diagnosis.
- Mode of onset
- Duration
- Pain
- Discharge
- Associated disease
- Age of the patient

Protocol for description of the ulcer
Position
Color
Tenderness
Temperature
Shape
Size
Specific to the ulcer:
• Base
• Edge
• Depth
• Discharge
• Relationship to other structures
• Lymph nodes

DIFFERENTIAL DIAGNOSIS

Traumatic Ulcer

- Sharp edge of a fractured tooth
- Over extended denture
- Thermal and chemical burns
- Iatrogenic—including radiotherapy/chemo-therapy.

Infective Ulcer

- Bacterial (TB, ANUG, syphilis)
- Viral (HSV, HZ, CMV, HIV, HHV8, coxsackie),
- Fungal (histoplasmosis, mucormycosis, cryp-tococosis, blastomycosis, candidiasis).

Neoplastic Ulcers

- Squamous cell carcinoma
- Kaposi's sarcoma
- Non-Hodgkin's lymphoma
- Malignant melanoma
- Malignant salivary gland tumors.

Systemic Ulcers

- Mucous membrane pemphigoid
- Pemphigus
- Erythema multiforme
- Lichen planus
- SLE
- Gastrointestinal disorders (Crohn's disease, ulcerative colitis)
- Hematological disorders (anemias, neutrope-nias, and leukemia)
- Radiation-induced necrotic ulcer (Fig. 16.2).

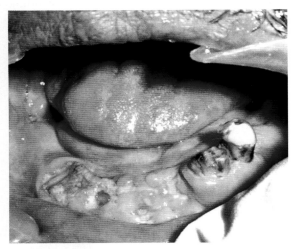

Fig. 16.2: Necrotic ulcer postradiotherapy

Miscellaneous

- Bechet's syndrome
- Necrotizing sialometaplasia
- Recurrent aphthous stomatitis (Fig. 16.3)
- Drug-induced, e.g. gold injections for rheumatoid arthritis.

CAUSES OF ORAL ULCERS

Traumatic

Ill fitting dentures, poorly finished restorations and rough edges to teeth may all cause oral ulcers.

Chemical and Temperature

Can lead to burn ulcers; aspirin and eugenol are known to produce ulcers. Thermal burns and cryotherapy have similar effects.

Recurrent Oral Ulceration (Fig. 16.3)

- Most recurrent oral ulceration (ROU) is of unknown etiology but in a few people there appears to be a related hematological disorder. This is ill defined, however, and causal relationships are difficult to establish
- ROU includes anemia, cyclic neutropenia, suggested haematinic deficiencies including iron, zinc, folate and vitamin B_{12}

- Other factors important in the assessment of the patient include lifestyle factors and stress, smoking, the relationship with food and the relationship with the menstrual cycle
- Evidence of immunodeficiency and granulocytopenia, is important as is family history. There are suggested HLA associations including HLA-A2, B_{12}, and Aw-29.

Neoplastic (Figs 16.4 to 16.6)

Oral squamous cell carcinoma often presents as an ulcer with a deep indurated crater and sometimes with associated cervical lymphadenopathy. The variant leukemia, mycosis fungoides infiltrates submucosally and may cause epithelial ulceration.

Connective Tissue Disease

- Systemic lupus erythematosus and rheumatoid arthritis may have oral ulcers as part of the symptom complex
- Bechet's syndrome has four described clinical subtypes; mucocutaneous, arthritic, neurological and ocular. Oral ulceration is typically part of the mucocutaneous syndrome but may occur in any of the other variants. Bechet's syndrome is rare and affects males more frequently than females in a ratio of about 3:1. The diagnosis requires oral ulceration and at least two other lesions.

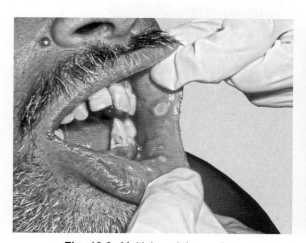

Fig. 16.3: Multiple aphthous ulcer

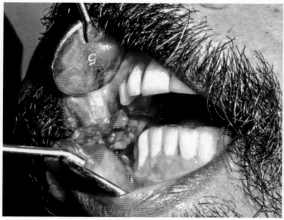

Fig. 16.4: Carcinomatous ulcer

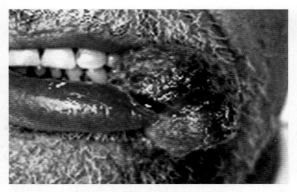

Fig. 16.5: Carcinomatous ulcer

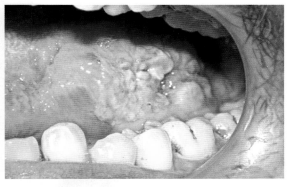

Fig. 16.6: Carcinomatous ulcer

Iatrogenic

- Lasers, cryotherapy, diathermy, topical agents such as eugenol and drugs such as aspirin may all cause accidental oral mucosal breach, subsequent ulceration and inflammation
- Nonsteroidal anti-inflammatory agents (NSAID) and cytotoxic drug therapy are potentially complicated by oral ulceration
- Lichenoid reactions to antihypertensives and gold injections are also described
- Radiotherapy related mucositis and ulceration is well documented.

Factitious

Occasionally, patients present with ulcers that defy diagnosis and by a process of careful exclusion, self inflicted ulceration may be diagnosed.

BIOPSY

Definition of Biopsy

Removal of tissue from a living individual for diagnostic examination.

Indications for Biopsy

- Any lesion that persists for more than 2 weeks with no apparent etiologic basis
- Any inflammatory lesion that does not respond to local treatment after 10–14 days

- Persistent hyperkeratotic changes in surface tissues
- Any persistent tumescence, either visible or palpable beneath relatively normal tissue
- Inflammatory changes of unknown cause that persist for long periods
- Lesion that interfere with local function
- Bone lesions not specifically identified by clinical and radiographic findings
- Any lesion that has the characteristics of malignancy.

Characteristics of Lesions that Raise the Suspicion of Malignancy

- *Erythroplasia*—lesion is totally red or has speckled red appearance
- *Ulceration*—lesion is ulcerated or presents as an ulcer
- *Duration*—lesion has persisted more than 2 weeks
- *Growth rate*—lesion exhibits rapid growth
- *Bleeding*—lesion bleeds on gentle manipulation
- *Induration*—lesion and surrounding tissue is firm to the touch
- *Fixation*—lesion feels attached to adjacent structures.

Principles and Techniques of Biopsy

- It is important to develop a systematic approach in evaluating a patient with a lesion in the oral and maxillofacial region (Figs 16.7 to 16.10).

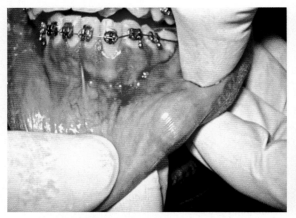

Fig. 16.7: Excisional biopsy step I

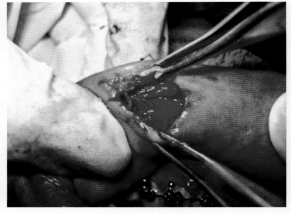

Fig. 16.8: Excisional biopsy step II

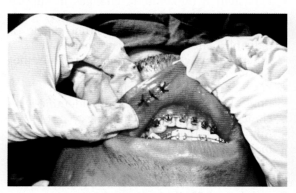

Fig. 16.9: Excisional biopsy step III

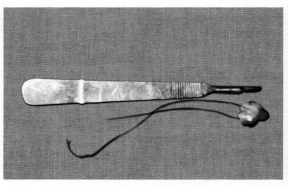

Fig. 16.10: Excised specimen

- These steps include:
  - A detailed health history
  - A history of the specific lesion
  - A clinical examination
  - A radiographic examination
  - Laboratory investigations
  - Surgical specimens for histopathologic evaluation (Figs 16.10 to 16.12).

Health History

- An accurate health history may disclose predisposing factors in the disease process or factors that affect the patients management

- Up to 90 percent of systemic diseases can be discovered through history taking
- The same can be true of oral lesions when one is familiar with the natural progression of the more common disease processes.

Medical Conditions that Warrant Special Care

- Congenital heart defects
- Coagulopathies
- Hypertension
- Poorly controlled diabetics
- Immunocompromised patients.

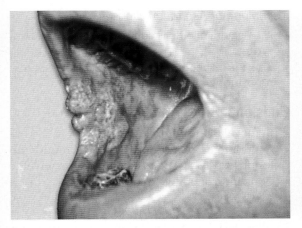

Fig. 16.11: Lesion indicated for incisional biopsy

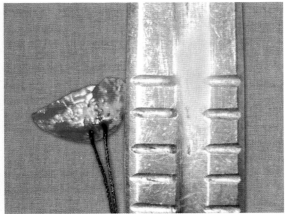

Fig. 16.12: Excised portion of the lesion

Historical Reasons for the Lesions

- Trauma to the area
- Recent toothache
- Habits.

Clinical Examination

The clinical examination should always include when possible:

- Inspection
- Palpation
- Percussion
- Auscultation.

Clinical Evaluation

- The anatomic location of the lesion/mass
- The physical character of the lesion/mass
- The size and shape of the lesion/mass
- Single versus multiple lesions
- The surface of the lesion
- The color of the lesion
- The sharpness of the boundaries of the lesion
- The consistency of the lesion to palpation
- Presence of pulsation
- Lymph node examination.

Radiographic Examination

- The radiographic appearance may provide clues that will help determine the nature of the lesion

- A radiolucency with sharp borders will often be a cyst
- A ragged radiolucency will often be a more aggressive lesion
- Radiopaque dyes and instruments can help differentiate normal anatomy.

Laboratory Investigation

- Oral lesions may be manifestations of systemic disease
- If a systemic disease is suspected it should be pursued.

Types of biopsy
Oral cytology
Aspiration biopsy
Incisional biopsy
Excisional biopsy
Needle biopsy

Oral Cytology

- Developed as a diagnostic screening procedure to monitor large tissue areas for dysplastic changes
- Most frequently used to screen for uterine cervix malignancy

- May be helpful with monitoring postradiation changes, herpes, pemphigus
- The disadvantage of oral cytological procedures include:
  - Not very reliable with many false positives
  - Expertise in oral cytology is not widely available
  - The lesion is repeatedly scraped with a moistened tongue depressor or spatula type instrument. The cells obtained are smeared on a glass slide and immediately fixed with a fixative spray or solution.

Aspiration Biopsy

Aspiration biopsy is the use of a needle and syringe to penetrate a lesion for aspiration of its content (Fig. 16.13).

Indication of Aspiration Biopsy

- Aspiration should be carried out on all lesions thought to contain fluid or any intraosseous lesion before surgical exploration a fluctuant mass in the soft tissues should also be aspirated to determine its contents
- Any radiolucency in the bone of the jaw should be aspirated to rule out a vascular lesion that can cause life threatening hemorrhage.

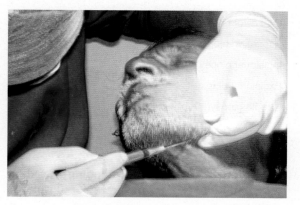

Fig. 16.13: FNAC procedure

Technique of Aspiration Biopsy

- A 18-gauge needle is connected to a 5 or 10 mL syringe
- The tip of needle may have to be repeatedly repositioned to locate a fluid center.

Excisional Biopsy

- Removal of the entire lesion
- A perimeter of normal tissue surround the lesion is also excised to ensure total removal
- Constitute definitive treatment.

Indication of Excisional Biopsy

Smaller lesions(<1 cm in diameter) that, on clinical examination, appear to be benign.

Principle of Excisional Biopsy

The entire lesion, along with 2–3 mm of normal appearing surrounding tissue, is excised.

Incisional Biopsy

- Samples only a particular or representative part of the lesion
- Lesion is large
- Lesion has different characteristics at different location.

Indication of Incisional Biopsy

- Extensive size (>1 cm in diameter)
- Hazardous location
- A great suspicious of malignancy.

Principles of Incisional Biopsy

- Representative areas of lesion should be incised in wedge fashion
- Selected in an area that shows complete tissue changes (the lesion extends into normal tissue at the base and/or margin of the lesion)
- Necrotic tissue should be avoided
- Taken from the edge of the lesion to include some normal tissue
- A deep, narrow biopsy rather than a broad, shallow one.

Anesthesia

- Block local anesthesia techniques are employed when possible
- The anesthesic solution should not be injected within the tissue to be removed, because it can cause artificial distortion of the specimen
- When blocks are not possible, infiltration of local anesthesia may be used locally, but the solution should be injected at least 1 cm away from the lesion.

Tissue Stabilization

- Tongue or soft palate
  - Heavy retractive sutures
  - Towel clips.
- Lip
  - Assistant's finger pinching the lip on both sides of the biopsy area.

Identification of Surgical Margins

- Marked with a silk suture to orient the specimen for the pathologist
- If the lesion is diagnosed as requiring additional treatment, the pathologist can determine which margin, if any had residual lesion
- Identification of surgical margins
- One must be certain to illustrate the orientation of the lesion and the method with which the specimen was marked in the pathology data sheet.

Hemostasis

- Avoid suction device
- Gauze wrapped over the tip of the low volume suction device
- Simple gauze compression.

Specimen Care

- Immediately placed in 10 percent formalin solution that is at least 20 times the volume of surgical specimen
- Totally immersed in the solution

- Care should be taken to be sure that the tissue has not become lodged on the wall of the container above the level of the formalin.

Surgical Closure

- Primary closure of the elliptic wound is usually possible
- *Palatal biopsy*: Best managed postoperatively with the use of an acrylic splint
- *Dorsum or lateral border of the tongue*: Sutures to be placed deeply and at frequent intervals into the substance of the tongue to retain closure.

INTRAOSSEOUS OR HARD TISSUE BIOPSY TECHNIQUE AND SURGICAL PRINCIPLES

Aspiration Biopsy of Radiolucent Lesion

- Any radiolucent lesion that requires biopsy should undergo aspiration biopsy before surgical exploration, which provides valuable diagnostic information regading the nature of the lesion
- Brisk, pulsating—vascular lesion
- Straw colored fluid—cyst
- Air—maxillary sinus.

Mucoperiosteal Flaps

- Most hard tissue lesions approached
- Through mucoperiosteal flaps
- Full thickness flaps, incision through mucosa, submucosa and periosteum
- Dissection to expose bone is done sub periosteally.

Osseous Window

Lesions within jaws (central lesions) require the use of cortical window.

Removal of Specimen

Most small lesions that have a connective tissue capsule can be removed with their entiret.

17

Cancer Biology

INTRODUCTION

Cancers are caused by abnormalities in the genetic material of the transformed cells. These abnormalities may be due to the effects of carcinogens, such as tobacco smoke, radiation, chemicals, or infectious agents. Abnormalities found in cancer affect two general classes of genes, cancer-promoting oncogenes and tumor suppressor genes. The heritability of cancers is usually affected by complex interactions between carcinogens and the host's genome. In addition, histologic grading, the presence of specific molecular markers can also be useful in establishing prognosis, as well as in determining individual treatments.

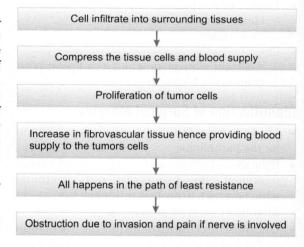

MODES OF TUMOR SPREAD

- Local infiltration
- Lymphatics
- Bloodstream
- Along the natural passages
- Through serous cavities
- By inoculation
- Perineural spread.

Local Infiltration

Local Infiltration in Soft Tissues is by Centrifugal Manner

- Microscopically connective tissue then muscle break-up and destroy and ultimately replace the tissue involved. Also added factor which destroy muscle is *local inflammatory reaction* sometimes with marked lymphocytic infiltration, e.g. malignant melanoma.
- Local *fibrotic* response that is a stromal reaction induration and loss of mobility
- Bone involvement shows *endosteal reactive bone formation* characterized by lymphocytic and macrophages and osteoclastic infiltration (moth-eaten appearance)
- Marrow fibrosis, fatty hematopoietic marrow replaced by loose connective tissue,
- In older mandible there may be avascular necrosis (atheroma of IA artery).

Spread by Natural Passages

- In this tumor cells are implanted in epithelial surface and forms new growth
- For example, bronchus, bowel, ureter, also upper lip to lower lip.

Spread through Serous Cavities

Transcelomic spread passive transfer in cranial cavity (malignant glial tumor cells shed into ventricals and sub arachnoid space throughout CSF).

Implantation/Inoculation

In course of the operation in surrounding tissues.

Spread by Lymphatics

Wall of lymphatic vessel is breached.

Lymphatic Permeation

Lymph vessel lamina, cancer cell grow within vessel to reach regional lymph nodes.

Embolic Spread through Lymphatics

- Cancer cells form emboli that is carried along with lymph to reach regional lymph nodes
- Remain attached to the site and obstruct lumen
- May extend up to draining lymph node
- Spread along the whole group.

Growth of Cancer Cell in Lymph Nodes

Distribution of metastasis
- Tongue has rich pattern of lymph vessels also lymph flow is increased by muscular activity
- Hard palate has relatively less lymph vessels and absence of mobility hence low nodal metastasis
- Towards front of the mouth sub mandibular lymph nodes involve first
- Back in the mouth spread is straight to deep jugular chain, usually first to jugulo-digastric
- Nodes of posterior triangle are almost never involved in primary intraoral tumor
- Deep jugular chain mediastinal lymph nodes
- Internal jugular vein is in intimate contact with the nodes than the carotids and it becomes involved first by local infiltration, fixation and ultimate invasion of its lumen by tumor.

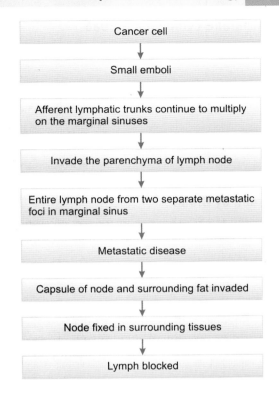

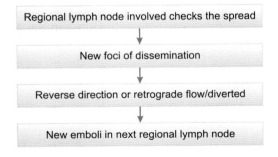

The Dissemination of Cancer from Metastasis

Examples
- Carcinomas of glandular epithelium metastasize through both lymphatics and blood stream.
- Carcinomas of breast metastasize early by lymphatics and late by blood stream.
- Epitheliomas of skin and oral mucosa spread through lymphatics.

Retrograde Lymphatic Spread

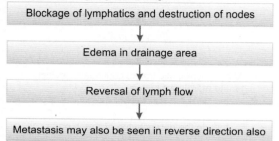

Blockage of lymphatics and destruction of nodes

↓

Edema in drainage area

↓

Reversal of lymph flow

↓

Metastasis may also be seen in reverse direction also

Spread by Blood

- Willis (1930) showed incidence of systemic metastasis is not dependent on blood supply.
  - Liver 41 percent
  - Lung 30 percent
  - Skeletal muscles 1 percent
- Spread to blood from
  - Jugular chain via thoracic duct
  - Direct invasion of blood vessel.
- Veins are invaded more than arteries because they are thin walled.
- Invasion of tumors of the major veins of the neck in systemic metastasis.
- Thrombus formation in vessels for the nutrients for the tumor cells.
- Extravasation mechanically block the channels attach to vascular endothelium survival and growth of metastatic deposits depends on PDGF, FGF, TGF-β, VEGF factors.

Differences in Lymphatics and Hematogenous Spread

Lymphatics spread	Hematogenous spread
Carcinomas more common because epithelial cells are larger	Sarcomas more common because close proximity to blood vessels
Detected early	Detected late
Less serious and localized	More serious as it involves multiple organs
Excision offers good prognosis	Poor prognosis

Retrograde Venous Spread

Due to peculiarities in blood flow on vertebral venous plexus cancer in which pressure variation in the thorax and abdomen cause temporary reversal of blood flow.

Examples
- Vertebral metastasis of thyroid carcinoma.
- Carcinoma of nasopharynx from spine to base of skull
- Carcinoma prostate spine and pelvic bones.

Perineural Spread

Sometimes tumor spread along the perineural space. Involved nerves are greater palatine and inferior alveolar nerve in oral carcionomas and also minor salivary gland tumors like adenoid cystic carcinoma.

PROCESS OF BONE METASTASIS

The spread of malignant neoplasms to bone is not a random process but rather a cascade of specific molecular events orchestrated through complex interactions between neoplastic cells and their environment. Certain malignancies exhibit osteotropism or anextraordinary affinity to target and proliferate in bone.

The cascade of events (bone metastasis)
Tumor cell detachment
Tumor cell motility
Interaction with the extracellular matrix
Interaction with endothelium
Direct effect on bone
Osteolitic metastasis
Osteoblastic metastasis

The primary sites of metastatic deposits to jaw bones in females is the breast followed by the adrenals, colorectum, female genital organs and thyroid. For males it is the lung, followed by the prostate, kidney, bone, and adrenals. Blood flow has traditionally been accepted as the only determinant of the site of a metastasic deposit, solid tumors metastasize most frequently to the vascular areas of the skeleton, and especially red bone marrow site.

BIOLOGY OF INVASION AND METASTASIS

Clonal Evolution Theory

- Nowell (1976) proposed clonal evolution theory
- This model is built on theory of natural selection and posits of cancer cells to develop strategies to survive hostile environment (tissue barriers, immune response, programmed cell death) and use host resource (e.g. oxygen and nutrients) to grow and proliferate
- Carcinogens bring about change usually at genetic or epigenetic level.

Molecular Progression Model

- Van der Riet and coworkers proposed Molecular Progression Model
- It is the accumulation of genetic events and not the specific ordering of events that appears to be associated with phenotypic progression.

Field Carcinogenesis

Slaughter (1953) hypothesized that because of constant carcinogenic pressure the multiple genetic events occurred through out the involved mucosa, allowing the development of multiple molecularly distinct lesions.

Competing Theory

It states that rather than several molecularly distinct lesions that arise independently, a single group of molecularly similar transformed progenitor cells migrates to distant sites, thus explaining the appearance of multiple primary lesions, second primary lesions and recurrent lesions.

Genetic Basis for Cancer

Genes have been classified as
Oncogenes, e.g. RAS genes
Tumor-suppressor genes, e.g. RB gene, TP53 gene
Various genes for tumor progression (angiogenesis, apoptosis, invasion, and metastases)

Oncogenesis

After the initial neoplastic transformation tumor cells under go progressive proliferation that is accompanied by further genetic changes and development of heterogeneous tumor cell population with varying degree of metastatic potential.

Angiogenic Switch

As the tumor grows the central tumor becomes more hypoxic and the tumor initiates the recruits its own blood supply which involves secretion of various angiogenic factors and removal of angiogenesis inhibitors.

Clonal Dominance and Invasive Phenotype

- Continued genetic alterations in tumor cell population results in selection of tumor cell clones with distinct growth advantage and acquisition of an invasive phenotype.
- Invasive tumor cells down regulate cell to cell adhesion, alter their attachment to extra cellular matrix by changing integrin expression profiles and proteolytically alter the matrix. These changes result in enhanced cell motility and the ability of the cells to separate from the primary tumor mass.

Survival in the Circulation

Once the tumor cells and tumor cell clumps (emboli) have reached the vascular or lymphatic compartments, they must survive a variety of hemodynamic and immunological challenges.

Tumor Cell Arrest

After the survival in circulation tumor cell must arrest in distant organs or lymph nodes, by size trapping on the in flow side of the microcirculation, or by Adherence of tumor cells through specific interaction with capillary or lymphatic endothelial cells, or by binding to exposed basement membrane.

Extravasation and Growth at the Secondary Site

After exiting the vascular or lymphatic compartments metastatic tumors may proliferate in response to paracrine growth factor or become dormant.

Angiogenesis in Metastatic Foci

The development of neovascular network at the metastatic site enhances the metastatic potential of the cells just as it does for primary tumor.

Evasion of Immune Response

Metastatic foci of tumor cells must evade eradication by immune responses that may be non-specific or targeted directly against the tumor cells.

Oncogenesis

- Metastasis and tumorigenesis are under separate genetic control, genetic analysis of different stages of tumor progression resulted in the multistep theory of tumorigenesis, which involves activation of oncogenes, inactivation of tumor suppressor genes and identification of host of tumor associated molecules (cancer markers)
- Thorgeirsson et al was first to demonstrate that transfection of activated Ras oncogene sequences into the fetal mouse fibroblast results in acquisition of a metastatic phenotype when these cells are implanted in the nude mouse
- In addition the adenovirus 2E1A gene was shown to suppress Ras gene induction of the metastatic phenotype without alteration in tumorigenecity or inhibition of soft agar colony formation
- This demonstrates clear suppuration between tumorigenicity and metastatic phenotype
- Candidate effector genes include those associated with:
  - Cellular adhesion to ECM component as well
  - As proteases, motility factors, angiogenic factors, and growth regulation

- Candidate suppressor genes include genes associated with:
  - Enhanced cell attachments
  - Phosphatase activity that regulate focal adhesion assembly
  - Angiogenesis inhibitors
  - Factors that suppress cell migration and growth.

Angiogenesis: Balance of Positive and Negative Effectors

- Judah Folkman and colleagues in 1970s demonstrate tumor cells release soluble factors that induce angiogenic response. For example, it includes platelet factor-4, interferon-α, thrombospondin and protease inhibitors
- Angiogenesis inhibitors is the identification of cryptic inhibitors that are revealed by proteolytic modification of ECM components, for example, 29 kD fragment of fibronectin, 16 kD fragment of prolactin, angiostatin released from plasminogen and endostatin.

Tumor Heterogeneity and Clonal Dominance

- Fidler et al first demonstrated the concept of heterogeneity of primary neoplasm
- It suggested that not all tumor cells in the primary tumor population share the same propensity to form metastases and the formation of metastatic foci selects for an aggressive subpopulation of tumor cells out of primary tumor
- This dominance arises secondary to a selective growth advantage in the metastatic cells responding to local growth factor.

Defining the Invasive Phenotype

- Extensive changes occur in quantity, organization and distribution of subepithelial basement membrane
- Invasive carcinoma is characterized by loss of basement membrane around the invasive tumor cells in the stroma

- Quantity and location of tumor cells that have escaped the primary tumor once the basement membrane barrier is compromised is difficult to determine.

Cell-cell Adhesion Suppresses or Facilitates Metastasis Formation

- Varieties of cell surface receptor that mediate the interactions include cadherins, integrins, immunoglobulin superfamily CD44
- Tumor cells must decrease the cell and matrix adhesive interactions to escape from the primary tumor, at later stages in the metastatic cascade, however, tumor cells may need to increase adhesive interactions with cells and ECM
- E-cadherin is a transmembrane glycoprotein that has five extracellular homologous domains, single membrane spanning region and a cytosolic domain
- E-cadherins is physically anchored to the actin cytoskeleton by cytoplasmic proteins termed *Catenins*
- Any disruption of the intracellular E-cadherin-catenin complex results in loss of adhesion
- This would include changes in E-cadherin expression or function, as well as genes other than E-cadherins that are required for complex formation and function
- *Lochter* et al reported that E-cadherin function can be disrupted by degradation of E- cadherins extra cellular domains by stromelysin-1 a member of MMP
- In normal cells β catenin is sequestered in the intracellular adhesion complex with cytoplasmic domain of E-cadherin, α catenin, γ catenin and p120
- Loss of cell-cell adhesion results in disruption of adhesion complex and free β catenin. Free β catenin is bound adhenomatous polyposis coli (APC) gene product
- In many cancer tumor suppressor gene APC is nonfunctional
- This leads to high levels of cytoplasmic β catenin that can be subsequently trans located

to the nucleus. The WNT-1 proto-oncogene initiated signaling pathway which includes frizzled (FRZ) and disheved (DSH) gene product, can block the activity of GSK3 β, which also can result in accumulation of β catenin

- In nucleus free nonphosphorylated β catenin can bind to the members of TCF (tissue coding factor)/ LEF-1 [lymphoid enhancer-binding factor 1] family of transcription factor. Catenin activates transcription from the cyclin D1 promoter and contributes to neoplastic transformation by causing accumulation of cyclin D1
- Other type of molecules facilitate metastasis formation, i.e. during tumor cell arrest and extravasations immunoglobulin super family members-nerve adhesion molecule and vascular cell adhesion molecule-1
- Role of vascular cell adhesion molecule-1 is in endothelial cell is cytokine inducible counter receptor for VLA-4 (very late antigen-4) integrin
- VLA-4 is expressed on leukocytes and in attachment to endothelial cells VLA-4 is expressed on tumor cells in malignant melanoma and metastatic sarcoma but not in adhenocarcinomas.

Cell-extracellular Interaction in Tumor Progression

During the process of metastases the cell must interact with interact with ECM (subepithelial basement membrane of tissue origin, stromal elements of tissue origin, sub endothelial basement membranes during extravasations, stromal and basement membrane of organs.

Role of CD 44 in tumor invasion
A transmembrane glycoprotein with large ectodomain and a small cytoplasmic domain
Involved in cell adhesion to hyaluronan (HA)
Gene encoding CD44 is on short arm of chromosome 11 has constant and variable exons
Differentially spliced forms of CD44 can be generated

Role of Integrins in Tumor Invasion

- Integrins are dimeric transmembrane proteins that are formed by the noncovalent association of α and β subunits.
- Integrins bind to individual matrix proteins, such as laminin, fibronectin, vitronectin and collagens
- Direct integrin signaling starts after engagement of integrin with ECM ligands
- Lateral clustering of integrin receptors, and the interaction of the integrin cytoplasmic domain to form complexes the proteins that link to cytoskeleton. This results in organization of cell structure known as focal adhesions (FAK)
- The decreased expression of alpha 5, beta 1 and alpha 2, beta 1 integrin is associated with cellular transformation and tumorigenesis .

Cellular Migration: New Insight

- Assembly of cytoskeleton elements to form membrane ruffles, lamellipodia, filopodia and pseudopodia accomplishes cell movement integrin connection to the ECM provides adhesive traction and contraction of the actin filaments results in forward propulsion of cell body
- As the cell moves new projection occur at the leading edge and are anchored to new focal adhesions. As the cell moves forward, the focal adhesions appear in the retrograde fashion on cell surface
- When cell moves on the rigid surface more restraining force is exerted to prevent movement of the focal adhesion
- The last step in integrin mediated cell migration is the release of the ECM integrin-cytoskeletal attachment at the trailing edge of the cell.
  - Release of integrin from the cell surface (integrin release has been observed in fibroblast migration)
  - Destabilization of the cytoskeletal linkages intracellularly.

Proteases in Tumor Cell Invasion

- Matrix proteolysis is key part of tumor cell invasion. Matrixins or MMPs matrixins and their specific inhibitors TIMPs
- Twenty matrixins and 4 TIMPs have been recognized
- These have signal peptide sequence, a pro peptide domain; a catalytic domain (zinc ion) and a hemopexin–like domain. TIMP also contain 12 absolutely conserved cysteine residue that are involved in intermolecular disulphate bond
- Amino-terminal domain for inhibitory site/ carboxy terminal domain other binding interaction
- Many matrixins are initial protease cleavage of prodomain by another matrixins or serine, such as plasmin or by urokinase type plasminogen activator the bond brakes and prodomain released and active site for catalysis is freed. In 1980, MMP secreted from a melanoma cell line that was able to degrade basement membrane collagen
- MMP have shown to degrade plasminogen to angiostatin, the angiogenesis inhibitor.

Invasion, Extravasation, and Orthotopic Effect

Tumor cell Extravasation

Tumor cell extravasation is quantitated by using polymerase chain reaction amplication of human specific alu genomic DNA sequences of tumor cells present in chorioallantoic membrane. These demonstrate:
- MMPs
- Urokinase type plasminogen activator
- Urokinase type plasminogen receptors are involved in tumor cell intravasation.

Extravasation

Eighty percent of the circulating tumor cells remain viable in circulation and extravasate up to

3 days after there introduction in the circulation and the process is not protease dependant.

Local Environment of Target Organ

Local environment of target organ may profoundly influence the growth potential of extravasated tumor cells the importance tissue micro environment (host) on the growth of primary tumor is well-known and is referred to as orthotopic effect

Occult Metastases

A proportion of patient with no evidence of systemic dissemination will develop recurrent disease after primary therapy these patients had occult systemic spread of disease that was undetectable by methods routinely employed.

Methods used for detection of occult metastases
Immunohistochemisty
Molecular methods
Flow cytometry
Prognostic markers

Immunohistochemistry: Monoclonal antibodies to detect occult metastatic cells are antibodies to epithelial specific antigens.

Molecular methods: Reverse transcriptase-polymerase chain reaction (RT-PCR) which differentiates gene expression between and lymphoid cells to identify epithelial cancer cells.

Flow cytometry
- To detect cancer cells in bone marrow and blood
- Extremely sensitive (1 in 1,000,000 cells).

Prognostic markers
- *Clinical*: Size, grade, vascular invasion, nodal invasion
- *Molecular*: Expression of oncogene by cells, CD44 molecule, estrogen receptor, epidermal growth factor receptor, angiogenic growth factor and degree of neovascularization, expression of metastases associated gene or nucleic acid in DNA.

SUMMARY

- Integrins are a family of heterodimeric, cation-dependent cell membrane adhesion molecules which mediate cell-cell and cell-matrix interaction. They play a fundamental role in the maintenance of tissue integrity and in oral squamous cell carcinomas there is variable loss or reduced expression of beta 1 integrins and of alpha 6 beta 4, which correlates to loss of basement membrane proteins and is most extensive inpoorly differentiated lesions
- Integrins are also involved in regulating the activity of proteolytic enzymes that degrade the basement membrane—the intial barrier to surrounding tissue
- Integrins are essential for cell migration and invasion not only because they directly mediate adhesion to the extracellular matrix
- Integrins not only send signals to the cell in responce to the extracellular environment, but also they respond to intracellular cues and alter the way that they interact with the extracellular environment
- Integrin binding to legends in the extracellular matrix initiates several proservival mechanisms to prevent apoptosis.

Surgical Treatment Plan for Oral and Maxillofacial Cancers

18

INTRODUCTION

Surgery for oral cancer can be mutilating and disfigurement is a problem for patient, as head and neck is an important component of body image. Patients must cope not only with loss of structure and function as a result of operation, many aspects of health related quality of life are affected. Failure to deal with issue of appearance can lead to distress such as avoiding social contacts, alcohol misuse aggression, etc.

Technique of reconstruction of head and neck and mid-face has remained a challenge in the field of maxilla facial surgery microvascular reconstruction technique in head and neck cancer surgery are well-established, reconstruction with free flap, radial fore arm flap, composite radial fore arm flap, iliac crest flap or fibular flap, latissimus dorsi flap are few to name available options.

The most important considerations
Suitability of the flap to replace excised tissue
Mobility at the donor site
Facility and ability to operate as a teamwork
Reliability of transfer tissue

EPIDEMIOLOGY

- *Oral cancer*: Sixth most common malignancy in the world is 30 percent of all head and neck cancers. Squamous cell carcinoma: 95 percent of all oral cancers

- *Age*: Over the age of 40 years: 95 percent of patients Average age: 60 years
- *Sites*: Lateral border of middle-third and ventral surface of tongue: most common sites of oral cancer
- *Lower lip cancer:* Significant reduction in cancer incidence during the last few decades reflect the increased use of sun screens
- *Tongue cancer:* Greatest increase in frequency.

TNM DEFINITIONS

Primary Tumor (T)

- TX: Primary tumor cannot be assessed
- T0: No evidence of primary tumor
- Tis: Carcinoma *in situ*
- T1: Tumor 2 cm or less in greatest dimension
- T2: Tumor more than 2 cm but not more than 4 cm in greatest dimension
- T3: Tumor more than 4 cm in greatest dimension
- T4: (lip) Tumor invades through cortical bone, inferior alveolar nerve, floor of mouth, or skin of face, i.e. chin or nose.

Regional Lymph Nodes (N)

- NX: Regional lymph nodes cannot be assessed
- N0: No regional lymph node metastasis
- N1: Metastasis in a single ipsilateral lymph node, 3 cm or less in greatest dimension
- N2: Metastasis in a single ipsilateral lymph node, more than 3 cm but not more than 6 cm

in greatest dimension; or in multiple ipsilateral lymph nodes, none more than 6 cm in greatest dimension; or in bilateral or contralateral lymph nodes, none more than 6 cm in greatest dimension
- N2a: Metastasis in a single ipsilateral lymph node, more than 3 cm but not more than 6 cm in dimension
- N2b: Metastasis in multiple ipsilateral lymph nodes, none more than 6 cm in greatest dimension
- N2c: Metastasis in bilateral or contralateral lymph nodes, none more than 6 cm in greatest dimension
- N3: Metastasis in a lymph node more than 6 cm in greatest dimension.

Distant Metastasis (M)
- MX: Distant metastasis cannot be assessed
- M0: No distant metastasis
- M1: Distant metastasis.

MANAGEMENT

Prognostic Factors
- Stage (Table 18.1)
- Size of lesion
- Nodal involvement
- Tumor thickness
- Perineural invasion
- Intralymphatic invasion
- Vascular invasion.

Selection of Initial Treatment
- Surgical treatment of the regional lymph node for CA oral cavity is based on understanding of the regional lymphatic, lymph nodes metastasis
- When regional metastasis are clinically palpable, comprehensive clearance of the lymph nodes should be done
- Classical radical neck dissection remains gold standard of surgical management of clinically apparent metastatic lymph nodes

Table 18.1: TNM staging

Stage	Tumor (T)	Node (N)	Metastasis (M)
0	Tis	N0	M0
I	T1	N0	M0
II	T2	N0	M0
III	T3	N0	M0
	T1	N1	M0
	T2	N1	M0
	T3	N1	M0
IV A	T4	N0,N1	M0
	Any T	N2,N3	M0
	Any T	Any N	M1
IV B	Any T	N3	M0
IV C	Any T	Any N	M1

Surgery ladder of reconstruction
Primary closure
Free grafts
Skin
Bone
Flaps

Lip
- T1: WE + primary closure
- T2: External beam radiation (50 g in 15 fractions)
- T3: RT + prophylactic neck RT
- T4: Surgery + postoperative RT.

Anterior 2/3rd of Tongue
- T1 and T2: Interstitial implant
- Tip: Surgical excision
- T3: Implant and external beam including ipsilateral lymph node drainage
- T4: Surgery along with postoperative RT.

Buccal Mucosa
- T1 and T2: External beam RT
- T3 and T4: Surgery and postoperative RT
- Large lesions: Treated by surgery or radiation therapy or combination of these.

Floor of Mouth
- T1: Interstitial implants morbidity is rare as small volume of tissues is irradiated
- T2: Implant and external beam RT to include ipsilateral lymph node drainage. Beam arrangement uses anteroposterior oblique field
- T3 and T4: Surgery and post RT.

Assessment of mandibular invasion
Tumor adjacent to but not fixed to the mandible-inner table of the periosteum to be removed
Tumor fixed to the periosteum—marginal mandibulectomy
Bony infiltration—segmental resection

Lower Alveolus
- Because of proximity to mandible, invasion occur at an early stage,
- Detected by CT scan or MRI or OPG
- T1 and T2: external beam radiation
- Extensive bone involvement—surgery followed by postoperative RT.

Retromolar Triangle
- Tumor at this site spread along the mandibular ramus and tract superiorly into the pteryoid fossa.
- T1 and T2: external beam RT
- Advanced stages—surgery.

Upper Gingiva and Hard Palate
- Most small lesions are treated surgically as invasion in the bone is common
- Reconstructed with obturator.

Treatment Option for Lymph Nodes

Clinically Negative Node
- T1: No dissection
- T2: Supraomohyoid or modified radical neck dissection of carcinoma of floor of the mouth, tongue, buccal mocosa
- Radiotherapy if recurrence is less than 2 cm outside the irradiated area.

Node Positive Neck
Surgery: Neck dissection—radical neck dissection or modified radical neck dissection or selective neck dissection.

Ipsilateral Mobile Nodal Finding
- T1: Radiation
- T2: Modified radical or radical neck dissection
- Radiotherapy: Extracapsular rupture of tumor metastasis.

Bilateral Nodal Disease
- First neck dissection of side less involved
- Attempt to preserve the IJV
- Fixed nodal disease—CT scan

Indications for Classical Radical Neck Dissection
- N3 disease
- Multiple gross metastasis involving multiple levels
- Recurrent metastasis in previously irradiated neck
- Extranodal spread
- Involvement of accessory chain lymph node.
  There are multitudes of surgical accesses for the facial skeleton based on the concept of modular osteotomies.

MAXILLARY APPROACH

Transfacial Approach

The term transfacial is used to describe any procedure that mobilizes the mid facial skeleton through a facial (skin) incision, irrespective of the extent of midface disassembly used. One of the most commonly used transfacial approaches to the midface for the resection of maxillary tumors is the Weber-Fergusson (WF) maxillectomy incision.

Weber-Fergusson Incision (Figs 18.1 and 18.2)
This approach was first described by Weber in the German literature and was later modified by Fergusson in the English literature.

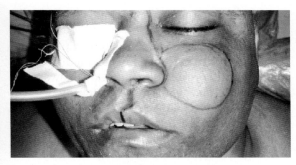

Fig. 18.1: Weber-Fergusson maxillectomy incision. Modification marking

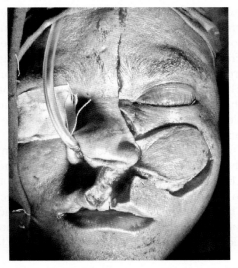

Fig. 18.2: Weber-Fergusson maxillectomy incision

Advantages
- It allows for improved access to the maxilla and for unimpeded resection of tumors affecting the anterior and superior aspects of the maxilla
- It may also be used to aid in swinging the maxilla laterally while pedicled to the cheek flap. The lateral maxillary swing is used routinely in accessing the nasopharynx for the resection of nasopharyngeal carcinomas.

Drawback
When the tumor involves the posterior aspect of the maxilla and/or the pterygoid plates, the approach does not improve the access.

Modifications
Altemir's incision—straight line incision in the lip is moved from the midline and placed on the philtrum.

Technique
- This is accomplished by placing the incision along the philtrum, carrying the lip extension with a slight step away and with an option of placing a chevron in the vermillion portion of the incision
- The superior extent of the lip incision should be performed into the nasal sill and then extend out along the base of the ala and in a cephalad direction
- The lateral nasal incision should be raised and placed in the nasal side wall at the junction of the nasal subunit. Once the medial canthal region is approached, the incision may be extended laterally inferior to the lower eyelid in one of the creases (as in the Dieffenbach modification) or extended superiorly into a Lynch incision
- A full-thickness flap is then elevated while maintaining sound oncologic margins
- The bony osteotomies are made as the tumor dictates
- At the conclusion of the resection and reconstruction, the flap is reapproximated, taking care to have correct anatomic closure so as to minimize the postoperative scar.

Mid-face Degloving Technique

This approach requires familiarity with closed rhinoplasty techniques. The technique incorporates the use of vestibular and intranasal incisions to lift or "deglove" the facial skin from the facial skeleton, improving the access to the maxillary tumor.

Posterior Maxillary Approach

- Large tumor that extends anteriorly, superiorly, and posteriorly with extension toward the pterygoid plates or the infratemporal fossa, it may be advantageous to use two approaches
- The Weber-Fergusson approach may be combined with a lip-splitting mandibulotomy

approach so that the posterior aspect of the tumor can be resected in a more direct fashion. The combination of the two techniques was first reported by Dingman and Conley using a lateral mandibular osteotomy, and it was later modified by Lawson and colleagues by moving the osteotomy to a midline mandibulotomy

- Obwegeser's approach to the posterior maxilla and the retromaxillary and/or infratemporal space.

Transmandibular Approach

Lip-split Mandibulotomy Approach

- The mandibulotomy approach is typically used in combination with a lip split
- The first description of a lip-split technique was by Roux in the middle of the nineteenth century. Since then, there have been a multitude of variations to the lip-splitting incision
- The 3 classic incisions most often used are:
  - The Roux incision, whereby a straight-line incision is made from the midline of the lower lip, extending through the chin and connecting to the neck incision
  - The McGregor incision (Figs 18.3 and 18.4), which extends in a vertical fashion from the midline of the lip toward the chin,

circumventing the chin along the chin and/ or labiomental groove
  - The Robson incision, which is placed on a relaxed skin tension line medial to the commissure and descends down toward the neck to meet with the neck incision.

- Hayter and colleagues recently published a modification of the McGregor incision that incorporates a chevron into the vermillion margin and the midline lip incisions to improve closure, thereby improving the final esthetics. The incision is marked in the midline of the lower lip, with or without a chevron, and extended to the labiomental crease. Once the crease is reached, the incision is extended to the ipsilateral side of the along the mental crease toward the midline submental region; from there, the incision to the neck incision
- The placement of the circum-mental incision on the ipsilateral side rather than the contralateral side of the neck dissection is to decrease the possibility of ischemic necrosis of the chin
- Once the flap is elevated, the osteotomy is then marked anterior to the mental foramen
- The osteotomy is completed first, taking care to elevate the lingual mucosa and protect it. The osteotomy is completed, and the mucosa incision is performed on the floor of the mouth along the lingual mucosa. A cuff is left for later

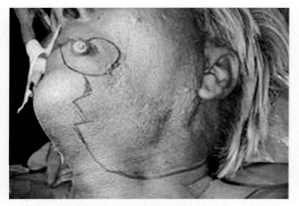

Fig. 18.3: Hayter and colleagues modification of the McGregor incision marking

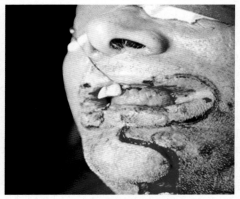

Fig. 18.4: Hayter and colleagues modification of the McGregor incision

closure if possible, or a gingivosulqular incision is placed to reflect a lingual mucoperiosteal flap. The mucosal incisions through the buccal and lingual gingival mucosa should be stepped away from the bone cuts so that the soft tissue closure does not lie directly over the osteotomy site

- With the osteotomy and mucosal incision completed, the mandible is then able to be reflected laterally, providing a clear view of the tumor and allowing for uncompromised resection. This lateral "swinging" of the mandible is why this technique is at times referred to as the mandibular swing approach. Once the resection and reconstruction are completed, the fixation is reapplied and the incisions are closed. When the incisions are closed with attention to the careful alignment of tissues, the postoperative scar is imperceptible

- The use of a non-lip-splitting mandibulotomy is most commonly employed to improve access to the parapharyngeal space and the infratemporal fossa. In some circumstances, however, it may be used to improve access to the oral cavity. This approach incorporates two osteotomies: one at the parasymphyseal area and another at the ramus region. The approach of Attia and coworkers uses a parasymphyseal and horizontal ramus osteotomy above the lingula and swings the segment in a superior direction. As described by Attia and coworkers, this procedure involves a lip-splitting incision

- The concept of ill-continuity resection has been around for many years. The rationale for this approach lies in the possibility of a tumor focus in the lymphatics between the primary and the cervical nodes. To that end, proponents of this theory advocate that the resection should remove the primary, the intervening lymphatics, and the cervical nodes in one block specimen. The technique was first described by Scheunemann in 1975 and was later modified by Stanley. The pull-through operation is performed by making a releasing incision on the lingual aspect of the gingival and the elevation of a mucoperiosteal flap. The dissection is performed until the mylohyoid

muscle is encountered, taking care to leave a small cuff of muscle attached to the mandible to aid in closure. Similarly, the genioglossus and geniohyoid muscles are detached, and the contents of the oral cavity are then pulled into the neck, allowing for a more direct resection through unimpeded visual and tactile feel of the tumor. Devine and colleagues compared their experience between the lip-split mandibulotomy and the mandibular lingual releasing access and found that patients with lingual release reported more problems with speech, swallowing, and chewing.

Visor Flap

- An alternative to the pull-through technique is the visor flap. This flap is mostly used in the resection of tumors involving the anterior oral cavity; however, at times, it may also be used in the resection of lateral tongue and floor of the mouth tumors

- The incision for the flap is performed from the mastoid process on one side and is extended toward the contralateral mastoid or to the mandibular symphysis on the unaffected side

- The flap is elevated as usual, taking care to identify and preserve the marginal mandibular branch of the facial nerve. Once the inferior border of the mandible is encountered, a periosteal incision is made along the exposed mandible. An intraoral incision is made along the gingivobuccal sulcus, and a mucoperiosteal flap is elevated and reflected toward the inferior border of the mandible. The two dissections are then connected

- The flap is tethered to the mandible only at the mental foramen region. The mental nerve is incised, and the flap is then mobilized in a cephalad direction with the aid of two rubber drains. With the drains secured, the surgeon has an unimpeded view of the oral cavity to proceed with the tumor extirpation

- One of the obvious drawbacks of this technique is the sacrifice of the mental nerve, leading to anesthesia of the lip and chin. The benefit is that the surgeon is able to remove the tumor without the need for a lip-splitting incision.

Some More Access Approach (Figs 18.5 to 18.10)

Surgical Procedure for Neck Dissection and Hemiglossectomy (Figs 18.10A to Z and 18.10AA to DD)

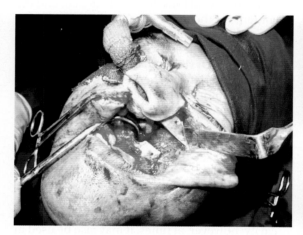

Fig. 18.5: Showing LeFort-I down fracture—access surgery

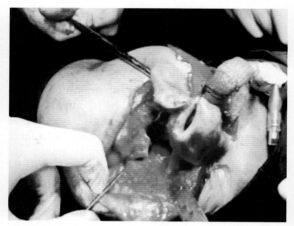

Fig. 18.6: Showing LeFort-I down fracture—lesion removal (*Courtesy* of Figures 18.1 to 18.6: Dr Vikram Shetty)

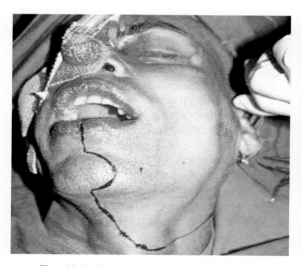

Fig. 18.7: Lip split access surgery marking

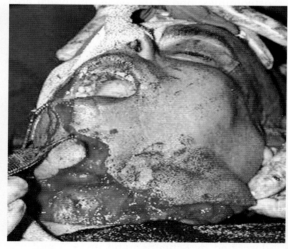

Fig. 18.8: Lip split access surgery

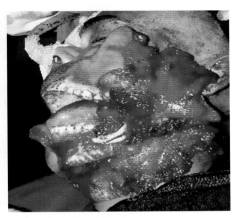

Fig. 18.9: Lip split access surgery—lesion removal

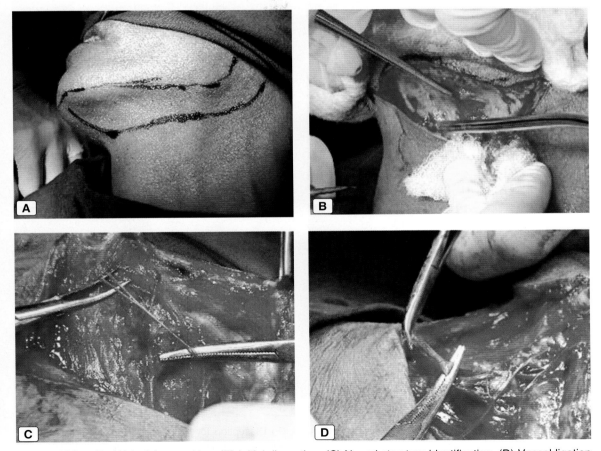

Figs 18.10A to D: (A) Incision marking, (B) Initial dissection, (C) Neural structure identification, (D) Vessel ligation

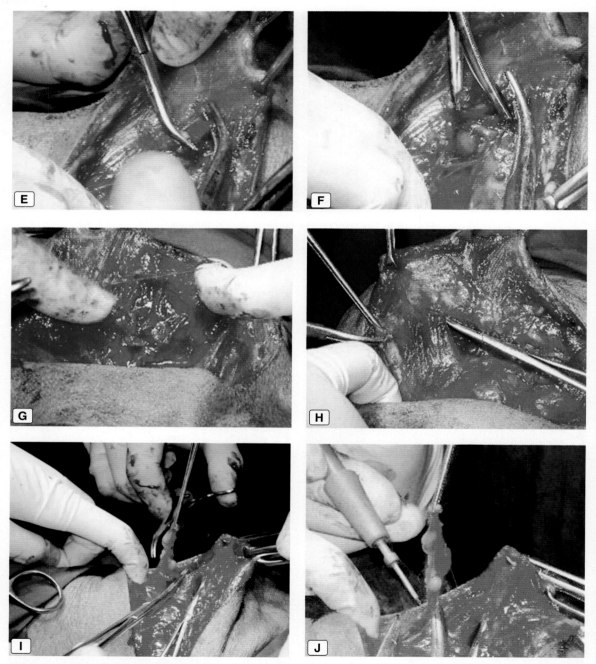

Figs 18.10E to J: (E) Identification of vascular structure, (F) Dissection for lymph node, (G) Neural structure identification, (H) Dissection (I) Identification of lymphatic channel, (J) Lymph node group dissection

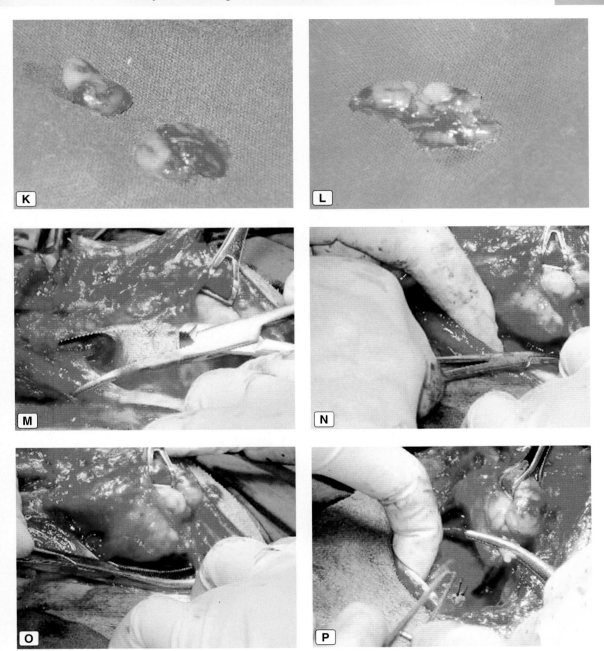

Figs 18.10K to P: (K and L) Dissected lymph nodes, (M) Dissection, (N) Identification of deeper lymph node, (O and P) Dissection for deeper lymph node

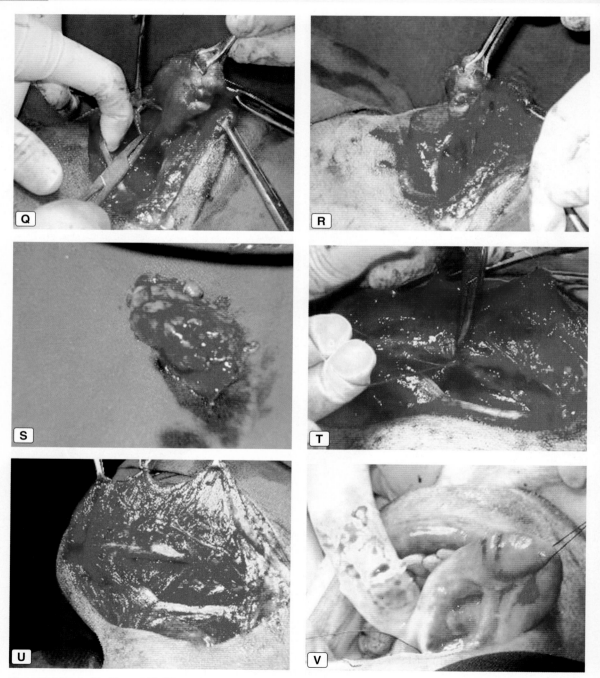

Figs 18.10Q to V: (Q and R) Dissection for deeper lymph node, (S) Dissected lymph node. (T) Ligated vascular structure, (U) Hemostasis achieved after neck dissection, (V) Holding tie

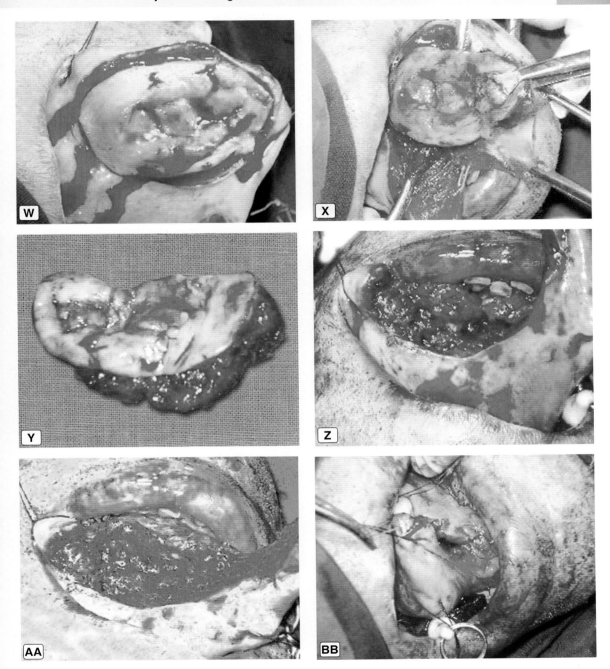

Figs 18.10W to BB: (W) Areas marked for dissection, (X) Glossectomy dissection, (Y) Excised lesion of the part of tongue, (Z) Tongue after hemiglossectomy, (AA) Hemostasis achieved after glossectomy, (BB) Closure after hemiglossectomy

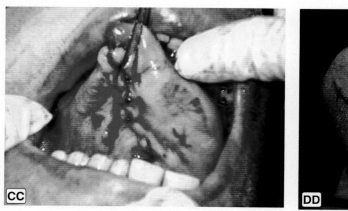
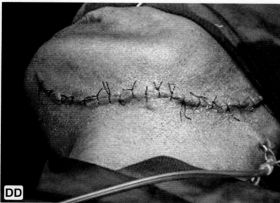

Figs 18.10CC and DD: (CC) Closure after hemiglossectomy, (DD) Incision closure

Management of Neck in Oral and Maxillofacial Carcinoma

19

INTRODUCTION

Oral and maxillofacial surgeons frequently encounter neck masses in adult patients When adult patients presents with neck mass, malignancy is the greatest concern. Accurate diagnosis of neck mass requires good medical history, knowledge of normal anatomy. Lymph nodes are located throughout the head and neck, fixed, firm, or matted lymph nodes larger than 1.5 cm require further evaluation, Biopsy should be considered for neck masses with progressive growth, location within the supraclavicular fossa or size greater than 3 cm. Biopsy also should be considered if a patient with neck mass develops symptoms. Frozen section of the mass followed by neck dissection should be performed if the mass proves to be metastatic. Hence, the single most important prognostic factor in squamous carcinoma of the maxillofacial region is the status of the cervical lymph nodes.

HISTORY

20th Century

- 1951: Martin advocates radical neck dissection after analysis of 1450 cases
  - Advocated RND for all cases
  - Standardized the radical neck dissection
- 1952: Suarez describes a functional neck dissection
  - Preservation of SCM, omohyoid, submandibular gland, IJV, XI.
  - Enables protection of carotid.

- 1989, 1991, and 1994: Medina, Robbins, and Byers – classification of neck dissection.

ANATOMICAL DIVISIONS

Fascial Layers of the Neck

- Superficial cervical fascia
- Deep cervical fascia
  - Investing or outer layer
  - Visceral or middle layer
  - Internal layer.

Deep Cervical Fascia—Investing Layer

- Splits to contain 2 muscles and 2 glands
- Forms carotid sheath
- Nerves embedded in the fascia
  - Glossopharyngeal
  - Accessory
  - Hypoglossal
  - Ansa hypoglossi.

Deep Cervical Fascia— Middle or Visceral Layer

- Forms pretracheal fascia
- Surrounds pharynx, larynx, esophagus, and trachea.

Deep Cervical Fascia—Internal Layer

- Forms prevertebral fascia
- Nerves superficial to prevertebral fascia
  - Cervical sympathetic trunk

- Nerves deep to prevertebral fascia
  - Cervical plexus
  - Phrenic nerve
  - Brachial plexus.

Head and Neck Lymphatics

- Waldeyer's internal ring
  - Collection of lymphoid aggregates in pharynx
- Superficial lymph node system
  - Occipital, post auricular, parotid, preauricular, facial nodes
- Deep system
  - Junctional nodes
  - Upper cervical nodal group
  - Middle cervical nodal group
  - Lower cervical nodal group
  - Spinal accessory group
  - Nuchal nodes
  - Visceral nodes
  - Nodes in upper mediastinum.

Patterns of Cervical Lymph Node Metastases

- Predictable and sequential progression of metastatic spread from each primary site
- Select group of regional lymph nodes
- are at risk for initial involvement
- Skip metastases are rare.

Lymph Node Levels in Neck

- Lymph node levels
  - Sloan Kettering nomenclature
  - Subgroups.
- Common nodal drainage patterns.

Lymph Node Levels in Neck

- Level Ia: Submental
  Level Ib: Submandibular
- Level II: Upper jugular
- Level III: Middle jugular
- Level IV: Lower jugular
- Level V: Posterior triangle
- Level VI: Anterior compartment/visceral/central compartment
- Level VII: Superior mediastinum (nodes in tracheo-esophageal groove).

Level I

- Submental triangle (Ia)
  - Anterior digastric
  - Hyoid
  - Mylohyoid.
- Submandibular triangle (Ib)
  - Anterior and posterior digastric
  - Mandible.

Marginal Mandibular Nerve

- Most commonly injured in dissection of level 1b
- Landmarks:
  - 1 cm anterior and inferior to angle of mandible
  - Mandibular notch
- Subplatysmal
- Deep to fascia of the submandibular gland
- Superficial to facial vein.

Hypoglossal Nerve

- Lies deep to the IJV, ICA, CN IX, X, and XI
- Curves 90 degrees and passes between the IJV and ICA
- Lateral to hyoglossus
- Deep to mylohyoid.

Level Ia

- Chin
- Lower lip
- Anterior floor of mouth
- Mandibular incisors
- Tip of tongue.

Level Ib

- Oral cavity
- Floor of mouth
- Oral tongue
- Nasal cavity (anterior)
- Face.

Level II

- Upper jugular nodes
  - Anterior: Lateral border of sternohyoid, posterior digastric and stylohyoid
  - Posterior: Posterior border of SCM

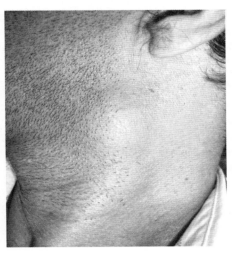

Fig. 19.1: Lateral neck swelling

- – Skull base
- – Hyoid bone (clinical landmark)
- – Carotid bifurcation (surgical landmark).
- Level IIa anterior to XI
- Level IIb posterior to XI
  - – Submuscular recess
  - – Oropharynx is greater than oral cavity and laryngeal meets (Fig. 19.1)
- Spinal accessory nerve relationship with the IJV.

Level II Range

- Oral cavity
- Nasal cavity
- Nasopharynx
- Oropharynx
- Larynx
- Hypopharynx
- Parotid.

Level III

- Middle jugular nodes
  - – Anterior: Lateral border of sternohyoid
  - – Posterior: Posterior border of SCM
  - – Inferior border of level III

- Cricoid cartilage lower border (clinical landmark)
- Omohyoid muscle (surgical landmark)
  - – Junction with IJV.

Level III Range

- Oral cavity
- Nasopharynx
- Oropharynx
- Hypopharynx
- Larynx.

Level IV

Lower Jugular Nodes

- Anterior: Lateral border of sternohyoid
- Posterior: Posterior border of SCM
- Cricoid cartilage lower border (clinical landmark)
- Omohyoid muscle (surgical landmark)
  - – Junction with IJV
- Clavicle.

Phrenic Nerve

- Sole nerve supply to the diaphragm
- C3-5
- Anterior surface of anterior scalene
- Under prevertebral fascia
- Posterolateral to carotid sheath.

Thoracic Duct

- Conveys lymph from the entire body back to the blood
- Begins at the cisterna chyli
- Enters posterior mediastinum between the azygous vein and thoracic aorta
- Courses to the left into the neck anterior to the vertebral artery and vein
- Enters the junction of the left subclavian and the IJV.

Level IV Range

- Hypopharynx
- Larynx
- Thyroid
- Cervical esophagus.

Level V

Posterior Triangle of Neck

- Posterior border of SCM
- Clavicle
- Anterior border of trapezius
- Va → Spinal accessory nodes
- Vb → Transverse cervical artery nodes
  - Radiologic landmark
    - ♦ Inferior border of cricoid
- Supraclavicular nodes.

Spinal Accessory Nerve

- Penetrates deep surface of the SCM
- Exits posterior surface of SCM deep to Erb's point
- Traverses the posterior triangle on the levator scapulae
- Enters the trapezius about 5 cm above the clavicle.

Level V Range

- Nasopharynx
- Oropharynx
- Posterior neck and scalp.

Level VI

- Anterior compartment
  - Hyoid
  - Suprasternal notch
  - Medial border of carotid sheath.
- Perithyroidal lymph nodes
- Paratracheal lymph nodes
- Precricoid (Delphian) lymph node.

Level VI Range

- Thyroid
- Larynx (glottic and subglottic)
- Pyriform sinus apex
- Cervical esophagus.

Natural History of Malignant Neck Disease

- Drainage patterns apply in nonviolated neck, hence, supraomohyoid neck dissection suitable in previously untreated neck

- Lymph node biopsy alter lymphatic drainage for 1 year
- Extensive surgery and RT lead to shunting of lymph and opening of abnormal channel.

Prognostic nodal factors
Clinical status
Size
Number
Extranodal spread
Level of involvement
Tumor emboli

Risk in "N_0" neck
High tumor stage
High grade tumor
Local depth of infiltration
Site of lesion

Treatment options for N_0 neck
Elective neck dissection SOHND
Sentinel node biopsy
Elective neck radiotherapy in the event of clinically evident cervical neck metastasis
Wait and watch

VARIOUS INCISIONS FOR NECK DISSECTION (FIGS 19.2 TO 19.9)

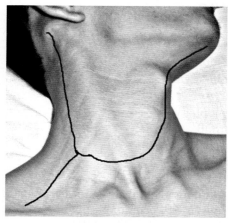

Fig. 19.2: Apron incision

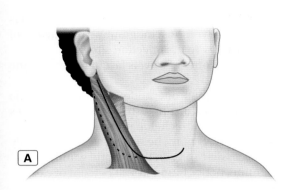

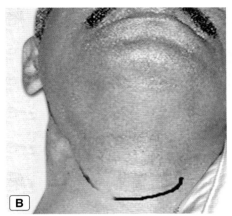

Figs 19.3A and B: Half apron incision

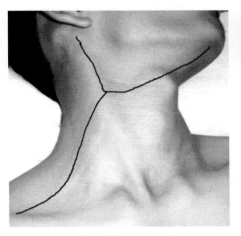

Fig. 19.4: Conley incision

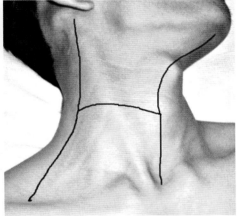

Fig. 19.5: H-incision

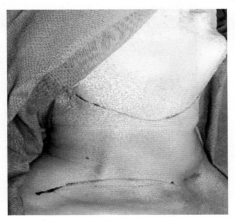

Fig. 19.6: MacFee incision

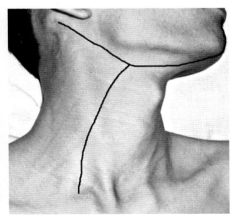

Fig. 19.7: Y-incision

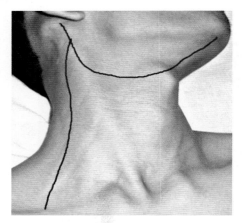

Fig. 19.8: Schobinger incision

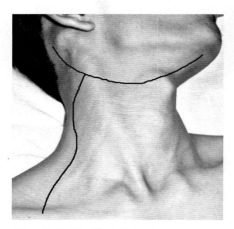

Fig. 19.9: Modified Schobinger incision

SENTINEL NODE BIOPSY

If the first draining lymph node had no evidence of micro metastasis on histopathological examination, there was <5 % incidence of micrometastases to the remaining lymph node basin

Sentinel Lymph Node Concept

- Tumor spreads via lymphatics to a primary node
- Examination of primary echelon nodes for tumor directs the need for surgical management of the nodal basins

- Difficulties of lymphatic mapping in head and neck.
  - It is difficult to visualize lymphatic channels using lymphoscintigraphy because of proximity to the injection site
  - The radiotracer travels fast in the lymphatic vessels
  - If more than one node is visible, it can be difficult to distinguish first-echelon nodes from second-echelon nodes
  - The SLN may be small and not easily accessible (e.g., in the parotid gland).
- Sentinel nodes found in >90 percent of cases.
  - Experience matters
  - Surgeons with less than 10 cases—56 percent success in SLNB.
- Lymphoscintigraphy revealed unexpected bilateral or contralateral disease in about 14 percent of patients.

CLASSIFICATION OF NECK DISSECTIONS

- Comprehensive neck dissection
- Selective neck dissection.

COMPREHENSIVE NECK DISSECTION

All surgical procedures on the lateral neck which comprehensively remove cervical lymph nodes from level I to level V (Figs 19.10 to 19.31).

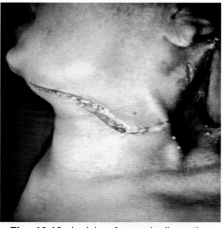

Fig. 19.10: Incision for neck dissection

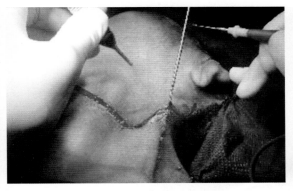

Fig. 19.11: Electrosurgical dissection (I)

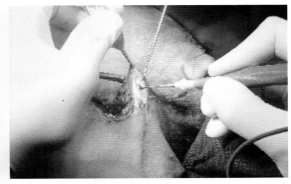

Fig. 19.12: Electrosurgical dissection (II)

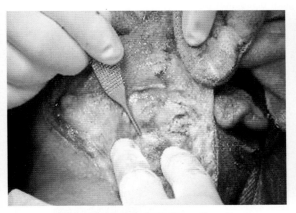

Fig. 19.13: Surgical dissection (I)

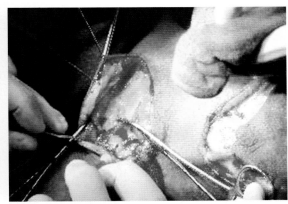

Fig. 19.14: Electrocautery (I)

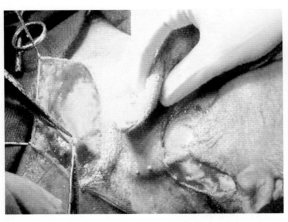

Fig. 19.15: Electrocautery (II)

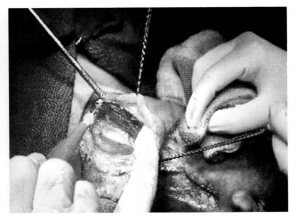

Fig. 19.16: Electrosurgical dissection (III)

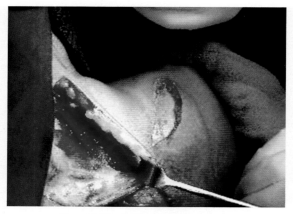

Fig. 19.17: Surgical dissection (II)

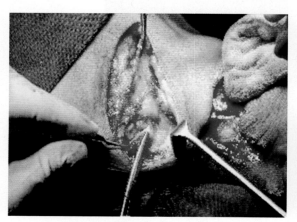

Fig. 19.18: Surgical dissection (III)

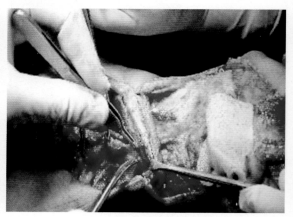

Fig. 19.19: Surgical dissection (IV)

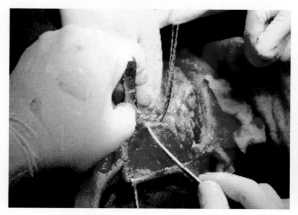

Fig. 19.20: Surgical dissection (V)

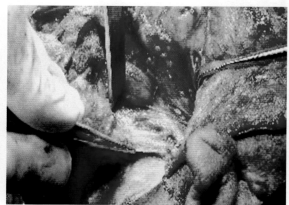

Fig. 19.21: Surgical dissection (VI)

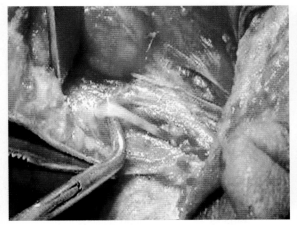

Fig. 19.22: Identification of neural structure

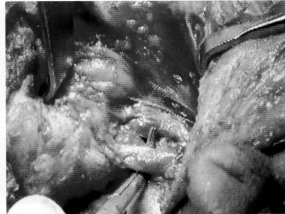

Fig. 19.23: Identification of vascular structure

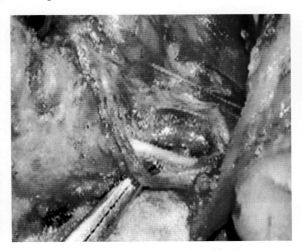

Fig. 19.24: Carotid artery identification

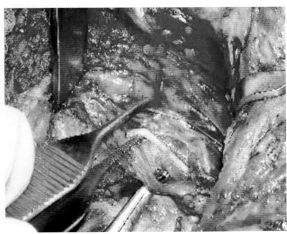

Fig. 19.25: Identification of neural structure

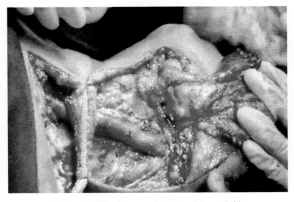

Fig. 19.26: Hemostasis achieved (I)

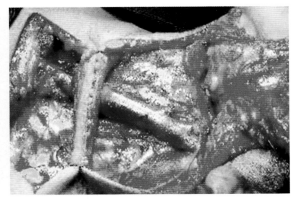

Fig. 19.27: Hemostasis achieved (II)

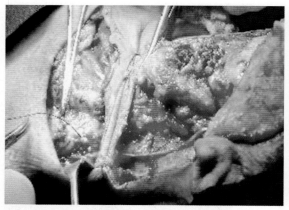

Fig. 19.28: Lymph node dissection (I)

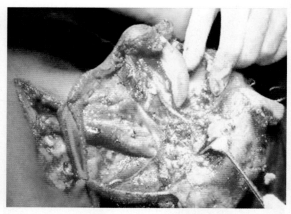

Fig. 19.29: Lymph node dissection (II)

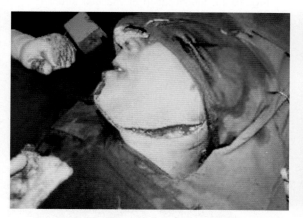

Fig. 19.30: Modified lip split approach for submandibular lymph node step I

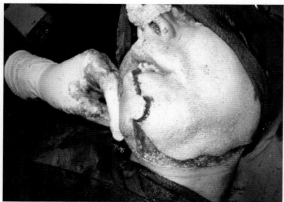

Fig. 19.31: Modified lip split approach for submandibular lymph node step II

Comprehensive neck dissection
Classical RND
Extended RND (Additional regional lymph nodes/cranial nerves, muscles, skin)
MRND type 1: Selectively preserves spinal accessory nerve
MRND type 2: Preserves spinal accessory nerve and SCM/IJV
MRND type 3: Preserves spinal accessory nerve, IJV, and SCM

Radical Neck Dissection

- Removal of all ipsilateral cervical lymph node groups extending from the inferior border of the mandible to the clavicle; medially, the midline; and posteriorly, the anterior border of the trapezius muscle
- Included are all lymph nodes from levels I through V
- The SAN, IJV and SCM are also removed.

Indications

- N3 disease
- Recurrent metastatic disease in previously irradiated neck
- Grossly apparent extranodal spread with invasion of spinal acc N/IJV at the base of skull
- Access prior to pedicled flap reconstruction.

Contraindications

- Untreatable primary tumor
- Unfit for major surgery
- Distant metastasis
- Significant B/L neck disease
- Inoperable neck disease
- RND Structures excised.

Extended RND

- RND plus additional lymph node groups/non lymphatic structures/both
- Retropharyngeal lymph nodes
- Parotid nodes
- Lymph node levels 6,7.

Nonlymphatic Structures

- Mandible
- Parotid gland
- Mastoid tip
- Prevertebral fascia
- Musculature
- Digastric muscle
- Hypoglossal nerve
- ECA
- Skin.

Indications

- Neck disease invades nonlymphatic structures
- Primary tumor of parotid, pharynx

$$\downarrow$$

Retropharyngeal LN dissection
- Transglottic and subglottic CA
- Carcinoma cervical esophagus-paratracheal, pretracheal, anterior compartment nodes
- Carcinoma thyroid.

Modified RND

- MRND refers to the excision of all lymph nodes routinely removed by the RND with preservation of one or more nonlymphatic structures (i.e. the SAN, IJV and SCM) (SAN = Spinal accessory nerve; IJV = Internal jugular vein; SCM = Sternocleidomastoid muscle)
- The structure(s) preserved should be specifically named.

SELECTIVE NECK DISSECTION (SND) (FIGS 19.32 TO 19.34)

Selective neck dissection refers to cervical lymphadenectomy in which there is preservation of one or more of the lymph node groups that are routinely removed in the radical neck dissection.

Supraomohyoid Neck Dissection (Level I–III)

- T1-T4, No
- Oral cavity.

Extended SOHND (Level I–IV)

- Primary Ca lateral border of oral tongue
- Skin CA (SCC and melanoma) anterior to line of tragus.

Lateral Neck Dissection (Level II–IV)

- T2-T4 No
- SCC larynx, oropharynx, hypopharynx.

Posterolateral (Level II–V)

- Postauricular, suboccipital nodes
- Skin CA posterior to the line of tragus.

SND for Primary Treatment of N⁺ Neck

Efficacy of leaving levels IIb and V undisturbed in oral carcinoma.

SND for Salvage of Neck Persistence/ Early Recurrence

- SND: Persistant stable adenopathy post-RT
- Progressive neck disease after RT: Comprehensive neck dissection (l–V)

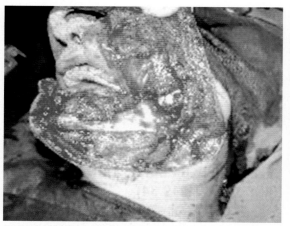

Fig. 19.32: Exposure for segmental mandibulectomy

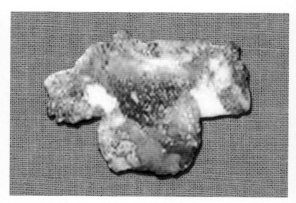

Fig. 19.34: Resected specimen Courtesy of Figures 19.10 to 19.34: Dr BR Prasad)

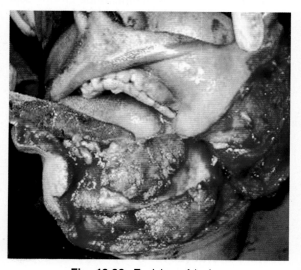

Fig. 19.33: Excision of lesion

Fixed Nodes

- Overall poor prognosis
- Extracapsular spread present
- Resectability dependant on the anatomic structure to which fixed, e.g. mandible, larynx, sternocleidomastoid muscle.
- R+ resection common
- 5-year survival—15 percent, if surgery + postoperative RT

Complication of neck dissection
Infection and festula formation
Shoulder dysfunction
Airleak through wound drain
Chylous fistula (1–2.5%)
Facial and cerebral edema
Bleeding and postoperative hematoma under the flap
Apnea
Jugular vein thrombosis
Blowout of carotid
Neuroma
Brachial plexus injury
Cervical plexus injury
Lingual nerve injury
Cervical symphathetic chain injury
Hypoglossal nerve injury
Phrenic nerve injury
Vagus nerve injury

- Preoperative radiotherapy with salvage surgery—no improvement in survival.
- Skin fixity—wide excision of skin with resurfacing and postoperative RT—better long-term survival.

Role of Chemotherapy and Radiotherapy in Oral and Maxillofacial Carcinoma

20

INTRODUCTION

The standard protocol in the treatment of oral malignancies is surgery, radiation and chemotherapy. Cancer is one of the major causes of death. The treatment of cancers after so many years of research and experience is still unsatisfactory due to certain characteristics of the cancer cells-like capacity for uncontrolled proliferation, invasiveness and metastasis. Recently targeted treatment in form of monoclonal antibodies with antiangiogenesis, epidermal growth factor inhibitors and tyrosin kinase inhibitor are use along with chemotherapy and radiation. The main aim of this is to eliminate the residual cells which are resistant to the major modalities of treatment like chemo therapy or radiation.

The newer monclonal antibodies are
Transtuzumab
Cetuximab
Bevacizumab
Gefitinib
Erlotinib

Phases of Cell Cycle (Fig. 20.1)

- Four phases of the cell cycle are G_1, S, G_2, and M
- G_1 is the presynthetic phase and the duration is variable
- During the S phase the synthesis of DNA occurs and hence the activity of replicating enzymes like DNA and RNA polymerases, topoisomerases, thymidine kinases and dihydrofolate reductases are maximum at this phase of 12 to 18 hours duration
- G_2 is the postsynthetic phase (1–8 hr) and in the M phase (1–2 hr) the mitosis takes place.

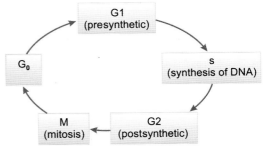

Fig. 20.1 Phases of cell cycle

Cell cycle specific drugs	Cell cycle nonspecific drugs
S phase: Antimetabolites, doxorubicin, epipodophyllotoxins, vinca alkaloids	Alkylating agents Anticancer antibodies
G2 and M phases: Bleomycin	Cisplatin
M phase: Taxanes, vinca alkaloids	Procarbazine, camptothecins

The daughter cells may start dividing or may enter into a dormant phase called G_0

- The knowledge of cell cycle may be used for staging and scheduling treatment because different drugs act at different stages of the cell cycle. However, some drugs are cell cycle non-specific

Common Adverse Effects to Anticancer Drugs

Since most anticancer drugs act on the rapidly multiplying cells, they are also toxic to the normal rapidly multiplying cells in the bone marrow, epithelial cells of skin and mucous membranes, lymphoid organs and gonads. Thus, the common adverse effects are:

Bone Marrow Depression

Results in leukopenia, anemia, thrombocytopenia and in higher doses—aplastic anemia. In such patients, infections and bleeding are common.

Other Proliferating Cells

- GIT—stomatitis, esophagitis, glossitis and proctitis can be painful. Diarrhea and ulcers along the gut are common
- Alopecia (loss of hair)—partial to total alopecia is seen following treatment with most anticancer drugs but it is reversible and the hair grows after the chemotherapy is completed
- Reduced spermatogenesis in men and amenorrhea in women (due to damage to the germinal epithelium) can occur, for example, men treated with mechlorethamine for 6 months can become infertile.

Immediate Adverse Effects

Nausea and vomiting are very common with most cytotoxic drugs. They result from the stimulation of the CTZ and start about 4–6 hr after treatment and may continue for 1–2 days. Prior treatment with powerful antiemetics is required.

Hyperuricemia

Rapid tumor cell lysis can result in an increased plasma uric acid levels and may precipitate gout.

Teratogenicity

All cytotoxic drugs are teratogenic and are therefore contraindicated in pregnancy.

Carcinogenicity

Cytotoxic drugs themselves may cause secondary cancers, e.g. leukemias may follow the treatment of Hodgkin's lymphoma.

Measures to prevent adverse effects to anticancer drugs (Table 20.1).

Table 20.1: Measures to prevent the adverse effects of anticancer drugs	
Toxicity	*Measures*
Naysea, vomiting	Antiemetics: Ondansetron, granisetron, metoclopramide
Hyperuricemia	Allopurinol
Methotrexate toxicity	Folinic acid (10 mg)—dose as per blood methotrexate levels
Cystitis due to cyclophosphamide and Ifosfamide Myelosuppression	Mesna IV; n-acetyl cysteine—bladder wash
Anemia	Iron, blood transfusion
Leukemia	Erythropoietin
Thrombopoietin	G-CSF, GM-CSF
Nephrotoxicity due to cisplatin	Thrombocytopenia
Xerostomia due to radiation	Amifostine

Oral complications of chemotherapy
Ulceration and mucositis
Xerostomia
Generalized oral pain
Lymphadenopathy
Necrotizing ulcerative gingivitis
Hemorrhage
Oral mucositis

- Due to chemotherapy, interference with cellular mitosis decreases the regenerative ability of oral mucosa
- Common sites—labial mucosa, buccal mucosa, soft palate, floor of mouth and central surface of tongue.

Treatment (Table 20.2)

- Elimination of mechanical irritants
- Pain can be controlled by viscous xylocaine, benadryl

Table 20.2: Classification of drugs used in cancers
Alkylating agents
• *Nitrogen mustards* – Mechlorethamine, cyclophosphamide, Ifosfamide, chlorambucil, melphalan • *Ethylenimines* – Thiotepa • *Alkyl sulfonate* – Busulfan • *Nitrosoureas* – Carmustine, streptozotocin • *Triazine* – Dacarbazine
Antimetabolites
• *Folate antagonist* – Methotrexate, pemetrexed • *Purine Analogs* – mercaptopurine, thioguanine, pentostatin, fludarabine, cladribine • *Pyrimidine analogs* – 5-fluorouracil, fioxuridine, capecitabine, cytarabine (cytosine arabinoside) gemcitabine
Natural Products
• *Antibiotics* – Actinomycin-d (dactinomycin), daunorubicin, doxorubicin, bleomycin, mitomycin-C, mithramycin • *Epipodophyllotoxins* – Etoposide, teniposide • *Camptothecins* – Topotecan, irinotecan • *Taxanes* – Paclitaxel, docetaxel • *Vinca alkaloids* • Vincristine, vinblastine, vinorelbine
Miscellaneous
• Hydroxyurea, procarbazine, mitotane, 1-asparaginase, cisplatin, interferon alpha, imatinib
Hormones and their antagonists
• Glucocorticoids, androgens, antiandrogens, estrogens, antiestrogens, progestins, aromatase inhibitors

- Systemic analgesics—codeine, morphine
- Antibiotics
- Xerostomia
- Promotes the accumulation of oral bacteria which initiates dental caries
- Treatment—Sialagogs
- Replacing lost secretions—rehydration.

Radioactive Isotopes

- Some radioactive isotopes can be used in the treatment of certain specific cancers
- Radiophosphorus P^{32} is used in polycythemia vera. It is taken up by the bone where it emits β rays and has a half-life of about 14 days
- Strontium chloride emits β rays and has a longer half-life in the bony metastases. It is used to alleviate pain in painful bony metastases
- Radio active iodine I^{131} is used in the treatment of thyroid cancers.

BIOLOGICAL RESPONSE MODIFIERS

- Several agents are used to beneficially influence the patients' response to treatment and to overcome some adverse effects. These have also been termed biological response modifiers. They are as follows:
  - Hematopoietic growth factors like erythropoietin and myeloid growth factors like GM-CSF, G-CSF, M-CSF and thrombopoietin are used to treat bone marrow suppression
  - Interferons like interferon alpha are used in hairy cell leukemia, Kaposi's sarcoma and condylomata acuminata
  - Monoclonal antibodies are immunoglobulins that react specifically with antigens present on the cancer cells. Allergic reactions are common. Trastuzumab also enhances host immune responses and is useful in breast cancers. Rituximab attaches to antigens on the B cells causing lysis of these cells. It is used in B cell lymphomas
  - Aldesleukin is recombinant interleukin-2. It enhances cytotoxic activity of T-cells, induces activity of natural killer cells and also induces interferon production.

- Tretinoin (alltransretinoic acid) induces differentiation in leukemic cells and the leukemic promyelocytes loose their ability to proliferate. It is useful to induce remission in acute promyelocytic leukemia
- Amifostine has been designed to offer selective cytoprotection to normal tissues from the effects of cytotoxic drugs. Amifostine activates an enzyme in the normal tissues which can inactivate the active form of cisplatin and radiation. It has also been shown to stimulate the bone marrow in some bone marrow disorders. Amifostine is used to prevent toxicity due to cisplatin and radiation induced xerostomia (Table 20.3).

GENERAL PRINCIPLES IN THE TREATMENT OF CANCERS

Chemotherapy in most cancers (except the curable cancers) is generally palliative and suppressive. Because of the ability of cancers for recurrence. To avoid this it is essential to kill all the cells or as many cells as possible during treatment—to achieve what is known as 'Total cell kill'. Chemotherapy is just one of the modes in the treatment of cancer. Combination of drugs is preferred for synergistic effect, to reduce adverse effects and to prevent rapid development of resistance. Drugs which do not depress bone marrow are useful in combination regimens to avoid overlapping of adverse effects. With appropriate treatment, cure can now be achieved in a few cancers. Maintenance of good nutrition, treatment of anemia, protection against infections, adequate relief of pain and anxiety and good emotional support—all go a long way in the appropriate management of these dreaded diseases.

COMPONENTS OF CHEMOTHERAPY

Components of chemotherapy
Induction or Neo adjuvant chemotherapy
Adjuvant chemotherapy
Concurrent chemotherapy

Table 20.3: Choice of drugs in malignancies	
Malignancy	*Preferred drugs*
Acute lymphatic leukemia	Vincristine + prednisolone + L- asparaginase maintenance - Mercaptopurine/methotrexate, cyclophosphamide
Acute myeloid leukemia	Cytosine arabinoside + daunorubicin
Chronic lymphatic leukemia	Fludarabine/chlorambucil + prednisolone
Chronic myeloid leukemia	Hydroxyurea, busulfan Imatinib; interferons
Hodgkin's disease	MOPP M-Mechlorethamine O-Oncovin (vincristine) P-Procarbazine P-Prednisolone ABVD A-Adriamycin (doxorubicin) B-Bleomycin V-Vinblastin D-Dacarbazine
Non-Hodgkin's lymphoma	Cyclophosphamide + doxorubicin + vincristine (oncovin) + Prednisolone (CHOP)*
Multiple myeloma	Melphalan + prednisolone/vincristine + doxorubicin + dexamethasone
Carcinoma of the head and neck	Fluorouracil + cisplatin
In; CHOP, 'H ' stands for doxorubicin formerly called hydroxydaunomycin	

Induction or Neoadjuvant Chemotherapy

Use of chemotherapy in newly diagnosed patients without metastatic disease before primary surgery or radiotherapy.

Objectives

- Better drug delivery because of intact vascular bed
- Reduction of tumor bulk, to allow earlier application of definitive radiation
- Early eradiation of micrometastasis
- Higher doses and improved tolerance of chemotherapy with possibility that chemotherapy sensitive tumors may be cured with less aggressive surgery.

Disadvantage

- Delays potential curative surgery/radiotherapy in tumors non responsive to chemotherapy
- Noncompliance to surgery or radiation in patients who respond initially to chemotherapy and may loose the chance for cure
- Increased therapy related morbidity, cost and duration of treatment.

Drugs Used

Methotrexate, fluorouracil and leucovorin.

Adjuvant Chemotherapy

Chemotherapy given following definitive primary treatment like surgery and radiotherapy.

Objectives

- To eradicate the sub clinical persistent disease after surgery/radiotherapy and decrease the rate of loco-regions and distant relapse
- Has improved overall survival in locally advanced squamous cell carcinoma of head and neck but its role is unclear.

Concurrent Chemotherapy

Chemotherapy given along with radiotherapy.

Objectives

- To prevent the emerging of radioresistant colonies
- To inhibit the development of drug resistance
- To irradiate distant micrometastasis.

Drugs Used

Fluorouracil, bleomycin, mitomycin, methotrexate, cisplatin, carboplatin, hydroxyurea.

Disadvantages

- Administration of chemotherapy along with radiation increases toxicity and often necessitates interruption in radiotherapy
- Prolongation of total treatment has been adversely affecting the success of radiotherapy in squamous cell carcinoma of head and neck
- To overcome this problem, chemotherapy is administered in two different ways
- Chemotherapy + radiotherapy administered at full or nearly full dosage (split course radiotherapy)
- Chemotherapy and radiotherapy administered in rapid alteration interrupting one modality at the time while administrating the other.

Drugs Used

- Cisplatin (100 mg/m^2 every 3 weeks for 3 doses)
- Carboplatin (45 mg/m^2 for 5 days during weeks 1,3,5 and 7)
- Gemcitabine (150 mg/m^2/ week infusion).

Chemotherapy Both as Single Agent and Combination

Single Agent

- Palliative
- Used mostly in head and neck cancer of squamous cell carcinoma
- Response is of short duration averaging 3 months
- Patients benefits from less pain, better ability to swallow and having prolonged survival.

Drugs used

- Methotrexate (standard single agent for oral cancer)
- *Dose*: 40 mg/m^2 and 3 g/m^2 weekly for short treatment.

Other drugs

- Bleomycin, cisplatinum, fluorouracil, vinblastin.

Combination Therapy

- Used in recurrence of tumor after initial treatment with surgery/radiotherapy (Figs 20.2 and 20.3)
- Used for palliation of symptoms
- Prolong life.

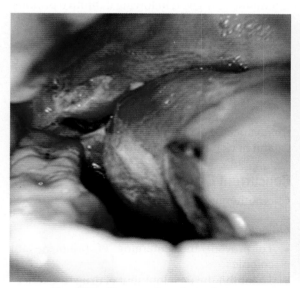

Fig. 20.2: Preoperative chemotherapy

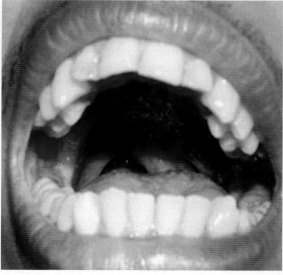

Fig. 20.3: Postchemotherapy

Drugs used
- Combination of cisplatin + methotrexate + bleomycin
- Combination of cisplatin + fluorouracil.

CASE STUDY

- Female aged 33 years
- Reported with painful swelling in right side of the face since 20 days
- Small painful swelling in right submandibular region (Fig. 20.4)
- After 10 days she consulted a local doctor
- Incision and drainage was tried
- The swelling rapidly grew to present size
- No contributory medical and dental history
- No history of drug allergy
- Personal history: Occasional tobacco chewer.

Clinical Examination

General Physical Examination
- Moderately built and nourished
- Vital signs within normal limits.

Extraoral Examination
- Gross facial asymmetry
- Solitary diffuse swelling noted over the right side of the face (Fig. 20.5)
- Measuring 15 × 15 cm.
- Periorbital edema (Fig. 20.6)
- Skin over the swelling appeared erythematous in areas.

Intraoral Examination
- Restricted mouth opening
- No signs of swelling noted intraorally
- Pericoronitis noted in relation to 48.

To summarize.........
A 33 years old female with a solitary, tender, rapidly growing diffuse inflammatory swelling, soft to firm in consistency, on the right side of the face since 20 days.
Provisional diagnosis: Fascial cellulitis?

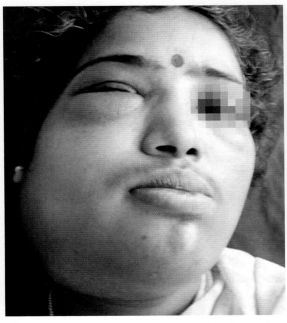

Fig. 20.4: Diffuse swelling over right side: Front view

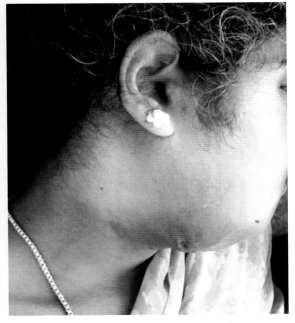

Fig. 20.5: Diffuse swelling over right side: Lateral view

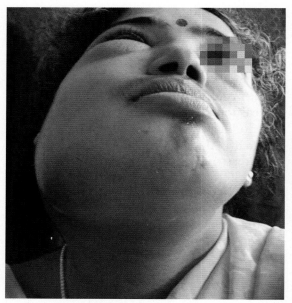

Fig. 20.6: Facial asymmetry with periorbital edema

PANORAMIC RADIOGRAPH (FIGS 20.7 TO 20.14)

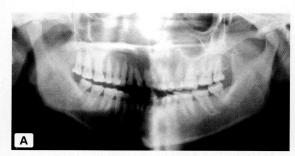

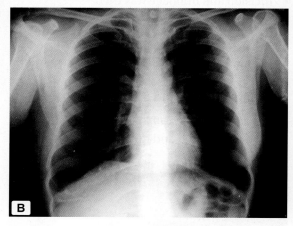

Fig. 20.7A and B: Chest X-ray

Differential Diagnosis

- Infected right fascial spaces?
- Infected sarcoma?
- Metastasis from supraclavicular primary tumor?
  - Thyroid
  - Salivary gland
- Metastasis from infraclavicular primary tumor?
  - Lung
  - Esophageal.

Routine Blood Investigations

Raised neutrophil count.

Differential Diagnosis

- Infected sarcoma
- Malignant salivary gland tumor
  - Culture results negative.

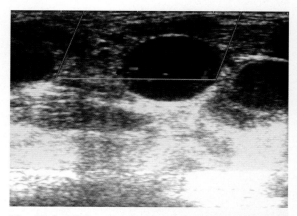

Fig. 20.8: USG—color doppler showing increased soft tissue mass

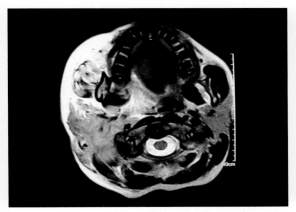

Fig. 20.9: MRI axial showing extensive homogenous hypotense mass

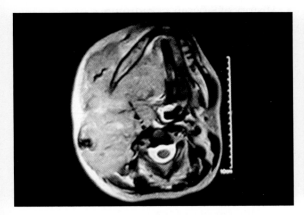

Fig. 20.10: Coronal View hypotense mass

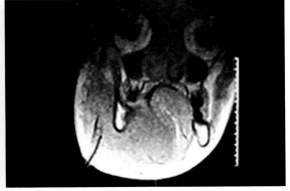

Fig. 20.11: ELISA HIV negative

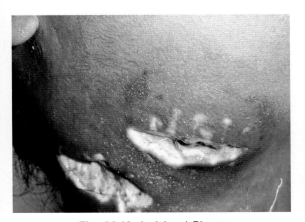

Fig. 20.12: Incisional Biopsy

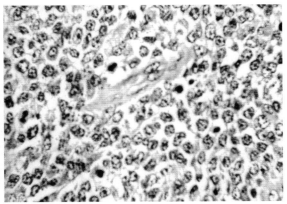

Fig. 20.13: Histopathology (I)

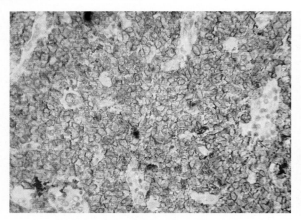

Fig. 20.14: Histopathology (II)

Immunohistochemistry

- CD-20:Positive
- CD-3: Negative

Summary

- Rapidly growing soft tissue swelling in 33 yr female
- Not responding to antibiotics
- No obvious odontogenic cause
- USG increased soft tissue mass
- MRI extensive homogenous hypointense mass
- Histopathology: immature lymphoblast.

Final Diagnosis

Extranodal non-Hodgkin's lymphoma ANN-ARBOR stage II E.

Management

Chemotherapy

CHOP regimen: 4 drugs
1. Cyclophosphamide.
2. Doxorubicin.
3. Vincristine.
4. Prednisone.

Post-chemotherapy

- Lymphomas are a heterogenous group of neoplastic disorders originating from the lymphoreticular system

- Lymphomas account for 4–5 percent of all neoplasms
- Non-Hodgkin's lymphoma accounts for 65 percent
- Incidence is low in Asia.

Williams et al, Hematology 4th edition 1991
Shohat et al Oral Surg, Oral Med, Oral pathol 2004:97:328-31.

ETIOLOGY

Unknown.

Predisposing Factors

- Exposure to drugs or infectious agent
- History of Sjögren's syndrome
- Immunosuppression
- Previous irradiation
- Williams et al. Hematology 4th edition 1991
  Stenson et al. Am J of Otolar 1996;17(4);276-80.

PATHOGENESIS (FIG. 20.15)

Clinical Presentation

- Males
- 5th–7th decades
- Tonsil- Waldeyers ring (34%) followed by salivary glands (15%)
- Swelling or mass (59%)
- Pain and dysphagia (7%)
- Primary osseous lymphoma accounts for 4% of all ENH
- Mandible is most common site presenting as osteolytic lesion
- Hart et al. Clinical Oncology 2004;16;186-92
- Bryan et al. The Lancet Onc 2004:5:341-53
- Gusenbauer et al. J O M S 1990;46;409-15.

CLASSIFICATION

Working Formulation

Low Grade

- Small lymphocytic
- Follicular small cleaved cell
- Follicular mixed cell

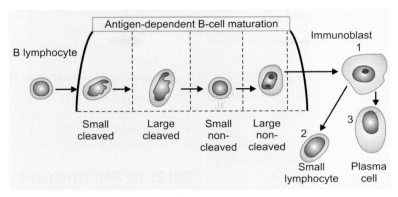

Fig. 20.15: Pathogenesis of cancer cell

Intermediate Grade
- Follicular large cell
- Diffuse mixed cell
- Diffuse large cell

High Grade
- Immunoblastic
- Lymphoblastic
- Rosenberg et al Cancer 1982;49;2112-35.

REVISED EUROPEAN-AMERICAN LYMPHOMA [REAL]

B-Cell Neoplasms
- Precursor b-cell neoplasms
- Peripheral B-cell neoplasms
- Mental cell lymphoma
- Follicle cell lymphoma
- Marginal zone b-cell lymphoma
- Hairy cell leukemia
- Lymphoplasmacytoid lymphoma
- Diffuse large B-cell lymphoma
- Burkitt's lymphoma.

T Cell and NK Cell Neoplasms
- Precursor T cell neoplasms
- Peripheral T cell neoplasms
- Mycosis fungoides
- Peripheral T cell lymphoma
- Angiocentric lymphoma

- Angioimmunoblastic T cell lymphoma
- Anaplastic large cell lymphoma.

Hodgkin's Disease
Harris, et al Blood 1994;84(5);1361-92.

Staging
- ANN-ARBOR staging
- *Stage I:* Involvement of a single lymph node region or of a single extranodal organ or site (IE)
- *Stage II:* Involvement of two or more lymph node regions on the same side of the diaphragm, or localized involvement of an extranodal site or organ (IIE) and one or more lymph node regions on the same side of the diaphragm
- *Stage III:* Involvement of lymph node regions on both sides of the diaphragm, which may also be accompanied by localized involvement of an extranodal organ or site (IIIE) or spleen (IIIS) or both (IIISE)
- *Stage IV:* Diffuse or disseminated involvement of one or more distant extranodal organs with or without associated lymph node involvement.

Systemic Symptoms
- A-No symptoms
- B-Weight loss >10% in 6 months, fever, night sweats
- Carbone et al. Cancer Res 1971;31;1860.

RECOMMENDED PROCEDURE FOR STAGING

General

1. History and physical examination.
2. Pathologic diagnosis from biopsy specimen with review by an experienced hematopathologist.
3. Laboratory studies: complete blood count, blood chemistry, LDH ,beta-2 microglobulin, uric acid, renal and liver function HIV testing.
4. Bone marrow aspiration and biopsy .
5. Chest X-ray, CT scan of chest, abdomen, and pelvis.

Additional

1. Ultrasonography and MRI to clarify CT scan abnormalities.
2. Gallium scan in large masses.
3. Lumbar puncture.
4. Gastrointestinal studies.
5. CT scan or MRI of brain.
6. MRI to detect bone marrow involvement.

Swan et al. J Clin Oncol 1989;7:1518–27.

SPREAD OF ORAL LYMPHOMA

- Lymphatic spread via cervical lymph nodes to extranodal organs
- Contiguous spread to adjacent organs
- Blood-borne distant metastases
- Takahashi et al. J Oral Max Surg 1990;46;409-15.

TREATMENT OPTIONS

Radiotherapy

- 2000–2500 cGy—palliative therapy
- 4500–5000 cGy—curative therapy.

CHEMOTHERAPY

- CHOP-Cyclophosphamide: 750 mg/m^2 IV
  - Oncovin: 1.4 mg/m^2 IV
  - Adriamycin: 50 mg/m^2 IV
  - Prednisone: 100 mg

- **MOPP**- Nitrogen mustard-6 mg/m^2 IV
  - Oncovin-1.4 mg/m^2 IV
  - Prednisone-40 mg/m^2
  - Procarbazine-100 mg/m^2
- Williams et al. Hematology 4th edition 1991.

Monoclonal Antibodies - Bryan et al.
- Rituximab-anti CD-20 antibody
- Tositumomab-anti CD-20 antibody
- Alemtuzumab-anti CD-52 antibody.

ROLES OF RADIOTHERAPY

Madam Curie discovered radium in 1878. Same year it was used for treatment of cancer.
Alexander Grahambell wrote a letter to Dr Sowers in 1903 to try placing radium into very heart of tumor.

Introduction

The main aim of delivering radiation in treating malignancies is to treat the tumor and spare normal tissues. In this direction medical technology has revolutionized the way radiation was delivered using deep X-ray and the present use of advanced medical linear accelerators with sophisticated computer software.

- Radiation therapy may be used alone for the treatment for head and neck cancer, or it may be used before/after surgery for the combined modality treatment of patients with high-risk cancers
- Many advanced but resectable head and neck cancers require both surgery and radiation therapy for optimal control
- For early to intermediate cancers, either radiation therapy or surgery alone may lead to equivalent control
- For most early oral cavity cancers, a functional outcome is best achieved by resection and reconstruction, if needed
- In contrast, small glottic tumors located near the commissures are more expediently treated and have better functional outcomes with radiation therapy.

Types of Radiation

- X-rays produced electrically are the primary modality used in radiation therapy for head and neck cancer. Other modalities for external radiation therapy (teletherapy) are electrons, also produced electrically, and gamma rays, which are derived from cobalt-60 sources
- Radioactive sources such as cesium 137, iodine 125, or iridium 192 also produce gamma rays and can be placed directly into (interstitial brachytherapy) or next to (intracavitary brachytherapy) a tumor
- Less commonly used and highly specialized external modalities
- Gamma rays and X-rays behave identically both physically and biologically once they are formed both are photons (packets of energy without mass or charge).

Definitive	Radiotherapy alone for early larynx cancer
Preoperative	Radiotherapy before neck dissection for a fixed nodal mass
Postoperative	Postoperative radiotherapy after composite resection of oral cancer
Palliative	Radiotherapy for massive incurable head or neck cancer causing pain or bleeding
Benign	Radiotherapy for refractory keloids of the skin

- The only difference is the origin. X-rays are made electronically from some type of X-ray machine, whereas gamma rays are emitted from the disintegration of unstable radioactive isotopes (radioactive decay)
- The energies of all therapeutic radiations are sufficient to break chemical bonds in critical targets primarily DNA within tumor cells, leading to cellular death.

Pro-surgery	Pro-radiotherapy
Relatively quick, expeditious treatment	Avoids prolonged general anesthesia; few medical contraindications
Ability to assess prognosis through pathologic assessment of specimen (e.g. margins) and alter treatment accordingly (e.g. add postoperative radiotherapy or additional surgery)	Lower risk of systemic complications (e.g. sepsis, pneumonia, pulmonary embolism, acute treatment mortality)
Avoids risk of permanent radiation xerostomia and other late dental or oral complications	Ability to more easily treat a larger volume of potential occult microscopic disease (e.g. both sides of neck, base of skull, supraclavicular fossa)
Preserves the ability to use radiotherapy in the future, if needed	Ability to preserve normal anatomic structure, cosmesis, and often function
Avoids the risk of radiation carcinogenesis (thyroid, sarcoma) in young patients	Treatment can usually be given on an outpatient basis, and many patients can continue to work during treatment

X-ray Energy: Orthovoltage and Megavoltage

- In diagnostic X-ray machines, the electrons are accelerated toward the target by being placed within a large potential difference, they are attracted to the positively charged anode and accelerate toward it proportionate to the potential difference applied across the circuit. A target is placed at the anode
- This is a highly inefficient process, as more than 99 percent of energy is lost to heat
- This technique limits the maximal velocity achievable by the electrons and thus limits the maximal energy of the X-rays that are created. This energy range up to hundreds of kilovolts is sufficient for diagnostic imaging and was used historically for orthovoltage Xx-ray therapy; it is now used only for selected skin cancers
- X-rays for modern radiation therapy are made by a linear accelerator, which uses microwaves for electron acceleration. Microwaves are nonionizing electromagnetic radiations. The electrons can be conceptualized as being accelerated by riding the crests of the microwaves

- Electron velocity approaches 90 percent of the speed of light. This is a much more efficient process and leads to X-rays with energies measured in the millions of megavoltage radiation
- Lower-energy X-rays deposit their maximal energy at or near the skin surface, leaving little energy for greater depths
- This makes them efficient for use in the treatment of cutaneous lesions but extremely inefficient for the treatment of nodal or mucosal carcinomas at depths beyond 2 cm from the skin surface
- Higher-energy X-rays beams deposit their maximal energy below the skin surface (skin sparing) and penetrate more deeply
- An additional disadvantage of lower energy X-rays is that they interact with tissues dependent on the atomic number (number of protons) of the tissue, raised to the third power (photoelectric effect). Because the difference between the atomic number of soft tissue and of bone is approximately two, this means that diagnostic and orthovoltage X-ray energy, in principle, is absorbed up to eight times more by bone than by soft tissue
- This is highly undesirable for treatment of mucosal head and neck cancers, however, because the surrounding bones of the jaw and skull would absorb far more energy than the tumor
- There are three main advantages of megavoltage radiotherapy:
  - The higher-energy X-rays deposit at greater depths, allowing for a more homogeneous dose in the treatment of tumors at any head and neck location and at any internal depth
  - The maximal energy is deposited approximately 1 cm deep to the skin surface. Thus megavoltage radiation therapy is skin sparing. Even though patients may develop bothersome skin reactions during megavoltage radiation therapy, they are much less severe than the reactions occurring with orthovoltage treatment
  - Megavoltage radiation therapy is bone sparing. Megavoltage radiation is absorbed differently in tissues owing to the Compton effect, which is independent of atomic number. Therefore, bone and soft tissue within the irradiated volume absorb approximately the same doses.

Steps Involved in clinical radiation therapy
Consultation, including decision to irradiate.
Preradiation work-up, including staging, dental evaluation, nutritional assessment
Simulation, including immobilization of the area to be irradiated
Dosimetry (calculation of radiation dose to tumor and normal structures)
Setup or final quality assurance planning session
Radiation treatments, including on-treatment visits by the physician(s)
Conedown(s) if applicable: repeat of steps 3 through 6
Postradiation follow-up visits

Radiation Therapy Simulation, Treatment Planning, and Dosimetry

- "Simulation" process is designed to place the radiation field and its dose where the tumor is, while excluding as much of the surrounding normal tissue as possible
- In order to aim the radiation beam, a diagnostic X-ray energy machine called a simulator is used. The simulator is mechanically and optically identical to the treatment linear accelerator, except that it allows for fluoroscopy and uses diagnostic energy X-rays instead of a megavoltage X-ray. The resulting diagnostic-quality images facilitate aiming of the beam by visualizing internal structures
- The majority of treatment fields are set up isocentrically. This means that the patient is positioned so that the center of the tumor target volume corresponds to a point in space representing the intersection of the center of the radiation beam coming from the head of

the machine and a line through the center of the axis of the rotation of the gantry

- Because the radiation gantry moves in a 360-degree circle around the patient, the isocentric technique guarantees that the center of the radiation field always corresponds to the center of the tumor target volume. This allows radiation to be delivered in multiple beams from any angle; they intersect and deliver an additive dose to the tumor while traversing different normal tissues, thereby minimizing their dose accumulation and consequent risk for toxicity and injury.

Beam Angles and Fields

- Once a patient is immobilized, the radiation oncologist determines the specific beam angles to be used. Critical normal structures in the entry-exit path have a major impact on beam selection
- The entire neck from the lower limit of the clavicle to the skull base requires treatment for most patients. Because opposed anterior and posterior fields do not allow for selective shielding of critical structures such as the eyes or spinal cord, it is common to use right and left lateral opposed fields
- Wedge pair for lateralized tumors confines radiation and its toxicities, especially mucositis and xerostomia, to one side with a wedge-shaped dose distribution
- It is the role of radiation dosimetry to determine the appropriate number of radiation pulses or monitor units required to deliver the prescribed daily dose for a specifically sized and shaped radiation field for an individual patient, accounting for his or her size, shape, surface contour, thickness, and tissue homogeneity
- As a result of this process, graphic representations of radiation dose distribution (dose range and homogeneity) within a treatment volume, called isodose plots, are generated
- With segmental imaging techniques of CT and MRI, radiation oncologists began using more unusual beam angles

- This requires reliance on the imaging and computerized planning system for both placement and verification of radiation ports. The ability to use unusual field angles shaped by highly conformal shielding blocks represents three-dimensional or conformal, treatment planning
- The main advantage of these techniques is the potential for the delivery of higher radiation doses to the tumor with the goal of improving control, while minimizing dose and toxicity to critical normal structures
- X-ray fields are rectangular, and the borders are defined by collimators. These X-ray fields are set up for individual patients at the time of simulation. Fluoroscopy allows for rapid placement of fields and verification with diagnostic-quality X-ray films, called simulation films
- The radiation oncologist can further customize the shape of the port within the rectangular radiation treatment field by the addition of shielding blocks made of a lead alloy called cerrobend. This allows for the protection of sensitive normal structures not at cancer risk.

Course of Radiation Therapy and its Toxicities Risks and Potential Complications

- A typical course of radiation therapy for head and neck cancer is delivered 5 days per week, Monday through Friday, over 7 weeks for 35 fractions. Each individual treatment takes a few minutes
- There are no immediate side effects for most patients. There is one exception: about 5 percent of patients develop a self-limited parotitis after the first fraction that spontaneously resolves in 1 to 2 days
- Toxicities that occur during or shortly after the completion of radiation therapy are called acute effects, and those that occur several months or longer after completion of radiation therapy are called late effects
- The acute effects generally start after 2–3 weeks, and include dermatitis, swelling, mucositis,

permanent xerostomia, and usually temporary loss of taste

- Irradiation does not appreciably affect tissue temperature, but the acute skin reaction resembles a suntan or, if severe, a burn. The skin adnexa are also affected, leading to epilation and dryness
- Mucositis is manifested by pain, odynophagia. Weight loss
- Temporal bone radiation may lead to serous otitis media, which is generally self-limited but may require myringotomy
- Nasal radiation leads to crusting. There will be temporary hoarseness if the larynx is irradiated
- Xerostomia begins within the first week of radiotherapy, progresses, and is generally permanent. Studies indicate a 35 percent to 50 percent decrease in stimulated salivary flow at the end of the first week of radiotherapy. This increases to an 80 percent to 90 percent decrement by the end of radiotherapy. Serous acini are more radiosensitive, so patients are left with more scant and viscid secretions
- Excretion was maintained in all salivary glands exposed to 25 Gy or less, and in about 50 percent of salivary glands at doses of 25–45 Gy. Recent studies suggest that pilocarpine and amifostinell may either palliate or reduce xerostomia. Dilute salt and baking soda oral irrigations help dissipate radiation-induced thick secretions
- Expected late effects include chronic skin changes such as mild altered pigmentation, epilation, telangiectasia, edema, and subcutaneous induration
- The severe form of bone damage is osteoradionecrosis (ORN). Meticulous pretreatment evaluation is required so that patients with dental problems can have bad teeth restored or extracted. All teeth maintained must receive adequate lifetime dental prophylaxis, including daily fluoride treatment and a rigorous hygiene program
- ORN can occur in any cancellous bone but is seen most often in the mandible. ORN of the mandible is defined as an area of gingival dehiscence lasting more than 6 months in which nonvital bone is exposed and does not heal with local wound care
- ORN occurs sporadically and spontaneously in half of cases but occurs more predictably as a result of trauma
- If dental extraction or invasive surgery is required after radiotherapy, hyperbaric oxygen (HBO) therapy has been shown to decrease the risk of ORN from about 30–5 percent
- The spinal cord is irradiated in many head and neck setups. If the dose exceeds the tolerance a complication is possible. Acute transient radiation myelopahty (ATRM), or Lhermitte's syndrome, is characterized by shock-like tingling paresthesias radiating to the extremities
- ATRM is thought to be a result of transient demyelination of the posterior columns
- It usually starts 1–3 months following radiation and is thought to be self-limited, lasting 1–9 months
- Transverse myelopathy generally starts 6–18 months following radiotherapy and represents irreversible lower motor neuron injury. This is probably the most feared of all radiation complications, as it may progress to the loss of all spinal cord function
- The generally accepted tolerance of the spinal cord is 45–50 Gy
- If the thyroid is irradiated, at least one-third of patients will develop abnormally high thyroid-stimulating hormone levels. Patients may not become symptomatic for some time, but this overstimulation may lead to the development of thyroid nodules and tumors. Screening for hypothyroidism is part of routine surveillance.

Shrinking Field or Cone-down Technique

- Radiation therapy is fractionated over many weeks, and the beam angles, field sizes, and techniques of delivery are altered to maximize a differential effect on the tumor while limiting the effects on normal tissue

- The larger the deposit of tumor cells, the greater the dose of radiation therapy required for control. Grossly visible tumor requires at least the full prescribed radiation dose, whereas microscopic disease several centimeters away may be eradicated with a 10–20 percent lower dose
- Other regions "at risk" even farther from the gross and microscopic tumor may require an even smaller dose because of an even smaller tumor cell infestation. This allows the radiation oncologist to use a shrinking field or conedown technique in which newer, smaller fields are used successively during the course of radiation therapy
- A constant radiation dose per fraction is administered, but to progressively smaller volumes. This technique allows for reducing the volume of normal tissues, especially mucosa, exposed to the highest doses of radiation therapy, thereby limiting toxicity
- Additionally, changing beam angles to traverse different areas of normal tissue. spreads out the entry-exit path dose so that the same normal tissue areas surrounding the treatment volume do not receive the cumulative dose
- The reality of cure for an individual patient is dependent on the elimination of the last tumor cell. A constant proportion of tumor cells is killed with each fraction of radiation therapy. This may vary from less than 40–60 or more
- There is no absolute resistance to radiation therapy, unlike the potential for tumor cell survival with chemotherapy
- This is because whereas the cell membrane may be an absolute barrier to the entry of, or a mechanism for eliminating, chemotherapy drugs, the cell membrane is not a barrier to ionizing radiation therapy
- Clinically, there can be relative resistance to specific doses of radiation therapy for individual tumors, and in some cases, the total dose required for cure exceeds that which the surrounding normal tissue can tolerate
- In principle, almost all tumors can be controlled by radiation therapy if a sufficiently high dose is delivered. It is the normal tissue tolerance that limits the dose prescribed.

Brachytherapy

- Brachytherapy represents an alternative technique for a final cone down boost. The radioactive source may be placed directly into tumors, called interstitial brachytherapy (e.g. for tongue or floor of the mouth tumors), or adjacent to tumors, called intracavitary brachytherapy (e.g. for nasopharynx tumors)
- The advantage of brachytherapy is based on the inverse square effect described earlier, in which an extremely high dose of radiation is delivered to the tumor while delivering a much lower dose to the surrounding normal tissue. Effective brachytherapy requires surgical skills and appropriate resources
- Brachytherapy is established and indicated as a boost for early nasopharynx cancers, is considered by most a requisite for definitive treatment of early oral tongue and floor of the mouth cancers, and is used commonly for base of the tongue cancers. Brachytherapy can, in principle, be applied to any other head and neck site and is limited only by the imagination of the therapist.

Fractionation

- *Fractionation* refers to the schedule on which the radiation dose is administered
- Standard radiotherapy is administered daily, 5 days a week, with weekends off. In an effort to maximize damage to the more rapidly dividing tumor cells while sparing normal tissues as much as possible, fractionation schedules have been altered
- It is now well recognized that there is a clinical advantage to multiple-exposure therapy. Multiple fractions controlled tumors better than single larger doses, and, paradoxically, normal tissues tolerated repeated small doses better than single large doses
- *Accelerated fractionation* refers to an overall reduction in treatment time accomplished by giving two or more daily dose fractions of close to conventional size.
- *Hyperfractionation* implies that the overall treatment time is conventional or slightly

	Table 20.4: Site specific radiotherapy	
Site	Indication	Technique
Oral tongue/floor of mouth	Radiotherapy (mandatory boost)	Interstitial: Implant via submental approach
Base of tongue	Radiotherapy boost or for palliation after local failure	As for oral tongue
Nasopharynx	Radiotherapy boost or for palliation after local failure	Intracavitary: Insertion using nasogastric or endoracheal tube
Neck	Postoperative radiotherapy after incomplete resection	Interstital: Temporary catheter implant or permanent iodine 125 seed placement into operative bed

reduced, but an increase in total dose is achieved by giving two or more small-dose fractions on each treatment day. Each of these regimens is associated with varying degrees of early and late toxicities

- For example, some clinicians feel that long-term effects such as osteoradionecrosis are increased with hyperfractionated schedules, especially when combined with concomitant chemotherapy
- The radiobiologic principles explaining why fractionation allows for tumor control without local necrosis are the "four R's":

"Four R's"
Repair
Reoxygenation
Repopulation, and
Redistribution

- *Repair* is a series of enzymatic processes of intracellular mechanisms for healing intracellular radiation damage. Patients who lack enzymes that are important for DNA repair are extraordinarily sensitive to radiation injury
- *Reoxygenation* The sensitivity of tumor cells to the lethal effects of radiation varies with the local oxygen concentration. There may be as much as a 2.5–3-fold ranges of sensitivity to cell killing, depending on oxygen concentration
- There is a gradient of oxygenation and hypoxia within a tumor. When a fraction of radiation is applied, the more radiosensitive oxygenated cells will be killed, and there will be relative sparing of hypoxic cells

- Reoxygenation represents the process by which the oxygen gradient is restored to the remaining hypoxic cells in the interval between radiation therapy fractions, restoring the potential for further cell killing
- It has also been suggested that more hypoxic tumors would be more radioresistant. Recent data on several human tumors suggest that oxygen measurements made by an interstitial needle, the Eppendorf probe, may predict tumor behavior and response to treatment
- In general, more hypoxic tumors have lower local control and a greater probability for the development of distant metastases, independent of whether treatment is with surgery or radiation therapy
- More recently, the hypoxic toxin tirapazamine has been shown to augment radiation response in experimental models by selectively killing hypoxic cells not killed by radiation exposure *Repopulation*, which refers to the ability of various cell populations to divide in the interval between radiation therapy fractions.
- Accelerated repopulation may occur in tumors during radiotherapy, so it is important to complete any planned course as quickly as possible (i.e. minimizing unscheduled interruptions)
- Some fractionation schedules are designed to get the total dose even more quickly (accelerated fractionation) to minimize the effect of tumor regrowth

Redistribution this reflects the relative variability of cell radiosensitivity throughout the cell cycle. In some cell lines, relative radiosensitivity can vary threefold from one part of the cell cycle to another.

- In general, the cells are considered to be the most radiosensitive during the mitotic phase (late G2) and most radioresistant in late S-phase.
- Clinical radiotherapy represents the balance among the four R's for tumor versus normal tissue.

Fractionation schedules can be defined by
Dose per fraction
Number of fractions per day
Overall treatment time
Total cumulative radiation dose

Radiosensitization and Radioresistance

- In clinical radiation therapy, it is noted that some tumors shrink more rapidly than others during a course of radiation therapy. The rate of relative tumor regression can be described as its Radioresponsiveness. The rate of tumor regression depends on the time to expression of its lethal injury
- It is generally accepted that most irradiated head and neck squamous cancer cells undergo a mitotic death, or loss of clonogenicity. A tumor cell with a lethal injury may live for some time but must attempt to divide before expressing that injury. In other words, a tumor cell "does not know it is dead, until it tries to divide"
- Thus the underlying rate of tumor cell turnover that determines the rate of tumor regression, or radioresponsiveness
- There is no absolute relationship between the rate of tumor response and its ultimate control. Radiation-induced cell killing may even persist for many weeks after the completion of radiation therapy

- Although it is possible to achieve control of some tumors when a mass persists at the end of radiation therapy, this is uncommon in practical terms. For carcinomas that are not cleared toward or by the end of radiation therapy, durable control is uncommon
- Radiosensitizers are agents that enhance the radiation effect without having any necessary direct antitumor effects
- The strongest radiation sensitizer ever discovered is oxygen. Many early experiments with radiosensitizers involved various modes of oxygen delivery or the use of drugs that mimicked the effect of oxygen.

Preoperative and Postoperative Radiation Therapy

- Many patients with stage III and IV head and neck cancer are at high risk for local regional recurrence even after gross total resection of their cancers. The combination of surgery and radiation therapy can improve local regional control and perhaps survival
- The most common approach involves the use of postoperative radiation therapy. This allows the surgeon to operate on tissues unaffected by radiation therapy, it allows for surgical staging to identify areas at highest risk.

The indications for postoperative radiation therapy include
Large infiltrating tumors
Compromised margins of surgical resection
Perineural spread
Extension of the tumor into the deep soft tissues or bone
Multiple lymph nodes
Large lymph nodes
Extracapsular nodal spread

Generally, postoperative radiation therapy is initiated 4–6 weeks after surgery, or earlier if practical.

- This is based on several retrospective studies suggesting that further delays may compromise tumor control and survival. There is a suggestion that the overall treatment package time from the time of surgery until the completion of radiation therapy may also be an important factor for tumor control and possibly survival. This is based on the concept of accelerated repopulation of tumor clonogens
- It is therefore important that patients undergo oral medicine evaluation very early. If dental restorations or extractions are required, these must be done at or close to the time of ablative surgery so that all surgical wounds can heal during the same interval, avoiding a delay in starting radiation therapy
- Planned preoperative radiation therapy has been used in the past for tumors thought to be unresectable or at high-risk for incomplete resection

- This technique has generally fallen out of favor because it is now believed that if a tumor is initially unresectable, preoperative radiation therapy will not make it so
- Radiation therapy may be helpful, however, for borderline resectable tumors, particularly large neck nodes
- Theoretical advantages of preoperative radiation therapy are that blood supply may be better than after surgery, leading to improved oxygenation, and that tumor seeding during surgery may be decreased
- Major disadvantages of preoperative radiation therapy are the loss of definitive tumor staging and the lower doses given because of concern about an increase in surgical morbidity
- Many tumors will regress within 6–8 weeks of RT. Preoperative RT has been limited to 45–50 Gy in total dose to avoid incidence of postoperative complications (Figs 20.16A to C)

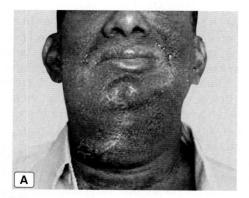

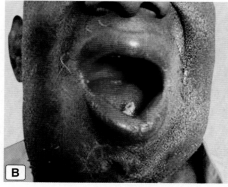

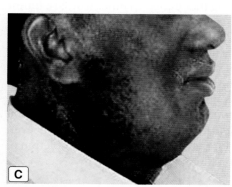

Figs 20.16A to C: Postradiotherapy skin changes

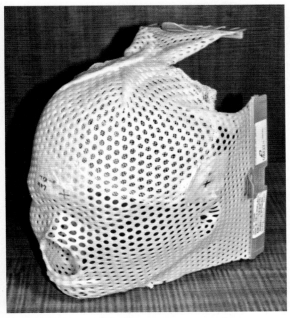

Fig. 20.17: Radioprotective shield

- Planned preoperative radiation therapy usually involves a lower dose of radiation therapy 50–60 Gy using a protective shield (Fig. 20.17) and is followed by surgery in approximately 4–8 weeks.
- There is a "window of opportunity" for surgery when the acute inflammation of radiation is optimally resolving but the chronic sequelae of fibrosis and vascular changes that impede wound healing are not pronounced
- Salvage surgery, in contrast, is performed on an unplanned basis generally months to years after the completion of full dose (65–70 Gy) radiation therapy
- This is done for recurrent or persistent cancers that are associated with poorer outcomes with respect to tumor control and greater normal tissue complications because of more pronounced late effects
- The main use of postradiation surgery involves management of the neck when there is initial gross nodal disease. Lymph nodes less than 2 to 3 cm can generally be well controlled with radiation therapy alone. Although radiation therapy may control larger nodal masses, the frequency and reliability of this control are lower
- It is therefore accepted that when radiation therapy is selected as the modality to control the primary tumor, neck dissection may be added if there is an initial gross lymph node independent of the response to radiation therapy
- Even with complete clinical tumor clearance, studies have shown that up to 40 percent of neck dissection specimens harbor tumor cells thought to be viable.

Radiation Therapy: Sites and Subsites (Fig. 20.18)

Carcinoma Oral Tongue

- Exophytic T1 and T2 superficial lesions of the anterior 3rd and tip without deep muscle invasion best treated with wide local excision
- T1 and T2 lesions of middle 3rd and which require more extensive resection up to hemiglossectomy are better treated by radical RT
- Posteriorly seated tumors with infiltration into tongue base are better treated EBRT or with surgery and postop RT
- Extension into gingiva or mandible is contraindicated for RT alone as subsequent ORN may develop.

Carcinoma Floor of Mouth

- For tumors more than 4 cm, brachytherapy is a relative contraindication because an interstitial implant will result in local soft-tissue ulceration and risk of ORN due to the decreased distance between gingival mucosa and bone (Fig. 29.19)
- Interstitial implant is suitable for small tumors (T1 lesions with well-demarcated borders). For T3 or T4 lesions, combined EBRT (preoperative or postoperative) and surgery is appropriate.

Buccal Mucosa

In small superficial T1 tumors, surgery and RT can be used. In lesions larger than 1 cm, neck dissection is preferred to EBRT with the primary treated with brachytherapy.

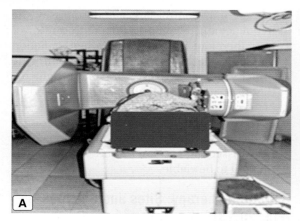
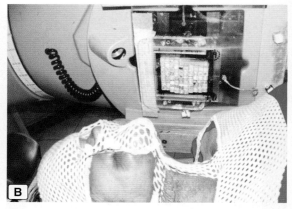

Figs 20.18A and B: Cobalt radiotharapy unit

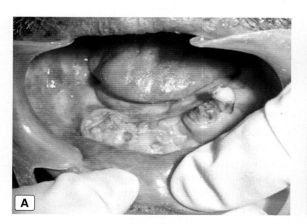
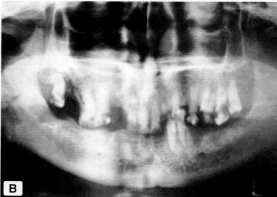

Figs 20.19A and B: Case of osteoradionecrosis post-radiotherapy

Maxillary Tumors

- Tumors of the maxilla are generally first treated with surgery postoperative RT is indicated in all except small lesions resected with wide margins. The retro maxillary prevertebral space is generally included to cover lymphatic drainage
- In tumors of the antrum, the orbit is not included in the treatment volume. Shielding of the orbital contents is mandatory
- Tumors of the PNS need an extended irradiation volume to include the medial border of the contralateral sinus. The ethmoid sinuses are also included.

Management of Neck

- In large and less well differentiated. tumors of the tongue, floor of the mouth, gingiva, buccal mucosa without clinical involvement of the lymph node, elective (adjuvant) RT is performed
- Combined RT and neck dissection is the procedure of choice in for N1 and N2 neck after the primary lesion is controlled. Postoperative RT is also indicated in patients with extracapsular extension in the histospecimen.

Salivary Gland Tumors

Indication
Perineural invasion of tumor
Locoregional LN mets
Incomplete or marginal resection
High-grade malignancy
Extraparotid extension of tumor
Tumor cell spill during surgery
Enucleation of tumor

Advances in Radiation Therapy

- Other particles that can be used for the treatment of head and neck cancer include protons and neutrons. Neutrons and protons have equivalent masses of approximately 2000 times the mass of an electron. Neutrons have no charge, and protons have a unit charge of +1. The use of neutrons has been mainly experimental, except in the treatment of unresectable salivary neoplasms
- The main advantage of neutrons is enhanced biologic efficiency. For any unit distance traveled by a neutron, there is a higher degree of ionization than with most other forms of radiation therapy. Neutrons cause substantially more ionizing damage than X-rays, protons, or electrons. This deposition of energy per unit length or density of ionization is called linear energy transfer (LET). The advantage of neutrons is based on their high LET characteristics. A given dose of neutrons thus leads to greater tissue damage in both tumors and normal tissue than does the same dose of photons. The goal, as always in radiation therapy, is a therapeutic index. Neutrons are thus said to have a greater relative biologic effect (RBE)
- Protons and other heavy charged particles have a unique way of depositing their doses. Toward the end of their deceleration process deep in tissue, protons stop abruptly and rapidly deposit their energy in what is called the, Bragg peak. This limits the ionization process to a well-defined area near the terminal range of the proton
- The biologic qualities LET and RBE of protons are very similar to those of photons. The major advantage of protons is this physical property. The use of protons allows for the placement of a tightly defined three dimensional volume of dose deposition while sparing the surrounding normal tissue. This is particularly helpful in central locations, for example, at or near the optic apparatus and pituitary region. Protons and electrons deposit their energies at opposite ends of their paths: electrons earlier, and protons later
- The main aim of delivering radiation in treating malignancies is to treat the tumor and spare normal tissues. In this direction medical technology has revolutionized the way radiation was delivered using deep X-ray and Tele cobalt machines in 60s and 70s and the present use of Advanced medical linear accelerators with sophisticated computer software.

3D CRT

- Telecobalt machines, with Co-60 as the source of radiation, were first installed in the early 1950s. They become highly popular and continued to dominate the radiotherapy scenario till the 70s when Medical Linear accelerator was installed
- The treatment was given two dimensionally where normal tissues and the tumor was irradiated as a conventional treatment
- But the main goal of radiotherapy is to deliver high radiation dose to the tumor with as less as possible dose to the normal tissues
- During the past two decades, advances in radiological imaging and computer technology have significantly enhanced our ability to achieve this goal through the development of Three-dimensional -image based conformal radiotherapy (3D CRT) (Figs 20.20 and 20.21)

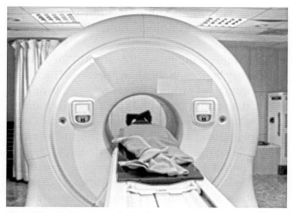

Fig. 20.20: The ring gantry-based platform combines integrated CT imaging with conformal radiation therapy

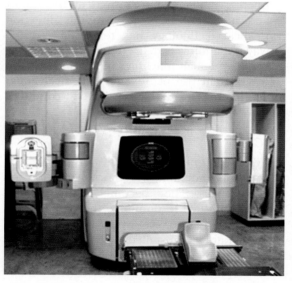

Fig. 20.21: linear accelerator radiotherapy machine

- Three-dimensional conformal therapy is a method of irradiating target volume defined by a set of X-ray beams individually shaped to conform the two dimensional beams eye view projection of the target
- In 3D CRT the target and non-target structures are delineated from patient specific 3-D image

data sets primarily CT more recently often supplemented with Magnetic resonance imaging (MRT). From these inputs the planned dose distributions are then calculated and displayed by advanced treatment planning systems

- In the delivery of 3D CRT Computer controlled radiation machines with multileaf collimators (MLC) and treatment verification with electronic portal images, are increasingly used.

Intensity Modulated Radiation Therapy

- Intensity modulated radiation therapy (IMRT) is an advanced method of 3D CRT (super conformal therapy) that utilizes sophisticated computer controlled radiation beam delivery to improve the conformality of the dose distribution to the shape of the tumor
- The radiation beam can be made to bend the way you want it treating the tumor and sparing the normal tissue like spinal cord. This is a medical revolution in technology. This is achieved by the use of multileaf collimator capable of dynamic beam delivery or multiple static beams sequentially altered in shape by the MLC
- Both 3DCRT and IMRT utilizes sophisticated strategies for patient immobilization and positioning and computer enhanced treatment verification
- The treatment planning steps for IMRT are similar to 3DCRT during initial and final stages but the diverge in the middle. In IMRT the treatment planner would not specify the MLC settings as these would be calculated by the computer. Once all relevant tissues have been delineated and beam direction specified, the Radiation oncologist specifies the desired doses to tumor and normal tissues. From these specifications treatment planning system adjust beam shapes and intensities so as to best meet these dose criteria. When the treatment plan has been accepted, all planning data's are transferred to linear accelerator to deliver the

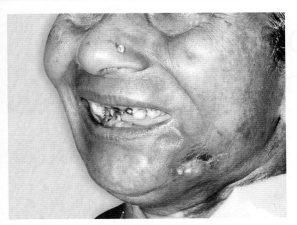

Fig. 20.22: Post-radiotherapy cutaneous fistula and dental caries

desired X-ray intensities The medical physicist must perform dosimetric and QA tasks to verify that all equipments is functioning properly and that of the dose prescription and treatment plan are accurately delivered to the patient on a daily basis (Fig. 20.22).

Image-guided Radiotherapy

- Image-guided radiotherapy (IGRT) is an advanced method of IMRT. In modern RT modalities the volume of the irradiated normal tissue must be reduced in order to limit acute and late injury
- The reduction of safety margin around the tumor plays a decisive role in limiting toxicity
- The main limitation in margin reduction are setup errors and organ motion issues. The only way to reduce the safety margins is the accurate daily localization of the target volume with image guided techniques. For these two couples of X-ray images and acquired for setup correction and verification in order to evaluate residual target localization errors and intra-fraction motion. The process of target position correction and verification takes about 5 minutes. The delivery of treatment will be there while tumor tracking in the same position. IMRT is an art of precise Treatment planning and IGRT is an art of precise Treatment delivery.

Reconstructive Options in Oral and Maxillofacial Cancer

21

INTRODUCTION

- Reconstructive surgery has a leading role in the management of Maxillo-Facial Cancer. The role of free tissue transfer has revolutionized the resection. The surgical challenge in the reconstruction of the Face and jaws uniquely involves the restoration of the facial skeleton as well as the soft tissues of the face and mouth. Stereo lithography has recently added a new dimension in the planning of complex facial and orbital defects after cancer resection

- Oral and Maxillo-Facial region reconstruction after tumor resection is most challenging problem since mandible play a major role in airway protection, support of the tongue, muscles of floor of the mouth, dentition, mastication, articulation, deglutition and respiration

- During reconstruction, continuity and contour of the lower third face should be kept in mind, otherwise it results in deviation of mandible towards the resected side due to unopposed pull of remaining muscles of mastication, contraction of soft tissue and scar formation

- While undertaking reconstruction of deformity, restoration of soft tissue, or bony continuity should not be the only criteria. Maxillary defects are inherently complex because they generally involve more than one component of mid-face and most of them are composite in nature

- A number of local flaps, pedicle flaps, and Microvascular free flaps have been employed for reconstruction of defects. Function of chewing, swallowing, articulation and lip competence must also be addressed. Ultimate goal is to restore function, bony continuity, tongue movement and restoration of sensation

- With the advent of newer modalities of treatment and multimodality approach it is now possible to decrease morbidity and has given a wide scope of reconstructive surgeries

- The soft tissue component of the radial forearm flap is now the favored method of reconstructing the soft tissues of the mouth and pharynx. This flap can be made sensate by incorporating the antebrachial nerve of the forearm and anastamosing this nerve to a donor nerve in the oral region. The improved sensation can help initiate the swallow reflex and improve overall oral function. Reconstruction of the mandible is necessary in about 30% of oral cancer resections. Techniques include the use of the fibula, iliac crest and scapula flaps and, in selected cases, the immediate placement of implants in the grafted bone enabling rapid rehabilitation of oral function

- Maxillectomy defects, which may be so extensive as to include evicerated eye, may be treated by obturation with prosthesis to fill the large defect which communicates between the eye socket and the oral cavity. a combination of intraoral and extraoral implants (for example in the supraorbital rim) offer considerable advantages in these situations

- However, the restoration of the excised bone and soft tissues with a vascularised graft from the iliac crest, incorporating one of the muscles that lie in the abdominal wall, may be a better option for many patients. This allows the patient to wear a denture which can be supported by implants in the reconstructed maxilla and the eye can be restored with a separate implant-retained orbital prosthesis
- Maxillofacial reconstructive techniques are not as yet able to restore the function of tissues to normal that they replace with the exception of the mandible. For example, tissue to replace the tongue can never fulfill the functions of speech, taste and swallowing so important to a patient's quality of life. Although it is technically possible to transplant a tongue with its nerve and blood supply, further research will have to be carried out to assess the function of such techniques. On the other hand, we can replace the structure and function of the mandible by transferring bone and soft tissue and then placing osseointegrated implants to which a prosthetic appliance can be attached to restore the function of chewing as well as restore a patient's appearance and smile.

Principles of reconstruction
Minimal morbidity of recipient and donor site
Replace like with like
Functional reconstruction
Esthetic consideration
Adequate vascularity

A MULTIDISCIPLINARY APPROACH

- Reconstructive surgery is part of the multidisciplinary team
- Adequate reconstruction is the first step in rehabilitation
- Maximize the quality of life for the patient
- Restoration of form and function of tissues.

GOALS OF RECONSTRUCTION

- To replicate the function and appearance of the resected tissue
- Normal speech, mastication, swallowing, and oral continence
- Replace with 'like tissue'
- Minimize donor site deformity.

TIMING OF RECONSTRUCTION

Immediate Reconstruction

- Is ideal
- Prevents retraction and fibrosis of the defect
- Allows adjuvant therapy
- Minimizes number of surgical procedures
- Favors psychological rehabilitation.

Delayed Reconstruction

- Easier identification of recurrence
- Better appreciation of the defect by the patient.

Types of defects
Surface defects
• Mucosa
• Skin
Full thickness defects
Bony defects
Composite defects

Reconstruction options
Primary closure
Skin graft
Local flaps
Regional flaps
Distant flaps
Free flaps

CURRENT APPROACH

- Choose a reconstructive method which best provides with the ideal reconstruction (Fig. 21.1)
- Small defects does not necessarily require reconstruction.

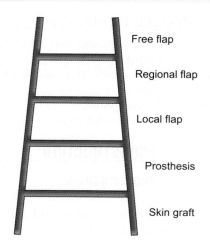

Free flap

Regional flap

Local flap

Prosthesis

Skin graft

Fig. 21.1: Reconstruction ladder

PRIMARY CLOSURE

- Should be done without much distortion or tension
- V- excision ideal for lip and eyelids.

SKIN GRAFTS

Advantages
- Useful for surface defects: mucosa, skin.
- Well vascularized bed is must
- Full thickness graft for small defects.

Disadvantages
- Graft contraction
- Does not resemble original tissues.

Split Thickness

- Includes epidermis and part of dermis
- Thickness varies from thin to thick
- A higher percentage of "take" (survival) is more likely with a thinner graft
- Recipient site wound contraction is less with a thicker graft.

Uses
- Large areas of skin loss
- Granulating tissue beds
- May be meshed to allow increased area of coverage

- Donor site—Heals by epithelialization from wound edges and from skin appendages.

Full Thickness

- Includes epidermis and all dermis
- Provides better coverage but is less likely to "take" than a split skin graft because of greater thickness and slower vascularization
- Donor site is full thickness skin loss and must be closed primarily or with a split thickness skin graft.

Uses
- Usually on the face for better color match
- On the finger to avoid contractures
- Anywhere that thick skin or less contraction of the recipient site is desire.

Decision making in oral cavity reconstruction is depicted in Flowchart 21.1.

FLAPS

- The term "flap" originated in the 16th century from the Dutch word "flappe," meaning something that hung broad and loose, fastened only by one side
- The flap is a full thickness segment of tissue that has its own blood supply.
- Flaps differ from grafts in that they maintain their blood supply as they are moved.

Criteria for choosing a flap
Adequate amount of skin or mucosa
Adequate bulk
Good location and color match
Predictable blood supply
Distance from irradiated sites
Low donor morbidity

Classification of flaps
By the arrangement of their blood supply
Configuration
Location
Tissue content
Method of transferring the flap

Flowchart 21.1: Decision making in oral cavity reconstruction

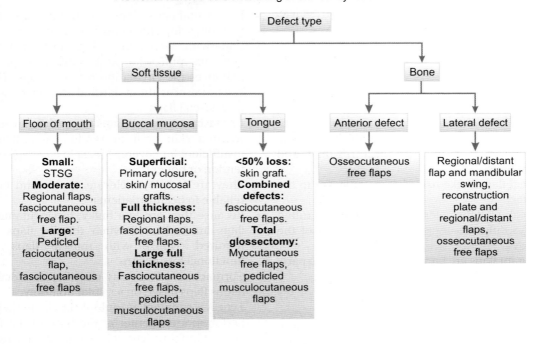

Definition

A flap is a unit of tissue that is transferred from one site (donor site) to another (recipient site) while maintaining its own blood supply or from an anastomised vessel.

Arrangement of Blood Supply

These include random pattern, axial pattern, and pedicle flaps.

Random Flaps

Are supplied by the dermal and subdermal plexus alone and is the most common type of flap used for reconstructing facial defects.

Has limited length to width ratio (1.5–2:1).

Axial Pattern Flaps

- Are supplied by more dominant superficial vessels that are oriented longitudinally along the flap axis
- Greater length possible than with random flap.

Axial pattern flaps (Facial/faciocutaneous)
Submental
Temperoperital
Deltopectoral

Mathes and Nahai Classification

- One vascular pedicle (e.g. tensor fascia lata)
- Dominant pedicle(s) and minor pedicle(s) (e.g. gracilis)
- Two dominant pedicles (e.g. gluteus maximus)
- Segmental vascular pedicles (e.g. sartorius)
- One dominant pedicle and secondary segmental pedicles (e.g. latissimus dorsi).

Pedicle Flaps

- Are supplied by large named arteries that supply the skin paddle through muscular perforating vessels.
- Can be

– Peninsular — skin and vessel intact in pedicle
– Island — vessels intact, but no skin in pedicle.

Free Flaps

Refers to flaps that are harvested from a remote region and have the vascular connection reestablished at the recipient site.

Location

Classification by the region from which the tissue is mobilized. This includes local, regional, and distant flaps:

- Local flaps make use of tissue adjacent to the defect
- Regional flaps refer to those flaps recruited from different areas of the same part of the body
- Distant flaps are harvested from different parts of the body.

Configuration

Flaps are often referred to by their geometric configuration. Examples of these flaps include bilobed, rhombic, and Z-plasty.

Tissue Content

The layers of tissue contained within the flap can also be used to classify a flap.

- Cutaneous flap refers to those flaps that contain the skin only
- Fasciocutaneous flap refers to those flaps that contain the fascia and skin
- Myocutaneous flap refers to those flaps that contain the skin, subcutaneous tissue, and muscle. Blood supply of skin and fat comes from blood vessels perforating the muscle.

Muscle/Myocutaneous
Pectoralis major
Latismus dorsi
Reapezius
Masseter
Platysmus
Infrahyoid

Fasciocutaneous Flaps

- Fasciocutaneous flaps are tissue flaps that include skin, subcutaneous tissue, and the underlying fascia. Including the deep fascia with its prefascial and subfascial plexus enhances the circulation of these flaps. They can be raised without skin and are then referred to as fascial flaps
- Use fasciocutaneous flaps to provide coverage when a skin graft or random skin flap is insufficient for coverage (e.g., in coverage over tendon or bones)
- They are simple to elevate, quick, and fairly reliable in healthy patients
- Because they are less bulky, fasciocutaneous flaps are indicated when thinner flaps are required. Unlike with muscle flaps, no functional loss occurs
- Cormack and Lamberty classified fasciocutaneous flaps based on vascular anatomy.
  Type A is supplied by multiple fasciocutaneous perforators that enter at the base of the flap and extend throughout its longitudinal length. The flap can be based proximally, distally, or as an island.
  Type B has a single fasciocutaneous perforator, which is of moderate size and is fairly consistent. This flap may be isolated as an island flap or used as a free flap.
  Type C is based on multiple small perforators that run along a fascial septum. The supplying artery is included with the flap. It may be based proximally, distally, or as a free flap.
  Type D is an osteomyocutaneous flap, similar to Type C but including a portion of adjacent muscle and bone. It may be based proximally or distally on a pedicle or used as a free flap.
- Cormak and Lamberty also introduced a new classification based on clinical applications.
  Type A has a fascial plexus,
  Type B has a single perforator, and
  Type C has multiple perforators and a segmental source artery.
- Mathes and Nahai likewise classified fasciocutaneous flaps as Type A (with a direct cutaneous pedicle to the fascia), Type B (with a

septocutaneous perforator), and Type C (with perforators from a musculocutaneous source

Myocutaneous/Muscle Flap

- Myocutaneous flap is a composite soft tissue flap in which skin portion provided wound closure while the muscle mass merely served as a carrier for the essential blood supply
- Muscle flap contains only muscle with its blood supply, if required further covered with skin graft

Types of muscle flaps
Type I—One vascular predicle
Type II—Dominant vascular predicles and minor vascular pedicles
Type III—Two dominant pedicles
Type IV—Segmental vascular pedicles
Type V—One dominant vascular pedicle and secondary segmental vascular pedicles

Advantages

- Rich blood supply with distinct vascular pedicle
- Vascular pedicle is often located outside the surgical defect owing to the arc of rotation and length of the muscle
- Muscle provides bulk for deep, extensive defects and protective padding for exposed vital structures
- Muscle is malleable and can be manipulated to produce a desired shape or volume
- Well vascularized muscle is resistant to bacterial inoculation and infection
- Reconstruction using muscle or musculocutaneous flap is often a one stage procedure.

Disadvantages

- Donor defect may lose some degree of function
- Donor defect may be esthetically unacceptable to the patient
- Sometimes these flaps may provide excessive bulk, leaving an esthetically unacceptable rersult
- Flap may eventually atrophy and fail to provide adequate coverage.

Method of Transfer

The most common method of classifying flaps is based on the method of transfer.

- Advancement flaps are mobilized along a linear axis toward the defect
- Rotation flaps pivot around a point at the base of the flap
- Transposition flap refers to one that is mobilized toward an adjacent defect over an incomplete bridge of skin. Examples of transposition flaps include rhombic flaps and bilobedflaps
- Interposition flaps differ from transposition flaps in that the incomplete bridge of adjacent skin is also elevated and mobilized. An example of an interposition flap is a Z-plasty
- Interpolated flaps are those flaps that are mobilized either over or beneath a complete bridge of intact skin via a pedicle. These flaps often require a secondary surgery for pedicle division
- Microvascular free tissue transfer from a different part of the body relies on reanastomosis of the vascular pedicle.

Advancement Flaps (Figs 21.2A and B)

- Flap directly moves forward into a defect without any lateral movement
- Advancement flaps have a linear or rectangular configuration. Advancement flaps are subclassified as simple, single pedicle, bipedicle, and V-Y flaps.

V–Y Flap

This flap is unique among advancement flaps in that it is pushed rather than stretched into the defect. The donor flap, which usually is triangular, is advanced, and the resulting donor defect is closed in a straight line. This approach results in a suture line with a Y configuration.

Pivotal Flaps

Pivotal flaps are moved about a pivotal point from the donor site to the defect. Pivotal flaps include rotation, transposition, and interpolation flaps.

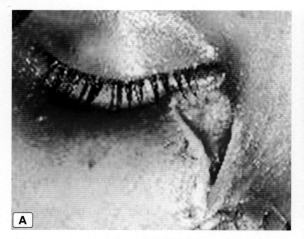
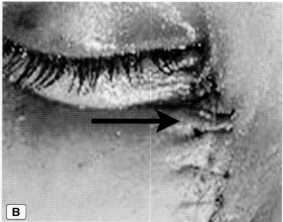

Figs 21.2A and B: Advancement (*Courtesy:* Dr Vikram Shetti)

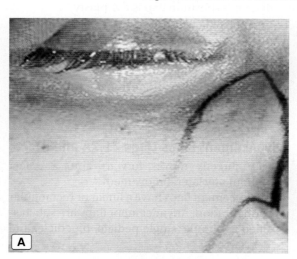
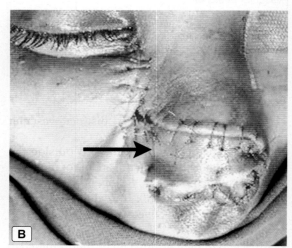

Figs 21.3A and B: Rotation and transposition (*Courtesy:* Dr Vikram Shetti)

Rotation Flaps (Figs 21.3A and B)

Rotation flap is a semicircular flap that rotates about a pivot point to fill the defect.

Causes of Flap Complications

Preoperative
- Poor flap design
- Under estimation of recipient requirements
- Premorbid condition of the patient.

Intraoperative
- Technical errors
- Design errors
- Poor choice of recipient vessels
- Judgment errors.

Postoperative
- Extrinsic
- Pedicle kinking/pressure
- Infection

- Vascular thromboses
- Intrinsic
- Distal ischemia.

Improving Skin Flap Survival

- Improve the blood flow to the flap
- By pharmacologically
- Changing the rheological properties of blood
- Improve the flap's ability to tolerate ischemic insult
- Avoidance of infection
- Prevention of hematoma
- Avoidance of raw areas.

Tests of skin flap circulation
Subjective tests
• Color
• Capillary blanching
• Warmth
• Bleeding from stab wound
Objective tests
• Metabolic tests
• Photoelectric tests
• Temperature tests
• Vital dye
• Quantitative tests
• Clearance tests

Local Flaps

- Forehead flap
- Nasolabial flap
- Cervical flap
- Submental flap
- Tongue flap.

Tongue flap
Advantages
• Perforator from Ipsilateral lingual vessels
• Intraoral defects
• Anterior and posterior based
• Provide bulk
Disadvantages
• Two stages
• May affect speech
• Field change
• Decrease mobility of tongue
• Limited arc of rotation

Regional Myocutaneous Flaps

- Pectoralis major flap
- Deltopectoralis flap
- Sternocleidomastoid flap
- Trapezius myocutaneous flap
- Latissimus dorsi myocutaneous flap
- Temporalis flap
- Masseter flap
- Platysma flap .

Free Flaps

- Radial forearm
- Iliac crest with rectus abdominalis muscle
- Fibula
- Scapula.

Nasolabial Flap

- Earliest description by *Sushrutha* in 700 BC
- *Dieffenbach 1830* superiorly based nasolabial flap for nasal alae rec
- *Von Langenbeck 1864* Used nasolabial flap for nasal recon
- *Esser 1921* used inferiorly based nasolabial flap for palatal fistula closure
- The nasolabial flap is an arterialised local flap in the head and neck region
- Axial blood supply provided either by the facial artery (inferiorly based) or by the superficial temporal artery through its transverse facial branch and the infraorbital artery (superiorly based)
- It is used in a variety of situations including reconstruction of the lower eyelid and small defects of the nose, lips and oral cavity
- In cancer treatment its major role is for reconstruction of the floor of the mouth, palate and ala of the nose. The recent innovation of folding the flap has further expanded its role, as it is now able to provide lining and cover for a full thickness commissural defect.

Forehead Flap

- First described in Indian literature
- Kazanjianin 1946 described the median forehead flap for nasal repair

- This flap was based on supratrochlear vessels and occasionally, the supraorbital artery
- Used to cover the defects below the level of the eye.
- Bridge segment is not tubed as they can cope up with raw surface without causing sepsis
- There is a depression if the frontalis muscle is involved it can be countered by beveling the margin or grafting after 10 days so that some amount of granulation tissue is formed
- Width to length is 5:1
- Esthetic deformity.

Submental Flap (Figs 21.4 to 21.7)

- First described by Martin et al
- Submental flap has been described for reconstruction of intraoral defects, cutaneous defects of lower and middle third of face, cervical esophagus and laryngeal defects
- Axial pattern flap
- Based on submental branch of facial artery
- Venous drainage—submental vein which drains into the common facial vein
- 2 mm in diameter at its origin
- Pedicle length—8 cm
- The maximum dimension that can be reliably harvested is 15 × 7 cm, this must be individualized to each patient based on the laxity that dictates the amount of skin that can be harvested without compromising a primary closure.

Tongue Flap (Fig. 21.8)

- Described for use in intraoral reconstruction of a soft palate defect *(Kloop and Schurter 1956)*

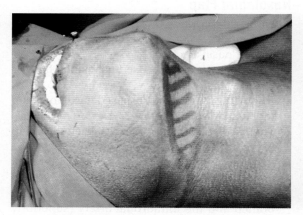

Fig. 21.4: Submental flap marking

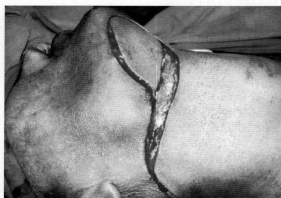

Fig. 21.5: Submental flap incision

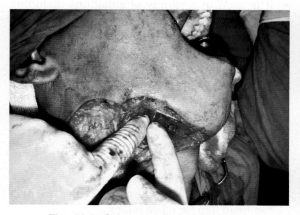

Fig. 21.6: Submental flap transposition

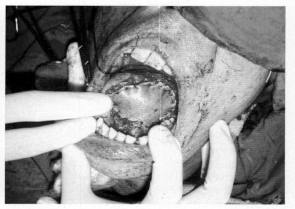

Fig. 21.7: Submental flap for tongue reconstruction
(*Courtesy:* Rajendra Prasad)

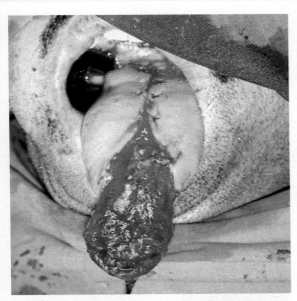

Fig. 21.8: Tongue flap (*Courtesy:* Vikram Shetty)

- Variants of flap design for temporary or definitive coverage of small defects
- Correction of lip deformities and reconstruction for treatment of electrical burns
- Closure of palatal fistulas
- Anteriorly or posteriorly based
- Midline or lateral
- Useful for small intra-oral defects
- Donor site closed primarily
- Two stage procedure
- Base of flap should measure 2.5–3.0 cm wide
- Length of flap should be sufficient to avoid tension on the pedicle from the motion of the tongue
- Length may be extended 5–6 cm
- Vasculature.
- Lingual artery from the external carotid gives 4 branches
  - suprahyoid artery
  - dorsal lingual artery
  - deep lingual artery
  - sublingual artery.

Advantages
- Excellent blood supply
- Low morbidity
- Reinnervation from the adjacent host tissue
- Can provide 90–100 cm of mucosal tissue for rotation can be used in patients post radiotherapy also.

Limitation
Size of flap and the defect.

Abbe Flap (Figs 21.9 to 21.11)

- When more than 30 percent width of lip is resected reconstruction requires mobilization of flap from the opposite lip
- When 2/3rd lip is excised reconstruction done by borrowing tissue equivalent to half of surgical defect
- Popularised by Abbe for reconstruction of upper lip and Estlander for lower lip
- The upper lip defect is usually shaped as an inverted V but if it is central and must fit into the phitral area it may end up as an inverted W
- The flap is then designed on the lower lip to correspond in shape through a flap initially cut as a V-may be converted into a W-ay by splitting the tip if the W is narrow one.

Karapandzic Flap

- The Karapandzic manuver depends on the creation of paired lip flaps based on branches of the facial artery. The skin incisions parallel the lip margin at a distance equal to the depth of the defect
- The principle is mobilization and utility of skin, soft tissues, mucosa of lower portion of nasolabial region, which are shifted medially
- The superficial muscles of facial expression are divided but sensory and motor nerves which run in close proximity to main arterial channels are spared

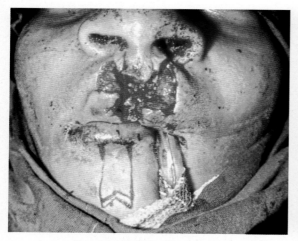

Fig. 21.9: Abbe flap marking

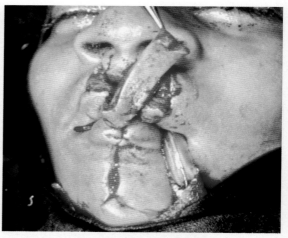

Fig. 21.10: Abbe flap transposition

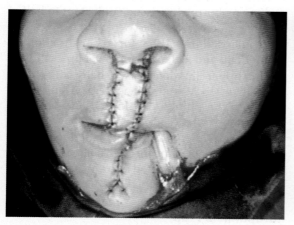

Fig. 21.11: Abbe in position for upper lip construction
(*Courtesy:* Rajendra Prasad)

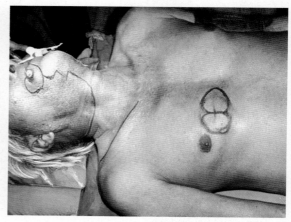

Fig. 21.12: PMMC flap marking (*Courtesy:* Rajendra Prasad)

- For reconstruction of defects of lower lip where 80 percent or more of lower lip is resected in its central part leaving the lateral ends near commisure intact.

Pectoralis Major Myocutaneous Flap (Figs 21.12 to 21.15)

- Workhorse for head and neck reconstruction
- First described by Ariyan 1977
- Broad, flat fan shaped muscle that covers pectoralis minor, subclavius, serratus anterior and intercostal muscles.

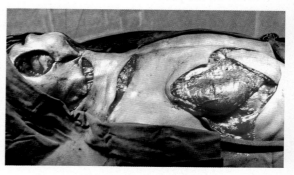

Fig. 21.13: After incision

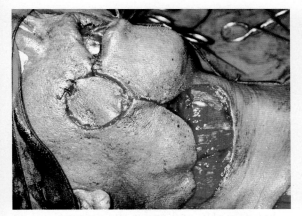

Fig. 21.14: Buccal defect closed with flap

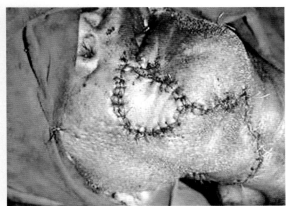

Fig. 21.15: After suturing (*Courtesy:* Rajendra Prasad)

Based on

- Thoraco-acromial artery (axillary artery)
- Internal (thoracic) mammary artery
- Lateral thoracic artery (subclavian artery)

Can be harvested
- As a muscle paddle
- As an island
- As a bipedal.

Advantages
- Non-delayed, one-stage procedure
- Highly reliable success rate of more than 95%
- Technically easy and quick to perform
- Primary closure of the donor site
- May be used along with other flaps
- Change of position of patient not required during surgery
- Skin coverage, muscle bulk and good blood supply.

Disadvantages
- Excessive bulk and thickness may compromise its blood supply
- Hair bearing area

- Shoulder disability
- Blood loss is more as compared to other faciocutaneous flaps
- Avoid twisting, torsion and tension.

Pectoralis Major Flap: Island Type
- Very reliable limited arch of rotation
- Entire muscle may be elevated or divided from the lateral portion of the muscle
- Tunnelized to defect and fixate
- Primary closure of donor site.

Pectoralis Major Flap: Paddle Type
- Island flap is not long enough to cover defect
- Skin of the flap is not directly attached to the muscle
- Increase arch of rotation
- Pectoralis major flap: gemini type
- Bilobular island flap
- When defects require closure of the oral mucosa and overlying skin
- Manipulate as a single island flap, after transposition: fold the muscle on itself so each island covers the appropriate defect.

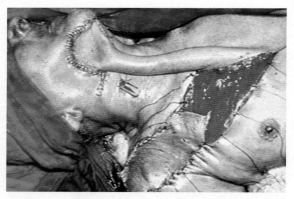

Fig. 21.16: Deltopectoral flap

Deltopectoral Flap (Fig. 21.16)

- Outlined along the inferior border of the clavicle, medially the sternum extending to the lateral acromion process returning at the level of 5th rib
  Lateral to medial elevation beneath the level of the pectoralis muscle fascia
- Base: 2 cm from the lateral sternal border
- Axial pattern flap
- Perfused by intercostal perforating branches of the internal mammary artery
- Useful for cheek, chin and neck defects
- Two stage procedure
- Donor site requires split thickness skin graft
- Horizontal flap design with round tip
- Excellent reliability in head and neck defects, but color match and texture not satisfactory.

Sternocleidomastoid Flap

- First described by Owens in 1955

Blood supply
Superior : branches of occipital artery
Middle : branches of the superior thyroid artery
Inferiorly : Branches of the thyrocervical trunk

- Can be used as a muscle flap only, myocutaneous flap or as a composite flap
- Can be based superiorly or inferiorly
- The superior thyroid vessels should be preserved at all times

- The vascularization from the occipital artery is additionally supplied by preserving the platysma during preparation of the SCM flap
- Mainly used for intraoral and pharyngeal reconstruction
- Can be used for mandibular reconstruction if taken along with clavicle
- Limited rotational angle.

Latissimus Dorsi Flap

- First described by Tansini in 1895
- Not as versatile as pectoralis major myocutaneous flap but certain qualities such as the hair free skin and donor site scar make it an invaluable alternative
- Indicated when large amount of tissue is required
- Arterial supply based on thoracodorsal artery
- Venous drainage from thoracodorsal vein
- Motor nerve innervation potential with thoracodorsal nerve.

Advantages

- Large flap with long pedicle (artery 2–3 mm, vein 3–5 mm, length: 7–10 cm)
- 2nd largest skin paddle
- Possibility for "axillary megaflap"
- Multiple skin paddles
- Low donor site morbidity
- Possibility of muscle reinnervation via thoracodorsal nerve.

Disadvantages

- Difficult positioning and two team harvest
- Postoperative seroma formation
- Bulky flap
- Unable to tube.

Trapezius Flap

- Based on transverse cervical artery
- Useful for floor of mouth, skull base.

Anterolateral Thigh Flap

- First described by Song et al 1984
- First used in head and neck by Koshima and Kimata et al

- Fasciocutaneous/Myocutaneous/Chimeric
- Descending branch of Lateral circumflex femoral artery and its venae comitantes
- Musculocutaneous (60%)/septocutaneous (40%) perforators
- Fasciocutaneous flap
  - Soft tissue defects of head and neck region
  - Can be thinned to line the tongue
  - Bi-paddled by excising skin bridge (preserve subdermal venous plexus)
- Fascial flap—for intraoral mucosal defects
- Musculocutaneous flap
- Sensate flap—in association with lateral femoral cutaneous nerve of thigh
- Chimeric flap—in association with other composite flaps.

Indications
- Soft tissue defects
- External defects in head and neck
- Oropharyngeal lining.

Vascular Anatomy
- Transverse pedicle anomaly (10%)
- Descending branch still exists, but small <1.5 mm
- Two to three muscular perforators—superior to inferior from quadriceps artery
- Superior perforator runs on medial edge of vastus lateralis muscle (15%)
- Arterial diameter 0.2–3.5 mm
- Two venae comitantes dia. 1.8–4.0 mm.

Advantages
- Versatility
  - Thickness is moderate and uniform
  - Can be thinned down/muscle can be added for bulk
- Reliable pedicle
  - Large diameter pedicle (arterial/venous)
  - Long pedicle (when rectus femoris and transverse branches ligated)
- Sensate flap
- Large area of skin paddle (upto 15 cm wide and 25 cm long)

- Primary closure possible at donor site
- Relatively low morbidity
- Esthetically compliant donor area
- Possible for 2 surgical teams operating simultaneously'.

Disadvantages
- Variability of vascular pedicle
  - Transverse branch anomaly
  - Predominance of musculocutaneous/ septocutaneous perforators
  - Relation of perforators to vastus lateralis
  - Difficulty in identifying LCFA with doppler probe
  - Skin color may not match
  - Hair growth in male patients.

Platysma Flap

> The cervical skin is supplied by a random anastomosing network located superficial to the platysma
>
> Platysma-cutaneous branches from the facial, sub-mental and submandibular arteries supply the an-terosuperior aspects of the platysma muscle and overlying skin

- Branches from the occipital and posterior auricular arteries supply the skin over the posterosuperior aspect of the muscle. The anterior midportion of the muscle and skin is supplied by a branch of the superior thyroid artery
- The venous drainage of the vertical flap mainly passes through the anterior facial vein or submental vein, and that of the transverse design mainly through the external jugular vein.

Advantages
- Reconstruction of lingual defects, because it is not bulky and preserves motor innervation
- The relative simplicity of raising the flap
- Lower postoperative morbidity
- Proximity to the oral cavity and face, being thin, pliable.

Disadvantages

- This flap has hair-bearing nature in males
- Due to postoperative swelling in the sub mandibular region flap necrosis can be seen
- Post operative chemo/radio therapy can lead to flap necrosis.

Temporalis Flap (Fig. 21.17)

Blood supply
Deep temporal fascia : middle temporal branch (superficial temporal artery)
Anterior deep temporal artery
Posterior deep temporal artery

- Orbital, skull base and small intraoral defects.
- Small scar with minimal cosmetic deformity
- Muscular flap only with a good rotational arch.
- Facial nerve injury is seen in few cases.

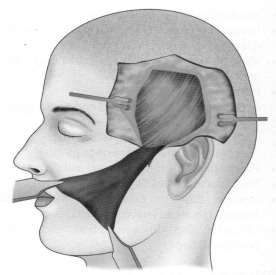

Fig. 21.17: Temporalis flap

Pedicle flaps: Disadvantages
Limited size and arc of rotation
Distal most flat: least vascular
Mobility limited by the pedicle
Gravitational pull, hence dehiscence
Bulky
Partial flap loss, complications up to 20%
Interfere with early lymph node detection

Free Vascularised Flaps

- Early 1900s Alexis Carrel-Free tissue transfer in animals (jejunum to neck)
- 1950s Jacobsen and Suarez—first anastomoses in animal
- 1959 Seidenberg—free jejunum segments to repair pharyngoesophageal defects
- 1972 McLean and Buncke—omental flap to cover a cranial defect
- 1973 Daniels and Taylor—first free cutaneous flap
- 1976 Baker and Panje—first free flap in head and neck cancer reconstruction—groin pedicled on the circumflex iliac artery.

Indications

- Bony defects >3 cm
- Defects that require considerable bulk and tissue
- Defects that require thin skin flaps with sensation
- Composite floor of mouth and tongue defects
- Defects that are not amenable to regional flaps.

Advantages

- Two team approach
- Improved vascularity and wound healing
- Low rate of resorption
- Potential for sensory and motor innervation
- Permits use of osseointegrated implants
- Wide variety of available tissue types tailored to match defect
- Wide range of skin characteristics
- More efficient use of harvested tissue
- Immediate reconstruction.

Disadvantages

- Technically demanding
- Increased operating room time
- Increased flap failure rate
- Functional disability at donor site.

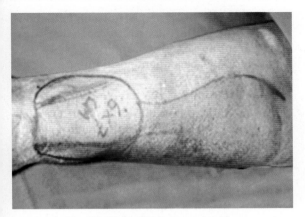

Fig. 21.18: Radial forearm free flap

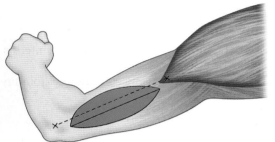

Fig. 21.19: Lateral arm free flap

Contraindications
- Severe medical illness who cannot withstand long surgery,
- Uncontrolled hypertension or diabetes,
- Severe atherosclerosis with vessel wall calcification and
- Very aggressive pathology with doubtful of resected margins.

Radial Forearm Free Flap (Fig. 21.18)
- Arterial source - radial artery
- Venous Source—paired vena commitantes and/or cephalic vein
- Fasciocutaneous (type-C)
- Ideal for intraoral soft tissue defects.

Advantages
- Thin, pliable skin with long,
- Large pedicle
- Easy positioning
- Potential for sensate flap
- Potential for unusual shapes
- Potential for vascularized bone
- Ease of preoperative evaluation.

Disadvantages
- Poorly esthetic donor site requires skin graft
- Potential for pathologic fractures
- Loss of hand function.

Lateral Arm Free Flap (Fig. 21.19)
- Arterial supply—posterior radial collateral artery from profunda brachii artery
- Venous supply—vena commitantes in spiral groove of humerus.

Advantages
- Low donor site morbidity (vertical scar)
- Easy positioning
- Potential for sensory innervation via posterior cutaneous nerve.

Disadvantages
- Short and smaller caliber artery (1.55 mm, up to 8-10 cm)
- Longer dissection than RFFF
- Thicker subcutaneous tissue
- Pressure dressing
- Risk to radial nerve.

Lateral Thigh Free Flap
- Arterial supply is from third perforator of profunda femoris artery
- Venous output from associated vena commitantes.

Advantages
- Large amount of thin, hairless skin
- Low donor site morbidity (primary closure)
- Easy positioning
- Sensation potential with lateral femoral cutaneous nerve.

Disadvantages

- Difficult dissection
- Retraction of vastus lateralis
- Short, variable pedicle 15 cm, 2–4 mm.

Rectus Abdominus Free Flap

- Arterial supply based on deep inferior epigastric artery
- Venous supply form vena commitantes joining external iliac vein.

Advantages

- Easy positioning and harvest
- Constant anatomy
- Long (8–10 cm) and large caliber vessel (average 3.4 mm)
- Donor site closed primarily
- Large flap obtained
- Anterior rectus sheath durable.

Disadvantages

- Often bulky
- No sensation potential
- Potential for hernia formation if dissection below arcuate line.

Scapular Free Flap

- Circumflex scapular artery and vein
- 14 cm of bone available (lateral aspect)
- Allows osseointegrated implants
- Long pedicle to axillary artery

- Multiple fasciocutaneous/musculocutaneous flaps available (scapular, parascapular, latissimus dorsi, serratus anterior)
- Major drawback: patient positioning.

Fibular Free Flap (Figs 21.20 and 21.21)

- The fibula is a long thin bone that has close proximity to the Peroneal artery and venae and can therefore be harvested on a single large pedicle. The length of the bone, consistent blood supply and relative ease of harvest make this donor one of the most useful when osseous reconstruction is required
- Consist of a large peroneal vessels and a long pedicle
- Approx 25 cm of bone can be harvested
- Arterial supply—peroneal artery
- Dual supply—endosteal and periosteal
- Venous supply—vena commitantes.

Advantages

- Longest and strongest bone stock (25 cm of bone)
- Cortical bone—weight bearing
- Straight—long bone defect
- Triangular cross section—resists angular and rotatory stress
- Can be a sensate flap—Lateral sural nerve
- Multiple osteotomies-precise contouring
- Skin for soft tissue defects
- Low donor site morbidity

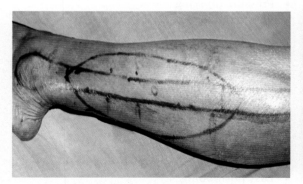

Fig. 21.20: Fibula free flap graft marking

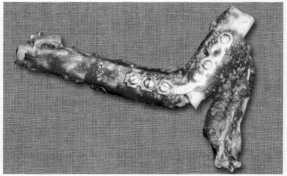

Fig. 21.21: Harvested graft

- Easy positioning
- Excellent periosteal blood supply (contoring)
- Support osseointegrated implants
- Bone union rapid.

Disadvantages

- High incidence of peripheral vascular disease
- Small cutaneous paddle
- Decreased ankle strength and toe flexion
- Small risk chronic ankle pain
- Requires invasive study for operative evaluation.

Conclusion

- Reconstruction is an integral part of treatment
- Should be done immediate
- Consider the safest and most reliable methods of reconstruction before embarking on more complex and time-consuming options
- Local and regional flaps are safe and reliable resources
- The pectoralis major myocutaneous flap is a time-proven method for reconstructing almost all defects of the oral cavity. But surpassed by microvascular free flaps
- The microvascular free flap has revolutionized the field of head and neck reconstruction in terms of preserved function and cosmesis. Reconstruction of oromandibular defects using osteocutaneous free flaps gives patients new hope in the face of historically devastating defects
- With all the tools available, a maxillofacial surgeon should repair many defects and give the patient a good, functional, and cosmetic outcome. These techniques include an increasing element of risk as you move up the reconstructive ladder. Therefore, it is always wise to start at the bottom and work your way up, trying the simplest technique that will work.

- Maxillofacial reconstruction is an extremely demanding process that needs continous improvements and refinements. Patients clinical condition should be managed with a team approach , including oncologists , radiotherapists, and reconstructive surgeon. Dispite the progress achieved in this field , challenges of maxillofacial reconstruction still remains elusive , because of the inability to attain complete functional and cosmetic recovery with current techniques.
- A competent maxillo-facial surgeon should be familiar with free-flap which is the workhorse in head and neck reconstruction. Of course every reconstruction has advantages and limitation with each technique knowing when and where to adopt particular procedure.
- Conservative surgical options including Mohs technique for skin cancers, newer endoscopic skull base tumor resection continue toward more organ sparing treatment plans.
- Transoral Robotic Surgery[TORS] for base of tongue neoplasm is a new emerging modality of surgery that may pave the road to more conservative surgeries. Reconstructive maxillo-facial surgeon should be aware of new surgical techniques and advances. Research is now progressing in the field of stem cell and osteosynthesis.
- The potential is that these research should provide rapid *de novo* bone growth which will eliminate the need for vascularized bone graft.
- Gene theraphy and immune system targeting are the newer treatment modalities entering in the battle against oral and maxillofacial cancer.

Reconstruction with Reconstruction Plate (Figs 21.22A to F)

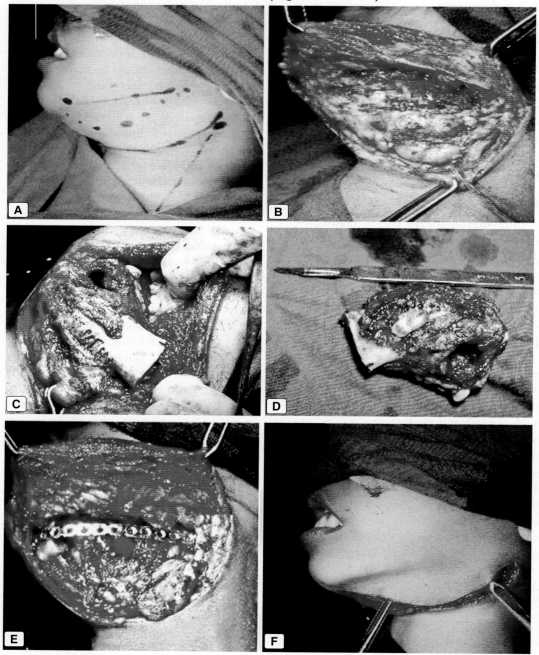

Figs 21.22A to F: Reconstruction with reconstruction plate (A) Marking of incision; (B) Exposure of surgical site; (C) Tumor mass detached from nearby tissues; (D) Excised tumor mass with portion of mandible; (E) Reconstruction plate *in situ*; (F) Approximation of tissue

Reconstruction with Free Fibula Graft (Figs 21.23A to J)

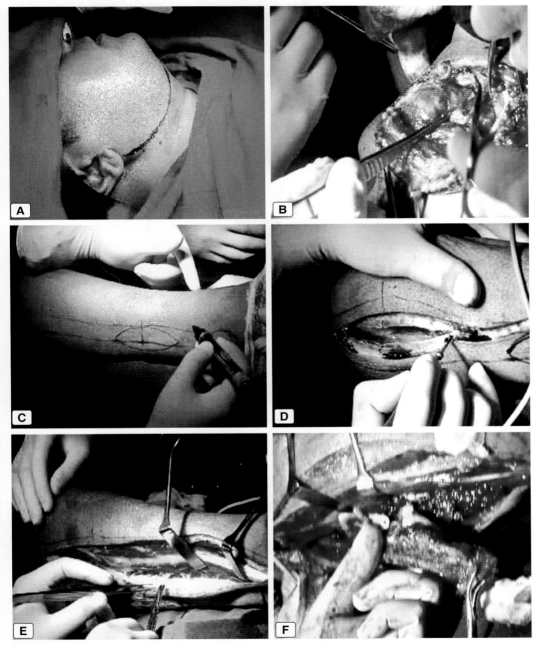

Figs 21.23A to F: Reconstruction with free fibula graft: (A) Marking of incision at recipient site; (B) Removal of pathology from recipient site; (C) Marking of incision at donor site; (D) Initial incision using electrosurgery at donor site; (E) Deep dissection for harvesting fibula graft; (F) Harvested fibula graft

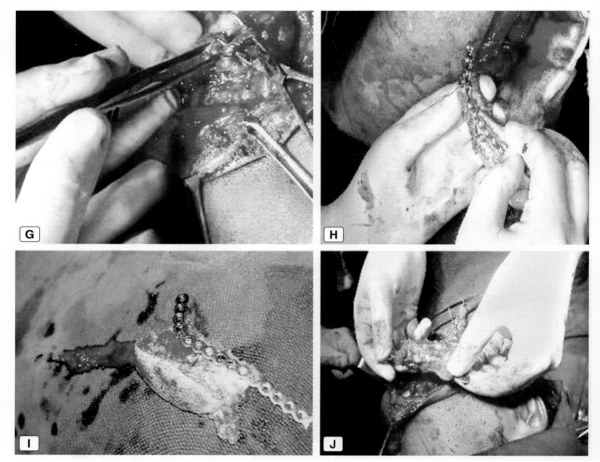

Figs 21.23G to J: (G) Preparation of recipient site; (H) Contouring of graft; (I) Contoured graft; (J) Placement of graft

Reconstruction with Submental Flap (Figs 21.24A to C)

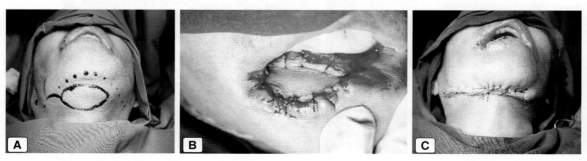

Figs 21.24A to C: Reconstruction with submental flap: (A) Marking of incision; (B) Flap *in situ* at recipient site; (C) Primary closure of donor site

Clinical Cases of Cancers of Oral Cavity

22

CASE NUMBER 1

A 50-year-old female patient complains of growth at the angle of the mouth since 2 months duration.

Intermittent discomfort while talking and chewing for 1.5 years.

History of Present Illness
- Intermittent pain while chewing and talking—1.5 years
- Small slowly progressive nodular growth in the angle of the mouth—2 months.

Medical
Patient is a known hypertensive for 4 years on regular medications.

Personal History
History of chewing betel (paan) leaf for 2 years for intermittent pain.

Systemic Examination
- Pallor +
- BP = 140/80 mm Hg.

Lymph Nodes
Not palpable in levels I–V.

Clinical Presentation: Extraoral Examination (Figs 22.1 to 22.3)
- 1 cm × 2 cm
- Pale pink induration on the lip medially

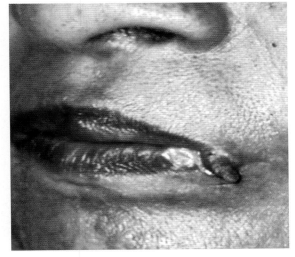

Fig. 22.1: Extraoral clinical picture

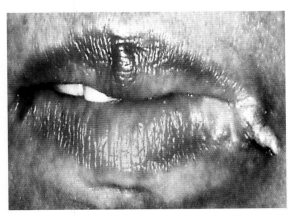

Fig. 22.2: Extraoral clinical picture frontal view

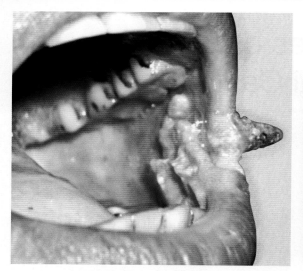

Fig. 22.3: Intraoral clinical picture

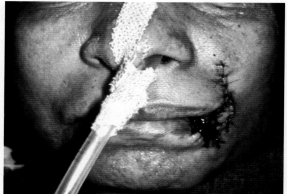

Fig. 22.4: Extraoral clinical picture postoperative

- Brown colored nodular growth from commissure = 1 cm
- Firm
- Indurated pyramidal shaped nodule
- Alteration of color and consistency up to 7 mm medial to the commissure.

T4a N0 MX LESION Left buccal mucosa, commissure of the lip and skin adjacent to the vermillion border of the lip.

Treatment Done

Wide excision and primary closure with local random rotational advancement flap under GA.

Postoperative

See Figures 22.4 and 22.5.

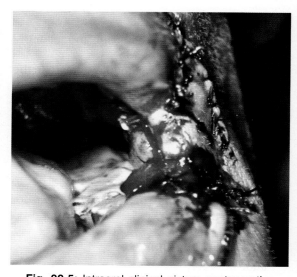

Fig. 22.5: Intraoral clinical picture postoperative

CASE NUMBER 2

60-year-old gentleman complains of ulcer on the tongue since 1 year.

History of Presenting Illness

- Ulcer at the lateral border of tongue
  - Since 1 year
  - Progressed to present size
- Associated with pain
  - Dull and intermittent
- Burning sensation of mouth
- No difficulty in speech and tongue movements.

Medical History

No relevant medical history.

Personal History

- Consumes mixed diet
- H/o paan chewing since 40 years 10–12 paans per day
- Consumes alcohol daily since 20 years
- Sleep normal
- Bowel and bladder habits normal.

General Physical Examination

- Conscious and cooperative
- Moderately built and moderately nourished
- Pallor present
- No signs of icterus, cyanosis, clubbing, edema
- Vital signs—normal.

Head and Neck Examination

- Eyes—no clinically detectable abnormalities
- Nose—no clinically detectable abnormalities
- TMJ—no clinically detectable abnormalities
- Mouth opening—34 mm.

Intraoral Examination

- Teeth present
  87654321 12345678
  87654321 12345678
- Calculus and stains present
- Mucosa is pale
- Depapillation of tongue is observed (Fig. 22.6).

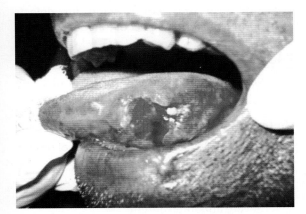

Fig. 22.6: Intraoral clinical picture of lesion on lateral border of tongue

Examination

Inspection

- No discharge noticed
- Floor covered with slough.

Palpation

Inspectory findings confirmed.
- Ulcer
  - Tender
  - Edges are raised and indurated
- Base
  - Indurated
  - Fixed to underlying tissue.

Lymph Node Examination

Submental lymph node
- Palpable
- 1 in number
- Not fixed
- Nontender
- Firm in consistency measuring approximately 1 cm in the longest diameter.

Left submandibular lymph node
- 1 in number
- Not fixed
- Nontender
- Firm in consistency measuring approximately 1 cm in the longest diameter.

Right submandibular lymph node
- 1 in number
- Not fixed
- Nontender
- Firm in consistency measuring approximately 1 cm in the longest diameter.

Investigations

- Routine blood investigations
- Histopathology
- FNAC of submental lymph node
- USG neck
- Chest radiograph
- MRI contrast study.

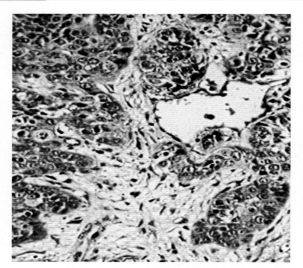

Fig. 22.7: Histopathology: Showing early invasive SCC: Deep elongation, branching off rete processses, and narrowing of junction of branches

Histopathology

Suggestive of early invasive squamous cell carcinoma (Fig. 22.7).

FNAC

Submental lymph node
- Nonspecific smear.

USG Neck

- No evidence of significant lymph node enlargement bilaterally
- Thyroid and Submandibular glands appear normal
- Neck vessels appear normal.

Final Diagnosis

- Squamous cell carcinoma of the tongue
- Grading and staging
  $T_2 N_{2C} M_X$
  Stage: IV A.

Management

- Resection of primary
- Adequate clearance

- Adequate node resection
- Reconstruction of defect
- Radiotherapy
- Chemotherapy.

Tumor Resection

Hemiglossectomy.

Neck nodes

- Left radical neck dissection
- Right extended supraomohyoid neck dissection.

Anterior Tongue Reconstruction

- Very difficult to reconstruct
- Complex intrinsic musculature and function
- Redundancy is advantageous
- Near hemiglossectomy does not significantly alter function.

Oral (Mobile) Tongue

- Speech and deglutition
- Mobility allows for:
  - Articulation of speech
  - Bolus manipulation in preparation for deglutition
- *Sensory functions:* proprioception, pain, taste
- Assists in mastication and bolus processing
- Defects < 50% can be closed primarily +/- STSG
- Larger or composite defects require more bulk (i.e. fasciocutaneous free flap)
- Lateral arm free flap is good for defects including posterior aspect of tongue/FOM.

CASE NUMBER 3

A 72-year-old gentleman complains of ulcer on the tongue since 3 months (Fig. 22.8).

History of Presenting Illness

- Ulcer on the left lateral posterior part of tongue
  - Since 3 months
  - *Progressed to present size*
- Associated with pain
  - Severe and intermittent
- Burning sensation of mouth
- No difficulty in speech and tongue movements.

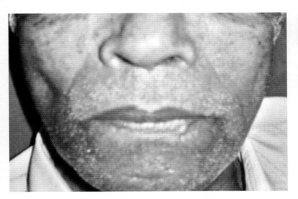

Fig. 22.8: Extraoral clinical picture

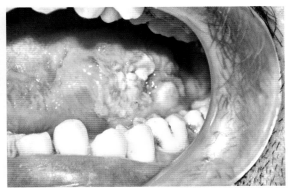

Fig. 22.9: Intraoral clinical picture of lesion on lateral border of tongue

Medical History

No relevant medical history.

Personal History

- Consumes mixed diet
- H/o paan chewing for 40 years 10–12 paans per day
- Habit of smoking cigarette and beedies 10–15 daily for 30 years
- Sleep normal
- Bowel and bladder habits normal.

General Physical Examination

- Conscious and cooperative
- Moderately built and moderately nourished
- Pallor present
- No signs of icterus, cyanosis, clubbing, edema
- Vital signs—normal.

Head and Neck Examination

- Eyes—no clinically detectable abnormalities
- Nose—no clinically detectable abnormalities
- TMJ—no clinically detectable abnormalities
- No gross facial asymmetry present.

Intraoral Examination (Fig. 22.9)

- Teeth present
  8754 321 12345
  87654321 12345

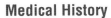

- Calculus and stains present
- Mucosa is pale
- Depapillation of tongue is observed.

Inspection

- No discharge noticed
- Floor covered with slough

Palpation

Inspectory findings confirmed

- Ulcer
  - Tender
  - Edges are raised and indurated
- Base
  - Indurated
  - Fixed to underlying tissue
- Floor
  - Covered with necrotic slough.

Histopathology

Suggestive of squamous cell carcinoma.

Final Diagnosis

- Squamous cell carcinoma of the tongue
- Grading and staging
  $T_3 N_0 M_X$
  Stage III.

Management

- Wide excision of primary lesion
- Ipsilateral mod type III neck dissection or
- Left extended supraomohyoid neck dissection
- Reconstruction of defect
- Radiotherapy
- Chemotherapy.

CASE NUMBER 4

A 65-year-old female was referred to the department with complains of mobility of teeth in lower left back region.

History of Presenting Illness

- Tooth mobility since 1 month
- Pain since 1 month, severe in nature, throbbing in nature, radiating to temporal region
- Mobility increased after tooth extraction
- Swelling in mandibular region for 15 days.

Past Medical History

- Undergone surgery in neck 18 years back (details unknown)
- Known asthmatic on medication
- Skin lesions for 2 years, not on medications.

Past Dental History

- Extraction of 45, 44 done, 1 month back, swelling increased since then

- Biopsy taken by a local doctor, report not collected.

Personal History

Paan chewing with tobacco 5–6 times a day for 30 years.

General Examination

- Moderately built and nourished
- Anemic
- Pallor present
- Lymph nodes positive
- Generalized skin lesions especially in bilateral legs.

Local Examination

Extraoral Examination

- Facial asymmetry present
- Swelling present in left mandibular region (Fig. 22.10)
- Size: 5 × 3 cm
- Extensions:
  Anteriorly: commisure
- *Posteriorly:* 2 cm anterior to angle of mandible
  Superiorly: 2 cm below the ala-tragal line
  Inferiorly: lower border of the mandible.

Intraoral Examination (Fig. 22.11)

- Poor oral hygiene, generalized tobacco stains
- *Mouth opening:* 38 mm.

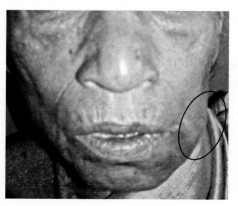

Fig. 22.10: Extraoral clinical picture showing swelling

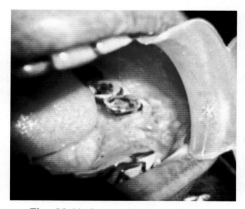

Fig. 22.11: Intraoral picture of lesion

Soft Tissue

- *Gingiva:* Generalized chronic gingivitis
- Ulceroproliferative growth in 34, 35 region
- Size 3.5 × 4 cm
- Extensions:
  Anteriorly: 34 area
  Posteriorly: Distal surface of 36
  Inferiorly: Gingivobuccal sulcus
  Superiorly: occlusal level of teeth on buccal mucosa
  Medially: involving the edentulous alveolar crest 1 cm sup to lingual sulcus
- *Teeth present:* 87654321 1234567
  87 4321 123 67
  Lymph nodes:
  Ipsilateral side:
- *Multiple nodes:* level 1b, single, 2 cm, firm, fixed, tender
- *level 2a node:* single, mobile, nontender
- *Level 3 node:* 0.5 cm single, mobile, nontender
- *Level 5 node:* single, mobile.

Contralateral Side

Level 1b node: 1 × 1 cm mobile, nontender.

Provisional Diagnosis

- Carcinoma lower alveolous/buccal mucosa
- Traumatic ulcer.

Clinical Staging

T4a N2c Mx, Stage IV A (operable disease).

Investigations

- OPG (Fig. 22.12)
- Incision biopsy.

Management

Multimodal Therapy

- Surgery: wide excision + hemimandibulectomy + MRND type 2 + reconstruction with PMMC
- Postoperative radiotherapy.

Newer Trends

Newer tumor specific medical therapies are anticipated to be less toxic while maintaining a high degree of efficacy. For resectable cancer, transoral laser microsurgery.

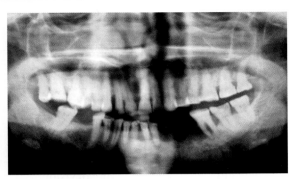

Fig. 22.12: OPG showing erosion of bone

CLINICAL CASE 5

A 17-year-old male presents with chief complaint of ulcer in the right retromolar region.

History of Presenting Illness

- Insidious in onset
- Initially noticed a small swelling measuring about 5 mm in size associated with pain and discharge since 4 months
- Gradually progressive in size and symptoms
- Pain radiating to lower jaw and ear
- Associated with yellowish discharge and foul smell
- Associated with difficulty in swallowing
- Not associated with fever or any other systemic symptoms.

Medical History

- Hospitalized 2 months back for the same complaint and biopsy was done
- Report—nonspecific ulcer.

Personal History

- Oral hygiene practice
- Mixed diet
- No addictive habits
- Normal bowel and bladder habits
- Disturbed sleep.

General Physical Examination

- Conscious and cooperative
- Moderately built and moderately nourished pallor present
- No signs of icterus, cyanosis, clubbing, edema
- Vital signs—normal.

Head and Neck Examination

- Eyes—no clinically detectable abnormalities
- Extraocular muscle movements—normal
- No proptosis, diplopia, blurring of vision
- Nose—no clinically detectable abnormalities
- TMJ—no clinically detectable abnormalities
- Mouth opening—restricted
- Lymph node examination.

Inspection

- Diffused swelling noticed below the angle of the mandible on right side (Fig. 22.13)
- Size—2 × 2 cm
- Involving right submandibular area
- No secondary changes noted.

Palpation

- Well defined, firm, tender, fixed swelling noticed
- Size 2 × 2 cm

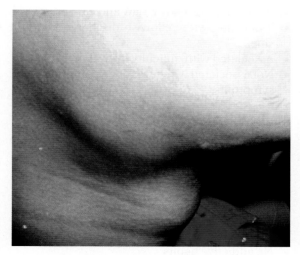

Fig 22.13: Clinical view showing swelling in submandibular region

- Involving right submandibular area
- Rt superficial cervical node palpable—single, firm, partially fixed, nontender, size—1 × 1 cm.

Intraoral Examination

Inspection

- Ulceroproliferative growth noticed involving right soft palate, faucial pillar, postpharyngeal wall, floor of the mouth, posterior ventrolateral surface of tongue, retromolar region (Figs 22.14 and 22.15)
- Size—4 × 5 cm
- Extensions
- *Anterior*—distal surface of right lower second molar
- *Posterior*—faucial pillar, soft palate and extending posteriorly into oropharynx
- *Lingually*—right postventrolateral surface of tongue and floor of the mouth
- Borders are ill-defined
- Surface appeared to be necrotic with erythematous areas.

Palpation

- Tender, ulceroproliferative growth noticed
- Size—4 × 5 cm
- Borders ill-defined and indurated
- Posterior extensions could not be made out
- Yellowish white discharge noticed.

To summarize.....

- A 17-year-old male with the c/o ulceration on the right posterior palatal region of 8 months duration associated with pain and pus discharge
- Extraoral examination revealed palpable lymph nodes in submandibular and superficial cervical region, two in no., firm, tender and fixed.

Intraorally, ulceroproliferative growth noted on posterior palatal, oropharyngeal and retromolar region, postlateroventral surface of tongue floor of the mouth with indurated ill defined borders, with the surface being necrotic. Blood investigation not significant except ESR slight increase with no bony involvement in radiograph. CT shows soft

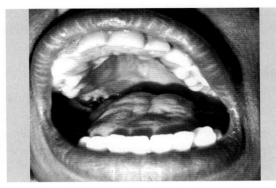

Fig. 22.14: Intraoral lesion at palatal region

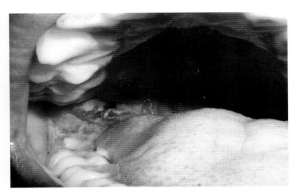

Fig. 22.15: Intraoral lesion

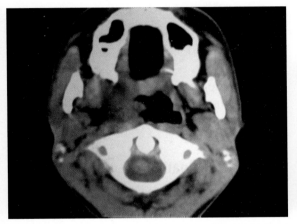

Fig. 22.16: Soft tissue growth involving the right lateral oropharyngeal extending inferiorly up to C4 level with no bony involvement

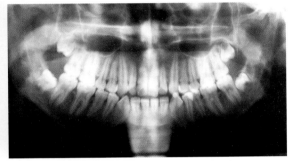

Fig. 22.17: No bony involvement in OPG

tissue growth involving right lateral oropharynx and extending inferiorly upto C4 level with no bony involvement (Figs 22.16 and 22.17).

Differential Diagnosis
- Carcinoma of minor salivary gland?
- Lymphoma?
- Carcinoma of soft palate extending to the oropharynx?

Investigations
- Exfoliative cytology
- Radiographs
- Routine blood investigations
- Incisional biopsy
- Microbial culture
- CT imaging
- Ultrasonography.

Routine Blood Investigations
- Hemoglobin—12.6 g/dL
- TLC—7800/cumm
- DLC—neutrophils—65%
- Lymphocytes—22%
- Eosinophils—13%
- Monocytes—5%

- Basophils—0%
- ESR—20 mm/hr
- Platelet count—3.62 lakhs/cumm
- RBC count—4.44 millions/dL.

CT Scan and Ultrasonography

Revealed multiple enlarged lymph nodes in RT submandibular region and bilateral deep cervical lymph node involvement.

Major salivary glands appears to be normal.

Final Diagnosis: Non-Hodgkin's Lymphoma

Treatment Options for Lymphoma

- Radiotherapy
  - 2000–2500 cGy—palliative therapy
  - 4500–5000 cGy—curative therapy
- Chemotherapy
  - CHOP—cyclophosphamide-750 mg/m^2 IV
  - Oncovin—1.4 mg/m^2 IV
  - Adrimycin—50 mg/m^2 IV
  - Prednisone—100 mg
- MOPP—nitrogen mustard-6 mg/m^2 IV
  - Oncovin—1.4 mg/m^2 IV
  - Prednisone—40 mg/m^2
  - Procarbazine—100 mg/m2
- Monoclonal antibodies
  - Rituximab—anti CD-20 antibody
  - Tositumomab—anti CD-20 antibody
  - Alemtuzumab—anti CD-52 antibody.

CASE NUMBER 6

A 58-year-male patient complains of swelling on the lower 1/3rd on the left side of face since one month.

History of Present Illness

Patient noticed a small swelling lateral to the angle of the mouth on left side. It was asymptomatic and nonprogressive, but since last one week the swelling showed a rapid progression in growth to present size.

Medical History

- Known hypertensive and under regular medication.
- Known asthmatic currently under medications
- Drug allergy—No relevant history
  Dental History—First dental visit
  Family History—No contributing factors.

Personal Habits

- Mixed diet
- Brushes teeth with coconut coir
- Smokes 15 bidis per day, stopped smoking 2 years back
- Chewing paan with betel nut, araca-nut with slaked lime since 30 years for 1 hour
- Alcohol consumption daily for a period of 20 years.

Physical Examination

General Physical Examination

- Patient is moderately built and nourished
- Cooperative
- Waddling gait
- Pallor—present
- Afebrile.

Extraoral Examination (Figs 22.18 to 22.20)

Inspection

- Facial asymmetry on the left side of the face due to the presence of swelling
- Mouth opening-2½ finger width (26 mm)
- Eyes, ear, nose—NAD
- Lips—NAD
- Skin—NAD.

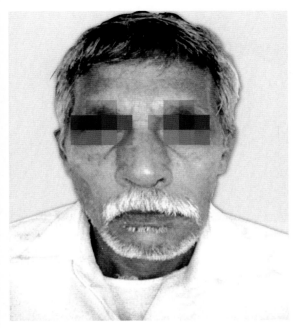

Fig. 22.18: Extraoral swelling: frontal view

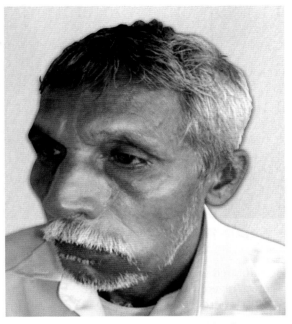

Fig. 22.19: Extraoral swelling: side view

Palpation
- Swelling is firm in consistency, tender, skin over the swelling is pinchable
- Two left submandibular lymph nodes palpable, tender 1.5 cm in diameter, partially fixed
- Submental lymph node palpable, mobile, nontender.

Intraoral Examination

Inspection
- A fissural indurated growth is noticed arising from the buccal mucosa approximately 3 cm in diameter, extending anteriorly to the canine region and posteriorly till the 1st molar region.
- Margins—well defined
- Floor—necrotic and filled with pus (Fig. 22.21).

Palpation
- The ulcer is tender
- No area of bleeding

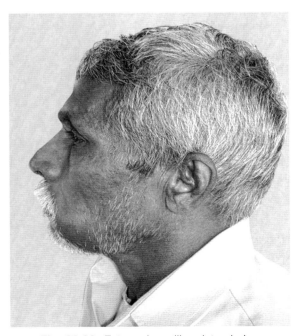

Fig. 22.20: Extraoral swelling: lateral view

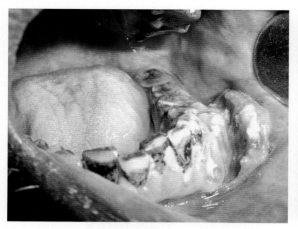

Fig. 22.21: Intraoral picture of lesion

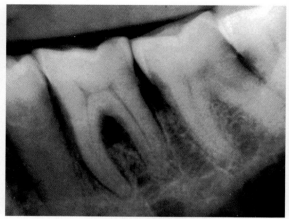

Fig. 22.22: Horizontal bone loss

- Indurated with everted margins felt on the left lower alveolus
- Base is hard.

Soft Tissue Examination

- Gingiva
- Generalized erythematous marginal gingiva
- Soft and edematous
- Generalized recession present.

Hard Tissue Examination

- Root stumps i.r.t 17, 47
- Missing 23.

Radiographic Examination (Figs 22.22 and 22.23)

- IOPA irt 36, 37, 38
- OPG
- Occlusal—mandibular.

Panoramic View Shows

- Normal anatomical landmarks
- Impacted 13
- Generalized horizontal bone loss.

Histological Examination

Biopsy specimen—The dimensions of the ulcer were measured and incisional biopsy was taken involving the normal and the affected tissue

FNAC was done of the left submandibular lymph node (Figs 22.24 and 22.25).

Extractions were carried out quadrant wise in a period of 15 days (Fig. 22.26).

Provisional Diagnosis

Ca of the left buccal mucosa.

Biopsy Report

- Submitted sections show dysplastic epithelium proliferating in form of islands into the connective tissue
- Dysplastic features like altered nuclear-cytoplasmic ratio, cellular and nuclear pleomorphism, prominent nucleoli, mitosis, individual cell keratinization and keratin pearl formation
- Surrounding connective tissue shows dense infiltration of lymphocytes, plasma cells, histiocytes and eosinophils.

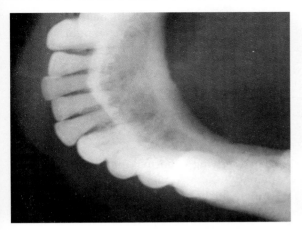

Fig. 22.23: No bony involvement is seen in the occlusal view

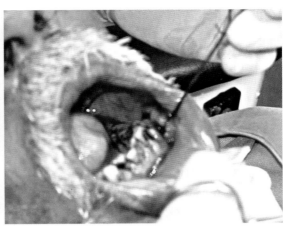

Fig. 22.24: Incisional biopsy of lesion

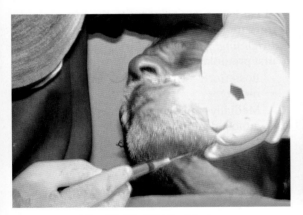

Fig. 22.25: FNAC of lesion

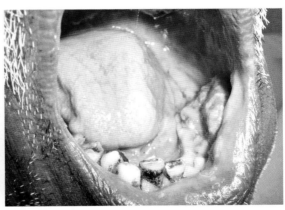

Fig. 22.26: Intraoral picture after extraction

Confirmed Diagnosis—Well-differentiated Squamous Cell Carcinoma

TNM staging- T3N1M0.

CASE NUMBER 7

- A 55-year-old female patient reported to the department with the complain of growth in the left lower back region of jaw since 6 months
- Also complains of mobile tooth in the lower back region of jaw since 2 months.

History of Present Illness

- Patient was apparently alright 6 months back, then she noticed painless growth over the left lower back region of the jaw, the lesion progressed gradually to the present size
- Associated with mild pain
- Decreased apatite
- History of weight loss
- History of mobile tooth adjacent to the lesion
- No history of increased salivation
- No history of paresthesia.

Medical History

- History of frequent episodes of cough with expectorant since 1 1/2 years—Diagnosed as having respiratory tract infection and is on medication
- Private physician advised investigation to rule out cancer of respiratory system
- Not a diabetic, hypertensive
- No history of drug allergy.

Personal History

Betel nut, arecanut, slaked lime consumption 8 times a day since 24 years, stopped 2 months back.

General Examination

- Poorly built, nourished, cooperative,
  - *Vitals*: A febrile
    - Pulse rate—80/min
    - Respiratory rate—20/min
    - Blood pressure—102/70 mm Hg
    - Weight—31 kg.
- Pallor—present
- Lympadenopathy present
- No icterus, cyanosis, clubbind, edema.

Systemic Examination

- Central nervous system, cardiovascular system – NAD

- Respiratory system—ronchi heard bilaterally over the lung field, but more on right side, and on right supraclavicular area.
- ? Wheeze present.

Extraoral (Fig. 22.27)

- Mild left side facial asymetry over the lower third of face present
- Extending from
- Skin overlying is normal, pincable, tender on palpation
- Underlying bony enlargement is present
- Mouth opening—50–52 mm.

Intraoral (Fig. 22.28)

- An ulceroproliferative lesion on buccal aspect of left lower jaw adjacent to the first molar to third molar.
- *Extending:* Anteriorly—mesial aspect of lower first premolar
  - Posteriorly—Up to distal aspect of third molar
  - Medially—involving the interdental gingiva, attached gingiva
  - Laterally—involving the buccal vestibule extending 1 cm of lower part of buccal mucosa.
- On palpation inspectory finding confirmed.

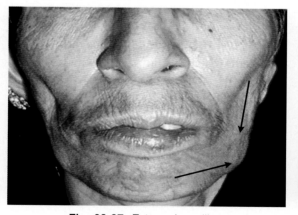

Fig. 22.27: Extraoral swelling

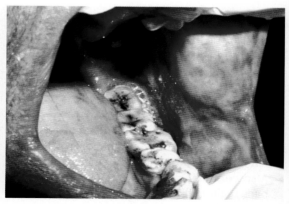

Fig. 22.28: Intraoral picture of lesion

- Mild tender
- Soft to firm in consistency
- Lesion not involving the lingual side of gingival and alveolar mucosa
- Adjacent teeth are mobile.

Lymph Nodes

Left submandibular, single node palpable, firm in consistency, mobile, nontender, measuring about 1.5–1.8 mm in diameter.

Investigations

- Radiographical (Figs 22.29 and 22.30)
  - IOPA
  - Mandibular occlusal
  - OPG (Fig. 22.31)
- Incisional biopsy done under local anesthesia.

Clinical Diagnosis

- Carcinoma lower alveolus adjacent to 36, 37, 38
- $CT_2 N_1 M_0$.

Treatment Plan

Surgical Management

Wide excision + left segmental mandibulectomy + Left modified radical neck dissection—type II + Primary closure.

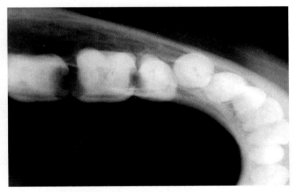

Fig. 22.29: Occlusal view showing radiolucency at buccal aspect

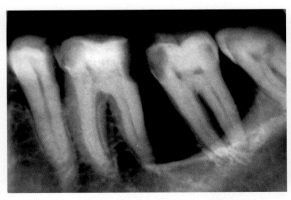

Fig. 22.30: Radiolucency bone loss

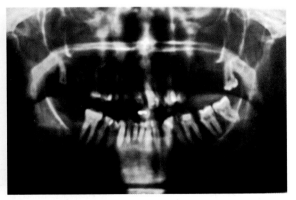

Fig. 22.31: OPG showing radiolucency

SOME MORE CLINICAL CASES (FIG. 22.32 TO 22.48)

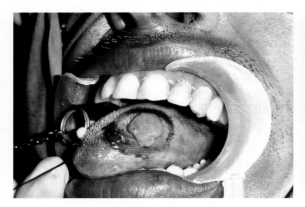

Fig. 22.32: CA tongue—lateral border

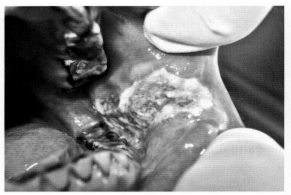

Fig. 22.33: CA buccal mucosa

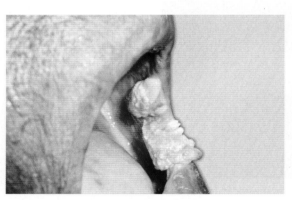

Fig. 22.34: Verrucous carcinoma—commissure area

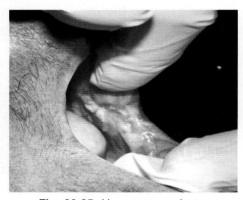

Fig. 22.35: Verrucous carcinoma

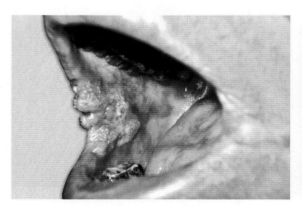

Fig. 22.36: Verrucous carcinoma

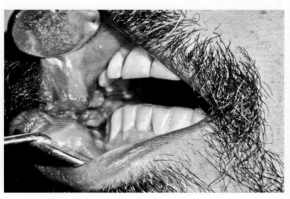

Fig. 22.37: CA buccal mucosa and commissure region

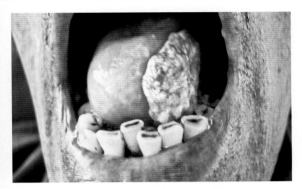

Fig. 22.38: CA lateral border of tongue

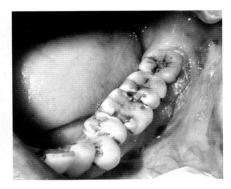

Fig. 22.39: CA gingival and alveolus—mandible

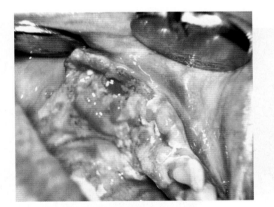

Fig. 22.40: CA alveolus

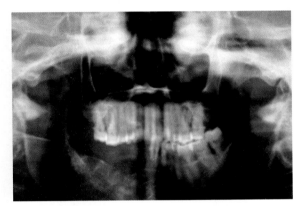

Fig. 22.41: CA alveolus showing of alveolar bone

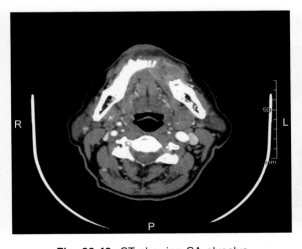

Fig. 22.42: CT showing CA alveolus

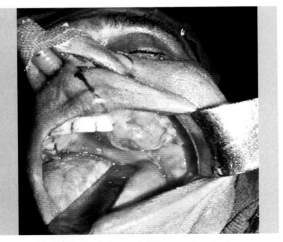

Fig. 22.43: Intraoral CA alveolus lesion

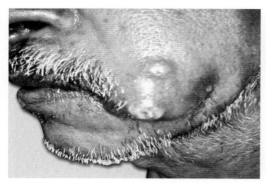

Fig. 22.44: CA buccal mucosa with extraoral fungating lesion

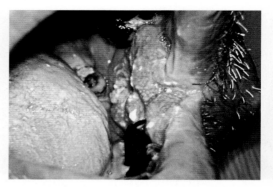

Fig. 22.45: CA gingival and alveolus—mandible

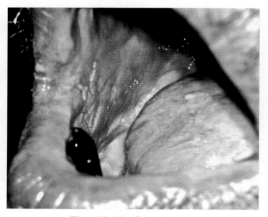

Fig. 22.46: CA alveolus

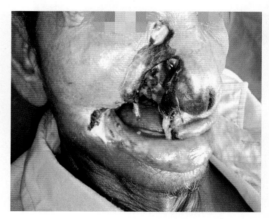

Fig. 22.47: CA alveolus showing erosion of alveolar bone

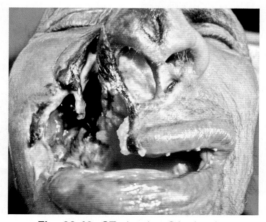

Fig. 22.48: CT showing CA alveolus

Section

4

Cysts and Tumors of Odontogenic Origin

Odontogenic Cysts

23

INTRODUCTION

Odontogenic cyst may arise in any of the soft or hard tissues in the area of the mouth and are frequently observed within the maxilla or mandible and quiet commonly have several origins few of them may arise in association with the tooth or tooth germ or it's primordial. Others arise from the reduced enamel epithelium of a tooth crown, epithelial rest of Mallassez, or the remnants of dental lamina. Some other arises from the extension of an inflammatory response in the pulpal tissue into the apical region and stimulates residual of Hertwigs sheath to proliferate. Still other group may be due to embryonic inclusions and injury

- "Cyst is an entity that constitutes an epithelium lined sac filled with fluid or semifluid material".
  —*Killey and Kay (1966)*

- A cyst is an abnormal cavity in hard or soft tissues which contains fluid, semifluid, or gas and is often encapsulated and lined by epithelium.
  —*Killey and Kay (1966)*

- A cyst is a pathologic cavity having fluid, semifluid or gaseous contents that are not created by the accumulation of pus; frequently, but not always, is lined by epithelium.
  —*Kramer (1974)*

CLASSIFICATION (FLOWCHART 23.1)

Classification—by World Health Organization (1992)

Intraosseous Cysts

Epithelial
- Odontogenic
  Developmental
  – Odontogenic keratocyst
  – Dentigerous (follicular) cyst
  – Lateral periodontal cyst
  – Calcifying odontogenic cyst
  – Inflammatory
    - Radicular cyst/apical/lateral periodontal cyst
    - Residual cyst
- Nonodontogenic cysts
  – Nasopalatine duct cyst (incisive canal/median anterior maxillary cyst)
    - Cyst of the incisive papilla
  – Palatal cyst of infants
    - Epstein's pearls
    - Bohn's nodules.

Nonepithelial/Pseudocysts
- Idiopathic bone cavity (Stafne's)
- Solitary bone cyst (traumatic)
- Aneurysmal bone cyst.

Flowchart 23.1: Classification of cysts of jaws, oral cavity, and fascial soft tissues

Cysts of the Maxillary Antrum

- Surgical ciliated cyst of maxilla
- Benign mucosal cyst of maxillary antrum

Soft Tissue Cysts

Odontogenic
- Gingival cysts
  - Adult
  - Newborn
- Eruption cyst.

Nonodontogenic
- Anterior median lingual cyst
- Nasolabial cyst (nasoalveolar cyst).

Retention cysts
- Salivary gland cysts
- Mucous extravasation cyst
- Mucous retention cyst
- Ranula.

Developmental/congenital cysts
- Dermoid and epidermoid cysts
- Lymphoepithelial cyst (cervical/intraoral)
- Thyroglossal duct cyst
- Cystic hygroma
- Trichilemmal cyst (pilar cyst).

Parasitic cysts
- Hydatid cyst
- Cysticercosis.

Heterotropic cysts: Oral cysts with gastric or intestinal epithelium.

Miscellaneous cysts
- Polycystic disease of parotid
- HIV-associated lymphoepithelial lesion.

Spurious cysts
- Globulomaxillary cyst
- Median mandibular cyst
- Median maxillary alveolar cyst.

Pathogenesis
- Cyst initiation
- Stimulus
- Inflammatory cysts—infection
- Others—predisposition to form cysts.

Cyst Formation

Formation of cavity lined by stratified squamous epithelium could occur by a number of mechanisms:
- Cleft produced by accumulation of purulent exudate in the form of a microabscess involved one of the proliferating strands of epithelium, and then the epithelial cells would be expected to line the cleft
- Stimulated epithelium proliferated to form a sphere of cells
- Epithelial cells become oriented in relation to their source of nutrition and the adjacent connective tissue. Thus in the normal situation they cover a surface and are finally desquamated
- Harris (1974a) suggests that the spongework of epithelial cells at the periphery of a granuloma plays a protective role, isolating the irritating and infected material in the center
- Valderhaug (1974) and Harris (1974b) also contend that the entire center of the granuloma becomes necrotic and after this the cell meshwork becomes consolidated into the epithelium- lined cyst
- Shear (1963) observes that the early developing periodontal cyst is surrounded by proliferating arcades and rings of epithelium, each with a vascular connective tissue core, and later this arcade pattern disappears.

Cyst Enlargement
- The attraction of fluid into the cystic cavity
- The retention of the fluid within the cavity
- The production of a raised internal hydrostatic pressure
- The resorption of surrounding bone with an increase in the size of the bone cavity.

Harris (1974) described the theories of cyst enlargement
- Mural growth
  - Peripheral cell division
  - Accumulation of cellular content
- Hydrostatic enlargement
  - Secretion
  - Transudation and exudation
  - Bone resorbing factor
- Livingstone (1927) estimated the annual increase in size of the periodontal cyst to be approxiamtely 5 mm in diameter per year
- Killey, Kay, and Seward (1977) estimated that in teenage and adult patients, approx. 10 yrs is required for the development of a cyst 2 cm in diameter
- Shear (1963) suggests that larger the cyst, the slower the yearly increase in diameter. The diameter of 2 cm is a crucial size beyond which it is likely that expansion of the jaw will be detected clinically.

Intraosseous Cysts

Developmental Odontogenic Cysts and Dentigerous Cyst

Defined as one which encloses the crown of an unerupted tooth and is attached to the neck.

Clinical features
- Age—2nd to 3rd decade
- Sex—Males > Females
- Race—Whites > Blacks
- Site—Mandible > Maxilla
- Mandibular III molar (D/d: Ameloblastoma)
- Maxillary canine (D/d: Adenomatoid odonto-genic tumor)
- Mandibular premolar, maxillary III molar, supernumerary.

Clinical presentation
- Slowly enlarging swelling
- Resorption of roots of adjacent teeth
- Bone expansion with facial asymmetry
- Displacement of teeth, pain.

Cyst contents
- Yellowish fluid containing cholesterol crystals

Pathogenesis: Accumulation of fluid between reduced enamel epithelium and tooth crown after crown formation is completed.

Radiographic features
- Radiolucent area associated with unerupted tooth crown
- Three varieties—lateral, coronal, circumferential
- Usually unilocular, rarely multilocular.

Potential complications
- Ameloblastoma
- Epidermoid carcinoma
- Mucoepidermoid carcinoma.

Treatment
- Enucleation
- Marsupialization.

Lateral Periodontal Cyst

Those cysts which occur in the lateral periodontal position and in which an inflammatory etiology and a diagnosis of collateral primordial cyst have been excluded on clinical and histological grounds. (Shear and Pindborg, 1975).

Clinical features
- Age—2nd to 7th decades
- Sex—Males > Females
- Site—Mandibular premolar area and anterior region of maxilla.

Clinical presentation
- Symptomless, discovered during routine radiographic examination
- Gingival swelling may occur on facial aspect. (D/d: Gingival cyst)
- Associated teeth—vital unless otherwise involved.

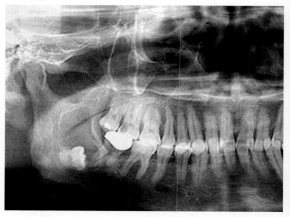

Fig. 23.1: OPG showing radiolucency associated with 48 sclerotic margin

Radiographic features
- Well defined round or oval radiolucent area with sclerotic margin (Fig. 23.1)
- Cyst lies between apex and cervical margin of tooth
- Mostly <1 cm in diameter; may be larger involving entire root length. (D/d: Collateral variety of primordial cyst).

Pathogenesis: From reduced enamel epithelium, remnants of dental lamina and cell rests of Malassez.

Histopathological features
- Cyst lining—nonkeratinized squamous or cuboidal epithelium 1–5 cell thick
- Presence of localized plaques in lining.

Treatment
- Surgical enucleation
Recurrence—None.

Botyroid Odontogenic Cyst

- Name proposed by Weathers and Waldron (1973), as the gross specimen resembles a cluster of grapes
- Radiologically and histologically similar to lateral periodontal cyst
- Microscopically seen as a multilocular lesion with very thin fibrous connective tissue septa.

Calcifying Odontogenic Cyst: Gorlin Cyst

- First described by Gorlin and associates (1962, 1964)
- Histologically resembles calcifying epithelioma of Malherbe
- Studies of Praetorius et al. (1981) conclude that this lesion comprises two entities—a cyst and a neoplasm.

Clinical presentation

- Symptomless, discovered accidentally.
- Swelling—most frequent complaint
- Peripheral or intraosseous lesion
- Intraosseous lesion produces hard, bony expansion
- Saucer shaped bony depression seen in cysts arising close to periosteum
- Displacement of teeth may be seen.

Radiological features

- When small, cyst seen between roots of teeth
- Periphery—well demarcated or irregular
- Usually unilocular
- Irregular calcified bodies of varying size and opacity maybe seen in radiolucent area
- Cyst maybe associated with a complex odontome or an unerupted tooth
- Resorption of roots of adjacent teeth maybe seen
- Cortical perforation maybe evident.

Pathogenesis

- Remnants of dental lamina, stellate reticulum
- Reduced enamel epithelium.

Epithelial lining has the ability to induce formation of dental tissues in the adjacent connective tissue wall.

Histopathology: Ghost cells seen which can evoke a foreign body reaction with the formation of multinucleated giant cells in the connective tissue wall.

Treatment: Enucleation.

Inflammatory Odontogenic Cysts

Radicular Cyst

- Is one which arises from the epithelial residues in the periodontal ligament as a result of inflammation
- Also referred to as:
  - Periapical (periodontal) radicular cyst
  - Lateral (periodontal) radicular cyst.

Clinical features

- Age—3rd to 4th decade
- Sex—Males > Females
- Site—Maxillary anterior teeth.

Clinical presentation

- Symptomless unless infected
- Associated with nonvital teeth
- May complain of slowly enlarging swelling
- Initially bony hard swelling, as cyst increases in size bony covering becomes thin and swelling exhibits *'springiness'*, later fluctuation.

Cyst content

- Uninfected cystic fluid is straw coloured or brownish containing cholesterol clefts
- Small amount of keratin flakes maybe seen
- In long—standing infection, a dirty white caseous material or frank pus maybe expressed.

Radiological features: Well-circumscribed unilocular radiolucency at apex or lateral aspect of tooth.

Histopathological features

- Inflammatory infiltrate of polymorphonuclear leucocytes seen in lining
- Epithelial lining may show presence of Rushton bodies, mucus or ciliated cells.

Treatment

- Enucleation with primary closure
- Associated nonvital teeth maybe extracted or endodontically treated
- Very small cysts can be removed through tooth socket
- Marsupialization and decompression.

Residual Cyst

Is a radicular cyst that remains behind in the jaws after the removal of the offending tooth.

Clinical features
- Site—greater in maxilla
- Typically seen in edentulous sites.

Clinical presentation
- Asymptomatic, discovered on radiographic examination
- Pathologic fractures or signs of encroachment on associated structures in case of large residual cysts.

Histopathologic features: Similar to underlying process that was present.

Treatment: Similar to radicular cyst.

Nonodontogenic Cysts

Nasopalatine Duct Cyst

Incisive canal cyst/Median anterior maxillary cyst.

Clinical features
- Age—4th to 6th decades
- Sex—Males > Females

- Site—within nasopalatine canal in soft tissues of palate, at the opening of the canal (cyst of the incisive papilla).

Clinical presentation
- Swelling in the anterior region of midline of palate or in the midline on the labial aspect of alveolar ridge
- 'Through and through' fluctuation maybe elicited between labial and palatal swellings.

Radiological features (Fig. 23.2 and 23.3)
- Well-defined cystic outline, between, or above the roots of the maxillary central incisors
- Maybe round, ovoid or heart-shaped
- Roots of central incisors may show divergence and intact lamina dura around tooth apices.

Histopathological features
- Cystic lining—varies at different levels
- Stratified squamous at a lower level; more superiorly pseudostratified columnar, cuboidal as well as ciliated
- Presence of mucous glands, goblet cells and cilia, nerves and blood vessels in the fibrous capsule.

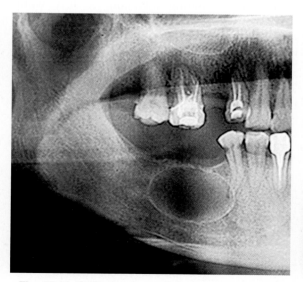

Fig. 23.2: OPG showing radiolucent area in molar region residual

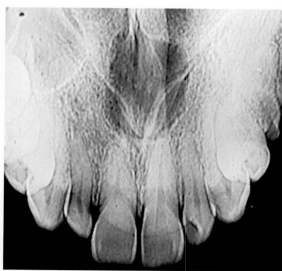

Fig. 23.3: Maxillary occlusal showing radiolucency in palatal region

Cyst contents: Mucous fluid content—maybe mucoid or purulent (if infected).

Treatment: Enucleation by raising a palatal flap.

Palatal Cyst of Infants (Fig. 23.3)

Epstein's pearls: Seen along the midpalatine raphe.

Bohn's nodules: Scattered on palate, especially at junction of hard and soft palate.

Clinical presentation: White or cream colored, number may vary from one to many, usually 5–6.

Pathogenesis: Epstein pearls-arise from epithelial inclusions at the line of fusion of the palatal folds and the nasal processes, which if not resorbed after birth, produce keratin containing microcysts.

Histopathological features
- Cysts are round or ovoid and may have a smooth or undulating outline
- Thin lining of stratified squammous epithelium with parakeratotic surface, and keratin fills cyst cavity.

Treatment: No indication for treatment.

Nonepithelial/Pseudocysts

Idiopathic Bone Cavity

Stafne's cavity/static bone cavity/latent bone cyst.

Etiology
- Due to failure of normal deposition of bone during development
- Developmental defects occupied by a lobe of salivary gland
- Close proximity of lobe of gland producing pressure atrophy of lingual surface of mandible.

Clinical features
- Site—Mandible—below inferior alveolar canal, approximately in line with the position of III molar tooth toward the inferior border of mandible
- Usually unilateral, bilateral defects maybe present

- Symptomless, nonprogressive lesions detected on routine radiographic examination.

Radiologic features
- Round or oval radiolucency, 1–3 cm in size, well demarcated by dense radio opaque line, below inferior alveolar canal, posterior to first mandibular molar
- Cortical perforation if lesion has extended to inferior border.

Histopathology
- No diagnostic tissue
- May contain salivary gland tissue, lymph node tissue or abnormal glandular tissue.

Treatment
- No surgical intervention required
- Regular radiological follow-up advised, as they constitute an area of weakness and pathologic fracture can occur.

Solitary Bone Cyst (Traumatic Bone Cyst/ Hemorrhagic Bone Cyst)

Similar lesions seen elsewhere in the skeleton, commonly at proximal ends of humerus and upper and lower portions of the femoral and tibial shafts, where it is known as unicameral cyst.

Etiology
- Trauma and haemorrhage with failure of organization
- Spontaneous atrophy of tissue in a central benign giant-cell lesion
- Abnormal calcium metabolism
- Chronic low-grade infection
- Necrosis of fatty marrow secondary to ischaemia
- Aberration in growth and development of local osseous tissue.

Clinical features
- Age—1st two decades
- Sex—Males > Females
- Site—Mandible—subapical region, above infe-rior alveolar canal, in cuspid and molar region.

Presentation
- Usually symptomless

- Cortex usually thinned but expansion occurs later on and may first involve lingual aspect below mylohyoid ridge
- Associated teeth vital
- Unerupted teeth maybe prevented from eruption.

Radiological features
- Cyst appears unilocular, which when it enlarges pushes up into the interdental bone to produce a scalloped outline
- Roots of related teeth maybe displaced, lamina dura is intact and no resorption.

Pathology
- Cyst cavities usually empty
- Loose vascular fibrous tissue membrane with hemosiderin pigment maybe seen with small multinucleat cells
- Adjacent bone may show osteoclastic resorption on its inner surface.

Cyst contents
- Deep yellow colored fluid contains plasma proteins and will clot, if left to stand
- Small cysts, heavily blood stained fluid or fresh blood maybe obtained
- Some cysts—empty. They may contain gas—nitrogen, oxygen and carbondioxide.

Treatment: Surgical exploration and gentle curettage.

Aneurysmal Bone Cyst
- First described by Jaffe and Lichenstein (1942)

- Usually seen in long bones and spine, rarely in jaws
- Previously described as atypical giant cell tumor, hemorrhagic osteomyelitis, ossifying hematoma or benign bone cyst.

Etiology
- Trauma
- Variation in hemodynamics of the area
- Sudden venous occlusion.

Clinical features
- No sex predilection
- Age—children, adolescents and young adults
- Firm swellings, with history of rapid enlargement
- Teeth maybe bisplaced, but vital
- Egg—shell crackling maybe exhibited
- Bruit not heard, lesion not pulsatile.

Radiological features (Fig. 23.4)
- Honey-comb or soap-bubble appearance
- Root resorption.

Cyst contents: Dark venous blood can be aspirated (Fig. 23.5).

Pathology
- Numerous blood-filled spaces of varying sizes in a fibrous connective tissue stroma
- Small multinucleate cells and scattered trabeculae of woven bone.

Treatment
- Curettage—recurrence rate of 26%
- Large lesions—local excision with bone grafting
- Radiotherapy contraindicated.

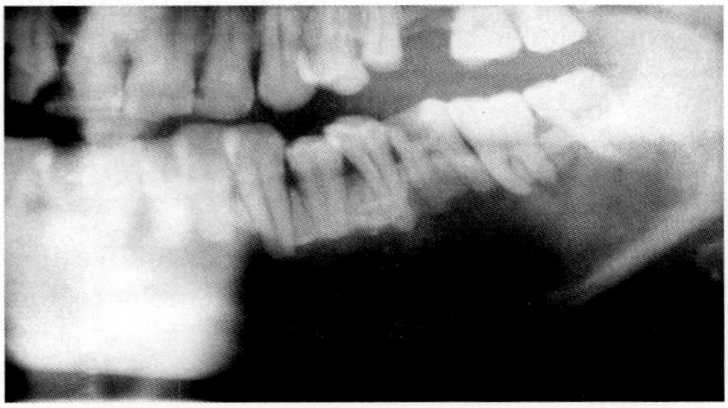

Fig. 23.4: OPG showing radiolucency in molar and premolar region

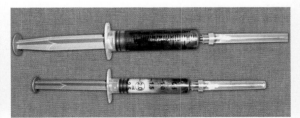

Fig. 23.5: Aspiration pump to aspirate from aneurysmal cyst lesion

Cysts of the Maxillary Antrum

Surgical Ciliated Cyst of the Maxilla

Iatrogenic—The cysts develop from the epithelial lining of the maxillary sinus, which was trapped in the surgical incision during closure following a maxillary surgical procedure that involved the maxillary sinus lining.

Clinical features: Patients complain of poorly localized pain or discomfort in the maxilla.

Radiological features: Well-defined radiolucency closely related to maxillary sinus.

Histopathological features: Cystic lining is pseudostratified ciliated columnar epithelium, with squamous metaplasia in infected areas.

Treatment: Enucleation.

Benign Mucosal Cyst of the Maxillary Antrum (Mucocele/Retention Cyst of Antrum)

Etiology

Infection and inflammation of ducts of mucous glands.

Clinical Features

- Age—3rd decade
- Site—Floor of sinus.

Presentation

- Discovered accidentally on radiographs
- Some complain of dull pain over antral region or a sense of fullness or numbness in the maxillary region
- Nasal obstruction
- Yellowish nasal discharge or postnasal drip
- Large cysts—produce swelling in maxillary region.

Radiological Features

Spherical, ovoid radiopacities in maxillary antrum, with smooth outline.

Pathology

- Pseudostratified ciliated columnar epithelium contains mucin
- Chronic inflammatory cells seen.

Treatment

- Large cysts removed through Caldwell-Luc approach, and drainage enhanced via cannulation through intranasal antrostomy
- Asymptomatic patient—conservative medical treatment.

Soft Tissue Cysts: Odontogenic Soft Tissue Cysts

Gingival Cyst of Adults

Etiology

- Remnants of dental lamina or rests of serres.
- Traumatic implantation cysts
- Enamel organ or epithelial islands of surface epithelium
- Glandular elements.

Clinical features

- Age—5th and 6th decades
- Site—Mandible > canine and premolar region, in the attached gingiva or interdental papilla on labial aspect.

Presentation: Painless, slow-growing swelling, with smooth surface and of normal color or bluish, soft in consistency and fluctuant.

Treatment: Surgical excision.

Gingival Cyst of Infants Eruption Cyst

- It is a dentigerous cyst occurring in the soft tissues
- It occurs when a tooth is impeded in its eruption within soft tissues overlying bone.

Clinical features

- Soft and fluctuant smooth swelling over erupting tooth which maybe color of normal gingiva, or blue.

- Painless unless infected
- Transillumination distinguishes eruption cyst from eruption hematoma.

Radiological features
- Cyst may throw a soft tissue shadow
- Dilated and open crypt seen.

Pathogenesis: Similar to dentigerous cyst.

Treatment: Marsupialization.

Nonodontogenic Cysts

Anterior Median Lingual Cyst
Clinical features
- Site—anterior 2/3rds of tongue
- Fluctuant swelling, present since birth.

Pathogenesis: Epithelium trapped between lateral tubercles of developing tongue.

Treatment: Enucleation.

Nasolabial Cyst
Clinical features
- Age—3rd to 5th decades
- Sex—Females
- Site—Above buccal sulcus under ala of nose, at the junction of globular, maxillary and lateral nasal processes.

Presentation
- Unilateral/bilateral swelling involving lip, that lifts up the nasolabial fold and obliterates the labial sulcus
- Difficulty in breathing, if it bulges into inferior meatus
- Fluctuant and painless unless infected Infected cysts discharge into nose or mouth.

Pathogenesis
- Remnants of nasolacrimal duct
- Lower anterior portion of mature nasolacrimal duct
- Mucous cysts arising from epithelial lining of floor of nose

- Mucous cysts within mucous glands in labial sulcus
- Sequestered epithelium from depths of groove between maxillary and lateral nasal process.

Cyst content: Straw colored or whitish mucinous fluid.

Treatment: Enucleation.

Retention Cysts (Figs 23.6 to 23.12)

Mucocele
Mucous extravasation cysts, mucous retention cysts.

Etiology
- Obstruction to salivary duct
- Trauma to salivary duct
- Trauma to secretory acini
- Congenital atresia of submandibular duct orifices
- Cystic type of papillary cystadenoma.

Clinical features
- Retention cysts more common in older patients
- Extravasation cysts common in younger age group
- Site—Except anterior ½ of hard palate, they can occur anywhere in the oral cavity, i.e. cheeks, ventral surface of tongue, floor of mouth, retromolar area
- Majority of mucoceles seen in lower lip.

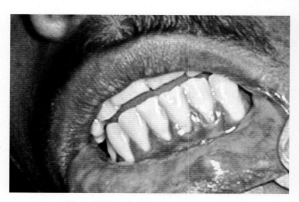

Fig. 23.6: Mucocele at lower lip

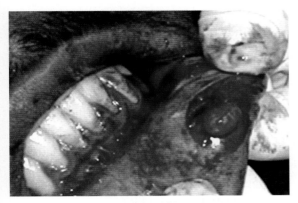

Fig. 23.7: Lesion after exposure

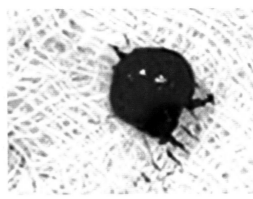

Fig. 23.8: Lesion removed

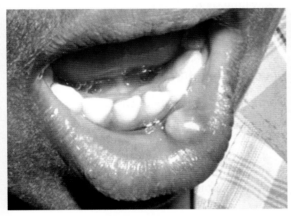

Fig. 23.9: Mucocele in a child

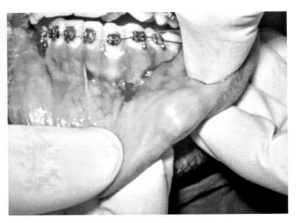

Fig. 23.10: Mucocele at lower lip

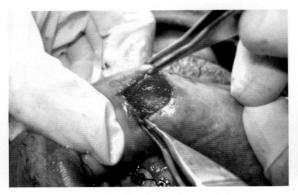

Fig. 23.11: Site after removal of lesion

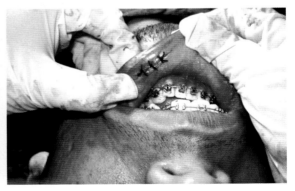

Fig. 23.12: After suturing

Presentation
- Small, painless, superficial, well circumscribed swelling on mucosa, 1–2 mm in size, not more than 1–2 cm.
- Fluctuant
- Color—translucent or bluish
- Rupture spontaneously with liberation of viscous fluid. Lesion reappears within weeks by fluid accumulation.

Pathology
- Extravasation cysts—no epithelial lining,
  - Poorly-defined pools containing eosinophilic mucinous material, vacuolated macrophages, granulation tissue, and condensed fibrous tissue
- Retention cysts—partly or completely lined by epithelium.

Treatment: Surgical excision together with associated minor salivary gland tissue and surrounding connective tissue.

Ranula
- Mucocele present in the floor of the mouth, beneath the tongue
- Two types—superficial ranula and plunging ranula.

Etiology
- Trauma to excretory ducts of sublingual salivary gland
- In plunging type, the extravasated mucus passes through mylohyoid muscle and gets collected in submandibular region
- Atresia of submandibular duct orifices.

Clinical features
- Dome-shaped bluish swelling located laterally in floor of mouth beneath tongue
- Tongue maybe raised or displaced as it enlarges
- Swelling may cross midline
- In plunging type extraoral submandibular swelling seen.

Treatment: Surgical removal of sublingual gland via intraoral approach.

Developmental/Congenital Cysts

Dermoid and Epidermoid Cysts
- Dermoid cysts are a form of cystic teratoma, lined by epithelium and contains skin appendages (Figs 23.13 to 23.15)
- Epidermoid cysts are lined by epithelium but do not contain appendages.

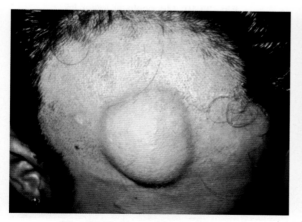

Fig. 23.13: Dermoid cyst scalp (I)

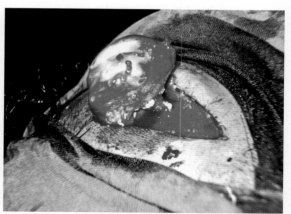

Fig. 23.14: Exposure of lesion

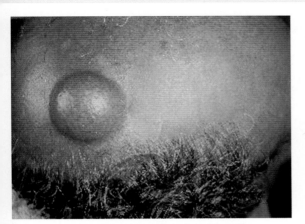

Fig. 23.15: Dermoid cyst scalp (II) (Figs 23.13 to 23.16
Courtesy: Dr Vikram Shally)

Pathogenesis
- From epithelial rests persisting in the midline after the fusion of mandible and hyoid branchial arches
- It is comprised of a combination of ectoderm, endoderm, and mesoderm elements
  The tissue elements may become malignant.

Clinical features
- Age—young adolescents
- No sex predilection
- Site—median dermoids—midline, floor of mouth, superior or inferior to geniohyoid muscle.
- Lateral dermoids rarely seen.

Presentation
- Midline or lateral swellings in floor of mouth or neck
- Those above geniohyoid, elevate tongue, causing difficulty with mastication and speech
- Those inferior to geniohyoid, cause submental swelling, causing a double-chin
- Small in infancy but enlarge to several cms in diameter
- On palpation, dough-like consistency.

Pathology
- Lined by keratinising str sq. epi. and contains keratin scales
- Dermoid cysts—appendages in its wall.

Treatment
- Surgical excision
- Cysts in floor of mouth—intraoral approach
- Large cysts inferior to mylohyoid—extraoral approach via a horizontal submandibular incision.

Implantation Keratinizing Epidermoid Cysts

Etiology
- Implantation following trauma or surgical intervention
- Site—face, neck scalp.

Pathology
Two types—Epidermal cyst
- Found on hands and fingers
- Lined by keratinized stratified squammous epithelium with prominent stratum granulosum.

Trichilemmal (Pilar) Cyst
- Occur on scalp, rarely on face
- No stratum granulosum
- Cyst content is low in sulfur-containing amino acids; thus, differs from hair cortex.

Lymphoepithelial Cysts/Branchial Cleft Cysts (Fig. 23.16 A and B)

Clinical features
- No age or sex predilection
- Site—close to angle of mandible, anterior to sternocleidomastoid muscle, less commonly in floor of mouth, ventral surface of tongue
- Other sites—soft palate, anterior palatine pillar, buccal vestibule.

Presentation
- Neck lesions—vary in size; seen as soft, fluctuant mass at or above cervical sites. They may develop fistulous tract and drain externally
- Intraoral lesions—1–10 mm in size; submucosal, freely mobile. May develop fistulous tract and drain intraorally.

Pathogenesis
- Epithelial remnants of branchial clefts and pouches

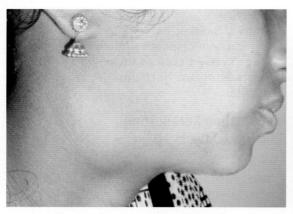

Fig. 23.16A: Branchial cyst presenting as neck swelling

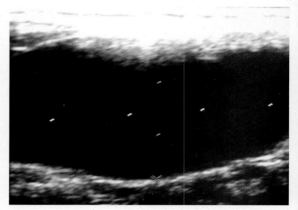

Fig. 23.16B: USG of branchial cyst

- Residual cervical sinus epithelium
- Salivary gland inclusions in parotid nodes which undergo cystic changes
- Cystic changes within cervical lymph nodes of epithelial inclusions. (Benign lymphoepithelial cyst).

Pathology
- Cervical cysts—lumen contains mucus and desquamated parakeratotic cells
- Intraoral cysts—lumen contains watery fluid. Lymphoid tissue envelops cystic lining.

Treatment: Surgical excision by cervical or intraoral approach.

Thyroglossal Duct Cyst

Clinical Features
- Age—highest in infancy and 2nd decade
- Site—anywhere in midline along course of embryonic thyroglossal duct
- Floor of mouth, area around hyoid, thyroid cartialge region—common sites.

Presentation
- Midline swellings; slight lateral positional variations maybe seen
- Soft, tender and movable
- Swelling moves with deglutition and protrusion of tongue

- Dysphagia, dysphoria or dyspnoea, at times
- Size—1–5 cm in diameter
- Sinus tract may develop due to infection.

Pathology
- Cysts above hyoid—lined by stratified squammous epithelium
- Cysts below hyoid—lined by ciliated respiratory or columnar epithelim
- Fibrous wall shows lymphoid tissue, thyroid tissue, or mucous glands.

Treatment
- Complete radical surgical excision
- Central part of hyoid, 1–2 cm may require to be removed during surgery.

Cystic Hygroma
- It is a type of lymphangioma
- It is a developmental abnormality in which cavernous lymphatic spaces communicate and form large thin-walled cysts that may grow to a large size.

Clinical Features
- Age—appear in 1st few months of life
- Site—in sites of primitive lymphatic lakes—on floor of mouth, under the jaw, neck and axillae, but may occur anywhere in the body.

Presentation

- Painless and compressible swellings, which may increase in size, remain static, or regress
- Overlying skin—bluish
- Transillumination—positive
- Sudden increase in size when there is an upper respiratory tract infection, causing respiratory obstruction, may require emergency tracheostomy or surgical extirpation.

Pathology: Dilated cystic spaces lined by endothelial cells.

Treatment: Early excision.

Parasitic Cysts

Rarely involves oral tissues.

Hydatid Cyst

- In hydatid disease or echinococcosis
- Hydatid disease is common in sheep-raising countries such as Australia, New Zealand, South Africa
- Maybe seen in the tongue as a painless swelling slowly increasing in size
- Cyst fluid—clear, albumin-free, contains 'hydatid sand', containing brood capsules and scolices.

Cysticercus Cellulosae

- Man develops cysticercosis through pork tapeworm—*Taenia solium*
- Larval forms penetrate intestinal mucosa and then distributed through blood and lymphatics to all parts of body, where they develop into cysticerci.

Site

- Lip, cheek, and skin.
- Harmless in oral tissues, but localization in brain, heart valves and orbit occurs producing important functional derangements.

Heterotropic Cysts

Oral Cysts with Gastric or Intestinal Epithelium

Clinical features
- Age—infants and young children
- Site—sublingual region, apex and dorsum of tongue.

Pathogenesis: In intrauterine life, in the 3–4 mm embryo, stomach lies in the midneck region, not far from the anlage of the tongue, thus it is possible that the ectodermal and endodermal epithelia fuse, which explains the cystic lesions in the oral cavity.

Pathology
- Cysts lined partly by stratified squammous epithelium and partly by gastric mucosa
- Gastric glands, goblet cells maybe seen.

Treatment: Surgical excision.

General Principles of Treatment

Reasons for Treatment of Benign Cysts of the Oral Cavity

- Cysts tend to increase in size
- Cysts tend to get infected
- Cysts weaken the jaw and can cause pathological fracture
- Some cysts can undergo malignant changes and it is not possible to be certain about a cystic lesion unless the tissue is examined histologically
- Cysts can prevent eruption of teeth.

Clinical Presentation

- Most cysts are discovered accidentally on radiographs
- In case of a smooth, rounded expansion of the jaw bones a cyst should be suspected until proved otherwise
- A change in the fitting of dentures in the presence of a swelling

- Absence of a tooth from its place in the arch
- Presence of a carious, discolored, fractured or heavily filled tooth related to the swelling, suggestive of apical periodontal cyst
- Tilting of the crowns of teeth suggests that their roots have been displaced by te expansion of a cyst or tumor
- On extraction of a tooth with a sizeable radicular cyst, cystic fluid may escape from the socket
- Infected cysts may present as painful, tender swellings and may have discharging sinuses
- Percussion of teeth overlying a solitary bone cyst produces a dull, hollow sound
- Fissural cysts are generally small in size
- Periodontal cysts may occur anywhere in the dental arch
- Dentigerous cyst is mainly associated with impacted third molars, canines and premolars
- Solitary bone cyst is virtually assigned to the mandible
- Static bone cavity is located beneath the inferior alveolar canal
- OKCs are most commonly in the lower III molar area and extending into the ramus
- Large cysts usually deflect the neurovascular bundle, paresthesia and anesthesia are rare
- Infected cysts may cause some degree of neuropraxia
- As a cyst enlarges, a smooth, hard, painless prominence is generally seen on the labial side
- Expansion of the lingual aspect alone can occur with an odontogenic cyst in the ramus or III molar region
- Expansion of both cortical plates is generally indicative of a lesion rather than a cyst
- *Egg-shell crackling* is a term used to descibe the fragile outer shell of bone that has thinned out due to the expansion and the sensation and sound produced on palpation is like egg-shell crackling
- Fluctuation is elicited when the cystic lining lies immediately beneath the mucosa.

Vitality of Teeth

- Preoperative and postoperative vitality tests should be performed on all teeth related to the cyst, regardless of the method of treatment
- Teeth adjoining OKC, fissural cyst, solitary bone cyst and other nonodontogenic cysts will have vital pulps, unless otherwise infected
- Apical periodontal cysts are associated with nonvital teeth
- Lateral periodontal cyst is associated with a vital tooth
- In infected cysts, there may be a temporary absence of a vital response in adjacent teeth because of pressure interference with sensory transmission from the pulp.

Radiographic Examination

- Periapical radiographs provide a clear and accurate image of small cystic lesions
- Occlusal films of the maxilla will disclose amoutn of palatal bone destruction by a cystic process
- Occlusal view of mandible will reveal expansion of inner or outer cortical plates
- Extraoral radiographs provide the full extent of the lesion and help in assessing the damage caused to the adjacent structures, e.g. lateral oblique views, OPG
- PA mandible view helps to reveal both lateral and medial expansion of the ramus
- Anterior cysts of the antrum are best visualized in the Water's projection
- CT scans maybe helpful in the assessment of large cystic lesions and multicystic lesions
- In multilocular lesions, D/d with other multicysti lesions such as giant cell lesions, myxomas, hemangiomas and ameloblastomas should be considered.

Radiopaque Dyes

- When the size and relations of a cyst are in doubt, its contents maybe aspirated and radiopaque dye injected prior to further radiography

- To follow the progress of regression of a marsupialized lesion
- Radiopaque dyes used—lipiodol, triosil.

Aspiration

- Valuable diagnostic aid
- Helps to distinguish:
  - Maxillary cyst from maxillary sinus.
  - Cystic lesion and solid tumor mass.
  - Aneurysmal bone cyst from central cavernous hemangioma
  - Helps to distinguish various cysts.

Biopsy

- Valuable diagnostic aid in the differential diagnosis of the nature cyst or its differentiation from tumor
- Biopsy prior to surgery is done for large lesions and when doubt exists.

Assessment: This includes:
- Estimation of the size of the cystic lesion
- Extent of bone loss
- Risk of pathological fracture
- Relationship of cyst to adjacent structures
- Vital teeth, having satisfactory periodontal condition should be preserved
- Nonvital teeth embedded in sound bone, should be treated endodontically and epicectomy done
- Nonfunctional, mobile, nonvital teeth, beyond restoration should be extracted
- If extensive bone loss expected, as in surgical excision, consent and preparation for rehabilitation methods such as reconstructive plates, bone grafts, etc. should be planned
- Acutely infected cysts should be treated with antibacterial drugs, or drainage should be done prior to surgery
- In case of multicystic lesions, possible syndrome should be ruled out

- Postoperative monitoring of teeth by vitality tests should be done until bone formation is complete.

Operative Procedures

Cysts of the jaws maybe treated by one of the following basic methods:

Marsupialization

- Partsch I
- Partsch II (combined marsupialization and enucleation)/Waldron's method
- Marsupialization by opening into nose or antrum.

Enucleation

- Enucleation and packing
- Enucleation and primary closure
- Enucleation and primary closure with reconstruction/bone grafting.

Marsupialization/Decompression

Principle

- It refers to creating a surgical window in the wall of the cyst and evacuation of its contents
- This decreases the intracystic pressure and promotes shrinkage of the cyst and bone fill.

Indications

- In young children with developing tooth germs
- In elderly, debilitated patient
- Proximity of cyst to vital structures
- When cyst impedes tooth eruption, marsupialisation facilitates the eruption of the unerupted tooth or any other developing tooth that have been displaced
- Large cysts, where enucleation could cause pathological fracture
- When apices of many adjacent erupted teeth are involved within a large cyst.

Advantages
- Simple procedure
- Spares vital structures
- Allows eruption of teeth
- Prevents, oronasal, oroantral fistulae
- Prevents pathological fractures
- Reduces operating time
- Reduces blood loss
- Helps shrinkage of cystic lining
- Allows endosteal bone formation to take place
- Alveolar ridge is preserved.

Disadvantages
- Pathologic tissue is left in situ
- Histologic examination of entire cystic lining cannot be done
- Prolonged healing time
- Prolonged follow-up visits
- Periodic irrigation of cavity
- Regular adjustments of plug
- Periodic changing of pack
- Inconvenience to patient
- Secondary surgery maybe needed
- Formation of slit-like pockets that may harbor foodstuffs
- Risk of invagination and new cyst formation.

Enucleation

Principle

Complete removal of cyst with cystic lining, and closure of cystic cavity by a mucoperiosteal flap, so that the space fills up with blood clot, which will eventually organize and form normal bone.

Indications
- Treatment of OKCs
- Cysts with high recurrence rate
- Small cysts.

Advantages
- Primary closure of wound
- Rapid healing
- Postoperative care reduced
- Thorough examination of entire cystic lining can be done.

Disadvantages
- In young persons the unerupted teeth associated with the cyst, will be removed with enucleation
- Pathologic fractures, when large cysts are enucleated
- Damage to adjacent vital structures
- Pulpal necrosis.

Complication of Cystic Lesions
- Pathological fracture
- Infection
- Postoperative wound dehiscence
- Loss of vitality of teeth
- Neuropraxia in infected cysts
- Postoperative infection
- Recurrence in some cysts
- Dysplastic, neoplastic or malignant changes.

Keratocystic Odontogenic Tumors

24

INTRODUCTION

Keratocystic odontogenic tumors (KCOTs) previously known as odontogenic keratocysts are aggressive intraosseous lesion with a recurrence rate of approximately 25–60%. World Health Organization (WHO) defined keratocystic odontogenic tumor as "a benign unicystic or multicystic, intraosseous tumor of odontogenic origin, with a characteristic lining of parakeratinized stratified squamous epithelium and potential for aggressive, infiltrative behavior." WHO recommends the term "keratocystic odontogenic tumor" [2005] as it better reflects its neoplastic nature of odontogenic keratocyst.

- KCOT was first described by Mikulicz in 1876 as a dermoid cyst
- Later, it was described as a cholesteatoma by Hauer, 1926
- In 1956, Philipsen separated jaw cysts from cholesteatomas occurring in other cranial areas. Because he thought that these were odontogenic cysts and not of inflammatory origin, he coined the term odontogenic keratocyst (OKC)
- In 1963, Pindborg and Hansen described the essential features of this cyst
- In the 2005 World Health Organization classification, the former odontogenic keratocyst is added to the benign odontogenic tumors category as "keratocystic odontogenic tumor"

(KCOT). The change in terminology was based on the observation that the odontogenic keratocyst behaves as a neoplasm and not like a benign cystic lesion.

PATHOPHYSIOLOGY

Several theories of the development of the KCOT have been presented. Most of the available evidence points to two main sources of the epithelium from which KCOT is derived:
  i. Remnants of the dental lamina.
  ii. Basal cell layer of the oral mucosal epithelium often referred to as basal cell hamartoma.

CLINICAL PRESENTATION

Site

It comprises approximately 11% of all jaw cysts. Approximately 65% of KCOTs occurs in the mandible with the predilection for the third molar-ramus region (73.2%). They always occur within bone, although a small number of cases of peripheral KCOT have been reported. The peripheral KCOT has the clinical features of a gingival cyst of adults but the histological characteristic is of a typical KCOT.

Gender

More frequently in males, the male: female ratio was 1.27:1 (Jonesetal; 2006).

Age

Occur over a wide age range, from the first to the ninth decades of life; the peak incidence is during the second and third decades of life.

SIGNS AND SYMPTOMS

Patients with KCOTs complain of pain (Fig. 26.1), soft tissue swelling, bone expansion, drainage and neurological manifestations such as paraesthesia of the lip.

Sometimes KCOTs are asymptomatic and are found incidentally during routine radiological examination or until they develop pathological fractures. This occurs because the KCOT tends to expand in the medullary cavity in an anterior to posterior direction so clinically observable expansion of the bone occurs late. The enlarging lesions may lead to displacement of the adjacent teeth.

Intraoral Presentation of KCOT

Distinctive clinical features include a potential for local destruction and a tendency for multiplicity, especially when the lesion is associated with nevoid basal cell carcinoma syndrome (NBCCS) or Gorlin-Goltz syndrome.

RADIOLOGICAL FEATURES (FIGS 24.2 TO 24.4)

- KCOTs appear as well defined radiolucencies with distinct sclerotic margins, which can be either unilocular or multilocular

- Unilocular lesions occurred with a greater frequency than multilocular variant
- Main (1970), classified OKCs, according to their position in the jaw:
  - Extraneous—usually in the ramus away from the existing teeth
  - Collateral—adjacent to the roots of teeth
  - Replacement—in place of normal tooth
  - Envelopmental—embracing existing adjacent unerupted tooth.

HISTOLOGICAL FEATURES (FIG. 24.5 AND 24.6)

- KCOTs are lined by stratified squamous epithelium which may be parakeratinized (80–90%) or orthokeratinized
- The epithelium is corrugated, with a regular thickness of about 5–8 layers
- Lack of rete ridge formation
- Well defined often palisaded, hyperchromatic, basal layer consisting of columnar or cuboidal cells or mixture of both
- The cells superficial to basal layer are polyhedral and often exhibit intercellular edema
- Mitotic figures are found in the basal layer but more frequently in the suprabasal layer
- Sometimes small satellite cyst, cords or islands of odontogenic epithelium may be seen within the fibrous wall

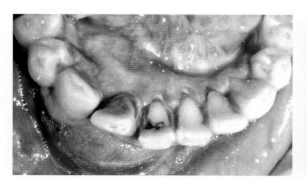

Fig. 24.1: Clinical presentation of anterior KCOT showing lingual buccal cortex expansion

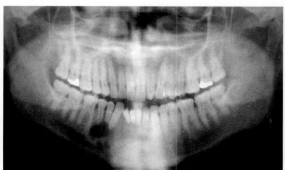

Fig. 24.2: OPG showing unilocular radiolucency

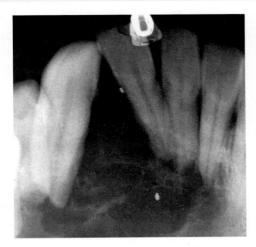

Fig. 24.3: IOPA showing multilocular radiolucency

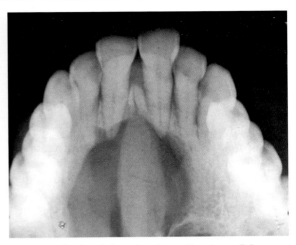

Fig. 24.4: Occlusal view showing unilocular radiolucency

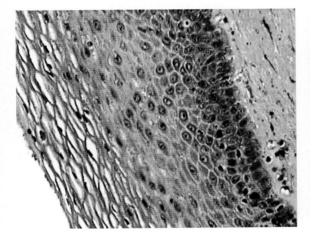

Fig. 24.5: Squamous parakeratinized epithelium, 8–14 layers, basal layer palasading and hyperchromatic cell

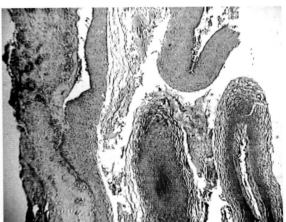

Fig. 24.6: Slit/gap between epithelium and connective tissue with extravasated RBC

- Generally devoid of inflammatory infiltrate in fibrous wall
- In the presence of inflammatory changes, the typical features of KCOT may be altered. The parakeratinized epithelial surface may disappear and the epithelium may proliferate to form rete ridges with the loss of the characteristic palisaded basal layer.

TREATMENT

Treatment modalities for KCOT
Enucleation
Marsupialization
Resection

Eyre and Zakrzewska in 1985, have stated the following treatment options for the KCOT:

- *Enucleation*
  - with primary closure
  - with packing
  - with chemical fixation
  - with cryosurgery.
- *Marsupialization*
  - only, or
  - followed by enucleation.
- *Resection:* Bramley in 1971, proposed a treatment plan for the keratinizing cystic odontogenic tumor due to its tendency to recur. He suggested:
  - Small single cysts with regular spherical outline—Enucleation with intra—oral approach
  - Larger or less accessible cysts with regular spherical outline—Enucleation with extraoral approach
  - Unilocular lesions with scalloped or loculated periphery and small multilocular lesions—Marginal excision
  - Large multilocular lesions with or without cortical perforation—Resection followed by primary or secondary reconstruction with reconstruction plates or bone grafting procedures.

Intralesional Adjunctive Therapy

- Chemical fixation with Carnoy's solution: mixture of absolute alcohol, chloroform, glacial acetic acid, and ferric chloride
- This mixture penetrates bone to a predictable and time-dependent depth without injuring the neurovascular structures
- A 5-minute application penetrates bone to a depth of 1.54 mm, nerve to a depth of 0.15 mm, and mucosa to a depth of 0.51 mm.

Recurrence

- KCOTs have a high recurrence rate of 25–60% (when associated with NBCCS, the recurrence rate is about 82%)
- It is believed that the parakeratinized variant (previously called primordial cyst is thought to have a higher recurrence rate than the orthokeratinized variant

- The possible reasons for its recurrence are:
  - Occurrence of satellite cysts (bud-like projection of basal cell layer into the connective tissue) which may be retained during the enucleation procedure
  - KCOTs have very thin and fragile lining which is difficult to enucleate particularly when the lesion is large. Hard portion of the lining maybe left behind and constitutes the source of recurrence
  - Enucleation in one piece may be more difficult when the lining has more scalloped margins. This may explain the higher recurrence rate than those with scalloped contours
  - An intrinsic growth potential in the epithelial lining of KCOTs which may be responsible for a higher recurrence rate
  - KCOTs may arise from proliferation of the basal cells of the oral epithelium.

CONCLUSION

Keratocystic odontogenic tumor has high recurrence rate and aggressive behavior. The potential for recurrence relates to the high proliferative activity of the keratocyst epithelium. Because of high recurrence, different treatment techniques can be chosen. The treatment includes:

- Conservative treatment generally includes simple enucleation, with or without curettage, using spoon curettes or marsupialization
- Aggressive treatment generally includes peripheral ostectomy, chemical curettage with Carnoy's solution, and resection
- Because of its agressivity its high recurrence and possible malignant transformation odontogenic keratocyst is added to the benign tumor category, the new term is keratocystic odontogenic tumor. This change in terminology was based on the observation that the cyst behaves as a neoplasm and not like a benign cystic lesion.

CASE PRESENTATION

A 31-year-old male complained of swelling in the right lower posterior tooth region since 6 months (Fig. 24.7).

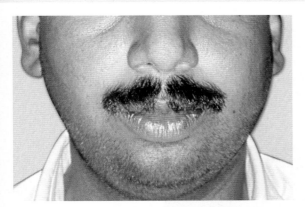

Fig. 24.7: Extraoral frontal view (*Courtesy*: Dr Rajendra Prasad)

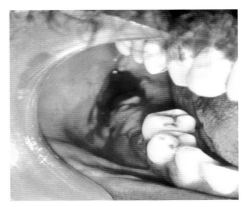

Fig. 24.8: Intraoral showing nonhealing ulcer and buccal swelling (*Courtesy*: Dr Rajendra Prasad)

History of Presenting Illness

The patient first had pain and swelling in the right posterior region of lower jaw 1 year back. Was diagnosed as impacted tooth and removal done under local anesthesia at Payannur. Six months later, patient had pain and swelling in same region for which tooth extraction was done under local anesthesia, but the swelling persisted was then referred from Periyaram Medical College for swelling suspected of being cyst.

Medical History

No relevant medical history reported, no history of any drug allergy.

Family History

No relevant family history.

General Examination

Patient is moderately built and nourished.

Examination of Head and Neck Region

No gross facial asymmetry.

Intraoral Examination (Fig. 24.8)

Inspection

- Swelling present in right side of mandible
- Involving the alveolus and buccal sulcus
- Minimal expansion of lingual cortex present in the region of 47,48

- Extraction socket of 46 and 48 visible. Extraction socket nonhealing.

Palpation

- Inspectory finding confirmed
- Discontinuity present in buccal cortex in the region of 47,48
- Extending onto the anterior border of ramus
- Adjacent tooth not mobile
- Missing teeth 48 and 46
- Mucosa with respect to 46 nonulcerated
- No discharge or discoloration noted
- Mouth opening is minimally reduced.

Provisional diagnosis

Residual cyst.

Differential Diagnosis

- Keratocystic odontogenic tumor
- Ameloblastoma.

Investigations (Figs 24.9 and 24.10)

Excisional biopsy.

Confirmed Diagnosis

Keratocystic odontogenic tumor.

Treatment Provided

Cyst enucleation + lateral decortication + chemical cauterization + reconstruction with reconstruction plate under general anesthesia.

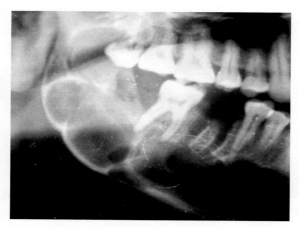

Fig. 24.9: Panoramic radiograph showing multilocular radiolucency (*Courtesy*: Dr Rajendra Prasad)

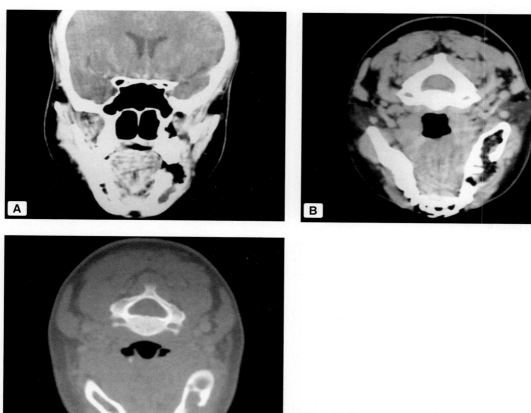

Figs 24.10A to C: Computed tomography (CT) scan showing perforation of outer cortex (*Courtesy for Figure 24.10A*: Dr Rajendra Prasad)

DISCUSSION

Philipsen in 1956 first described a cyst of the jaws lined by keratinizing epithelium which was known as odontogenic keratocyst. The knowledge regarding the treatment of the odontogenic keratocyst, now renamed as the Keratocystic Odontogenic Tumor (KCOT), is still a debate in oral and maxillofacial surgery. Various treatment modalities have been tried for the successful treatment of the KCOT, ranging from simple enucleation to resection, but none has been regarded as the ideal treatment. The KCOT behaves like a tumor in many ways, e.g. involvement of large areas of the bone, high recurrence rate, distinctive histopathological features of the lesion. On the other hand, successful treatment by marsupialization denies its tumor characteristics. Cases of carcinoma arising in KCOT have been reported.

Recurrence of the lesion has been reported in a bone graft.

Blanas et al. in 2000 have concluded that a simple enucleation results in an unnecessarily high recurrence rate when treating the KCOT. For a routine KCOT in a person who is likely to return for a follow-up treatment, Carnoy's solution appears to be the least invasive procedure with a lowest recurrence rate. If the lesion is very large, decompression of the cyst followed by enucleation will also have a low recurrence rate. Use of Carnoy's solution should also be considered at the enucleation stage. If the patient is unlikely to return for follow-up, the lesion should be resected.

Bradley and Fischer in 1975 have described the combined enucleation and cryosurgical treatment of the KCOT. Webb and Brockbank in 1984 have presented the treatment of the KCOT of the mandible using a combination of enucleation and cryosurgery. They have followed up the case for 5 years and have found no recurrence. Then suggest that cryosurgery, as an adjunct to enucleation, may prove to be a conservative and reliable method of treatment with a low recurrence rate.

According to Voorsmit RA et al. (1981) recurrence of the KCOT is 2.5% whereas according to Pindborg et al. (1963) to 62%. The possible mechanisms of recurrence have been described by Voorsmit et al. in 1981. They state that any lining epithelium left behind in the oral cavity may give rise to a new lesion formation. Daughter cysts, microcysts or epithelial islands can be found in the walls of the original cysts. New KCOTs may develop from epithelial offshoots of the basal layer of oral epithelium.

Conservative approach as well as aggressive approach has been advocated for the treatment of the KCOT. Conservative approach, however, has not gained much popularity, because complete removal of the KCOT can be difficult because of the thin friable lining, limited surgical access, skill and experience of the surgeon, and desire to preserve adjacent vital structures. The goals of treatment should involve eliminating the potential for recurrence while also minimizing the surgical morbidity.

Stoelinga in 2001 has concluded in a long term follow-up study that enucleation gave rise to a fairly low number of recurrences. Enucleation followed by chemical cauterization using Carnoy's solution along with excision of overlying attached mucosa is used for the treatment of KCOT. Peripheral ostectomy combined with Carnoy's solution may give good results.

Resection of the lesion supposedly gives the least recurrence rate out of all treatment modalities. Bataineh and Al Qudah in 1998 have advocated resection without continuity defects as a radical treatment, in which removal of the cyst, teeth and the overlying soft tissue is followed by packing of the cavity to minimize the risk of recurrence.

Nakamura et al. in 2002 have stated that marsupialization, as well as decompression, has the purpose of relieving the pressure within the cystic cavity and allowing the new bone to fill the defect. It saves the contiguous structures such as tooth roots, the maxillary sinus or the inferior alveolar canal can be saved from surgical damage. They have concluded that marsupialization was highly successful in reducing the size of the KCOT before surgery. It was more effective in the mandibular body than the ramus region. It did not adversely affect the recurrence tendency. The characteristics of the KCOT may become less aggressive during the course of marsupialization.

Stoelinga PJ (2003) states that complete elimination of recurrences is probably not possible for two reasons. Firstly, some cysts are still treated like ordinary odontogenic cysts because a preoperative diagnosis was not made and the cysts were not treated according to the suggested protocol. Secondly, despite excision of the overlying mucosa there may still be epithelial islands or even microcysts left behind in the mucosa, which develop into a new keratocystic odontogenic tumor.

Keratocystic odontogenic tumor may mimic the appearance of an endodontic lesion. In a case reported by Pace R et al. lesion was successfully treated by complete enucleation and application of Carnoy's solution.

In a retrospective study of 255 Chinese patients, Zhao YF et al. have concluded that KCOT treated with enucleation alone have a higher recurrence rate. Enucleation with adjunctive treatment can decrease recurrence rate. Radical excision has no recurrence but does have the highest morbidity rate and should be reserved for multiple recurrent cysts after conservative means.

Literature contains many reports regarding management of KCOT, debate still exists as to the most effective treatment for this lesion. According to Ghali as with any odontogenic lesion, initial evaluation must include a thorough history and physical examination, radiographic studies, and the development of a probable differential diagnosis. Depending on size, location, and behavior, the clinician should decide on an incisional versus excisional biopsy. Prior aspiration may be helpful. In patients with multiple KCOTs, evaluation for the presence of basal cell nevus syndrome should be undertaken.

Genetic studies have thrown light on new modalities of treatment of the KCOT at a molecular level. According to some studies, cyclopamine, a plant-based steroidal alkaloid, inhibits the cellular response to the Sonic Hedgehog signal. It is found that cyclopamine blocks activation of the Sonic Hedgehog pathway caused by oncogenic mutation making it a potential 'mechanism- based' therapeutic agent for human tumors whose pathogenesis involves excess Sonic Hedgehog pathway activity which is seen in keratocystic odontogenic tumor.

Nevoid Basal Cell Carcinoma Syndrome

- First reported by Jarisch, detailed description given by Gorlin
- Also known as Gorlin's syndrome.

Presenting Features

Facies
- Frontal and temporoparietal bossing
- Prominent supraorbital ridges in men
- Hypertelorism
- Mandibular prognathism.

Skeletal abnormalities
- Bifid, fused rudimentary ribs
- Occult spina bifida
- Bridging of sella tursica
- Shortening of metacarpals
- Calcification of falx cerebri.

Skin lesions
- Milia, around eyes
- Dyskeratosis (palms and soles)
- Epidermal cysts
- Basal cell nevi
- Basal cell carcinomas.

Cyst
- Fifty percent show multiple OKCs.

Soft tissue anomalies
- Ovarian fibromata
- Lipomas

SOME MORE CASES

See Figures 24.11 to 24.17.

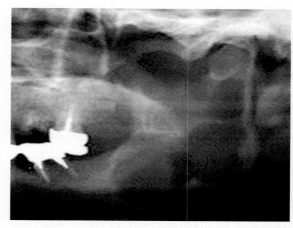

Fig. 24.11: OPG showing radiolucency involving ramus (I)

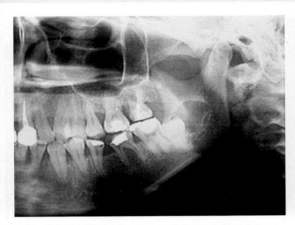

Fig. 24.12: OPG showing radiolucency involving ramus (II)

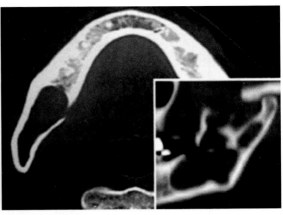

Fig. 24.13: CT showing radiolucency involving ramus

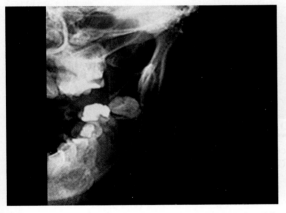

Fig. 24.14: PA mandible showing radiolucency involving body of mandible

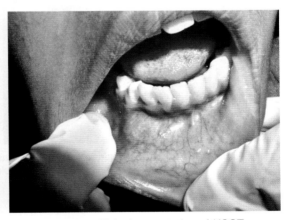

Fig. 24.15: Clinical presentation of KCOT

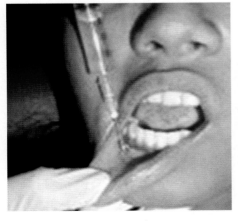

Fig. 24.16: Aspiration of cystic content

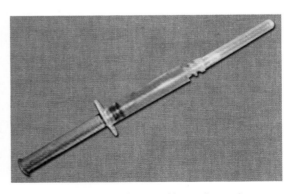

Fig. 24.17: Aspirate—golden yellow color

Basal Cell Nevoid Syndrome (Figs. 24.18A to D)

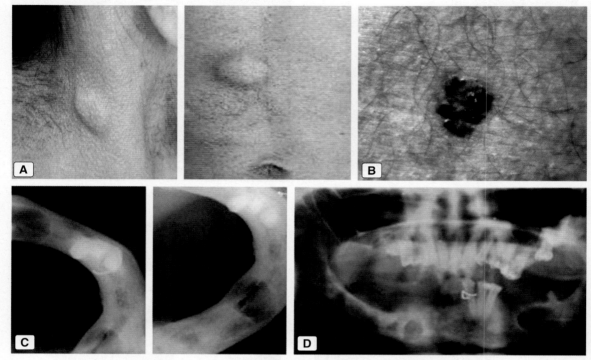

Figs 24.18A to D: (A) Epidermoid cysts; (B) Basal cell nevi; (C) Multiple KCOT-occlusal radiograph; (D) Multiple KCOT-OPG

Odontogenic Tumors

25

INTRODUCTION

Odontogenic tumors comprise an unusual groups of lesion of the jaws, derived from primordial tooth forming tissue and presenting in a large number of histologic patterns. Some of these lesions, particularly the odontomas, are now interpreted as developmental malformation or hamartomatous lesions rather than true neoplasms. Other lesions, such as ameloblastoma, are accepted as true neoplasm and must be diagnosed and treated as such.

Most odontogenic tumors are essentially benign lesions but infiltrate the adjacent bone between the spicules of the medulla. This form of bony infiltration, common to many benign tumors of bone, is not the true invasiveness of malignant tumors but represent a clinical problem in that the tumor can recur after surgical therapy if the bony margins still contain some of the tumor infiltration.

Generally, the odontogenic tumors tend to be more common in younger patients but can occur at any age. They originate in the jaws and usually are found in the tooth bearing sites. They are often associated with impacted or missing teeth. The common sites for odontogenic tumors are the mandibular molar region and the maxillary cuspid region. Odontogenic tumors are slow growing and asymptomatic (Fig. 25.1).

Pain is not a feature of benign tumors of the jaws but is a common symptom of malignant tumors of the jaws. The odontogenic tumors are expansile lesions and may expand the bony cortex, but usually do not invade or perforate it (Fig. 25.2).

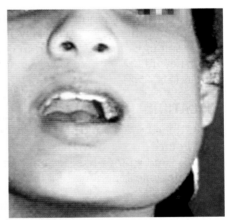

Fig. 25.1: Clinical presentation of odontoma as swelling on left side of face

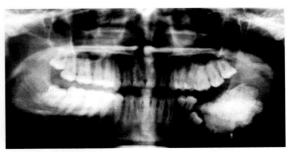

Fig. 25.2: OPG showing impacted tooth (radio-opacity in left molar region)

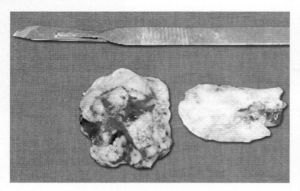

Fig. 25.3: Excised lesion

DEFINITION

"Lesions derived from epithelial, ectomesenchymal and/or mesenchymal elements that are, or have been, part of the tooth forming apparatus."

They are found therefore, exclusively in the jaw bones or soft mucosal tissue overly in occurs at any age. They infiltrate in the jaws, e.g. tooth-bearing areas (Fig. 25.3).

CLASSIFICATION

Approved at the editorial and consensus conference, Lyon, France in 2003 by WHO.

Neoplasms and tumor-like lesions arising from the odontogenic apparatus.

Benign

Odontogenic epithelium with mature, fibrous stroma; odontogenic ectomesenchyme not present
Ameloblastomas – • Solid/multicystic • Extraosseous/peripheral • Desmoplastic • Unicystic
Squamous odontogenic tumor
Calcifying epithelial odontogenic tumor
Adenomatoid odontogenic tumor
Keratocystic odontogenic tumor

Odontogenic epithelium with odontogenic mesenchyme with or without dental hard tissue formation
Ameloblastic fibroma
Ameloblastic fibrodentinoma
Ameloblastic fibro-odontoma
Complex odontoma
Compound odontoma
Odontoameloblastoma
Calcifying cystic odontogenic tumor
Dentinogenic ghost cell tumor

Mesenchyme and/or odontogenic ectomesenchyme (with or without occluded odontogenic epithelium)
Odontogenic fibroma
Odontogenic myxoma
Cementoblastoma

Malignant

Odontogenic carcinomas
Metastasizing or ameloblastic carcinoma
Primary
Secondary (dedifferentiated), intraosseous
Secondary (dedifferentiated), extraosseous
Primary intraosseous squamous cell carcinoma (PIOSCC)
PIOSCC solid type
PIOSCC derived from odontogenic cysts
PIOSCC derived from keratinizing cystic odontogenic tumor
Clear cell odontogenic carcinoma
Ghost cell odontogenic carcinoma

Odontogenic sarcoma
Ameloblastic fibrosarcoma
Ameloblastic fibrodentinoma and fibro-odontosarcoma

AMELOBLASTOMA

- Ameloblastoma is a *true neoplasm* of enamel organ type of tissue which does not undergo differentiation to the point of enamel formation
  - No reports of this lesion arising elsewhere in the body
  - Only craniopharyngioma resembles it histologically
  - The epithelium considerably resembles that seen in bell stage of enamel organ.
- Second most common odontogenic neoplasm
- Its incidence combined with its clinical behavior, makes ameloblastoma *the most significant odontogenic neoplasm* of concern to oral and maxillofacial surgeons.

Nomenclature

- Adamantinoma—Mallasez 1885
- Ameloblastoma—Churchill 1934
- First Reported—Guzack in 1826.

Definition

Robinson described it as a tumor that is unicentric, nonfunctional, intermittent in growth, anatomically benign and clinically persistent.
U: Unicentric
N: Nonfunctional
I: Intermittant in growth
A: Anatomically benign
C: Clinically persistant.

Pathogenesis

- *Field origin theory*: Neoplasm do not start as a propagation wave from a single cell, but rather areas of changed cells responsive to neoplastic inductive effects
- *Various theories*:
  - Cell rests of enamel organ, either remnants of Hertwig's root sheath or rests of Mallasez
  - Epithelium of odontogenic cysts—dentigerous and from odontomas
  - Developing enamel organ—disturbances
  - Basal cells of jaw-surface epithelium
  - Epithelium from other parts—pituitary.

Clinical Features

- Second most common odontogenic tumor
- Highest incidence in blacks
- Asian population most affected
- Gender distribution
  - Male   54.9
  - Female   45.1
- Average size of tumor 4.3 cm
- Around 80 percent in mandibular molar -ramus - angle
- Three times > other sites
- Incidence equal to all other odontogenic tumors combined.

Clinical Presentation

- Swelling
- Pain
- Local discomfort
- Purulent discharge
- Symptomless
- Paresthesia
- Discomfort
- Purulent discharge
- Delayed healing of extraction socket
- Tooth mobility.

Classification: Histological

- Follicular (simple) most common (Fig. 25.9)
- Plexiform
- Acanthomatous
- Granular cell ameloblastoma
- Basal cell ameloblastoma
- Desmoplastic.

  The growth pattern of the neoplasm, categorized as conventional or unicystic, is more important than the histopathologic subtype in treatment decision.

Clinical and Radiographic Presentation (Figs 25.4 to 25.15)

- Conventional/solid/multicystic   86%
- Unicystic   13%
- Peripheral   1%

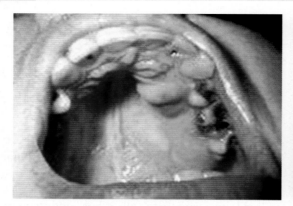

Fig. 25.4: Ameloblastoma—anterior palate

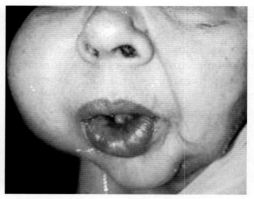

Fig. 25.5: Swelling resulting due to recurrent ameloblastoma—frontal view

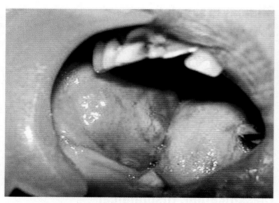

Fig. 25.6: Swelling resulting due to recurrent ameloblastoma— intraoral view (*Courtesy*: Dr Muralee Mohan)

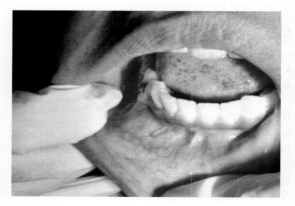

Fig. 25.7: Ameloblastoma anterior mandible intraoral

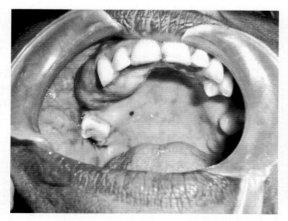

Fig. 25.8: Ameloblastoma—maxillary molar region

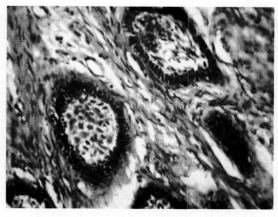

Fig. 25.9: Follicular ameloblastic island shows tall columnar cell with hyperchromatic nucleus and reverse polarity

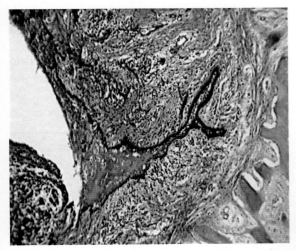

Fig. 25.10: Some islands are arranged in the form of long thin strands which gives enamel-like pattern with peripheral cuboidal cells and central hypercellular area

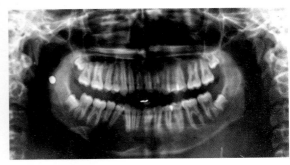

Fig. 25.11: Unicystic radiolucency

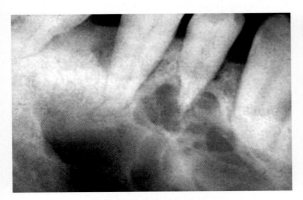

Fig. 25.12: Soap bubble

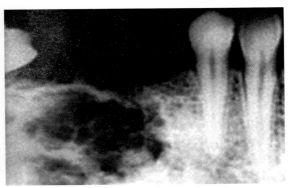

Fig. 25.13: Honeycomb appearance

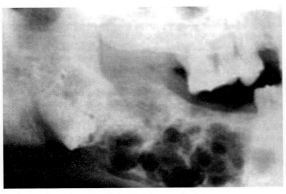

Fig. 25.14: Multilocular radiolucency

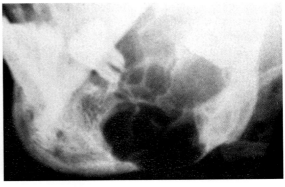

Fig. 25.15: Cortical resorption

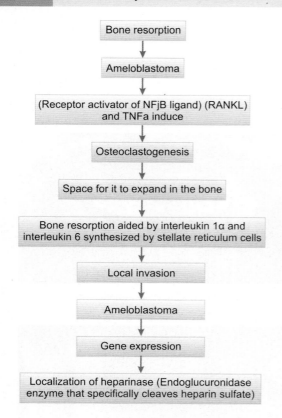

Radiographic Features

Multilocular radiolucency (septae are finer and more curved) (Figs 25.13 to 25.15)

Growth Relation to Inferior Alveolar Nerve Canal

- Unlike carcinomas, ameloblastomas are circu-mferentially delineated by a continuous basement membrane, and they tend to spread into tissue spaces by expanding their compartment volumes
- Therefore, they are theoretically unlikely to invade the nerve bundle
- Follicular ameloblastoma with more invasive tendency may infiltrate the cancellous marrow spaces and proliferate around the mandibular canal, later destroying the bony canal and infiltrating perineural tissue

- Destroying cell–cell and cell–matrix attachment and tumor cells to readily penetrate the ECM or BM
- Releases the bioactive molecules attached to heparin sulfate and have profound effects on cellular junction and proliferation.

UNICYSTIC AMELOBLASTOMA

- Second most common growth pattern
- Less frequently encountered
- Often associated with impacted teeth
- Commonly cited as 'dentigerous cyst'
- Important to identify due to better prognosis
- Bone resorption
- Local invasion

Clinical Behavior

- Ameloblastoma is locally benign invasive tumor
- It has an high tendency to recur, metastasize
- Even has a potential for malignant transformation
- Recurrences often present after fifteen years or more
- Thus the need for long-term periodic follow-ups.

Various Treatment Modalities

- Curettage
- Enucleation
- Chemical cauterization
- Carbolic acid
  - Concentrated carnoy soultion
  - Electrocauterization
- Enbloc resection
- Radical resection with continuity defect.

Radiotherapy

- Ameloblastomas are generally considered to be radio-resistant tumors
- Radiotherapy could reduce the size of an ameloblastoma, primarily that part of the tumor that has expanded the jaw or has broken into the soft tissues
- Recurrence rates of 42–72 percent have been reported.

General Principles

- Goal is total removal of tumor by whatever surgical procedure or combination of procedures
- Less than complete excision is equivalent to planned recurrence
- Treatment decisions are based on individual patient situation
- Surgical plan strongly based on affected jaw (highly cancellous maxilla facilitates spread)
- First procedure should be planned to be definitive and offer best opportunity for cure
- Aggressiveness of lesion
- Anatomic location
  - Maxilla versus mandible
  - Proximity to vital structures
  - Size of tumor
  - Intraosseous versus extraosseous
- Duration of lesion
- Reconstructive efforts
- Resection with or without continuity defect employed if:
  - Lesion is extensive for pathologic fracture
  - Satellite cyst
  - Frozen section
  - Inability for 1.5 cm resection margin distant to radiographic bone-lesion interface (Figs 25.16 and 25.17).

Surgical Management

- *Enucleation(with or without curettage):*
  - Most benign tumors
  - Direct contact with lesion
- *Resection (en bloc resection):*
  - No direct contact with lesion
- *Marginal/segmental:* No disruption of bone continuity
- *Sectional/partial resection:*
  - Aggressive benign tumors
  - Includes margins of uninvolved tissue to reduce recurrence
  - Full thickness removal of portion of jaw
  - Continuity defect may vary from small to hemimandibulectomy

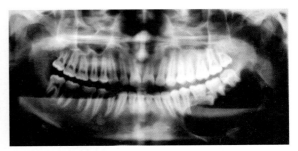

Fig. 25.16: Unicystic, clear radiolucency, with impacted supernumerary tooth, root resorption, thinning of inferior and post border of mandible

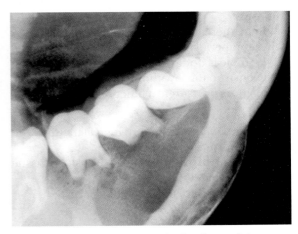

Fig. 25.17: Occlusal radiograph showing radiolucency, root resorption

- *Total resection:* Removal of involved bone (maxillectomy/mandibulectomy)
- *Composite resection:*
  - Includes removal of adjacent soft tisssue and dissection of lymph nodes
  - May also include radio, chemotherapy
  - Malignant tumors.

Specific Principles Intraosseous/Solid/ Multicystic

- Resection with or without continuity defect
- Inferior alveolar nerve sacrificed if it lies within the lesion

- Resection should be exterior to a tumor involved tissue plane
- Retention of an inferior border <1 cm thick may fracture, so resection with continuity defect performed
- Reconstruction
- If lesion microscopically infiltrates bone beyond tumor—bone interface seen in imaging.
- Margin 2 cm—solid/multicystic
- 1–1.5 cm—unicystic/peripheral
- Post treatment follow up for 15–20 years.
- Teeth immediately involved with ameloblastoma are removed with the tumor and a primary closure
- When there is perforation of cortical plates, a supraperiosteal dissection of the involved mandible is done
- Reconstruction without continuity defect enhances postsurgical function and esthetics.

Procedure
- *Intraoral incision*: Circumgingival incision and releasing incision on either side
  - Excision of overlying mucosal lesional tissue
  - Scar avoided
- *Extraoral*: Submandibular approach.

Reconstructive Options
- Stainless steel reconstruction plate
- Rigid titanium plate
- Ti mesh
- Autogenous free bone graft
- Iliac graft for contour in angle region
- Rib graft for facial convexity
- Reconstruction with patient marrow
- PRP
- Vascularised composite pedicle graft (Fig. 26.18G).

Clinical pictures showing surgical resection procedure (Fig. 25.18A to H).

Case Presentation (Fig. 25.19 to 25.23)

A 71-year-old female patient complain of swelling on the right side of face for 3 years.
- Progressive since 3 months
- Mildly tender

- Not associated with any symptom of paresthesia
- Associated with pain which is dull and intermittent in nature
- Pain radiates to parietal area of head
- Also complains of intraoral swelling for 6 months
- Insidious onset
- Gradually progressive
  Associated with pain and pus discharge.

Past Surgical History
- Patient underwent surgical excision for swelling present in the right mandibular area in 1982 which was then diagnosed as ameloblastoma
- In 1996 patient was operated again for recurrent ameloblastoma and right hemi mandibulectomy was done.
- In December 2003, excision of tumor was done on right pre auricular area and chin and was diagnosed as plexiform ameloblastoma.
- In February 2004, partial mandibular resection was done and implant placement was done and lesion was diagnosed as follicular ameloblastoma.
- In October 2004, infected implant removal was done.

Head and Neck Examination
- Facial symmetry—appears asymmetric due to the presence of a localized swelling on the right side of face
- Nose—nasal septum appears deviated to left side
- Lips—incompetent
- Enlargement and eversion of lower lip
- Drooling of saliva
- Sagging of chin and lower lip
- Pinna—raised
- Lymph nodes—not palpable.

Examination of the Swelling
- A solitary well-defined swelling noticed on the right side of face
- Size 10 × 10 cm roughly oval in shape

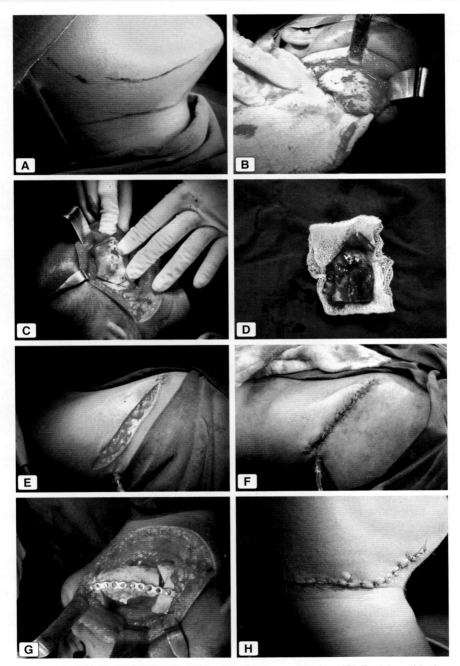

Figs 25.18A to H: (A) Incision marking; (B) Exposure of lesion; (C) Excision of lesion from nearby structures; (D) Excised lesion—iliac donor site; (E) Donor site incision; (F) Donor site closure with drain—reconstruction and closure; (G) Reconstruction with autogenous graft and reconstruction plate; (H) Closure and suturing

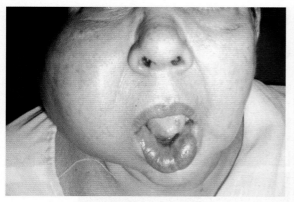

Fig. 25.19: Extraoral swelling (Front view)

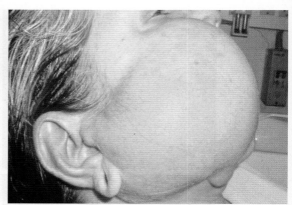

Fig. 25.20: Extraoral swelling (Side view)

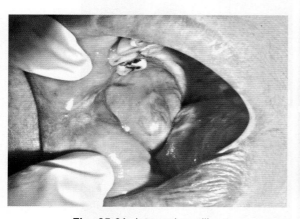

Fig. 25.21: Intraoral swelling

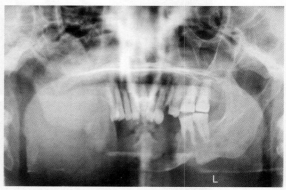

Fig. 25.22: Panoramic radiograph showing soft tissue infiltration with soft tissue shawdow shadow

- Anteroposteriorly from right nasolabial fold to the posterior auricular area
- Superor inferior from infraorbital margin to submandibular area
- Borders—well defined
- Overlying skin—mild signs of inflammation.

Palpation of the swelling
- Features found during inspection are confirmed
- Mildly tender
- No local raise in temperature
- Firm in consistency with well-defined borders
- Mildly fluctuant
- Skin over the swelling—non-pinchable
- Fixed to the underlying tissues
- No signs of paresthesia.

Intraoral Examination
- A solitary well-defined growth in the right buccal mucosa 6 × 7 cm
- *Extending*:
  - Anteriorly—2 cm from angle of mouth
  - Posteriorly—pterygomandibular space
  - Superiorly—extending beyond the line of occlusion of maxillary teeth
  - Inferiorly—lower buccal vestibule
- Complete obliteration of upper and lower buccal vestibule
- Surface appear smooth
- Pale pink in color with areas of bluish appearance
- Engorged veins seen on surface
- Spontaneous bleeding observed in the anteroinferior portion of the growth.

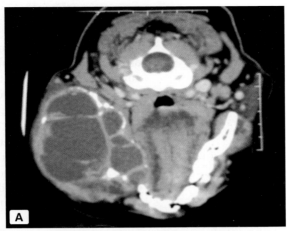

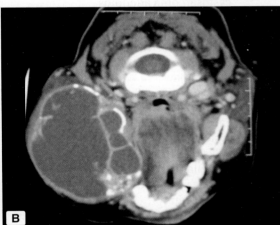

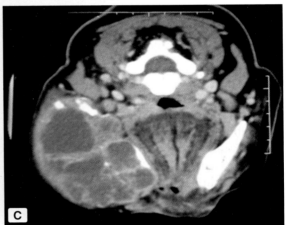

Figs 25.23A to C: CT showing extent of lesion

Palpation
- Features found during inspection are confirmed
- Mildly tender
- Smooth surface with well-defined borders
- Firm in consistency
- Fixed to the underlying tissues
- Nonfluctuant
- Noncompressible
- Nonreducible
- Pus discharge noticed.

Provisional Diagnosis

Recurrent ameloblastoma with soft tissue infiltration.

Differential Diagnosis
- Malignancy in ameloblastoma
- Sarcomatous—ameloblastic fibrosarcoma
- Carcinomatous
- Ameloblastic fibroma
- Lymphoma infiltration
- Fibrous histiocytoma
- Hemangiopericytoma.

Investigations
- Fine needle aspiration cytology
- Rim enhancing lesion with enhancing septae in right alveolar rim/ramus of mandible

- Extending up to zygomatic arch infiltrating the lateral wall of right maxillary sinus and the right parapharyngeal space
- Incisional biopsy of the lesion.

To Summarize

- A 71-year-old female complains of swelling on the right side of the face for 3 years
- Progressive 3 months
- Associated with pain which is dull and intermittent in nature
- Radiates to skull.

Clinically

- Solitary well-defined swelling
- Size 10 × 10 cm, roughly oval in shape
- Borders—well defined
- Overlying skin—mild signs of inflammation.

Intraorally

- A solitary well defined growth in the right buccal mucosa 6 × 7 cm
- Obliteration of upper and lower buccal vestibule
- Mildly tender
- Pus-like material discharge
- Smooth surface—pale pink in color with areas of bluish appearance
- Engorged veins seen on surface
- Spontaneous bleeding observed in the anteroinferior portion of the growth.

Radiographic Features

- Soft tissue shadow seen in right maxillary and mandibular area
- Computed tomography (CT)
- Rim enhancing lesion with enhancing septae in right alveolar rim/ramus of mandible
- Extending up to zygomatic arch infiltrating the lateral wall of right maxillary sinus and the right parapharyngeal space.

Radiographic Diagnosis

Recurrent ameloblastoma with soft tissue infiltration.

Review of Literature

Since the 19th century many terms have been used to describe the ameloblastoma. Hundreds of literatures have dealt with many facets of ameloblastoma.

- 1654: Scultet described –liquid tumors of jaw.
- 1746: Pierre Fauchard reported multicystic tumor.
- 1832: Dupuytren described clinically under the name of fibrous bodies of jaw (i.e. *corps fibreux de la machoire*)
- 1840: Forget described under curious name as cystic disease of the jaw.
- 1853: Weld called as cystosarcoma or cystosarcoma adenoids
- 1859: Robin described fibrous tumor arising from the dental follicle.
- 1868: Broca described as embroplastic odontome.
- 1876: Heath as cystic sarcoma or cystic disease of lower jaw
- 1877: Kolaczek as cystic adenoma
- 1877: Busch reported as cystic epithelioma.
- 1879: Falkson described initially as follicular cystoids.
- 1879: Falkson named as cystoma proliferrum folliculare.
- 1884: Malassez proposed it as epithelioma adamantin.
- 1885: Bernays named it as enamelogenous cyst.
- 1888: Bland–Suttan described as epithelial odontome.
- 1888: Audry as epithelioma oligokystique.
- 1889: Nasse called it as cystome central papadentair.
- 1890: Derujinsky suggested adamantinome.
- 1891: Bennecke called it as central solid epithelial tumor.
- 1893: Becker proposed central papilloma of the jaw.
- 1895: Tapie published excellent study of well documented cases of malignant degeneration and named as carcinoma adamantinum
- 1901: Blumm divided into:
  - Adamantinoma solidism
  - Adamantinoma cysticum

- 1902: Borst used the term cystadenoma adamantinum.
- 1904: Partsch-soft odontoma and multilocular cystoma.
- 1904: Pinkus- central cystadenoma.
- 1907: Ddreybladt-pseudo adenoma adamantinum.
- 1910: Galippe pointed out that adamantinoma was improper term and suggested a growth composed of enamel.
- 1929: *Ivy and Churchill pointed out that adamantinoma implies that neoplasm was calcified and proposed a new name ameloblastoma because the peripheral cells of tumor follicles were tall, columnar, polarized epithelial cells closely resembling ameloblast and center of the follicle structurally akin to stellate reticulum of enamel organ.*

The following terms have been recommended since Churchill's contribution:
- 1938: Cahn epithelioma of basal cell variety.
- 1946: Thoma and Goldman – adamantoblastoma.
- 1946: Byars and Sarnat-preameloblastoma.
- 1948: Willis – carcinoma of tooth germ residue.
- 1948: Fischer – Wasals – odontoma adamantinum.
- 1951: Schulenberg- basal celled carcinoma of the jaws.
- 1954: Mathis-epithelioma ameloblastoids.
- 1957: Treves termed as pre-ameloblastoma, metamorpho and pre-amelobotoma pro tomorfo.

Several other names were found in the world literature, but authors who originated was unable to trace.
- Multilocular cystic epithelial tumor
- Central epithelioma
- Chorioblastoma
- Cystodermoid
- Proliferating cyst of the jaw
- Proliferating mandibular cyst
- Adenoma adamantium
- Adamantine carcinoma
- Adamantinosarcome
- Adamantine tumor
- True ameloblastic tumor

- Enameloblastoma
- Adamantinoblastoma.

Today ameloblastoma and adamantinoma are widely used throughout the world

- *Robinson* described it as a tumor that is unicentric, nonfunctional, intermittent in growth, anatomically benign and clinically persistent.
- 2nd most common Odontogenic tumor
- Incidence—all other odontogenic tumors combined
- Highest incidence in blacks
- Asian population most affected
- Sex distribution of ameloblastoma
- Average size of tumor 4.3 cm.

Classification

Clinical and radiographic presentation:
- Conventional   86%
- Unicystic   13%
- Peripheral   1%
- *Others:* Pituitary ameloblastoma, rathke's pouch tumor, craniopharyngioma, adamantinoma of long bones, malignant ameloblastoma, ameloblastic carcinoma, desmoplastic Ameloblastoma.

Recurrent jaw lesions
- Conventional ameloblastomas infiltrate between the intact bony trabaculae at the periphery of the lesion before bone resorption becomes radiographically evident.
- Within the first 5 years.
- Around 15–25 percent after radical treatment.
- Around 75–90 percent after conservative treatment.

AMELOBLASTIC FIBROSARCOMA

- Ameloblastic fibrosarcoma (AFS) is an extremely rare malignant odontogenic neoplasm
- Ameloblastic dentinosarcoma and ameloblastic odontosarcoma are the same as AFS, because of the unvarying biological behavior of these neoplasms
- The AFS is composed of a benign epithelial component and malignant mesenchymal tissue. It has been reported that the epithelial component of AFS eventually becomes less prominent and may disappear altogether after local recurrences.

Pathogenesis

- *Field Origin theory*—neoplasms do not start as a propagation wave from a single cell, but rather areas of changed cells responsive to neoplastic inductive effects
- Two-thirds of ameloblastic fibrosarcoma seem to arise *de novo*, but the other has developed in recurrent ameloblastic fibromas or ameloblastic fibro-odontomas
- When reviewing the literature on ameloblastic fibrosarcoma, 63 cases have been reported up to 2003
- Malignant transformation of ameloblastic fibroma to ameloblastic fibrosarcoma: case report and review of the literature
- The AFS can present at any age
- Mean age is 33 years
- CD34 expressing ameloblastic fibrosarcoma arising in the maxilla—a new finding.

Clinical Presentation

- Ameloblastic fibrosarcoma may present as asymptomatic or as a painful swelling
- Intraosseous mass (2-6 cm) with occasional ulceration
- Malignant transformation of ameloblastic fibroma to ameloblastic fibrosarcoma:

Location

- Mandible (79%)
- Maxilla (21%)
- Most commonly affected site—posterior part of the mandible.

Radiographic Features

- May present as a well defined or irregular radio lucency
- May be unilocular or multilocular radio lucency.

Prognosis

- Ameloblastic fibrosarcomas are considered low grade lesions
- Rarely metastasize but are locally aggressive lesions.
- Around 20 percent of patients die of locally aggressive disease in 3 months to 19 years.

Lymphomas

- Primary malignancies of lymph node and peripheral lymphatics
- Most common site—hard palate or soft palate
- Appears as nonulcerated, diffuse, fleshy enlargements
- May cause mobility of teeth
- Fibrous histiocytoma
- Most common soft tissue sarcoma in adults.

Clinical Presentation

- More common in males
- Occurs in age group between 50–70 years.
- Oral lesion occurs in submucosa of tongue, floor of mouth and buccal mucosa
- Expanding mass
- May or may not be painful or ulcerated
- Tumors of nasal cavity and paranasal sinuses produce obstructive symptoms.

Pathogenesis

Similar to true neoplasm with continued and slow growth and a limited capacity for invasion.

Histopathologic Features

- Encapsulated masses of consisting of fascicles of fibroblastic cells with some histiocytic cells.
- Storiform – pleomorphic –most common
- Myxoid
- Giant cell
- Inflammatory
- Angiomatoid subtype
- Hemangiopericytoma
- Hemangiopericytomas are vascular tumours arising from mesenchymal cells with pericytic differentiation
- Ranges from benign to intermediate to overtly malignant.

Clinical Presentation

- Equal gender prediliction
- Peak incidence between age of 30–50 years
- Soft tissue mass with insidious growth
- Often contain pulsations or audible bruit
- Pain associated with enlarging mass
- Superficial lesions may develop pigmentation.

Some More Clinical Cause (Figs 25.24 to 25.35)

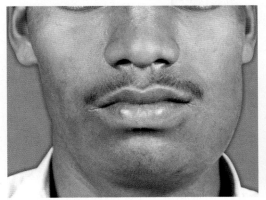

Fig. 25.24: Swelling on left side of face

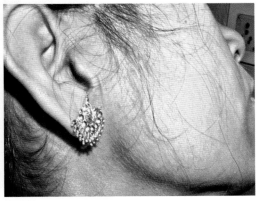

Fig. 25.25: Swelling on right side of face molar region

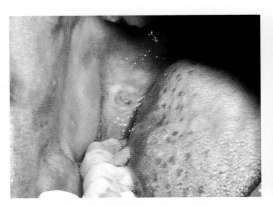

Fig. 25.26: Intraoral swelling

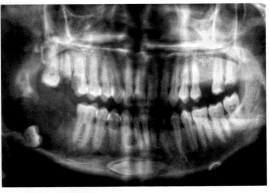

Fig. 25.27: OPG showing radiolucency in molar region

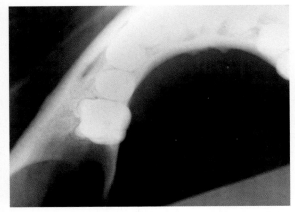

Fig. 25.28: Radiolucency in molar region with mild buccal cortex expansion

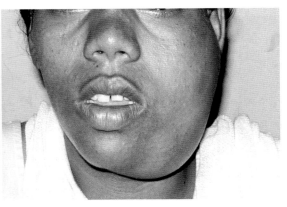

Fig. 25.29: Extraoral swelling on left side of face

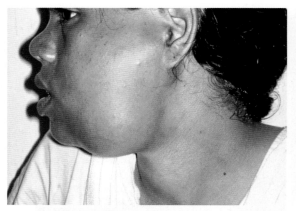

Fig. 25.30: Extraoral swelling on left side of face

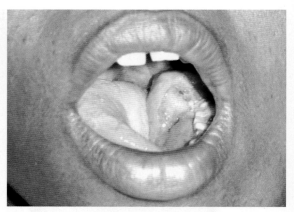

Fig. 25.31: Intraoral lingual sulcus obliteration and growth

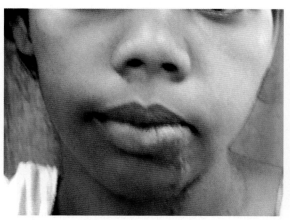

Fig. 25.32: Postoperative picture

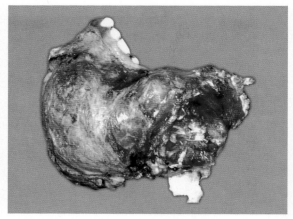

Fig. 25.33: Excised lesion

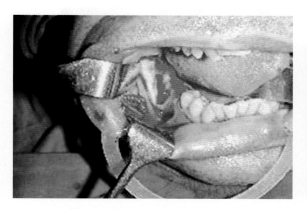

Fig. 25.34 Intraoperative picture

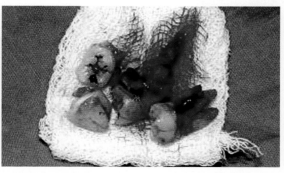

Fig. 25.35 Excised lesion with involved teeth

ODONTOGENIC MYXOMA

Superficial lesions may develop pigmentation.

The origin of odontogenic myxoma is believed to be the mesenchyme of a developing tooth or the periodontal ligament.

Myxoma of the jaws has been classified as a benign odontogenic tumor composed of odontogenic ectomesenchyme, with or without, included odontogenic epithelium. Myxomas usually present as a painless facial swellings, however, tumors of the maxilla tend to enlarge and often fill the maxillary sinus before presenting as a facial swelling. The destructive nature of the tumor can cause nasal obstruction or ocular changes even palatal swellings have been reported. Myxoma tends to affect the posterior part of the mandible more than the maxilla. Local recurrence is quite common (Figs 25.36 to 25.39).

Radiological Appearance

Odontogenic myxoma commonly shows multiple radiolucent areas of varying size separated by straight or curved bony septa (soap-bubble appearance). This appearance may be indistinguishable from that of an ameloblastoma. The CT images of the odontogenic myxoma shows osteolytic expansile lesions with a mild enhancement of the solid portion of the mass with expansion and thinning of the surrounding bony boundaries. The characteristic finding on CT scan may be the strands of fine lacelike density.

The tumor cells are small spindle shaped or stellate cells embedded in myxoid background, atypia and mitosis are rare, vascular invasion has not been reported. However, the tumor shows local infiltration, which explains the local recurrence in case of incomplete excision. The treatment of choice has traditionally been surgery because myxoma is radio-resistant. Adjuvant radiotherapy is generally not recommended in the treatment of odontogenic myxoma.

CASE PRESENTATIONS

Case 1

Chief Complaint

A 27-year-old female presents with a complaint of swelling in the right lower cheek region for past 6 months.

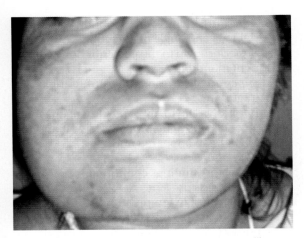

Fig. 25.36 Extraoral photograph showing swelling on right side of face

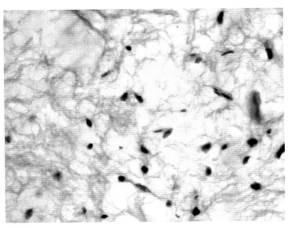

Fig. 25.37 Histological appearance showing myxomatous cells, fusiform stellate or tripolas

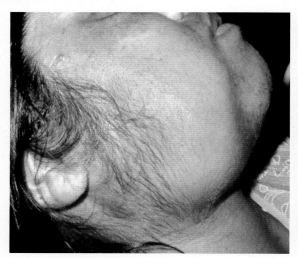

Fig. 25.38 Extraoral photograph showing swelling on right side of face

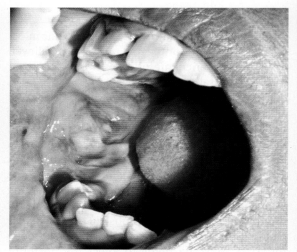

Fig. 25.39 Intraoral obliteration of buccal sulcus

History of Presenting Illness

History of similar swelling in the right lower face region 3 years back, which was much smaller than the present size.

Patient was advised extraction of the lower back teeth. She underwent extraction as well as excision of a lesion diagnosed as traumatic fibroma but the swelling failed to reduce.

She was referred to Dental College, where radiographs, CT and biopsy were advised.

The CT report was given as 'Expansile irregular mass involving the right mandible with erosion of ramus and body of the right mandible'.

She came back to another dentist at Nilgiris and was advised surgery. She was also told that the swelling would recur every 6 months and the surgery would have to be repeated.

She underwent surgery in early 2007 and a second one in early 2008.

The biopsy report taken in 2008 was suggestive of recurrent odontogenic myxoma of the right mandible.

The swelling started 6 months back and is associated with intermittent pain radiating to the ear.

Patient also complains of paresthesia of the lower lip intermittently mainly on the right side.

General Examination

- Appeared well built and well nourished
- No signs of pallor, icterus, cyanosis, clubbing, edema
- Vital signs—within normal limits.

Local Examination

- Facial asymmetry noticed because of a diffuse swelling in the right lower posterior of the jaw—8 × 5 cm
    - *Anteriorly*: Line corresponding from the right ala and angle of the mouth
    - *Posteriorly*: Up to the posterior border of the right mandible
    - *Superiorly*: Corresponding to the right ala-tragus line
    - *Inferiorly*: Up to upper 1/3rd of the neck involving the right lower border of mandible.
- Overlying skin appeared normal
- *On Palpation*:
    - Inspectory findings confirmed
    - Tenderness present
    - No local rise in temperature
    - Firm to hard consistency with ill-defined borders
    - Skin over the swelling—pinchable and moveable
    - Fixed to the underlying tissues.

Lymph nodes
- Left single submandibular lymph node palpable:
  - 1.5 cm size
  - Movable
  - Tender
- Mouth opening : 40 mm.

Intraoral Examination

On inspection: Well-defined expansile swelling 4 × 3 cm in size involving the right lower alveolus, right floor of the mouth, right buccal mucosa extending:
- Superiorly—1 cm below the right upper buccal vestibule to involve the right buccal mucosa
- Inferiorly—involving the lower right buccal vestibule
- Anteriorly—from the distal aspect of 44
- Posteriorly—up to the retromolar region
- Medially—involving the right lower alveolus up to 0.5 cm into the floor of the mouth
  Covering mucosa appeared pinkish and erythematous.

On palpation
- Tender
- Soft on palpation at the center of the swelling, firm otherwise
- Well-defined borders
- Fixed to the underlying tissues
- No bony crepitus or egg shell crackling noticed
- Nonfluctuant, noncompressible, nonreducible
- Tongue appeared to be shifted to the left.
  A well defined ulcer on the left posterior buccal mucosa—pale and covered with necrotic slough, tender suggestive of traumatic ulcer.

To Summarize

A 27-year-old female patient complain of swelling on the right lower posterior region of the jaw for the past 6 months. History of recurrence of the swelling every 6 months after a surgery.

Clinically
- Solitary ill-defined swelling of size 8 × 5 cm
- Extending from corner of mouth to posterior border of ramus
- Firm to hard.

Intraorally
- Well defined expansile swelling 4 × 3 cm in size involving the right lower alveolus, right floor of the mouth, right buccal mucosa
- Tender
- Soft on palpation at the center of the swelling, firm otherwise
- Well-defined borders
- Fixed to the underlying tissues
- Tongue appeared to be shifted to the left

Provisional Diagnosis
- Benign odontogenic tumor

Differential Diagnosis
- Ameloblastoma
- Ameloblastic fibroma
- Odontogenic myxoma

Investigations

Radiological investigations

Radiographically: Multilocular radiolucency A-P : Distal to root of 45 to the ramus S-I: Entire width of body destruction of the buccal cortical plate—Network of septae—at right angles—Sunray appearance (Figs 25.40 to 25.42).

Radiographic diagnosis: Benign odontogenic tumor.

Management

See Figures 25.43 to 25.45.

Case 2

A 45-year-old male, complain of swelling on the right lower posterior region of the jaw. Noticed since 10 years. Insidious onset, small and non-progressive, Rapid growth since last month. Not associated with any symptom of pain or paresthesia (Fig. 25.46).

Local Examination

Facial symmetry: Appears asymmetric due to the presence of a localized swelling on the right side posterior mandibular region.

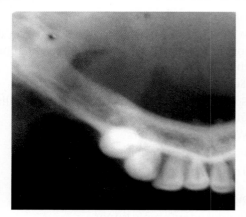

Fig. 25.40 Mandibular right occlusal with bicortical expansion

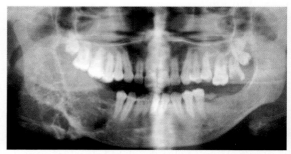

Fig. 25.41 Panoramic showing multilocular radiolucency at right molar region

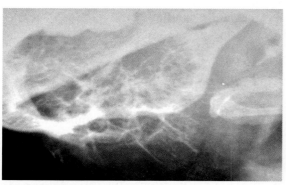

Fig. 25.42 Lateral oblique of right body of mandible radiolucency with network of septae

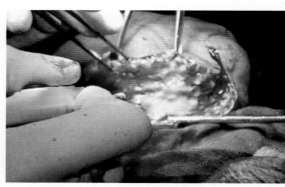

Fig. 25.43 Intraoperative electrosurgery and initial dissection

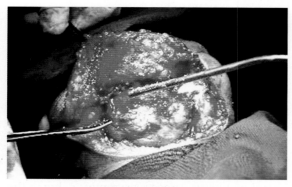

Fig. 25.44: Exposure of lesion

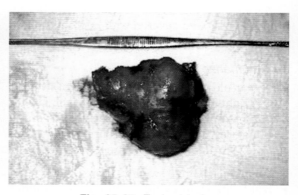

Fig. 25.45: Excised lesion

Neck Examination

Bilateral posterior cervical nodes were palpable
- Three in number
- Soft
- Nontender
- Mobile
- Measuring approximately 0.5 cm.

Examination of the Swelling

A solitary well-defined swelling noticed on the right side, lower posterior region of the mandible, Size 3.5 × 4 cm, roughly oval in shape (Fig. 25.47)
- Anteroposteriorly from corner of the mouth to angle of the mandible
- Superioinferior from ala tragal line to lower border of mandible.
- Borders—well defined
- Overlying skin—normal, without secondary changes

Palpation of the swelling
- Inspectory features confirmed
- Nontender
- No local raise in temperature
- Bony hard consistency with well-defined borders
- Skin over the swelling—pinchable and moveable.
- Fixed to the underlying tissues
- No signs of paresthesia.

Intraoral examination

A solitary ill-defined swelling arising from the buccal sulcus area extending into the occlusal surface of 46, 47, 3.5 × 2.5 cm with an ulceration at the center (Fig. 25.48).

Extending
- Anteriorly: Upto 44 region
- Posteriorly: Involving the anterior border of ramus.

The swelling due to soft tissue growth arising from the buccal sulcus was extending towards the occlusal surface of 46,47 region. Complete obliteration of buccal vestibule. Covering mucosa appears pale.

Ulceration noted with relation to 47 buccaly
- Size—1 × 1 cm
- Edges—ill-defined

- Margins—irregular
- Ulcer covered with necrotic slough.

Inspectory features confirmed
- Minimally tender
- Firm to hard in consistency
- Well-defined borders
- Fixed to the underlying tissues
- No bony crepitus or egg shell crackling noticed
- Non fluctuant
- Non compressible
- Non reducible
- Base of the ulcer—indurated
- Pus discharge noticed from the ulcer.

To Summarize

A 45-year-old male complains of swelling on the right lower posterior region of the jaw having no associated symptoms for past 10 years.

Rapid growth since one month. Intraoral pus discharge.

Clinically
- Solitary well-defined swelling of size 3.5 × 4 cm.
- Extending from corner of mouth to anterior border of ramus
- Minimal buccal expansion
- Bony hard.

Intraorally
- The swelling arising from the buccal sulcus was extending towards the occlusal surface of 46,47 region
- Complete obliteration of buccal vestibule
- 48 displaced distally
- No egg shell crackling noticed
- Non tender, Non fluctuant, non mobile
- Ulceration noted with relation to 47 buccaly
- Pus discharge.

Provisional Diagnosis

Benign odontogenic tumor malignancy

Differential Diagnosis
- Ameloblastoma
- Ameloblastic fibroma
- Odontogenic myxoma
- Ossifying fibroma

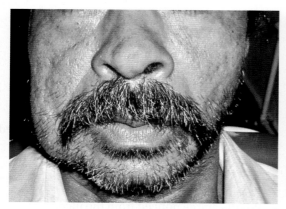

Fig. 25.46: Extraoral swelling at right side of face

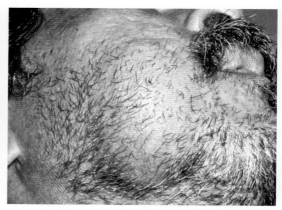

Fig. 25.47: Extraoral swelling at right side of face at molar region

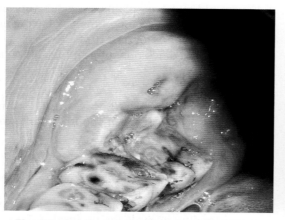

Fig. 25.48: Intraoral swelling and obliteration of buccal sulcus

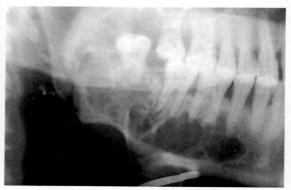

Fig. 25.49: OPG showing radiolucency at molar region

- Central giant cell granuloma
- Rareties
- Ameloblastic fibrosarcoma
- Osteogenic sarcoma

Investigations

- Hazy multilocular radiolucency
- Corticated margins
- Destruction of buccal cortical plate
- Soft tissue shadow noted

Odontogenic Myxoma

Site: Mandibular molar region

Clinical Features

- Slow, painless swelling, firm swelling
- Expansion of jaw
- Mobility/ displacement of teeth
- Occasionally causes ulceration.

Radiological Features

- Unilocular or multilocular radiolucent (Fig. 25.49)
- Well defined/irregular margins
- Straight etched septa
- square or triangular compartments
- Tennis racket appearance
- No root resorption

- Displacement of teeth
- Scalloping between the roots
- Maintains cortical outline

Ameloblastic Fibroma

- *Age*: 5–20 years also seen in adults
- *Gender*: Female and male ratio is equal
- Site mandibular molar region

Clinical Features

- Painful/ Painless swelling
- Hard swelling
- Associated with unerupted teeth
- Expansion of jaw
- Mobility of teeth

Radiological Features

- Unilocular or Multilocular radiolucent
- Well defined/irregular margins
- Curved indistinct septa
- No root resorption
- Displacement of teeth
- Maintains cortical outline

Ameloblastoma

- *Age*: 10–90 years (mean -40 years)
- *Gender*: Female and male ratio is equal
- Site mandibular molar region.

Clinical Features

- Painless swelling
- Expansion of jaw
- Mobility of teeth
- Egg shell crackling
- No paresthesia.

Radiological Features

- Unilocular or multilocular radiolucent
- Well-defined corticated borders
- Septa are coarse and curved
- Extensive root resorption

- Displacement of teeth
- Usually maintains cortical outline.

Ossifying Fibroma

- *Age*: Occur at any age
- *Gender*: Female and male ratio is equal
- *Site*: mandibular molar region

Clinical Features

- Painless slow growing swelling
- Asymptomatic swelling
- Minimal expansion
- Displacement of teeth.

Radiological Features

- Mixed radiolucent or radiopaque
- Sclerotic margins
- Wispy trabeculae
- Displacement of teeth
- Root resorption.

Central Giant Cell Granuloma

- *Age*: Occur at young age
- < 20 years
- *Gender*: Female and male ratio is equal
- Site mandibular anterior region

Clinical Features

- Painful rapidly growing swelling
- Painless slow growing swelling
- Overlying mucosa appear purplish
- Minimal uneven expansion.

Radiological Features

- Unilocular/Multilocular radiolucent
- Well-defined margins
- No evidence of cortication
- Displacement of teeth
- Irregular root resorption
- May cause destruction of cortical plate.

Ameloblastic Fibrosarcoma

- *Age*: 3–83 years
  - Mean age: 33 years
- *Gender*: Male-female ratio is 1.6:1
- *Site*: Mandibular molar region

Clinical Features

- Ameloblastic fibro sarcoma may present as asymptomatic or as a painful swelling
- Intraosseous mass (2–6 cm) with occasional ulceration.

Radiological Features

- May present as a well defined or irregular radiolucency
- May be unilocular or multilocular radio lucency.

Osteogenic Sarcoma

- Only 7 percent of osteosarcomas
- *Age*: Jaw lesions – peak at 4th decade
- *Gender*: Male and female ratio is 2:1
- *Site*: Mandibular angle and ramus region.

Clinical features

- Rapid swelling
- Very painful
- Ulceration
- Hemorrhage
- Trismus
- Paresthesia.

Radiological features

- R/L or mixed R/O
- Cotton ball/honeycomb pattern
- Ill defined borders
- No evidence of peripheral cortication
- Displacement and destruction of periostium
- Hair on end appearance
- Displacement of teeth
- Irregular Root resorption
- Destruction of cortical plate.

CASES OF ODONTOGENIC MYXOMA (FIGS 25.50A TO J)

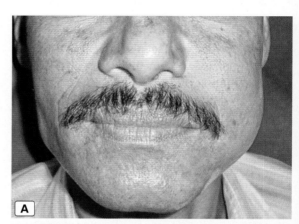

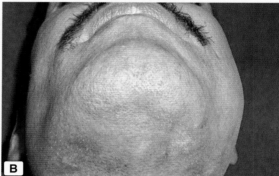

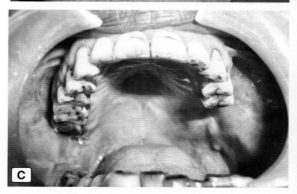

Figs 25.50A to C: (A) Extraoral picture showing swelling; (B) Basal view showing swelling; (C) Intraoral swelling in molar region

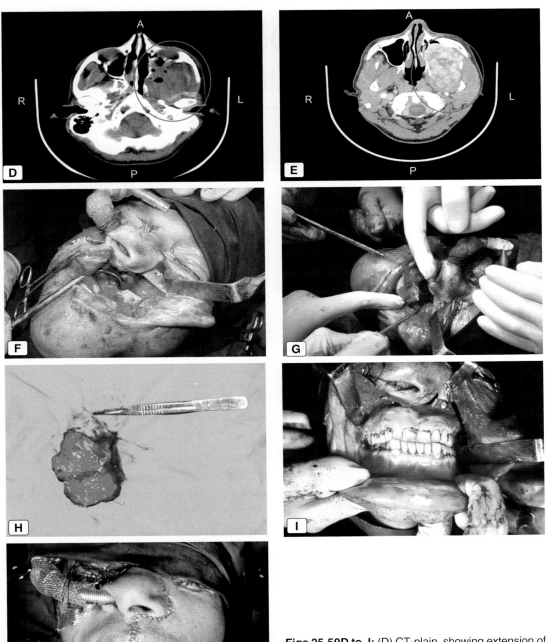

Figs 25.50D to J: (D) CT-plain showing extension of the lesion; (E) CT-contrast showing extent of lesion; (F) Donor site closure with drain-reconstruction and closure; (G) Exposed lesion; (H) Excised lesion; (I) Maxillary segment refixed with miniplates; (J) Closure and suturing (*Courtesy:* Dr Muralee Mohan)

Clinical Cases of Odontogenic Cysts and Tumors

26

CASE NUMBER 1

- A 22-year-old female patient with presented to the department with chief complaint of pus discharge from lower right back teeth region noticed since 6 months
- Not associated with any symptom of pain or swelling
- No history of trauma
- Prior to 15 days visited a dental clinic where:
  - Radiographs were taken
  - Biopsy done, extracted 48
  - Reported as ameloblastoma
  - Referred for surgery to our institution.

Extraoral Examination (Figs 26.1 and 26.2)

Facial asymmetry noticed.

Lymph Node

Right submandibular lymph node palpable
- One in number
- Soft
- Nontender
- Mobile
- Measuring approx 1 cm.

Intraoral Examination (Fig. 26.3)

- A solitary ill defined swelling in the right posterior mandibular region extending anteriorly from 47 to posteriorly involving the anterior border of ramus.

- Minimal bicortical expansion.
- Partially obliterating buccal vestibule.
- Mucous membrane normal
- Associated extraction socket filled with pus and necrotic slough
- Well defined borders
- Nontender
- Bony hard
- No bony crepitus or egg shell crackling noticed
- Not fluctuant
- Not compressible
- Not reducible
- No teeth mobility
- Heat vitality test revealed vital 46 and 47.

Radiological investigations (Fig. 26.4 to 26.7)
- Unilocular radiolucency
- Well defined
- Extending : Anteroposteriorly : Distal root of 46 to the ramus.

Superoinferiorly: Entire width of body
- Corticated margin.
- Lower border of the mandible thinned.
- Hazy radiolucency.
- Mandibular canal not displaced.
- Third molar displaced distally.

Histopathological diagnosis: Ameloblastoma
Final diagnosis: Ameloblastoma with secondary infection.

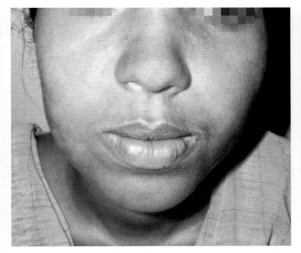

Fig. 26.1: Extraoral picture showing facial asymmetry

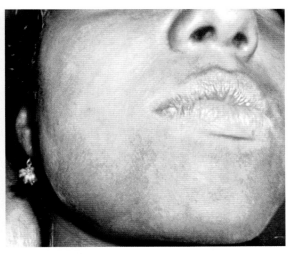

Fig. 26.2: Extraoral picture showing swelling at molar region

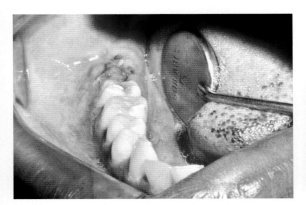

Fig. 26.3: Intraoral picture showing nonhealing socket

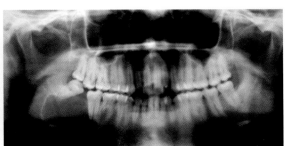

Fig. 26.4: OPG unilocular socket

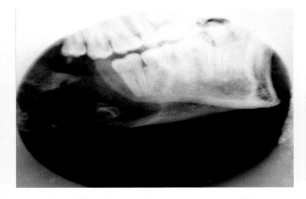

Fig. 26.5: Lateral body view of mandible

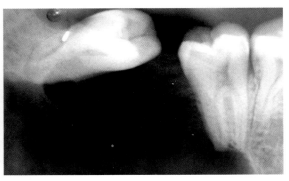

Fig. 26.6: IOPA (I)

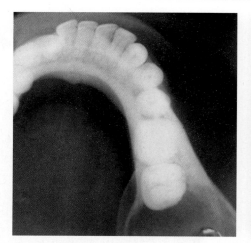

Fig. 26.7: Occlusal view showing bicortical expansion

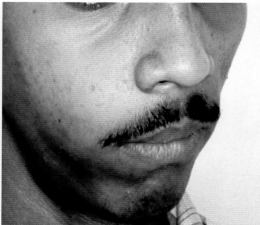

Fig. 26.8: Clinical photograph illustrating right-side facial swelling

CASE NUMBER 2

- An 18 years old male patient complaining of swelling in right side of face (Fig. 26.8)
- Complains of throbbing type of pain since 2 months.

History of Present Illness

Swelling noticed 2 months back. No increase in size of swelling.

Past Dental History

Patient had swelling in right side of face and undergone treatment

Medical History

No relevant history

Personal History

History of tobacco chewing since 5 years (4 packets/day)

General Examination

- Moderately built and nourished
- No systemic abnormality.

Local Examination

Extraoral

- Facial asymmetry present -

Swelling present on right side measuring approx. 2×2 cm

Intraoral (Fig. 26.9)

- Gingiva erythematous
- Swelling present
- No decayed tooth
- Clinically missing canine.

Palpation

- Hard swelling obliterating buccal vestibule extending from 11 to 16
- Gingiva soft and edematous
- Bony expansion present on buccal side.

Investigations

IOPA (Fig. 26.10)

- Shows impacted canine (13)
- Periapical radiolucency.

OPG (Figs 26.11 and 26.12)

- Shows well-defined unilocular radiolucent area extending from 11 to 16
- Impacted canine (13)
- Root resorption i.r.t 15 and 16.

Aspiration of lesion

- Straw colored fluid aspirated with cholesterol crystal present

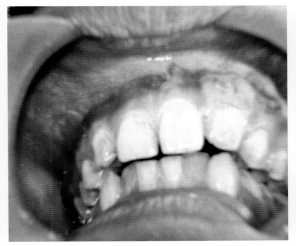

Fig. 26.9: Intraoral picture showing buccal swelling

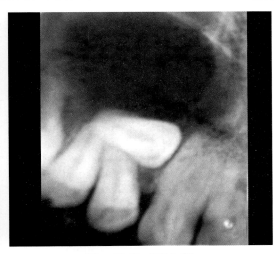

Fig. 26.10: IOPA (II)

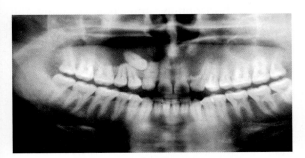

Fig. 26.11: OPG (I)

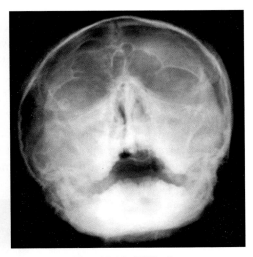

Fig. 26.12: PNS view

- Biochemical analysis of cystic fluid done
  - Total protein content – 9.2 gm/dL.

Provisional diagnosis
  - Dentigerous cyst.

Treatment
- Enucleation and primary closure
  Marsupialization.

CASE NUMBER 3

- A 26-year-old male patient with a complaint of swelling in the palatal region since 3 years
- Patient developed small swelling in the upper anterior palatal region which began insidiously 3 years back associated with pain only on palpation. It was nonprogressive in size, with no discharge associated. The swelling had

not regressed in size since then. History of exfoliation of the upper front tooth following mobility 4 years back.

Examination of the Swelling

- A Solitary diffuse swelling in the left middle third of the face adjacent to the ala of the nose measuring 2 cm in size causing obliteration of the left Nasolabial fold and was covered by normal appearing skin
- On palpation there is no local rise in temperature and it is mildly tender, with well-defined, solitary, bony hard in consistency, nonmovable swelling whose extent confirmed on palpation. The skin and soft tissue of the lip was freely movable over the swelling.

Intraoral Examination

- Partial vestibular obliteration noted with respect to 22, 23, 24, 25 due to a solitary well defined palatal swelling measuring 3 × 3 cm extending from
  - *Anterior* : 22
  - *Posterior* : 26
  - *Medially* : till the midline
  - *Laterally* : Mucogingival junction.
- Mucosa covering the swelling is normal in color, mildly tender, bony hard with fluctuance

noted; the mucosa was not movable over the swelling (Fig. 26.13).

Provisional Diagnosis

Dentigerous cyst with impacted 23.

Differential Diagnosis

- Adenomatoid Odontogenic Tumour irt maxillary left anterior quadrant
- CEOC irt maxillary left anterior quadrant.

Investigations

Radiographic

- IOPA (Fig. 26.14)
- *Maxillary occlusal radiograph*: shows right maxillary buccal cortical expansion (Fig. 26.15)
- *Panoramic radiograph*: A solitary large round radiolucent lesion in the left maxillary alveolus measuring 2 × 3 cm in size with well-defined corticated margins. Associated with a vertically impacted 23, whose cervical area is attached to the cystic margins along the posterior margin and a horizontally impacted 11 along the antero-inferior margins
- Internal structure appears mild hazy. The floor of the right maxillary antrum is superiorly displaced and intact (Fig. 26.16).

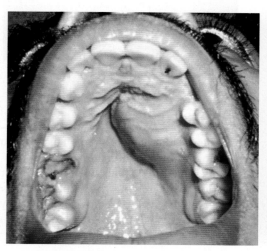

Fig. 26.13: Intraoral palatal swelling

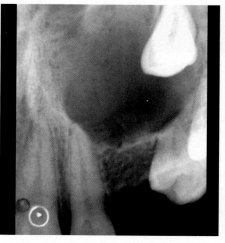

Fig. 26.14: IOPA showing radiolucency

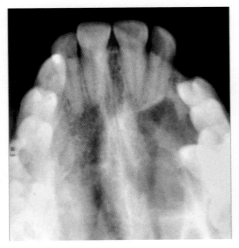

Fig. 26.15: Maxillary occlusal

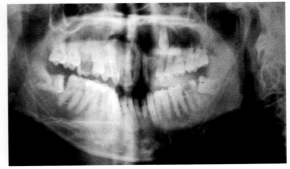

Fig. 26.16: OPG (II)

Histopathological Examination (Fig. 26.17)

It shows tissue composed of epithelial lining and connective tissue capsule with a lumen like cavity. Epithelial lining is 2–5 cell thick non- keratinized stratified squamous epithelium in most of the areas. However, in some areas: it is hyperplastic. Connective tissue capsule is made up of dense bundles of collagen fibers, some areas among which appear homogenized.

Impression

Suggestive of dentigerous cyst.

Confirmed Diagnosis

Dentigerous cyst.

CASE NUMBER 4

A 19 years old male patient with chief complaint of swelling in the lower left-side of the jaw for 5 months.

History

- Gradually increased to the present size associated with pain since 3 months
- Pain is moderate, intermittent, localized and presented only on chewing or biting hard food

- Slight numbness in the left lower corner of the lip area since 3 months
- Visited a general dental practitioner 2 months back who aspirated the contents of the swelling and 1 week back he was prescribed medicines for pain, but found no relief (Fig. 26.18)
- Unremarkable medical, drug, family and personal history.

General Examination

- Moderately built and nourished conscious and cooperative
- Normal vital and peripheral signs

Extraoral Examination

- Left solitary submandibular lymph nodes was palpable, enlarged, firm in consistency, mobile and measured 3 × 4 cm
- Gross facial asymmetry was seen due to the presence of a solitary diffuse swelling in the left lower 1/3rd of the face, 4 × 6 cms
- Swelling was firm–hard except the inferior border near the ramus of the mandible where it was soft
- Skin over the swelling was normal and taut. On palpation, there was local rise in temperature and tenderness.

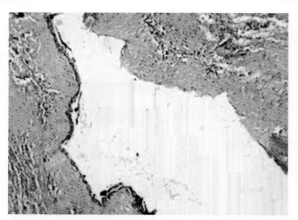

Fig. 26.17: Histopathologic view shows soft tissue lumen with epithelial lining thick, keratinized, stratified squamous epithelium

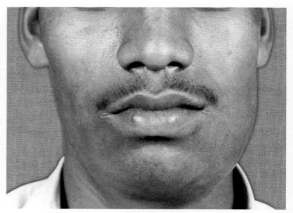

Fig. 26.18: Marked facial asymmetry

Intraoral Examination

- Swelling in the left buccal sulcus obliterating the buccal vestibule extending from the region of 35–38 (Fig. 26.19)
- Slight swelling was noticed in the lingual vestibule
- Swelling was firm in consistency and tender on palpation
- Grade I mobility was noticed in 34, 35, 36 and 37
- Aspiration yielded purulent fluid.

Provisional Diagnosis

Infected ameloblastoma.

Investigations (Figs 26.20 to 26.23)

- Radiographic
- Unicystic clear radiolucency with impacted supernumerary tooth, root resorption, thinning of inferior and post border of mandible.

Management

Lesion was marsupialized under GA.

CASE NUMBER 5

An 18-year-old girl with complains of painless swelling in the left lower third of the face since 2 years (Fig. 26.24).

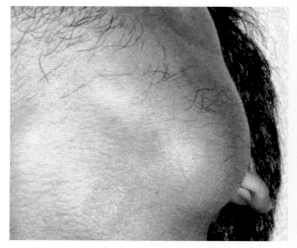

Fig. 26.19: Swelling at molar region

History of Presenting Illness

- Noticed a small swelling on the left side of mandible 2 years back, which gradually increased
- No history of pain, paresthesia, pus discharge associated with the swelling.

Past Medical and Family History

Unremarkable.

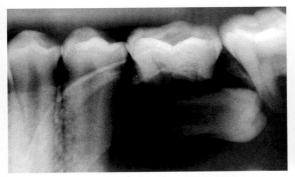

Fig. 26.20: IOPA marked root resorption

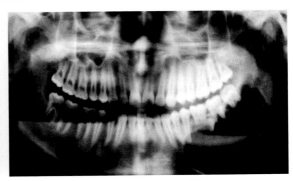

Fig. 26.21: OPG (III)

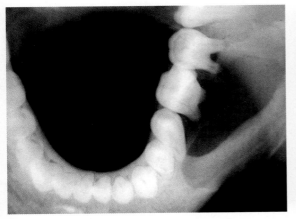

Fig. 26.22: Occlusal radiograph

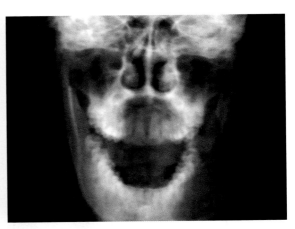

Fig. 26.23: PA skull

Extraoral Examination

- Solitary ill defined swelling noted in the left lower third of the face measuring approximately 4 × 5 cm
- Anteriorly: 3 cm from the midline
- Posteriorly: Angle of the mandible
- Superiorly: diffused
- Inferiorly: 1 cm into the submandibular region.
- No secondary skin changes noted.

On Palpation

- No local rise in temperature
- Nontender
- The margins were well-defined
- Surface was smooth

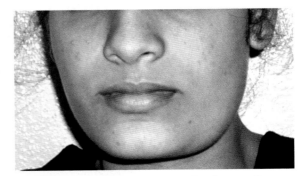

Fig. 26.24: Extraoral picture showing swelling

- Measuring approx—3 × 4 cm
- Bony hard in consistency
- Right submandibular lymph node was mobile, and soft in consistency.

Intraoral Examination (Fig. 26.25)

- Mouth opening was normal
- Left lower buccal sulcus was obliterated due to the swelling
- Extending from 35 to retromolar area
- Inferior extension of the swelling was not visible
- 36, 37 were missing
- Mucosa over the swelling was normal.

On Palpation

- Swelling was nontender.
- Bony hard in consistency.
- 34, 35, were not mobile, displaced.
- Very minimal expansion was palpated on lingual aspect.

Provisional Diagnosis: Odontoma? Radiographs (Figs 26.26 to 26.28) Differential Diagnosis

- Ameloblastoma
- Cemento-ossifying fibroma
- CEOT
- Complex odontoma.

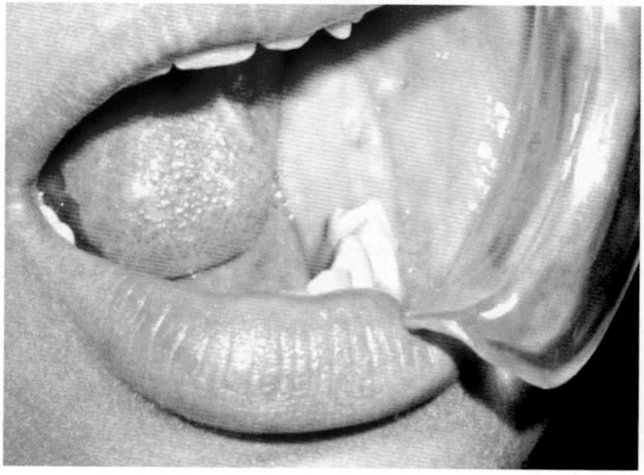

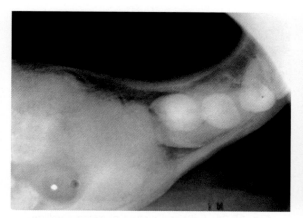

Fig. 26.25: Buccal sulcus obliteration

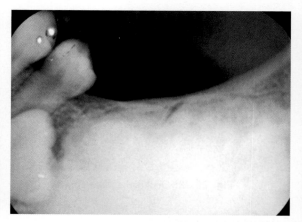

Fig. 26.26: Radiopacity indicative of odontome

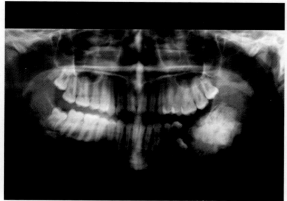

Fig. 26.27: Occlusal bicortical expansion due to extensive odontome

Fig. 26.28: OPG showing radiopacity in molar region

Excisional Biopsy: (Fig. 26.29 and 26.30)

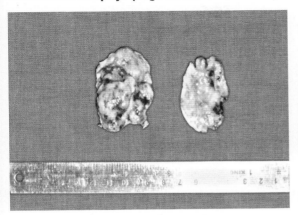

Fig. 26.29: Excised specimen

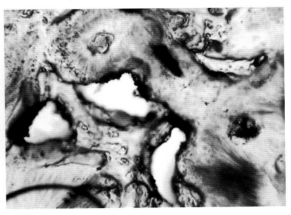

Fig. 26.30: Ground section of the biopsy showing mature tissues arranged in discrete tooth-like structure. (*Courtesy:* Dr Pushparaj)

5

Section

Maxillofacial and Cervical Swellings

Maxillofacial and Cervical Swellings: Differential Diagnosis

27

INTRODUCTION

Maxillofacial and cervical swellings are common. Most important considerations in an adult presenting with a lateral neck swelling is that it may represent a metastatic lymphadenopathy from a carcinoma of upper aerodigestive tract.

This is particularly true for patients aged more than 40 years and if they smoke and drink heavily, diagnosis of the primary tumor must be made without delay. In these patients diagnosis must be made without an open biopsy of the mass because the oncologic outcome may be compromised

Patients with neck mass should be examined systematically by maxillofacial surgeon. For this an accurate history should be taken and a thorough examination of the head, neck, and aerodigestive tract done. It could be with fiberoptic nasolaryngoscopy the most frequently seen swelling are enlarged lymph nodes, which could be bacterial viral or malignant or other rare causes

When a cervicofacial or neck presents with a swelling or mass, malignancy is the greatest concern. Differentiating benign or malignant mass can be difficult; a systematic approach will usually result in an accurate diagnosis and proper management. In this direction, framework for clinical decision-making for differential diagnosis should be made.

Accurate diagnosis of a maxillofacial and cervical swelling requires knowledge of normal anatomic structure. With good clinical, physical examination normal variations can be distinguished from true pathology without the need for additional diagnostic testing or imaging. Lymph nodes are located throughout the head and neck region and are the most common site of cervico-facial masses. Fixed firm or matted lymph nodes and nodes larger than 1.5 cm require further evaluation.

EMBRYOLOGY OF NECK

At Second Week of IUL

- Embryo has six branchial arches, five branchial clefts and five pharyngeal pouches
- Not parallel but come together at sixth arch
- Second pharyngeal pouch forms palatine tonsil.

At Fourth Week

Second branchial arch grows down to meet fifth arch enclosing third and fourth clefts forming "cervical sinus of His".

At Sixth Week

Branchial apparatus disappears having formed the ear, tongue, hyoid, larynx, tonsils and parathyroids.

Anatomy of Neck (Fig. 27.1)

A. Posterior belly of digastric muscle.
B. Sternocleidomastoid muscle.

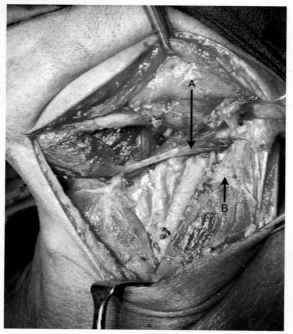

Fig. 27.1: Anatomy of neck muscle and vessels

Diagnosis of Neck Lumps

- First consideration—Age group (Table 27.1)
- Second consideration—Location
- Third consideration—Physical examination.

The common neck masses are depicted in Table 27.2.

Site of Neck Swelling

- It is essential to define the site of a lump in the neck. The neck is divided into two triangles
- The anterior triangle is bounded by the anterior border of the sternomastoid muscle, the lower edge of the jaw and the midline. Structures deep to sternomastoid are considered to be inside the anterior triangle

Table 27.1: Age group		
0–15 years	*16–40 years*	*> 40 years*
1. Inflammatory	1. Inflammatory	1. Neoplasia
2. Congenital/ developmental	2. Congenital / developmental	2. Inflammatory
3. Neoplasia	Neoplasia	3. Congenital/ developmental

Table 27.2: Common neck masses			
	Neoplastic	*Congenital/Developmental*	*Inflammatory*
M E T A S T A T I C	Known primary– Epidermoid carcinoma	Sebaceous cyst	Lymphadenopathy
	Unknown primary –	Brachial cleft cysts	• Bacterial
	Epidermoid carcinoma		• Viral
	Melanoma	Thyroglossal duct cysts	
	Adenocarcinoma	Lymphangioma/hemangioma	Granulomatous
	Thyroid	Dermoid cysts	• Tuberculosis
		Ectopic thyroid tissue	• Cat scratch
P R I M A R Y	Lymphoma		• Fungal
	Salivary	Laryngocele	• Sarcoidosis
	Lipoma	Thymic cyst	
	Glomus vagale		Sialadenitis
	Carotid body tumor		• Parotid
	Rhabdomyosarcoma		• Submandibular

- The posterior triangle is bounded by the posterior border of the sternomastoid muscle, the anterior edge of the trapezius and the clavicle
- To define the triangles, the patient must tense the neck muscles:
  - *Sternomastoid*: Put your hand under the patient's chin and ask him to nod his head against resistance. This tightens both sternomastoids
  - *Trapezius*: Ask the patient to shrug his shoulders against resistance.

Neck Swellings Derived from Unpaired Midline Structures

- These swellings tend to lie in the midline.
- The most common causes of a neck swelling derived from a midline unpaired structure are:
  - Ludwig's angina
  - Enlarged submental nodes
  - Thyroglossal cyst: Most common midline neck swelling and usually presents as a painless, rounded cystic lump which moves on swallowing or protruding the tongue. It can occur anywhere along the thyroglossal tract, i.e. from the foramen cecum to the thyroid isthmus, but is most commonly above the hyoid bone. The cyst is freely mobile and the majority transilluminate. Occasionally they become infected and present as a thyroglosal cyst.
  - Midline dermoid: These usually present as painless solid or cystic masses anywhere between the suprasternal notch and the submental region. The feature which distinguishes them from a thyroglossal cyst is that they do not move with protrusion of the tongue.
  - Pharyngeal pouch
  - Laryngocele
  - Subhyoid bursa
  - Carcinoma of the larynx, trachea and esophagus
  - Plunging ranula
  - Goiter of thyroid isthumus and pyramidal lobe
  - Enlarged lymph nodes and lipoma in suprasternal space of burns

- Retrosternal goiter
- Thymic swelling
- Bony swellings from manubrium sterni.

Neck Swellings Derived from Paired Lateral Structures

Found in the Anterior Triangle

- These swelling tend to lie laterally in the neck.
- The most common causes of a swelling derived from a lateral paired structure are:
  - Thyroid swellings
  - Branchial cysts
  - Pharyngeal pouch – unpaired on the left usually. Asymptomatic or may cause dysphagia and regurgitation
  - Salivary gland swellings
  - Lymph node enlargement (look for lymphadenopathy else where)
  - Carotid body tumor (tumors of the chemoreceptor apparatus at the carotid bifurcation. They tend to be oval and nontender, lateral mobility but cannot move them up and down.
  - Cervical rib (palpate this in the supraclavicular fossa and may be associated with neurological and vascular symptoms)
  - Sternomastoid tumor
  - Cystic hygroma
  - Carotid artery aneurysms
  - Arteriovenous fistula
  - Actinomycosis
  - Muscle tumors
  - Clavicular tumors
  - Spinal abscesses.

CLINICAL EXAMINATION OF NECK SWELLINGS

History

Examination of Swelling

- Size
- Site
- Shape
- Surface
- Consistency

- Compressibility
- Fixation
- Pulsatility
- Transillumination
- Bruit.

Inspect

- Scars
- Masses
- Patient swallowing
- Protruding tongue.

It is necessary to define information relating to the

- Site
- Mobility in relation to deep structures and with tongue protrusion/swallowing
- Relation to muscles
- Relation to trachea
- Relation to hyoid cartilage.

Palpate

- Mass (size, shape, consistency, and mobility)
- Lymph nodes
- Thyroid gland
- Parotid and submandibular
- While patient is swallowing.

Auscultation

Carotid mass.
Illuminate.

SUPERFICIAL SWELLINGS

Swellings or lumps, which are superficial to the underlying muscle and fascia are commonly caused by:

- Sebaceous cysts
- Lipomata
- Carbuncles
- Neurofibromata

Relation of neck swelling to muscles
Lumps in the neck should be palpated with muscles relaxed and then with them contracted
Lumps deep to a muscle will become impalpable when the muscle contracts

Relation of neck swellings to the trachea
If a swelling is fixed to the trachea then it will move when the trachea moves
The process of swallowing elevates the trachea
Observe the neck lump as the patient swallows

Relation of neck swellings to the hyoid cartilage
The hyoid cartilage ascends when the tongue is protruded. It moves only slightly during swallowing
If the swelling in the neck moves as the tongue protrudes then it must be fixed to the hyoid cartilage

INVESTIGATIONS FOR HEAD AND NECK MASSES

CT and MRI Imaging

Helps in determining the extent of disease and planning surgery.

MRI

T2- weighted images: helps identifying submucosal neoplastic disease as source of nodal disease in nasopharynx and tongue base.

Radionucleotide Scanning

Distinguishes between functioning/nonfunctioning tissue.

PET

- Differentiates recurrent cancer from post irradiation changes
- Helps to determine unknown primary sites
- Identifies concomitant distant metastasis
- Disadvantages
- High expense
- High false-positive rate due to background salivary activity.

Open Biopsy

Indicated only after complete head and neck examination using direct and indirect methods and inconclusive FNA biopsy.

Definite Indications

- Adult patient
- Progressively enlarging nodes
- Single asymmetric nodal mass
- Persistent nodal mass without signs of infection
- Actively infectious conditions not responding to conventional antibiotics.

Biopsy in Younger Age Group

- Solitary, asymmetric nodal mass
- Progressively increasing size
- Supraclavicular area – 60 percent malignant
- FNA—useful for sampling nodal mass
- FNA negative—follow up for other signs of neoplasia
- FNA showing lymphocyte predominance—studied by flow cytometry to aid in diagnosis of lymphoma.

Workup of Asymmetric, Unilateral "Nodal" Mass

- Complete repeated physical examination of:
  - Oral cavity
  - Nasopharynx
  - Hypopharynx
  - Larynx
  - Thyroid
  - Salivary glands
  - Skin of head and neck
- Needle biopsy (FNAC)
- Imaging
  - Chest
  - Upper aerodigestive tract/neck after FNA, if positive
- Pan endoscopy with guided biopsy based on nodal mass site
  - Nasopharynx
  - Base of tongue
  - Tonsillectomy
- Open biopsy of nodal mass with:
  - Frozen section
  - Epidermoid carcinoma, melanoma, upper neck adenoma – simult neck dissection
  - Lymphoma: close and stage before radiation therapy, chemotherapy, or both

- Adenocarcinoma: close; pursue primary lesion if supraclavicular
- Granuloma or inflammation: culture and close.

Pediatric neck mass (0–15 years)
• Congenital/ developmental
– Thyroglossal duct cyst
– Dermoid
– Laryngocele
• Inflammatory
– Adenitis
- Bacterial
- Viral
- Granulomatous
• Neoplastic
– Thyroid
– Lymphoma

Middle age neck masses (16-40 years)
• Congenital/developmental
– Branchial cyst
– Thymic cyst
• Inflammatory
– Sialadenopathy
- Parotid
- Submandibular
• Adenitis
– Bacterial
– Viral
– Granulomatous
• Neoplastic
– Thyroid
– Lymphoma

Metastatic	Primary
• Submandibular	• Carotid body
– Oral cavity	• Glomus
– Nasal sinus	• Hemangioma
– Face	• Neurogenic
• Upper jugular	• Neurilemoma
– Oropharynx	• Salivary
– Oral cavity	– Parotid
– Larynx	– Submandibular
• Lower jugular	
– Hypopharynx	
– Thyroid	

Old age neck masses (40+ years)
• Congenital/ developmental   – Lymphangioma

• Inflammatory
  – Adenitis
  – Bacterial
  – Viral
  – Granulomatous

• Neoplastic
  – Thyroid
  – Lymphoma

• Metastatic
  – Jugular
    - Posterior
    - Nasopharynx
    - Scalp

• Supraclavicular

UNKNOWN NECK MASS

Any neck mass (Fig. 27.2), particularly a *unilateral*, *asymptomatic* mass corresponding to known lymph node groups, must be considered a metastatic neoplastic lesion until proven otherwise.

BRANCHIAL CYST (FIG. 27.3)

Clinical Features

• *Site*: lateral neck deep to sternomastoid at junction of upper third middle third
• Fluctuant, transilluminant.

Pathophysiology (Figs 27.4 and 27.5)

• Develop from vestigial remnant of II branchial cleft
• Result of branchial epithelium entrapped in lymph node.

Diagnosis

USG and FNAC.

Histopathology

• Lined by squamous epithelium
• Thick, turbid fluid—cholesterol crystals.

Branchial Fistula (Fig. 27.6)

Clinical Features

• Unilateral/bilateral
• Represent a persistent II branchial cleft
• *Site*: external orifice: lower third neck near anterior border of sternomastoid
• *Internal orifice*: anterior aspect of posterior Faucial pillar behind tonsil.
• *Signs*: recurrent mucous/mucopurulent discharge.

Histopathology

Tract lined by ciliated columnar epithelium.

Treatment

Complete excision.

Cystic Hygroma (Lymphangiomas)

Clinical Features

• Neonate/early infancy occasionally at birth
• Neck, parotid, submandibular, tongue, floor of mouth, B/L also
• Soft, partially compressible, brilliant transilluminant, inc in size on crying/coughing.

Pathophysiology

Sequestration of jugular lymph sac from lymphatic system.

Histology: Filled with clear lymph and lined with single layer of epithelium.

Complication

• Expand rapidly—respiratory difficulty
• Infected
• Spontaneous regression.

Treatment

Defintive—surgical excision at early stage
• Sclerotherapy.

Sternocleidomastoid Tumor

Clinical Features

• Appears 10 days—2 weeks after birth
• Usually unilateral, rarely bilateral
• Lower third of sternomastoid muscle
• Disappears before 6 months of age

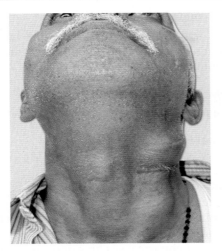

Fig. 27.2: Lateral neck swelling

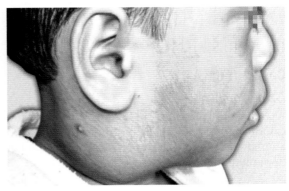

Fig. 27.3: Branchial sinus (*Courtesy:* Dr Vikram)

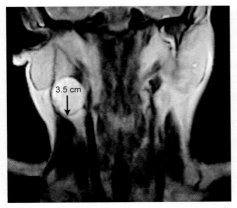

Fig. 27.4: MRI showing origin of sinus

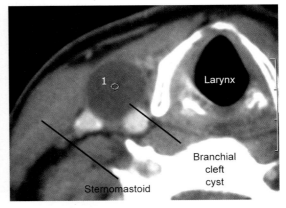

Fig. 27.5: Showing branchial cleft

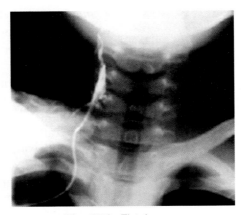

Fig. 27.6: Fistulogram

Etiology

Hematoma following birth trauma/vascular lesion

Complication: Permanent torticollis—manifest at 4 years.

CASE PRESENTATION

Case 1 (Fig. 27.7)

Chief Complaint

A 63 years old male patient hailing from Madikeri, Coorg reported to our Department in 2005 with a chief complaint of painless swelling in the left upper lateral part of the neck since 20 years.

History of Presenting Illness

Patient noticed a small swelling in the left sub mandibular region which appeared insidiously initially swelling started as small pea nut sized asymptomatic swelling which was slowly growing in size without any symptoms such as difficulty in swallowing or turning his head. He gives no history of trauma, weight loss; night sweats, persistent cough, or increase in size prior to having food.

Past Medical and Drug History

Patient gives no history of major illness, hospitalization, prolonged medication. No history of reported drug allergies.

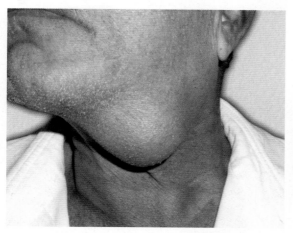

Fig. 27.7: Case of adenoma showing lateral neck swelling

Past Dental History

Patient had visited dentist 4 months back for extraction of carious teeth and the procedure was uneventful.

Family History

No history of familial, contagious, hereditary disease.

Personal History

Chewing pan 5/day for 20 years given up for 6 years

General Examination

- Moderately built and nourished
- Normal vital signs, with no pallor, icterus, cyanosis, clubbing, and edema noted
- No other abnormal swelling noticed elsewhere in the body.

Extraoral Examination

- Gross Facial asymmetry due to the presence of a solitary diffuse swelling in the left submandibular region
- Left submandibular lymph nodes were not palpable due to the swelling.

Examination of the Swelling

- Solitary well defined swelling in the left upper 1/3 of the neck, predominantly in the submandibular region measuring 3 cm (superoinferiorly) × 4 cm (anteroposteriorly), extending
- *Superior*: Mandibular lower border
- *Inferior*: 3 cm below lower mandibular border
- *Anterior*: 3 cm posterior to the symphysis
- *Posterior*: 1 cm anterior to the left angle of mandible
- The skin over the swelling appeared normal in color, without any secondary changes
- Palpation; there was no local rise in temperature nor the swelling is tender, surface is smooth with well defined borders
- The swelling was movable, without any areas of fluctuation and it was firm in consistency, it does not move with swallowing or during coughing.

Intraoral Soft Tissue Examination

- Normal mouth opening
- Normal oral mucosa—no other lesions noted intraorally
- No intraoral extensions of the swelling noted
- Normal buccal and lingual vestibules
- Normal salivary flow
- Generalized inflammation of the gingiva.

Summary of Findings

- A 63 years old male presented with asymptomatic slowly progressing swelling in the left Submandibular region of duration 20 years
- On examination, gross facial asymmetry was seen due to the presence of a solitary well defined swelling of 3 × 4 cm in the left submandibular region, skin over the swelling was normal without any secondary changes
- On palpation, non inflammatory nontender firm swelling, intraorally no extensions of the swelling were noted and there was no change in salivary flow and consistency.

Provisional Diagnosis

Benign adenoma of submandibular gland

Differential Diagnosis

- Warthins tumor
- Chronic Submandibular sialadenitis
- Mucoepidermoid carcinoma (low grade)
- Carcinoma expleomorphic adenoma.

Investigations

- Conventional radiographs
- Ultrasonography
- Incisional biopsy.

Conventional Radiographs

- *Mandibular occlusal view:* No calcifications noted in the region of the left submandibular gland (Fig. 27.8)
- *Panoramic:* No osseous changes in the mandible noted (Fig. 27.9).

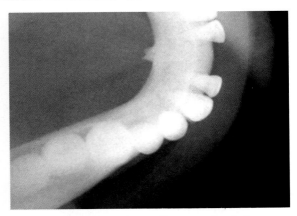

Fig. 27.8: Normal mandibular occlusal view

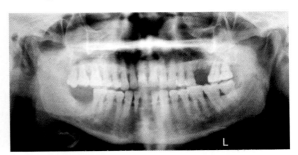

Fig. 27.9: OPG normal

Ultrasonography

- Showed a huge heterogeneous mass within the submandibular gland was noted, with well defined margins and internal echoes. Areas of anechoic, and hyperechoic fallowed by posterior attenuation was noted.
- Colour Doppler showed peripheral and central increase in vascularity (Fig. 27.10).

Histopathological Examination (Fig. 27.11)

Microscopy

- Showed the presence of epithelial and mesenchymal components, the epithelial cells were in clusters having round-oval nucleus. They were surrounded by coarse mesenchymal fibrils. The section was suggestive of pleomorphic adenoma
- *Impression:* Suggestive of pleomorphic adenoma of the submandibular salivary gland.

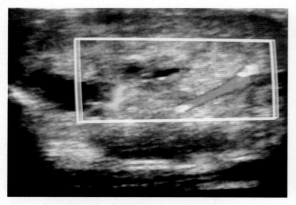

Fig. 27.10: Color Doppler of adenoma

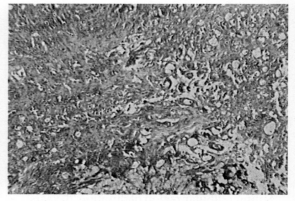

Fig. 27.11: Histopathology

Immediate Treatment Done

Left submandibular gland excision under GA.

Confirmed Diagnosis

Pleomorphic adenoma of the Submandibular salivary gland.

Case 2 (Fig. 27.12)

Chief Complaint

An 11-year-old boy with complains of swelling on left back region of face for 8 days.

History of Presenting Illness

- History of swelling for 8 days
- Sudden in onset
- Gradually progressed to present size
- Associated with pain for 5 days and fever for 2 days
- No change in the size of swelling while chewing/ eating.
- Pain is throbbing in nature, intermittent, radiating type and on taking food
- Pain relieved on taking medications
- Gives history of bilateral enlargement of tonsils for 8 days.

Past Medical History

- No relevant history
- No history of any drug allergies.
  - Drug history

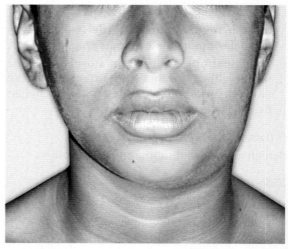

Fig. 27.12: Frontal view showing swelling on left side of face

  - Noncontributory
  - Past dental history.

Visited a dentist at Manjeshwar and was prescribed antibiotics and referred to our college.

  - Family history

No relevant history

Father is diabetic on medications.

Personal history

- Oral hygiene practice—brushes once daily with her toothbrush and tooth paste

- Mixed diet
- Normal bowel and bladder habits
- No H/o deleterious habits.

General Examination

- Conscious, cooperative, well oriented to time, place and person
- Moderately built and nourished
- Signs of pallor. No signs of icterus, cyanosis, clubbing, edema
- Vital signs—within normal limit.

Head and Neck Examination (Figs 27.13 and 27.14)

- Facial asymmetry
- TMJ—no clinically detectable abnormalities
- Lymph nodes –
- 2 cm swelling, oval in shape present near the left angle of mandible region
- 2 × 1 cm in level V
- 1 × 1 cm in level III
- Overlying skin appears normal
- Color – same as of skin.

Palpation

- Soft to firm in consistency
- Matted together
- Tender on palpation
- No local rise of temperature
- Overlying skin is pinchable.

Intraoral Examination

- No abnormality detected
- Normal salivary flow bilaterally
- No pus discharge
- No elevation of floor of mouth
  - Hard tissue examination
  No source of infection

Provisional diagnosis (Table 27.3).

Reactive Lymhadenitis Seconday to Tonsilitis

Differential diagnosis

- Tuberculosis lymphadenitis
- Infectious mononucleosis
- Hodgkin's lymphoma

Table 27.3: Hematological value profile

Parameter	Value
Hemoglobin	11.3 gm/dL
ESR	37 mm/hr
RBC	4.18 million/mm^3
Platelets	3,34,000/mm^3
Random blood sugar	118 mg/dL
Total leukocyte count	8600 cells/mm^3
Neutrophils	55%
Lymphocytes	37%
Eosinophils	5%
Atypical lymphocytes	3%

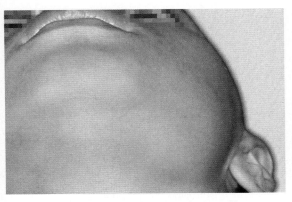

Fig. 27.13: Basal view showing swelling

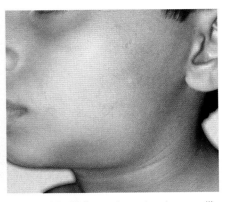

Fig. 27.14: Oblique view showing swelling

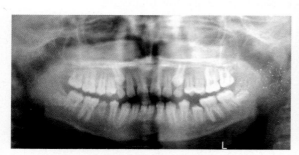

Fig. 27.15: OPG showing no source of infection

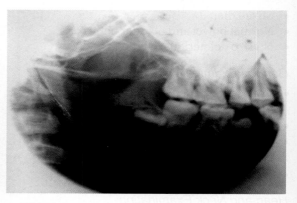

Fig. 27.16: Radiograph showing no source of infection

- Non-Hodgkin's lymphoma
- Acute lymphoblastic leukemia.

Investigation
- Radiographs
- Panoramic view (Fig. 27.15)
- Lateral mandible view (Fig. 27.16).

Peripheral Smear

Microcytic hypochromic anemia with occassional atypical lymphocytes seen.

USG Neck
- Evidence of multiple hypoechoic lesions of variable sizes noted in left submandibular, level II, III and V
- Largest lesion measuring about 22 × 17 mm in level II.

Pending Investigations
- Chest X-ray
- Mantoux test
- USG abdomen.

Salivary Gland Disorders

28

INTRODUCTION

Salivary tumors are uncommon. Any swelling near the ear is best considered a parotid tumor until proved otherwise. Parotid, submandibular and sublingual are major salivary glands.

Major salivary glands are characterized by an acinar and duct system saliva is produced in each acinus, which consist of prymidal cells grouped around a central lumen, this acinars cells may be serous (parotid), serromucous (submandibular), mucous (sublingual) or a combination (minor salivary glands). Salivary gland tumors vary in their histological and clinical features,and are challenging to diagnose and manage.

Major salivary glands	Minor salivary glands
Parotid glands	Lingual mucous glands
Submandibular glands	Lingual serous glands
Sublingual glands	Buccal glands
	Labial glands
	Palatal glands
	Glossopalatine glands

PAROTID GLAND

(Para—Near; Otis—Ear)
- Largest of salivary glands
- Weighs 20–30 g.
- Wedged between ramus of mandible and mastoid process and found below the external acoustic meatus
- It is irregular in shape, lobulated, yellowish mass.

Boundaries
- Anteriorly—Ramus of mandible
- Posteriorly—Mastoid process
- Superiorly—External acoustic meatus
- Medially—Styloid process
- Laterally—Parotid fascia.

Capsule
- Fibrous capsule derived from the investing layer of the deep fascia of neck
- Superficial layer (parotid fascia) is strong and adherent to the gland
- Deep layer continues inferiorly into the deep fascia of the neck
- Portion of the deep layer is thickened and is called the stylomandibular ligaments.

Shape
- Inverted three sided pyramid with
  Apex—pointing downwards posterior to angle of mandible
  Base—it is applied to the root of zygoma and neck of mandible.
- Three surfaces—
  – Superficial or lateral
  – Anteromedial
  – Posteromedial
- Lobes—
  Superficial and deep lobe connected by isthmus. The plane in between is known as faciovenous plane of the gland.
  Superficial lobe may separate to form the accessory parotid gland.

Superficial or lateral surface

It is covered with skin, superficial fascia with some fibers of platysma, parotid fascia, facial branch of greater auricular nerve, superficial parotid lymph node.

Anteromedial surface

- Has 'U' shaped groove to clasp the ramus of mandible
- Parotid duct emerge and five branches of facial nerve fan out over the face
- The terminal branches of the external carotid artery leave the gland.

Posteromedial surface

- Indented by masotid process and its attached muscle
- Lies against styloid process and its attached muscles
- External carotid artery enters
- Temporozygomatic and cervicofacial nerves enter

Structures Inside the Gland (Superficial to deep)

- Facial Nerve - Forms Pesanserinus (Goose foot pattern)
  Facial nerve forms a plexus of nerves within the gland and divides the gland arbitrarily into two lobes (not a true division) is known as parotid plexus.
- Retromandibular vein
- External carotid artery.

Parotid Duct (Stenson's Duct)

- 5 mm long and 5 mm in diameter
- Passes forward across the masseter and turns around its anterior border to pierce the buccal pad of fat, buccopharyngeal fascia, buccinator muscle, and finally in the mucous membrane
- Opens opposite to the upper 2nd molar.

Blood Supply

- External carotid and superficial temporal artery
- Venous drainage through retromandibular vein

Lymph Drainage

- Superficial and deep cervical lymph nodes
- 2 or 3 lymph nodes on and in the substance of the gland.

Nerve Supply

Parasympathetic fibers

- Preganglionic nucleus is the inferior salivatory nucleus
- Preganglionic nerve is the tympanic branch of the glosso-pharyngeal nerve to otic ganglion—ganglion of the relay
- Postganglionic branches are through auriculotemporal nerve.

Sensory Fibers

From gland it passes through the branches of great auricular nerve (C_2).

Sympathetic Fibers (Vasoconstrictor)

It comes from external carotid plexus after their relay in superior cervical ganglion.

Embryology

- The parotid anlagen are the first to develop, followed by the submandibular gland, and finally the sublingual gland
- Parenchymal tissue (secretory) of the glands arises from the proliferation of oral epithelium
- The stroma (capsule and septae) of the glands originates from mesenchyme that may be mesodermal or neural crest in origin
- Although the parotid anlagen are the first to develop, they become encapsulated after the submandibular gland and sublingual gland
- This delayed encapsulation is critical because after encapsulation of the submandibular gland and sublingual gland but BEFORE encapsulation of parotid, lymphatic system develops
- Therefore, there are intraglandular lymph nodes and lymphatic channels entrapped within the parotid gland
- Parotid gland is also unique because its epithelial buds grow, branch and extend around the divisions of the facial nerve

- The epithelial buds of each gland enlarge, elongate and branch initially forming solid structures
- Branching of glandular mass produces arborization
- Each branch terminates in one or two solid end bulbs
- Elongation of the end bulb follows and lumina appears in their centers, transforming the end bulbs into terminal tubules
- These tubules join the *canalizing ducts* to the peripheral acini.

Duct Canalization

- Canalization results from mitotic activity of the *outer layers* of the cord outpacing that of the inner cell layers
- Canalization is complete by 6th month postconception.

Acinar Cells

At around the 7–8th month in utero, secretory cells (acini) begin to develop around the ductal system.

Histological Structure

- Predominantly serous acini, many ducts
- Fat cells scattered between acini and ducts.

CLINICAL CASE OF PAROTID SWELLINGS (FIGS 28.1 TO 28.3)

Patient with swelling in the left parotid region of 2 days duration.

History of Presenting Illness

- Sudden in onset
- Rapidly progressive to the present size
- Associated with pain and fever for 2 days
- Pain is continuous, dull aching type. No aggravating and relieving factors
- Associated with difficulty in opening the mouth, swallowing and mastication for 1 day
- Not associated with dryness, pus discharge or any other secondary changes
- Not taken any medication
- H/o similar swelling associated with pain 1 month back.

Past Medical and Drug History

- Patient gives history of swelling in the neck since birth which was diagnosed as cystic hygroma
- It was surgically operated at the age of 10 months

General Physical Examination

- Moderately built and nourished
- No signs of pallor, icterus, cyanosis, clubbing or lymphadenopathy.

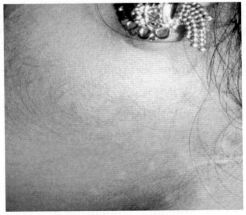

Fig. 28.1: Skin of preauricular region streched

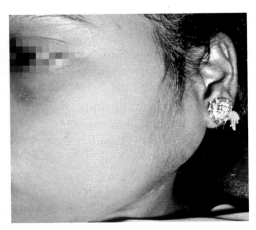

Fig. 28.2: Extraoral swelling in preauricular region

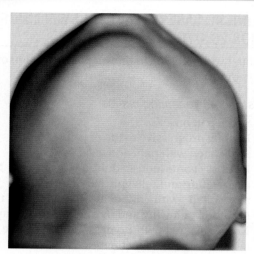

Fig. 28.3: Basal view showing swelling in preauricular region (*Courtesy*: Dr Vikram Shetty)

Extraoral Examination

- Mild facial asymmetry is noted due to a swelling present on left parotid region
- Pinna of ear is raised
- Mouth opening reduced to 2 finger breadth
- A scar is present on the left lateral part of neck
- Submandibular lymph nodes bilaterally palpable, single in number, 0.5–1 cm in size, soft, tender and mobile over underlying tissues.

Examination of the Swelling

Inspection

- Solitary well defined swelling, present on left parotid region measuring about 3 × 3cm in size, roughly oval in shape, raising the pinna of ear.

Extensions

- Anteriorly—1–2 cm from pinna of ear.
- Posteriorly—1 cm behind the ear
- Superiorly—up to zygomatic arch
- Inferiorly—up to the angle of the mandible.

Palpation

- Solitary well defined swelling, present on left parotid region measuring about 4–5 cm in size
- Roughly oval in shape, soft to firm in consistency, tender on palpation

- Raise in temperature is noted
- Skin over swelling is movable and pinchable. No signs of paresthesia noted
- Milking of parotid gland produces normal saliva with adequate flow rate. No pus discharge noticed from the duct.

Intraoral Examination Soft Tissues

Marginal gingiva in the lower and upper anterior region is inflamed and bleeds on probing.

Summary of Findings

- 19 years female patient with c/o swelling in the left parotid region of 2 days duration associated with pain and fever. H/o similar swelling 1 month back
- On extraoral examination, solitary well defined swelling on left parotid region measuring about 4–5 cm in size, tender and soft to firm in consistency noted. Milking of parotid gland produced normal saliva
- On intraoral examination, grossly decayed tooth present which was not tender to percussion
- Provisional diagnosis: Acute recurrent parotitis.

Differential diagnosis

- Chronic obstructive sialadenitis
- Pterygoid space infection
- Recurrent cystic hygroma
  Multiloculated hypoechoic lesion arising from the deep lobe measuring about 2.5 × 1.21 cm no calcification or solid component is noted. Submandibular and superficial lobe of parotid gland appears normal. Ultrasound of left parotid region is shown in Figure 28.4.

Immediate treatment: Antibiotics and analgesics for 5 days.

Submandibular Gland

- Second largest salivary gland, 8 – 10 g
- Mixed type *serous* and *mucous.*

Subdivision

- Large *superficial* and a small *deep* part
- United posteriorly around the free posterior margin of *mylohyoid.*

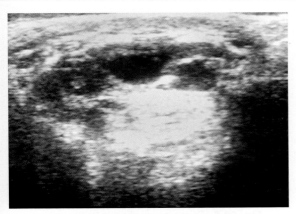

Fig. 28.4: USG of left parotid region

Fascia Covering

- Investing layer of deep cervical fascia splits to enclose
- Superficial layer is attached to the inferior border of mandible
- Thinner deep layer is attached to mylohyoid line.

Surfaces and Relations

Superficial part has 3 surfaces:
- Inferolateral surface
- Lateral surface
- Medial surface
   Deep part relations

Submandibular Duct (Wharton's Duct)

- 5 cm long, emerges from superficial part of gland
- It runs forward first between mylohyoid and hyoglosus, then between sublingual gland and geniohyoid to open into the floor of the mouth beside frenulum
- Duct opens through one to three orifice on a small sublingual papilla called *caruncula sublingualis* (sublingual caruncle).

Blood supply

- Branches from facial artery, few from lingual artery
- Veins drain into facial vein and lingual vein.

Lymphatic drainage: Submandibular lymph nodes

Nerve supply

- Parasympathetic secretomotor fibers arising from the superior salivatory nucleus run in the chorda tympani branch of the facial nerve and supply the gland after relaying in the submandibular ganglion
- Sympathetic (vasocontrictor) fibers come from the plexus around the facial artery.

Development

- The primordia bud off from the endodermal epithelium of floor of the mouth
- These buds branches extensively
- From the distal ends of these branches, alveoli differentiate
- A groove from the origin of the submandibular bud closes over to form the submandibular duct
- The submandibular gland arises from a series of buds each of which retains its own connection with the floor of the mouth and thus have several openings on the sublingual fold.

CLINICAL CASE PRESENTATION (FIGS 28.5 AND 28.6)

Chief Complaint

A 65-year-old male patient with the complaint of swelling in the lower right back face region for the past two months.

History of Presenting Illness

- The swelling was insidious in onset, had gradually increased in size over the past two months
- Associated with pain which was intermittent and dull in nature; no aggravating or relieving factors
- Not associated with any other systemic symptoms.

Past Medical History

Known hypertensive for the past 10 years and is under medication.

General Examination

- Moderately built and moderately nourished
- No signs of pallor, icterus, cyanosis, clubbing, edema

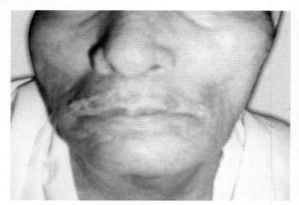

Fig. 28.5: Swelling in lower right back region

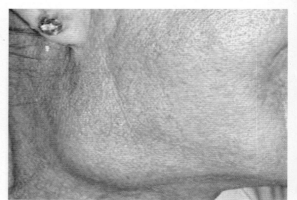

Fig. 28.6: Extraoral swelling in molar region

- Tremor of the arms and head were noticed
- Vital signs—within normal limits.

HEAD AND NECK EXAMINATION

- No facial asymmetry was noticed
- A diffuse swelling of 4/3 cm in size was noticed extending *anteriorly* about 3 cm from the midline, *posteriorly* up to the angle of the mandible, *superiorly* about 0.5 cm from the lower border of the mandible, *inferiorly* upto the middle 1/3rd of sternocleidomastoid muscle and extending behind it.

On palpation
- The inspectory findings were confirmed
- The swelling was firm, fixed to the underlying tissues and tender. Skin over the swelling was pinchable
- Lymph nodes—Right submandibular lymph nodes could not be palpated because of the extent of the swelling. The left submandibular lymph nodes were not palpable

Intraoral examination
- On inspection and palpation no abnormalities of the labial mucosa, buccal mucosa, tongue and palate were detected
- Gingiva was reddish, inflamed and soft in consistency with generalized gingival recession.

Summary of the Clinical Findings
A 65-year-old male with the complaint of swelling in the lower right back face region for the past two months.
- Associated with intermittent and dull pain
- Diffuse extraoral swelling at the right angle of the mandible region
- Firm, fixed and tender on palpation
- Grade 3 mobility of 46, 48.

Provisional diagnosis: Benign tumor of the right submandibular gland.

Differential Diagnosis
- Chronic lymphadenopathy of the right submandibular lymph node
- Hodgkin's and Non-Hodgkin's lymphoma
- Lymph nodal metastasis with unknown primaries.

Hematological Profile

Hemoglobin	15.4 g%
WBC count	6,300 /mm^3
Differential count	
– Neutrophils	69%
– Lymphocytes	26%
– Eosinophils	04%
– Monocytes	01%
RBC count	5.32 million/mm^3
ESR	60 mm/hr.

Radiographs
- Mandibular lateral occlusal
- Panoramic view.

Ultrasonography

Evidence of an ill-defined hypoechoic lesion 4.1/3.9 cm was noted in the right submandibular region. Right submandibular gland was not seen separately. No evidence of vascularity. The parotid and thyroid gland were found to be normal.

SUBLINGUAL GLANDS

- Smallest of the 3 major glands (2–3 g)
- Predominantly mucous
- Each almond shaped mass unite to form horseshoe shape, around the Lingual frenulum
- It raises the mucous membrane to form the sublingual fold.

Ducts
- Numerous small ducts *(Ducts of Ravinus)* about 8–20 opens into mouth on the sublingual fold
- Out of these one is larger called *Bartholin's duct*
- Half of the ducts open directly into submandibular duct.

Blood Supply
- Sublingual and submental arteries
- Veins drain into lingual and facial vein branches.

Lymphatic Drainage

Submandibular lymph nodes and deep cervical nodes.

Nerve Supply
- The nerves accompany those of submandibular gland to the sublingual gland
- They are derived from lingual and chorda tympani nerves and form the sympathetic (preganglionic) fibers
- Parasympathetic secretomotor (postganglionic) fibers arise from the parasympathetic ganglion (submandibular ganglion).

MINOR SALIVARY GLANDS

They are scattered throughout the oral mucous membrane attached to short ducts that open into the mouth. These glands are superficial lying beneath the mucosa.
- Lingual mucus glands
- Lingual serous glands *(von Ebner's gland)*
- Buccal glands
- Labial glands
- Palatal glands
- Glossopalatine glands.

Structure – Duct system of salivary glands
- Salivary glands are formed by the cells arranged in small groups around a central globular cavity called acinus or alveolus
- Central cavity is continuous with lumen of the duct
- Fine duct draining each acinus is called intercalated ducts
- Many intercalated ducts join to form intralobular ducts
- Two or more intralobular ducts join to form interlobular ducts which unite to form main ducts
- The gland with this type of structure and duct system is called *Racemose type* (bunch of grapes).

SALIVA

Volume: 1000–1500 mL/day
25% parotid gland, 70% submandibular, 5% sublingual
PH: 6.35 – 6.85 slightly acidic
Specific gravity: 1.002–1.012
Osmolality: Saliva is hypotonic to plasma.

Composition: 99.5% water, 0.5% solids (organic and inorganic substances).

Organic substance
- Salivary proteins—mucin and albumin
- Salivary enzyme—amylase (ptyalin), maltase, lysozyme, phosphatase, carbonic anhydrase
- Blood group components—antigens
- Free amino acids
- Nonprotein nitrogeneous substance like urea, uric acid, creatinine, xanthine and hypoxanthine

- Glucose is normally absent but in diabetic patient, glucose found in saliva
- *Inorganic substance:* Na, Ca, K, Br, Cl, F, P, bicarbonates
- *Gases:* O_2, CO_2, and N_2.

Salivary Secretions

- Saliva contains two major protein secretions
- Serous secretion that contains ptyalin (a amylase) for digesting starch (carbohydrates)
- Mucous secretion contains mucin for lubricating and for surface protecting purpose.

Salivary secretion is a two stage operation.
- Stage I: Acini secrete a primary secretion that contains ptyalin and/or mucin in a solution if ions
- Stage II: It takes place in salivary duct.
  Two major active transport process takes place that modify the ionic composition of fluid in saliva
- Na^+ actively reabsorbed, Cl^- passively reabsorbed, K^+ actively secreted
- Bicarbonate ions are secreted by ductal epithelium into the lumen of the duct; it is by active secretion and part by exchange of bicarbonate for Cl^-.

Functions of saliva
Preparation of food for swallowing
Appreciation of taste
Digestive function
Cleansing and protective function
Excretory function
Regulation of body temperature
Regulation of water balance

Regulation of Salivary Secretion

- Functions of parasympathetic fibers
- Functions of sympathetic fibers.

Reflex Mechanism of Salivary Secretion

Unconditional reflex

- This reflex is inborn and occurs immediately after birth
- The reflex does not need previous experience

- The flow of both resting and stimulated parotid saliva is reduced by blind folding or darkening the room. Light stimulate from the retina may induce sympathetic impulses to the salivary gland so that when these are absent the flow rate falls
- Unilateral stimulate produce a greater response on the stimulated side but some effect on the opposite side
- Saliva flow is independent of the number of masticatory strokes if it ranges between 40–80/minute. Below the rate of strokes the salivary flow diminishes and if exceeded flow increases.

Conditional reflex

- Occurs by sight, smell or thought of food due to impulse from eye, nose etc.
- It is an acquired reflex
- Needs previous experience.

CLINICAL EXAMINATION AND CLASSIFICATION OF SALIVARY GLAND DISEASES (TABLE 28.1)

1. Detection and examination of the patient's lesion.
2. Examination of the patient: chief complaint.
   a. Pain—inflammation/infection
      self mutilation – mucocele
   b. Burning sensation—xerostomia, vitamin deficiencies
   c. Xerostomia

Causes of xerostomia
Local inflammation
Infection and fibrosis of major salivary gland
Dehydration
Drug therapy
Autoimmune diseases
Post radiation changes
Psychosis
Alcoholism

Table 28.1: Classification of salivary gland diseases

Developmental
Aplasia
Atresia
Aberrancy
Ectopic—Stafne's cyst
Inflammatory
Viral: CMV, EBV, mumps, HIV
Bacterial
Allergic: rare (food, drugs, metals)
Radiation
Obstructive and traumatic
Sialolithiasis
Retention cyst
Atrophy
Functional disorders
Xerostomia
Sialorrhea
Autoimmune diseases
Sjogren's syndrome
Miculicz's disease
Neoplastic
Epithelial
Connective tissue
Metastatic

d. Sialorrhea
  - Psychosomatic—sight, thought, and smell
  - Denture
  - Teething
e. Swelling
  - Inflammation and infection
  - Cysts
  - Retention
  - Inflammatory hyperplasia
  - Benign/malignant tumor
f. Bad taste
  - Neurologic disorders
  - Medication
  - Decreased salivary flow
3. Onset and course
a. Masses which increase in size just before eating.

b. Slow growing masses (months to years)
  - Reactive hyperplasia
  - Chronic infections
  - Cysts
  - Benign tumors
c. Moderately rapidly growing (weeks to two months)
  - Chronic infections
  - Cysts
  - Malignancy
d. Rapidly growing (hours to days)
  - Abscess
  - Infected cysts
  - Salivary retention phenomena
  - Hematoma
e. Masses accompanying fever
  - Infection
  - Lymphomas
f. Re-examination of the lesion to evaluate
  - Fluctuation
  - Emptying
  - Blanching on pressure
  - Gas/liquid aspiration
  - Freely movable/ fixed to mucosa

Neoplastic
- Epithelial
  Benign
  – Pleomorphic adenoma
  – Warthin's tumor
  – Oxyphil adenoma
  – Bassal cell adenoma
  Malignant
  – Mucoepidermoid carcinoma
  – Adenocystic carcinoma
  – Papillary adenocarcinoma
  – Squamous cell carcinoma
  – Undifferentiated cell Ca
  – Ca in pleomorphic adenoma
- Connective tissue
  Benign
  – Hemangioma
  – Lipoma
  – Neurilemmoma
  – Fibroma

Malignant
- Malignant lymphoma
- Benign tumor may turn malignant
- Metastatic tumors.

Sialorrhea or Ptyalism

- Excessive salivation
- Can be mild, intermittent or continuous profuse drooling.

Etiology

- Aphthous ulcers
- Ill fitting dentures
- Gastroesophageal reflux disease—episodic
- Rabies
- Heavy metal poisoning
- Mentally retarded children
- Neurological disorder like cerebral palsy.

Clinical Features

- Drooling and choking
- Macerated sores around the mouth, chin and neck
- Social embarrasement to the patient.

Management

- Anticholinergic medications
- Transdermal scopolamine
- Surgical treatment includes:
  - Relocation of submandibular ducts (sometimes along with excision of sublingual glands
  - Relocation of parotid ducts
- Submandibular gland excision + parotid duct ligation
- Tympanic neurectomy + chorda tympani sectioning.

Hyposalivation

- Temporary hyposalivation occurs in emotional conditions like fear, fever and dehydration
- Permanent hyposalivation occurs in:
  - Sialolithiasis (Fig. 28.7)
  - Aptyalism or Xerostomia
  - Bell's palsy.

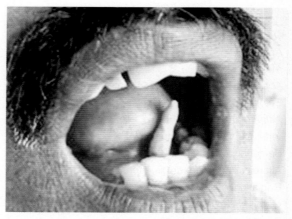

Fig. 28.7: Giant projecting sialolith (*Courtesy*: Pritam and BKS)

Xerostomia

- Subjective sensation of a dry mouth.
- Common problem
- Sex: women > men
- Age: more common in older people
- Incidence: 25% of older adults.

Etiology

Developmental
- Salivary gland aplasia

Water/metabolite loss
- Impaired fluid intake
- Hemorrhage
- Vomiting/diarrhea.

Iatrogenic
- Medications like anticholinergics, antihistamines, antidepressants, antipsycotics, antihypertensives
- Radiation therapy to the head and neck.

Systemic diseases
- Diabetes mellitus, diabetes insipidus
- Sjögren's syndrome
- Sarcoidosis
- Local factors
- Decreased mastication
- Mouth breathing.

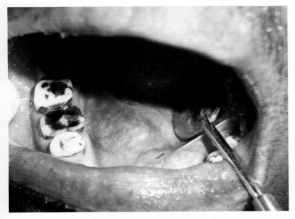

Fig. 28.8: Intraoral picture

Clinical Features

- Saliva appears either foamy or thick and ropey
- Tongue often is fissured and atrophy of filiform papillae
- Difficulty in mastication and swallowing
- Increased prevalence of candidiasis
- Xerostomia-induced caries (Fig. 28.8).

Management

- Artificial saliva
- Sugarless candy
- Systemic pilocarpine, cevimeline hydrochloride
- Maintenance of oral hygiene.

Effect of Drugs and Chemicals on Salivary Secretion

- Sympathomimetic drugs like adrenaline ephedrine stimulate salivary secretion.
- Paraympathomimetic drugs like acetylcholine, pilocarpine, muscarine, physostigmine increases salivation
- Histamine stimulates salivary secretion Sympathetic depressant like ergotamine and dibenamine abolish the salivary secretion
- Parasympathetic depressants like atroprine, scopolamine inhibit secretion

- Anesthetics like chloroform and ether stimulate secretion due to central inhibition.

Sialolithiasis

- It is the formation of salivary calculi in the salivary duct or gland resulting in obstruction of salivary flow
- 90% in the submandibular gland
- 80% radiopaque.
- More common in submandibular gland because of long, curved Wharton's duct, contains more calcium and also drainage is nondependent.

Clinical Features (Figs 28.9 to 28.12)

- Pain, swelling, tenderness in submandibular region
- Duct is inflamed and swollen
- Pain more during mastication
- When stone is in the duct, it is palpable as a tender swelling with features of inflammation in the duct.

Investigations

- Intraoral X-ray (occlusal films)
- Sialography
- Ultrasound
- Computed tomography.

Management

- Small sialoliths are treated conservatively by gentle massage of the gland
- Sialogogues, moist heat, and increased fluid intake
- Larger sialoliths are removed surgically
- If it is a ductal stone, removal of the stone is done intraorally, by making an incision on the duct
- If the stone is in the gland, excision of submandibular gland is done
- Lithotripsy may also help to fragment the stone.

External Lithotripsy

- Stones are fragmented and expected to pass spontaneously
- The remaining stone may be the ideal nidus for recurrence.

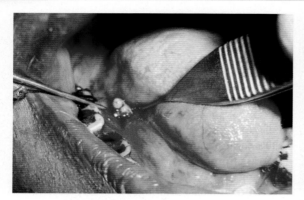

Fig. 28.9: Exposure of the sialolith

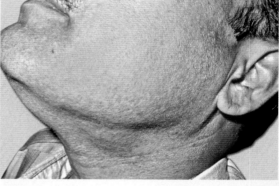

Fig. 28.10: Note swelling in submandibular region

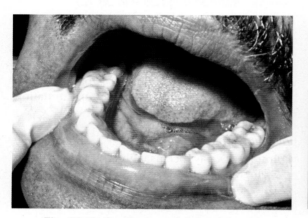

Fig. 28.11: Swelling presentation intraoral

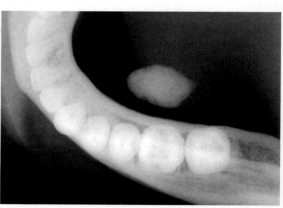

Fig. 28.12: Mandibular occlusal showing radiopaque mass lingual to premolars (*Courtesy:* Dr Subhas)

Interventional Sialendoscopy
- Can retrieve stones, may also use laser to fragment stones and retrieve
- Transoral versus extraoral removal
- If a stone can be palpated through the mouth, it can be removed transorally or if it can be visualized on a true central occlusal radiograph, it can be removed transorally
- Finally, if it is no further than 2 cm from the punctum, it can be removed transorally
- Floor of mouth (FOM) opened opposite the first premolar, duct dissected out, lingual nerve identified
- Duct opened and stone removed, FOM approximated.

Transoral advantages
- Preserves a functional gland
- Avoids neck scar
- Avoids risk to CN 7 and 12.

Case of Transoral Sialolithotomy of Submandibular Duct Sialolith (Figs 28.8 and 28.9)

Gland excision
Indications:
- Very posterior stones
- Intraglandular stones
- Significantly symptomatic patients
- Failed transoral approach

- Deeper submandibular stones (~15-20% of stones) may best be removed via sialadenectomy
- After submandibular gland excision, 3% cases have recurrence via retention of stones in intraductal portion or new formation in residual Wharton's duct
- No data regarding recurrence after parotidectomy
- While some believe that a gland with sialolithiasis is no longer functional, a recent study on submandibular glands removed due to sialolithiasis found, there was no correlation between the degree of gland alteration and the number of infectious episodes
- Fifty percent of the glands were histopathologically normal or close to normal
- A conservative approach to the gland/stone seems to be justified.

Classification of Salivary Gland Infections

Bacterial Infections
- Acute suppurative submandibular sialadenitis
- Acute bacterial parotitis
- Chronic recurrent submandibular sialadenitis
- Chronic recurrent parotitis
- Acute allergic sialadenitis (Radiological parotitis)
- Actinomycosis
- Cat scratch disease.

Viral Infections
- Epidemic parotitis (Mumps)
- Benign lymphoepithelial lesion (HIV disease)
- Cytomegalovirus

Fungal Infection

Mycobaterial infection
- Tuberculosis
- Atypical mycobacteria
- Parasitic infections.

Immunologically mediated infections
- Collagen sialadentitis (systemic lupus erythematous)
- Sjogren's syndrome

- Necrotising sialometaplasia
- Sarcoidosis.

Sialadenitis
- Inflammation of salivary glands is known as sialadenitis
- Viral, bacterial infections, allergic reactions and systemic diseases are the major causes
- It may be acute or chronic.

Viral Infections
- Mumps is the most common viral infection
- Caused by paramyxovirus
- Acute, contagious disease
- Parotid gland is usually affected.

Clinical Features
Prodromal symptoms
- Pain below the ear
- Sudden onset of firm, rubbery or elastic swelling of salivary glands
- Bilateral involvement
- Pain during mastication
- Trismus
- Lymphadenitis.

Investigations
- In acute phase, serum amylase level is raised
- Demonstration of mumps specific IgM antibody or four fold rise of mumps specific IgG titers.

Management
- Palliative in nature
- Antipyretics, analgesics.

Complications
- Meningitis, encephalitis
- Orchitis, epididymitis, oophoritis.

Bacterial Sialadenitis
- *Staph. aureus, Staph. pyogens, Strep. viridans, Pneumococcus* causes bacterial sialadenitis
- Children and older adults are usually affected.

Clinical Features
- Sudden onset of pain at the angle of jaw
- Affected gland is swollen
- Low grade fever, trismus
- Purulent exudate is observed from duct orifice
- Chronic sialadenitis caused by persistent ductal obstruction.

Investigations
- High leukocyte count
- Sialography demonstrates sialectsia proximal to area of obstruction.

Management
- Palliative
- Rehydration of patient
- Antibiotics
- Surgical drainage of pus.

Mucocele

- Swelling due to accumulation of saliva, as a result of obstruction or trauma to the salivary gland ducts
- Two types:
  - Extravasation type
  - Retention type

Clinical Features
- Dome shaped painless swelling
- Size—1 to 2 mm to several centimeters
- Most common in children and young adults
- Site—lower lip and tongue for extravasation type
- Palate, cheek, floor of mouth for retention type.

Treatment
- Surgical excision of the lesion
- Any adjacent minor salivary gland should be removed.

Ranula

- Mucoceles that occur in the floor of the mouth
- Rana (Latin word) means belly of frog
- Usually arises from trauma to sublingual gland
- Occasionally may arise from submandibular duct or from minor salivary glands in the floor of mouth.

Clinical Features
- Blue, dome shaped
- Fluctuant, nonpitting
- May be superficial or deep
- Large ranula can fill the floor of mouth and elevate the tongue
- Plunging or cervical ranula, occurs when the spilled mucin dissects through mylohyoid muscle and produces swelling within the neck.

Management
Removal of the feeding gland and/or marsupialization.

Benign Lymphoepithelial Lesion

- Also called mikulicz disease
- Age: In adults, mean age above 50 years
- Women > Men
- Site: 85% occurs in parotid gland
- Bilateral painless swelling of the lacrimal glands and all of the salivary glands
- Firm diffuse swelling
- Cases of parotid and lacrimal enlargement secondary to other disease are termed Mikulicz syndrome.

Sjögren's Syndrome

- Chronic, systemic autoimmune disorder
- Principally involves the salivary and lacrimal glands
- Two forms of disease—primary Sjögren's syndrome: also called sicca syndrome characterized by xerostomia and xerophthalmia
- Secondary Sjögren's syndrome: sicca syndrome + other autoimmune disorders like rheumatoid arthritis, systemic lupus erythematosus, scleroderma, polyarteritis nodosa or polymyo sitis
- Cause is unknown
- Viruses, such as EBV and HTLV may be responsible.

Clinical Features
- Age: above 40 years
- Female: male ratio = 10:1
- Xerostomia, altered taste
- Difficulty in swallowing

- Fissured tongue, denture sore mouth
- Angular cheilitis
- Diffuse, firm enlargement of the major salivary glands
- Nonpainful or slightly tender
- Bilateral presentation
- Xerophthalmia
- Keratocounjuctivitis sicca.

Investigations

- Sialography reveals fruit–laden branchless tree appearance
- Schirmer's test less than 8 mm wetting per 5 minutes
- Positive Rose Bengal staining of cornea or conjunctiva
- Elevated rheumatoid factor > 1:320
- Elevated antinuclear antibody > 1:320
- Prescence of anti-SSA or anti SSB antibodies
- Decreased parotid flow rate using Lashley's cups.

Treatment

Mostly supportive
- Sialogogues
- Artificial saliva and tears
- Sugarless candy
- Maintenance of oral hygiene.

Necrotizing Sialometaplasia

- Uncommon, locally destructive inflammatory condition of the salivary glands
- It mimics malignant process, both clinically and microscopically.

Etiology

- Traumatic injuries
- Dental injections
- Ill fitting dentures
- Upper respiratory infections
- Adjacent tumors
- Previous surgery.

Clinical Features

- Site: posterior part of palate
- Hard palate > soft palate

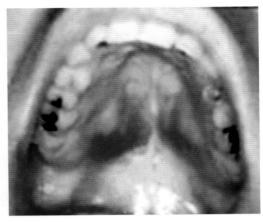

Fig. 28.13: Nonulcerated swelling in posterior palate after LA injection

- Two thirds of palatal cases are unilateral
- Age: mean age is 46 years
- Male : female = 2:1
- Begins as non-ulcerated swelling with pain (Fig. 28.13)
- Within 2–3 weeks, necrotic tissue sloughs out, leaving a crater like ulcer.

Investigations

Biopsy is indicated to rule out the possibility of malignant disease.

Management

- Debridement by hydrogen peroxide or saline
- Application of gentian violet
- Self limiting heals within 6–8 weeks.

CLASSIFICATION OF SALIVARY GLAND DISORDERS BY WHO

1. Salivary gland tumors
   - Pleomorphic adenoma
   - Myoepithelioma (myoepithelial adenoma)
   - Basal cell adenoma
   - Warthin tumor (adenolymphoma)
   - Oncocytoma (oncocytic adenoma)
   - Canalicular adenoma
   - Sebaceous adenoma

- Ductal papilloma
  - Inverted ductal papilloma
  - Intraductal papilloma
  - Sialadenoma papilliferum
- Cystadenoma
  - Papillary cystadenoma
  - Mucinous cystadenoma.
2. Carcinomas
  - Acinic cell carcinoma
  - Mucoepidermoid carcinoma
  - Adenoid cystic carcinoma
  - Polymorphous low grade adenocarcinoma (Terminal duct adenocarcinoma)
  - Epithelial-myoepithelial carcinoma
  - Basal cell adenocarcinoma
  - Sebaceous carcinoma
  - Papillary cystadenocarcinoma
  - Mucinous adenocarcinoma
  - Oncocytic carcinoma
  - Salivary duct carcinoma
  - Adenocarcinoma
  - Malignant myoepithelioma (myoepithelial carcinoma)
  - Carcinoma in pleomorphic adenoma (malignant mixed tumor)
  - Squamous cell carcinoma
  - Small cell carcinoma
  - Undifferentiated carcinoma
  - Other carcinomas
3. Non-epithelial tumors
4. Malignant lymphomas
5. Secondary tumors
6. Unclassified tumors
7. Tumor-like lesions
  - Sialadenosis
  - Oncocytosis
  - Necrotizing sialometaplasia (salivary gland infarction)
  - Benign lymphoepithelial lesion
  - Salivary gland cysts
  - Chronic sclerosing sialadenitis of submandibular gland (Küttner tumor)
  - Cystic lymphoid hyperplasia in AIDS

Incidence

3–4 percent of all head and neck neoplasms.

Cellular Origins of Salivary Gland

Multicenter Theory

- Each type originates from a distinctive cell type, e.g. Wharthin's/oncocytic: striated duct cells
- Acinic cell: acinar cells
- Mixed: intercalated and myoepithelial cells.

Bicellular Reserve Cell Theory

- All tumors arise from the basal cells of either the excretory or intercalated ducts
- These cells act as reserves, with the potential to differentiate into various epithelial cell lines, e.g. pleomorphic adenomas and oncocytic tumors: intercalated ducts
- SCC and mucoepidermoid tumors: excretory ducts.

Pleomorphic Adenoma

- Most common neoplasm of the salivary glands
- 10 times more common in the parotid than in the submandibular gland and it is very rare in the sublingual gland
- Age: 4th decade of life
- White persons have a slightly higher risk
- Though it is classified as a benign tumor, pleomorphic adenomas have the capacity to grow to large proportions and may undergo malignant transformation, to form carcinoma ex pleomorphic adenoma.

Clinical Features

- Presents as a slow growing, painless, soft, nodular mass
- Usually solitary
- Located at the back of the jaw just below the earlobe
- Almost all are asymptomatic, and they are usually brought to the attention of the physician when routine physical examination is performed
- It is usually mobile
- Facial nerve palsy and pain are rare
- Palate is most common site for minor salivary gland mixed tumors.

Gross Pathology

- Smooth
- Well-demarcated
- Solid
- Cystic changes
- Myxoid stroma.

Histology

- Mixture of epithelial, myopeithelial and stromal components
- Epithelial cells: nests, sheets, ducts, trabeculae
- Stroma: myxoid, chrondroid, fibroid, osteoid
- No true capsule
- Tumor pseudopods.

Treatment

- Surgical excision
- Superficial parotidectomy with identification and preservation of facial nerve
- Local enucleation should be avoided
- For tumors of deep lobe of parotid, total parotidectomy is usually necessary
- Submandibular tumors are best treated by total removal of the gland
- Tumors of hard palate are excised down to periosteum.

Warthin's Tumor (Fig. 28.14)

- Also called papillary cystadenoma lymphoma-tosum
- Most commonly found within the parotid gland
- Accounts for 4–15 percent of salivary gland neoplasms
- More common in men during their 6–7th decades
- Male predominance
- Smokers have 8 times increased risk of developing this neoplasm
- The etiology of Warthin's tumors is controversial and whether they are true neoplasms or developmental malformations continues to be debated.

Clinical Features

- Slowly growing painless, nodular mass

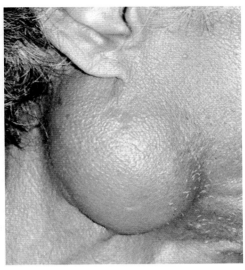

Fig. 28.14: Extraoral swelling at parotid region in Warthin's tumor (*Courtesy:* Dr Vikram Shetty)

- Swollen salivary gland, lump near back of lower jaw
- Firm or fluctuant to palpation
- Bilateral presentation
- Tinnitus, impaired hearing and earache.

Gross Pathology

- Encapsulated
- Smooth/lobulated surface
- Cystic spaces of variable size, with viscous fluid, shaggy epithelium
- Solid areas with white nodules representing lymphoid follicles.

Histology

- Papillary projections into cystic spaces surrounded by lymphoid stroma
- Epithelium: double cell layer
- Luminal cells
- Basal cells
- Sometimes oncocytes
- Stroma: mature lymphoid follicles with germinal centers (B lymphocyte).

Mucoepidermoid Carcinoma

- Most commonly occurring malignant neoplasm of the parotid gland.
- Second most common malignant neoplasm of the submandibular gland after adenoid cystic carcinoma.
- Represent about 5–10% of all salivary gland tumors.
- Age: 2nd–7th decades of life.

Clinical Features

- Painless, fixed, slowly growing swelling
- Tenderness, otorrhea, dysphagia, and trismus
- Facial nerve palsy may develop with high grade tumors
- Minor salivary glands constitute the 2nd most common site, especially the palate
- Asymptomatic swellings
- Blue or red color swellings that can be mistaken clinically for a mucocele (Fig. 28.15)
- Intraosseous tumors may also develop in the jaws.

Gross Pathology

- Well-circumscribed to partially encapsulated to unencapsulated
- Solid tumor with cystic spaces.

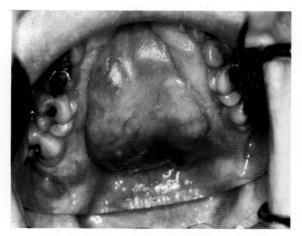

Fig. 28.15: Swelling in hard palate region

Histology

Low grade
- Mucus cell > epidermoid cells
- Prominent cysts
- Mature cellular elements.

Intermediate grade
- Mucus = epidermoid
- Fewer and smaller cysts
- Increasing pleomorphism and mitotic figures.

High grade
- Epidermoid > mucus
- Solid tumor cell proliferation
- Mistaken for SCCA
- Mucin staining.

Treatment

- Influenced by site, stage, grade
  Stage I and II
- Wide local excision
  Stage III and IV
- Radical excision +/- neck dissection +/- postoperative radiation therapy.

Adenoid Cystic Carcinoma

- It is one of the more common & best recognized salivary malignancies
- It was originally called cylindroma
- Approx. 50% develop within minor salivary glands
- Palate is the most common site. Remaining is found in parotid and submandibular
- Age: most common in middle aged adults
- Equal sex predilection.

Clinical Features

- Presents as a slowly growing mass
- Pain is common and important finding
- Patients often complain of a constant, low grade, dull ache which gradually increases in intensity
- Facial nerve paralysis may develop.

Gross Pathology

- Well-circumscribed
- Solid, rarely with cystic spaces.

Histology
- Tubular pattern
- Layered cells forming duct-like structures
- Basophilic mucinous substance.

Solid pattern: Solid nests of cells without cystic or tubular spaces.

Treatment
- Complete local excision
- Tendency for perineural invasion: facial nerve sacrifice
- Postoperative XRT.

Prognosis
- Local recurrence: 42%
- Distant metastasis: lung more common
- Indolent course: 5-year survival 75 percent, 20-year survival 13%.

Acinic Cell Carcinoma

- Second most common parotid and pediatric malignancy
- 5th decade
- F > M
- Bilateral parotid disease in 3 percent.

Presentation
- Solitary, slow-growing,
- Often painless mass.

Gross Pathology
- Well-demarcated
- Most often homogeneous.

Histology
- Solid and microcystic patterns
- Most common
- Solid sheets
- Numerous small cysts
- Polyhedral cells
- Small, dark, eccentric nuclei
- Basophilic granular cytoplasm.

Biopsy
- Fine needle aspiration biopsy (FNAC)
- Skinny needle biopsy
- Open biopsy.

Staging for Salivary Gland Cancer

(TNM classification accepted by the American Joint Committee for Cancer staging and end result, manual staging of cancer, Chicago, 1998)
- Staging is based on size of primary, spread to lymph nodes and metastases
- Staging is of clinical value
- It is based on clinical and radiographic examination and in some cases by surgical exploration.

T–tumor
- T_0 –No evidence of primary tumor.
- T_1 –Tumor—< 2 cm in greatest dimension.
- T_2 –Tumor—2–4 cm in greatest dimension.
- T_3 –Tumor—4–6 cm in greatest dimension.
- T_4 –Tumor—> 6 cm in greatest dimension.
  All categories are subdivided "a" no local extension. "b" local extension.
  Local extension is clinical/macroscopic invasion of skin, soft tissue, bone or nerve.

N-Node
- N_0 – No regional lymph node metastasis.
- N_1 –Single ipsilateral node < 3 cm in diameter.
- N_{2a} –Single ipsilateral node 3–6 cm in diameter.
- N_{2b} –Multiple ipsilateral node none > 6 cm in diameter.
- N_{2c} –Bilateral/contralateral nodes, none > 6 cm in diameter.
- N_3 –Metastatic lymph node > 6 cm.

M-Metastasis
- M_0 –No distant metastasis.
- M_1 –Distant metastasis.

Staging
Stage I
$T_1 N_0 M_0$
$T_2 N_0 M_0$

Stage II
$T_1 N_0 M_0$
$T_2 N_0 M_0$
$T_3 N_0 M_0$

Stage III
$T_3 N_0 M_0$
$T_4 N_0 M_0$
Any T (except T_4) $N_1 M_0$

Stage IV

T_4 Any N M_0

Any T N2/N_3 M_0

Any T Any N M_1.

Clinical History

- History of swellings/change over time?
- Trismus?
- Pain?
- Variation with meals?
- Bilateral?
- Dry mouth? Dry eyes?
- Recent exposure to sick contacts (mumps)?
- Radiation history?
- Current medications?

Examination

Inspection

- Asymmetry (glands, face, and neck)
- Diffuse or focal enlargement
- Erythema extraorally
- Trismus
- Medial displacement of structures intraorally?
- Examine external auditory canal
- Cranial nerve testing.

Palpation

- Palpate for cervical lymphadenopathy
- Bimanual palpation of floor of mouth in a posterior to anterior direction
- Have patient close mouth slightly and relax oral musculature to aid in detection
- Examine for duct purulence
- Bimanual palpation of the gland (firm or spongy/elastic).

Imaging of Salivary Gland Disorders

Role of conventional radiography

- Soft tissue swelling in the corresponding gland space
- It can pick up calcification within the lesion
- It can pick up adjacent bony involvement/ erosion
  - Use of contrast to overcome the inability to pickup the duct on plain radiograph— "sialography".

Disadvantages

- It cannot differentiate the type of soft tissue, i.e. blood, fluid—exudates/transudates or any other soft tissue
- Poor spatial resolution—superimposition of structures.

Sialography: It is Roentgenographic visualization of the ductal system of two of the paired major salivary glands this visualization is made possible by radiographic contact solution that is introduced into the duct.

- Radiopaque contrast infused (lipid soluble – ethiodol, nonlipid soluble—sinograffin)
- Scout film
- Ductal filling-tree limbs
- Acinar filling-tree comes to bloom.

Indications
Stone, stricture
To rule out autoimmune/radiation induced sialadenitis
Advantage
Visualizes ductal anatomy/ blockage
Disadvantage
Invasive, no quantification
Requires I-131 dye

Ultrasonography

- Painless, noninvasive, inexpensive and easy to perform
- Only real-time study, available.

Indication: Biopsy guidance, mass detection.

Advantage: Noninvasive, cost effective.

Disadvantage

- No quantification of function, observer variability
- Limited visibility of deeper portion of gland, no morphologic information.

Computed tomography (CT): Distinguishes both soft and hard tissue

Indication

- Tumor.
- Ruled out in calcified structure.

Advantage: Differentiates osseous structure from soft tissue.

Disadvantage: No quantification, radiation exposure, injection of contrast dye.

Magnetic resonance imaging
- Better soft tissue imaging, demonstrates vessels
- Demonstrates internal structures, regional extensions to adjoining spaces.

Advantage
- Excellent soft tissue resolution
- No radiation burden.

Disadvantage: Dental scatter, no quantification.

Contraindication: Pacemaker/metal implants.

Nuclear Medicine/Scintigraphy
- ^{99}Tc pertechnate IV is used which is secreted by the glands.
- Maximum concentration reached in 30–45 min

Indication
- Sialosis, tumor
- Ruled out in autoimmune sialadenites.

Advantage: Quantification of function.

Disadvantage: Radiation exposure, no morphologic information.

Radiographic features of Sjogren's syndrome
- Punctate sialectases distributed throughout the gland
- Large punctate sialectases are suggestive of main duct dilation and advanced autoimmune disease.

Radiographic modalities for cystic lesions
- Sialography: To see the displacement of
- ducts
- Ultrasound: Sharply marginated, echo free
- Radioisotope scan: cold spot
- CT: Well circumscribed low density areas HU 10–18.

Radiological features of pleomorphic adenoma
- Sialogram: Displaced ducts
- CT: Sharp margins
Round homogenous lesion.
Higher density than the adjacent glandular tissue.

- MRI: T-1 weighted images shows lower signal intensity (Dark areas).
- T-2 weighted images shows high intensity (Bright areas).
- On proton weighted images it shows as intermediate intensity.
- Scintigraphy: Cold spots

Radiological features of Warthin's tumor
- USG: Solid mass (hyperechoic).
- Scintigraphy: Intensely hot spots.
- CT and MRI: Not specific to this tumor.

Radiological features of malignant tumors
- Low-grade tumors present as benign salivary gland tumors.
- CT: Irregular and ill-defined margins.
- CT with intravenous contrast shows a sharply defined homogeneous mass
- MRI: T1-Weighted images have lower intensity (dark) than the surrounding structures.
- T2-Weighted more heterogeneous and intense (brighter) and slightly darker that the surrounding structures.
"Low intensity is suggestive of high-grade malignancy".
Benign and malignant tumor are characterized in Table 28.2.

NCCN Practice Guidelines in Oncology

Primary Treatment

T1 and T2 or untreated resectable clinically benign (< 4 cm)
- Complete surgical excision
- Benign and low grade – follow up
- Intermediate or high grade and adenoid cystic - post OP RT to tumor and neck.

Untreated resectable clinically >4 cm

CT/MRI: From base of skull to clavicle

Consider fine needle aspiration

Surgical resection

Benign—Follow-up

Table 28.2: Features of benign and malignant tumor	Benign	Malignant
Clinical feature	Slow rate of tumor growth. No symptoms	Carotid rapid growth rate. Pressure and pain. Facial neuropathy
Contrast sialogram	Pressure, shift of duct system, filling defect of gland parenchyma, stretching of duct in marginal region of pressure (ball in hand)	In addition to benign tumor; cut off of duct. Leakage of contrast medium
CT/CT sialogram	Clearly defined borders from surrounding tissue. Smooth tumor margin/oval shape	Unclear borders from surrounding margin. Irregular tumor margin

Malignant

Parotid superficial lobe

N0   parotidectomy

N+   parotidectomy + ND

Completely excised - follow up

Incompletely ⎤
Definitive   ⎬ excised
Gross residual disease ⎦ RT +

No further resection possible chemotherapy

Other salivary glands tumor

Clinically   N0 +   complete excision
                      No complete excision
                              +
                      Neck dissection

Partially Treated or Incompletely Resected

- Histopathology (FNAC + biopsy)
- MRI/CT
- CXR
- Negative physical examination –
- Adjuvant RT

Gross Residual Disease

- Surgical resection if possible
- If no surgical resection possible, then
  - Definitive RT or
  - Chemo + RT

Follow-up

- Physical examination
  - Every 1–3 months/1st year
  - Every 2–4 months/2nd year
  - Every 4–6 months/3-5 years
  - Every 6 months/> 5 years

- Chest X-ray annually
- TCH annually if thyroid irradiated.

Surgical Approach for Removal of Parotid Gland

Superficial parotidectomy
Superficial parotidectomy with partial deep lobe resection
Superficial parotidectomy with total deep lobe resection
Isolated deep parotidectomy
Extended total parotidectomy

Superficial Parotidectomy

- Superficial parotidectomy entails removal of the lateral portion of the parotid gland with preservation of the facial nerve
- It is the standard operation for masses that arise in the portion of the parotid gland lateral to the facial nerve, particularly when the histopathologic nature of the mass has not been confirmed
- Superficial parotidectomy is adequate treatment for benign tumors of the superficial parotid gland, such as pleomorphic adenoma, and for localized, well-encapsulated malignant tumors of low histologic grade which arise in the lateral lobe of the parotid gland.

Deep Parotidectomy

- To understand deep parotidectomy, the components of the deep gland need to be conceptualized. From a surgical dissection point of view, the deep parotid consists of three main parts:

Deep Parotid—Parts
The portion of the gland between cranial nerve VII and over the masseter muscle,
The gland deep to cranial nerve VII between the mandible and the mastoid/external auditory canal (greatest volume), and
The retromandibular gland that extends to or into the parapharyngeal space.

- The surgeon may individualize the extent of resection to involve some or all of these portions on the basis of the pathologic findings and presentation of the tumor. The major operations involving the deep parotid may include superficial parotidectomy combined with partial deep lobe parotidectomy, superficial parotidectomy with total deep lobe parotidectomy with or without resection of cranial nerve VII, isolated deep parotidectomy, deep lobe parotidectomy with parapharyngeal space extension, and extended total parotidectomy usually with resection of cranial nerve VII.

Superficial Parotidectomy with Partial Deep Lobe Resection

- This operation is commonly performed for benign tumors of the central deep parotid gland, such as pleomorphic adenoma involving the gland deep to the facial nerve. The surgeon may not always be able to predict the relationship of the tumor to the peripheral nerve from preoperative examination or imaging, and the decision to resect the deep gland may evolve during the operation after dissection of the superficial gland. This operation also may be performed for low-grade malignancies of the superficial gland for which the surgeon wants to include a portion of the deep gland to ensure an adequate margin of resection
- Rarely, this operation is performed in patients with refractory chronic sialadenitis in an effort to remove all chronically infected gland and prevent postoperative sialocele
- The operation also may be used for patients with mucosa-associated lymphoid tissue

(MALT) lymphoma of the parotid gland in the absence of other signs of lymphoma. This situation should be expected in patients with rheumatoid arthritis or Sjögren's syndrome who have development of nodular enlargement of the parotid gland.

Superficial Parotidectomy with Total Deep Lobe Resection

- Total removal of the superficial and deep parotid gland should be performed for malignant neoplasms with confirmed or suspected metastasis to the parotid lymph nodes, including the following situations: (i) metastasis to a superficial parotid node from a primary parotid tumor or an extraparotid malignancy, (ii) any parotid malignancy that indicates metastasis by involvement of cervical lymph nodes, and (iii) any high-grade parotid malignancy with a high risk of metastasis
- Total parotidectomy also is performed for primary parotid malignancies originating in the deep lobe and for primary malignancies that extend outside the parotid gland. The operation also is performed for multifocal tumors, such as oncocytomas, to ensure complete removal. The operation may involve sparing or sacrifice of the facial nerve branches or trunk depending on tumor extent to the nerve.

Isolated deep parotidectomy: Isolated removal of the deep parotid gland is most often performed for benign tumors of the inferior parotid gland deep to the facial nerve. This operation can be used for "dumbbell" tumors of the deep parotid gland that enter the parapharyngeal space through the stylomandibular tunnel. During this operation, the superficial gland is mobilized to aid in identification of the facial nerve, but it is not removed if not involved with tumor.

Extended Total Parotidectomy

Removal of the superficial and deep parotid gland also may be extended to involve adjacent structures such as the overlying skin, the underlying mandible, the temporal bone and external auditory canal, or the deep musculature of the parapharyngeal space. These extensions are dictated by tumor growth and behavior.

Surgical Technique

Preparation

- The operation is performed with the patient under general endotracheal anesthesia, and the endotracheal tube is positioned and taped to the oral commissure and cheek opposite to the lesion
- The patient is placed in a 45° reverse-Trendelenburg position or lounge-chair position with the head higher than the heart. The head is turned to the opposite side of the lesion, and the neck is extended
- If facial nerve monitoring is to be used, the nerve monitor is placed in the orbicularis oris and orbicularis oculi muscles to ensure upper and lower division monitoring
- Appropriate imaging studies and frozen-section review of the tissue should be available during the operation
- The risk of bleeding is low, and typing and cross-matching for blood transfusion are not needed during the operation
- Antibiotics are not routinely administered unless there are preoperative signs of infection.

Incisions and Flap Elevation

- The incision begins in the preauricular crease at the superior root of the helix and curves gently below the lobule, and then turns anteriorly to run horizontally in a skin crease approximately two finger widths below the angle of the mandible
- This limb of the incision should be oriented so that it could be extended into an incision that will accommodate dissection of the neck. The incision should not extend far posteriorly into the thin skin below the lobule over the mastoid tip
- In patients who are particularly concerned with scar camouflage, the incision can be placed

in the retrotragal area to hide the scar better. Although the exposure offered with this incision can allow full mobilization of the parotid gland, it is more difficult to incorporate neck dissection into the operation with this exposure. For this reason, postauricular incisions should be used only when the surgeon is convinced that the patient has benign disease

- The surgeon should raise the flap immediately over the parotid fascia, which is recognizable as a white fibrous layer deep to the subcutaneous fat and superficial musculoaponeurotic system layer
- Dissection should continue anteriorly over the fascia of the masseter muscle
- Branches of the facial nerve may be seen coursing toward the mid face just deep to this fascia. At the periphery, the parotid duct should not be looked for or isolated during this portion of the operation. Doing so could put the buccal branches of the facial nerve that accompany this duct at risk
- The anterior edge of the sternocleidomastoid muscle is identified, and the greater auricular nerve and external jugular vein, located just anterior to the nerve, are identified. The greater auricular nerve and its branches are the largest component of the upper surgical plexus. The nerve divides into mastoid, auricular, and facial branches, and the posterior branches can be preserved in some operations
- The greater auricular nerve should be followed distally beyond its branch point before division. It then can be divided at its branches and reflected inferiorly, thereby allowing for the potential for nerve grafting from the facial nerve trunk to distal branches if the facial nerve has to be sacrificed
- If possible, the external jugular vein should not be divided.

Deeper Dissection

- The parotid gland is next separated from the anterior sternocleidomastoid muscle by sharp dissection. The gland also is separated bluntly from the tragal cartilage

- After the parotid gland has been completely separated from the sternocleidomastoid muscle and the tragus, the posterior belly of the digastric muscle should be identified. The mastoid tip and the posterior border of the angle of the mandible serve as landmarks for the posterior digastric muscle. Once the muscle belly is identified immediately deep to the angle of the mandible, the remainder of the parotid gland is freed with blunt dissection.

Facial Nerve Mobilization

- The main trunk of the facial nerve exits the stylomastoid foramen immediately posterior to the styloid process
- The styloid process is rarely felt during superficial parotidectomy. The nerve gives off branches to the posterior belly of the digastric muscle and postauricular muscles before it turns anterolaterally and enters the parotid gland just anterior to the border where the digastrics muscle inserts into the mastoid. Tumors may thin the nerve or displace the trunk, but the position where the nerve enters the gland is constant
- Placing a finger on the mastoid tip, the surgeon uses the position of the cartilaginous tragal pointer and superior edge of the digastric muscle to identify the position of the facial nerve. It may be helpful to identify deeper structures such as the styloid process or tympanomastoid suture line to aid in nerve identification though these structures are not in view during this portion of the dissection. A small curved clamp is oriented perpendicular to the anticipated direction of the facial trunk to elevate tissues layer by layer. Scissors are never used for dissection down to the nerve, and no tissue is cut in this area until the nerve is seen. The tissue will separate with blunt dissection and traction before the nerve will tear, and this technique will prevent the surgeon from ever inadvertently cutting the facial nerve. Blunt dissection proceeds posterior to anterior until the surgeon identifies the nerve as a white cord 2–3 mm wide. The nerve is striking once

it is identified, and it will not be confused with other structures in the vicinity. Further mobilization is performed by separating gland from the nerve, proceeding anteriorly; often the assistant will notice some twitching of the face during this separation
- The only troublesome vessel in this area is the posterior auricular artery
- The posterior auricular artery travels posteriorly along the digastric muscle after it arises from the external carotid artery or, more rarely, the occipital artery. It usually lies inferior to the facial nerve trunk, but it may overlie it before sending branches to the mastoid and external auditory canal. The artery should not be divided until the facial nerve is identified. After identification of the trunk and during mobilization of the inferior parotid gland, the artery is ligated to prevent later hemorrhage.

Removal of the Superficial Gland

- The gland is separated at its edge, the temporal or marginal branches being followed to the periphery. Posteriorly superficial temporal vein and inferiorly posterior facial vein will be encountoured. The marginal branch usually passes directly anterior to posterior facial vein and the anterior facial vein. The cervical branch may be superficial or deep or have branches on both sides of this vein. The vein should be carefully ligated after identification and preservation of these branches
- The dissection progresses from posterior to anterior and either superiorly or inferiorly until the superficial gland has been completely separated from the facial nerve and the deep parotid gland. It may be necessary to dissect along the tumor capsule to separate it from the deep gland and facial nerve.
- The parotid duct is then divided and ligated.

Deep Parotidectomy

- The essence of deep parotidectomy is vascular control. The intraglandular segments of the external carotid artery and deep veins are ligated and divided. The superficial temporal artery and vein are ligated at the superior periphery of the gland

- The external carotid artery is isolated superior to the digastrics muscle before it enters the inferior surface of the gland. The surgeon may need to divide the digastric and stylohyoid musculature to gain adequate access. The transverse facial artery is divided at the superior anterior periphery of the gland
- After control of the intraglandular vessels is obtained, the facial nerve trunk and branches are mobilized off of the underlying tumor
- The gland is separated from the temporomandibular joint, bony ear canal, condyle of the mandible, and styloglossus and stylopharyngeus muscles
- The internal maxillary artery and adjacent veins will be encountered at the posterior mandibular ramus and need to be ligated and divided. The gland is now easily mobilized from superior to inferior and delivered from beneath the facial nerve trunk and inferior facial nerve division into the neck. The deep portion of the gland adjacent to the parapharyngeal space is mobilized with blunt dissection.

Total Parotidectomy with Facial Nerve Sacrifice

- In general, if facial nerve function is normal preoperatively, even in patients with malignancy, then the nerve can be preserved with careful dissection of the tumor off the nerve sheath. If the nerve is paretic or fully paralyzed preoperatively, then it is involved with tumor and is normally resected during tumor resection
- Nerve that is clearly invaded by high-grade malignant tumor should be resected with the specimen to negative proximal and distal margins. This may necessitate sacrificing peripheral branches, divisions, or even the main trunk of the facial nerve
- Intraoperatively, a nerve that is infiltrated with tumor will appear swollen and usually darker than the normal glistening white appearance of normal facial nerve

- After negative proximal and distal facial nerve margins are obtained, the nerve is reconstructed with primary neurorraphy or grafting. Mastoidectomy and nerve mobilization may be necessary to attain proper length of the facial nerve for tension-free anastomosis. Appropriate grafts include the ipsilateral greater auricular nerve if it is not involved with tumor or an ipsilateral sural nerve graft. The graft should be harvested with meticulous technique, freshened, and approximated without tension or redundancy with minimal use of well-placed 9-0 nylon sutures. If the proximal facial nerve is not suitable for grafting, peripheral branches can be grafted to the ipsilateral hypoglossal nerve by placement of an interpositional jump graft to preserve facial tone
- The surgeon may elect to perform additional procedures after resection of the facial nerve. The upper eyelid may be managed by placement of a gold-weight or temporary lateral tarsorrhaphy, the brow may be elevated with direct browlift, and the lower lid may be suspended with lateral canthoplasty and lid shortening
- Management of the lower face with suspension may be performed primarily or secondarily based on the surgeon's and the patient's expectations for facial nerve recovery
- The surgeon should be cautious in performing temporalis transfer after total parotidectomy because the deep and superficial temporalis vasculature has been compromised by division of the external carotid contributions.

Resection of Adjacent Structures and Reconstruction

- The goal is total tumor removal with negative margins. The operation may be extended to involve resection of adjacent structures that are involved with tumor. It may include lateral or subtotal temporal bone resection, partial mandibular resection, resection of the overlying skin, resection of portions or the entire auditory canal, and resection of surrounding musculature

- After complete removal of the parotid gland, the patient is left with a significant cosmetic defect. If the operation included resection of the facial nerve or adjacent structures, the patient may be left with a significant cosmetic or functional defect. Reconstruction of these defects depends on the patient's desires, age, additional treatment plans, and expected outcomes and on many other factors. In short, it is highly individualized to the patient
- Options for reconstruction include primary closure, dermal fat grafting, muscle transposition with locoregional flaps of the sternocleidomastoid or pectoralis muscles, and microvascular cutaneous, musculocutaneous, and innervated muscular flaps. Again, the reconstruction will be guided by the functional and aesthetic goals of the surgeon and patient.

Surgical Approach for Removal of Submandibular Gland

- Extraoral incision of 5 cm is made, which is parallel to the course of digastric muscle, platysma muscle is sectioned
- First structure encountered is facial vein, which is ligated and cut
- At the level of deep fascia, cervical ramus of 7th cranial nerve is encountered and is retracted posteriorly
- Blunt dissection between the pulley of digastric muscle and the gland will free anterior and inferior portions of the gland
- Dissection is continued around postero-inferior pole leaving superior and medial portions of gland attached
- Vital structures to be considered at this point are facial artery, lingual nerve and submandibular duct
- Facial artery can be located by prevascular and retrovascular lymph nodes, double ligate the artery
- Gland is then retracted posteriorly and detached from submandibular ganglionic connection
- Submandibular duct is noted passing superiorly and anteriorly over roof of mylohyoid muscle

- This muscle retracted anteriorly, the duct retracted posteriorly
- The gland may then be removed.

Excision of a Sublingual Gland Malignant Neoplasm

- The treatment of a malignant tumor of the sublingual gland usually includes the removal of the gland with a surrounding cuff of normal tissue (floor of mouth and lateral aspect of the oral tongue). This is due to the fact that the sublingual gland lies directly beneath the mucosal surface of the anterior floor of the mouth, and close to the inner aspect of the mandible. The development of a soft tissue cuff around a malignant tumor confined to the sublingual gland without extraglandular extension can be accomplished through excision of the mucosa (floor of mouth and small segment of tongue), the mylohyoid muscle, and the periosteum of the mandible. A careful bimanual palpation of the floor of the mouth and submental region with the patient under general anesthesia will often reveal its depth as well as its relationship to the surrounding structures. Although a ductoplasty may permit removal of small benign tumors through the oral cavity, most salivary gland cancers arising in the floor of the mouth are done in concert with at least level I neck dissection, thus removing the submandibular gland. More advanced or recurrent cancer of the sublingual gland is likely to require resection of the floor of the mouth along with a partial glossectomy, mandibulectomy, supraomohyoid structures, and the lingual and hypoglossal nerves
- The surgical techniques for resection of cancers of the sublingual glands do not differ significantly from those for removal of a floor of mouth squamous carcinoma

  Excision of sublingual gland cancer in association with the floor of the mouth and marginal mandibulectomy in continuity with neck dissection (Pull-through operation)

- Excision of moderately advanced sublingual malignant tumors usually implies in a wide exposure for access to the primary tumor and its satisfactory resection

- A lower cheek flap approach may be indicated depending on the extension of the primary tumor, particularly if a mandibulectomy (marginal or segmental) is needed. The lower cheek flap approach involves splitting the lower lip and the chin in the midline through its full thickness up to the symphysis of the mandible. The incision continues in the midline up to the thyrohyoid membrane, where it turns toward the ipsilateral neck along an upper skin crease
- This transverse component of the incision should be, at least, two fingerbreadths below the body of the mandible to prevent inadvertent injury to the mandibular branch of the facial nerve during elevation of the cheek flap
- The operative procedure planned for a moderately advanced sublingual gland cancer consists of ipsilateral neck dissection (extent of the procedure depends on the presence or absence of lymph node metastases) with resection of the sublingual gland and surrounding tissues (floor of mouth and lateral aspect of the tongue), usually in association with a marginal resection of the mandible
- The neck dissection is completed in the usual fashion except for level I, through which the specimen is attached to the primary tumor. All the attachments of the specimen inferior and deep to the digastric tendon are divided at this point. The upper neck flap is already elevated, with careful identification and preservation of the mandibular branch of the facial nerve.

Complications of Surgery

Intraoral approach
- Damage to lingual nerve
- Damage to Wharton's duct.

Extraoral approach
- Facial paralysis
- Auriculotemporal or Frey's syndrome
- Numbness of ear secondary to severance of greater auricular nerve.

Frey's Syndrome
- It is a condition in which sweating and flushing occurs in the area of skin supplied by auriculotemporal nerve
- Caused by stimulus to secretion of saliva.

Etiology
- Surgery of parotid gland and TMJ
- Injuries to this area of face.

Pathogenesis
Postganglionic parasympathetic fibers from otic ganglion become united to sympathetic fibers arising from superior cervical ganglion.

Clinical Features
- Pain in the auriculotemporal nerve distribution
- Associated gustatory sweating and erythema
- Flushing on the affected side of the face.

Investigations
- Positive minor starch iodine test
- Treatment options
- Antiperspirants and anticholinergics
- Radiation therapy
- Surgical procedures like auriculotemporal nerve section, tympanic neurectomy.

CLINICAL CASE PRESENTATION

Chief Complaint
A 63-year-old male patient reported to our department with a chief complaint of painless swelling in the left upper lateral part of the neck since 20 years (Figs 28.16 and 28.17).

History of Presenting Illness
Patient noticed a small swelling in the left sub-mandibular region which appeared insidiously, initially swelling started as small pea-nut sized asymptomatic swelling which was slowly growing in size without any symptoms such as difficulty in swallowing or turning his head. He gives no history of trauma, weight loss; night sweats, persistent cough, or increase in size prior to having food.

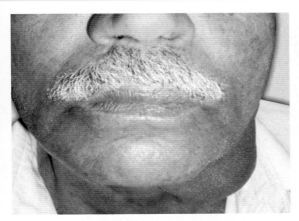

Fig. 28.16: Swelling in submandibular region: Front view

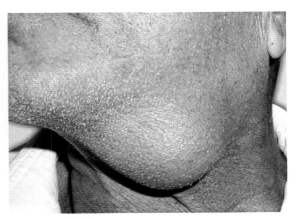

Fig. 28.17: Swelling in submandibular region: Lateral view

Past Medical and Drug History

Patient gives no history of major illness, hospitalization, prolonged medication. No h/o reported drug allergies.

Past Dental History

He had visited dentist 4 months back for extraction of carious teeth and the procedure was uneventful

Personal History

Chewing pan since 20 years .

General Examination

- Normal vital signs, with no Pallor, icterus, cyanosis, clubbing, and edema noted
- No other abnormal swelling noticed elsewhere in the body.

Extraoral Examination

- Gross Facial asymmetry due to the presence of a solitary diffuse swelling in the left submandibular region
- Left submandibular lymph nodes were not palpable due to the swelling.

Examination of the Swelling

- Solitary well defined swelling in the left upper 1/3 of the neck, predominantly in

the submandibular region measuring 3 cm (superoinferiorly) × 4 cm (anteroposteriorly), extending
- Superior: Mandibular lower border
- Inferior: 3 cm below lower mandibular border
- Anterior: 3 cm posterior to the symphysis
- Posterior: 1 cm anterior to the Left angle of mandible
- The skin over the swelling appeared normal in color, without any secondary changes
- Palpation: There was no local rise in temperature nor the swelling is tender, surface is smooth with well defined borders
- The swelling was movable, without any areas of fluctuation and it was firm in consistency, it does not move with swallowing or during coughing.

Intraoral Soft Tissue Examination

- Normal mouth opening
- Normal oral mucosa—no other lesions noted intraorally
- No intraoral extensions of the swelling noted
- Normal buccal and lingual vestibules
- Normal salivary flow
- Generalized inflammation of the gingiva.

Provisional Diagnosis

Benign adenoma of submandibular gland.

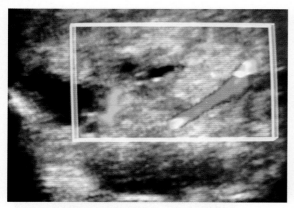

Fig. 28.18: Ultrasound color Doppler showing peripheral and central increase in vascularity

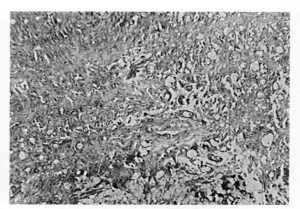

Fig. 28.19: Histopathological picture

Investigations

- Conventional radiographs
- Ultrasonography
- Incisional biopsy.

Conventional radiographs

Mandibular occlusal view: No calcifications noted in the region of the left submandibular gland

Panoramic: No osseous changes in the mandible noted.

Ultrasonography

- Showed a huge heterogeneous mass within the submandibular gland was noted, with well defined margins and internal echoes. Areas of anechoic, and hyperechoic fallowed by posterior attenuation was noted
- Color Doppler showed peripheral and central increase in vascularity (Fig. 28.18).

Histopathological Examination

Microscopy: Showed the presence of epithelial and mesenchymal components, the epithelial cells were in clusters having round-oval nucleus. They were surrounded by coarse mesenchymal fibrils. The section was suggestive of pleomorphic adenoma.

Impression: Suggestive of pleomorphic adenoma of the submandibular salivary gland.

Immediate treatment done: Left submandibular gland excision under GA.

Confirmed diagnosis: Pleomorphic adenoma of the submandibular salivary gland (Fig. 28.19).

SOME MORE CASES

Figures 28.20 to 28.27, 28.28 to 28.32, 28.33 to 28.36, and 28.37 to 28.40 depict four different clinical cases of lesions at submandibular regions. Their complete surgical management is shown in the figures.

CASES 1

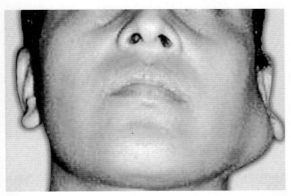

Fig. 28.20: Extraoral swelling note raised pinna

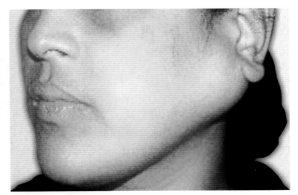

Fig. 28.21: Extraoral swelling in parotid region

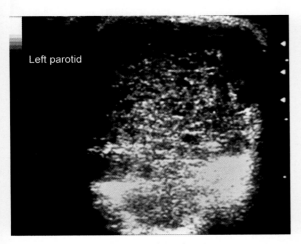

Left parotid

Fig. 28.22: USG of lesion

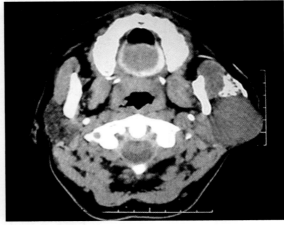

Fig. 28.23: CT plain showing the lesion

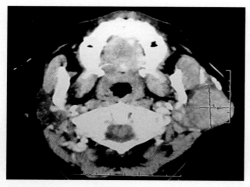

Fig. 28.24: CT contrast showing dimensions of the lesion

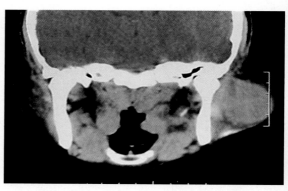

Fig. 28.25: CT plain showing the lesion

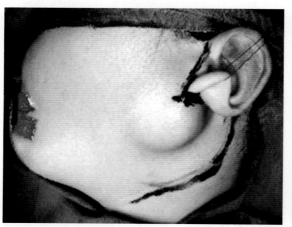

Fig. 28.26: Intraoperative marking of the lesion

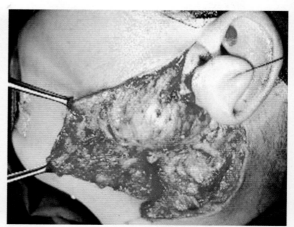

Fig. 28.27: Exposure of the lesion

Case 2

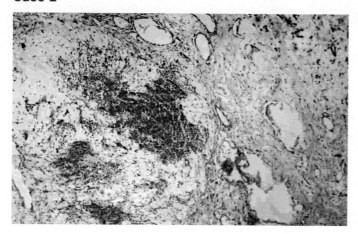

Fig. 28.28: Histopathological picture

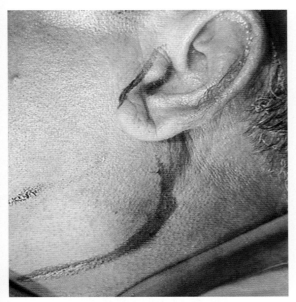

Fig. 28.29: Extraoral view showing swelling

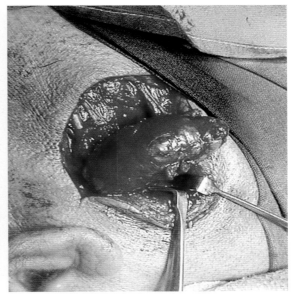

Fig. 28.30: Intraoperative exposure of lesion

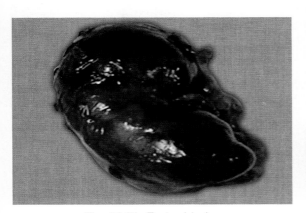

Fig. 28.31: Excised lesion

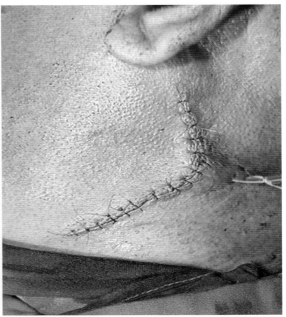

Fig. 28.32: Closed and suturing with drain *in situ*

Case 3

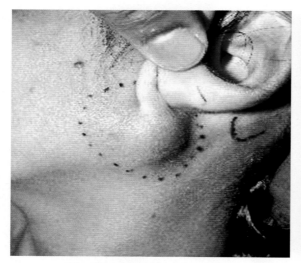

Fig. 28.33: Marking of a lesion

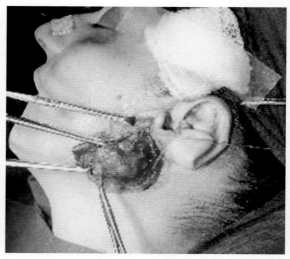

Fig. 28.34: Exposure of lesion

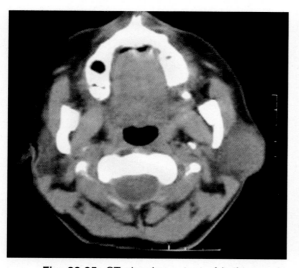

Fig. 28.35: CT showing extent of lesion

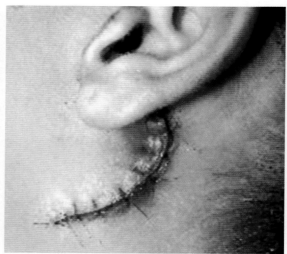

Fig. 28.36: Closure and suturing

Case 4

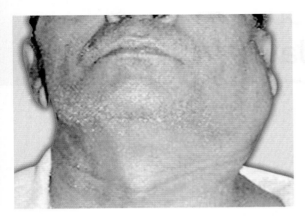

Fig. 28.37: Frontal view showing swelling

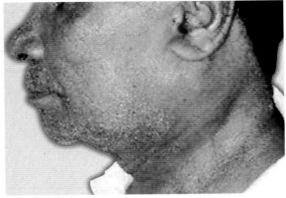

Fig. 28.38: Note the raised earlobe

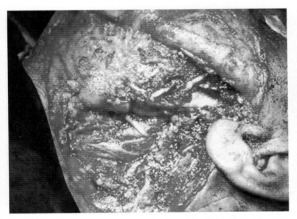

Fig. 28.39: Exposed lesion note the branches of facial nerve

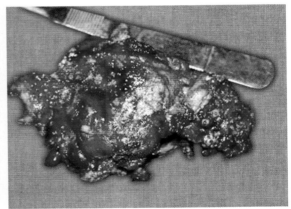

Fig. 28.40: Excised lesion (*Courtesy* for Figures 28.16 to 28.40: Dr R Prasad)

Fibro-osseous Lesions of Jaws

29

INTRODUCTION

Fibro-osseous lesions are a poorly defined group of lesions affecting the jaws and craniofacial bones. All are characterized by the replacement of bone by cellular fibrous tissue containing foci of mineralization that vary in amount and appearance. Benign fibro-osseous lesions are a collection of nonneoplastic intraosseous lesions that replace normal bone and consist of a cellular fibrous connective tissue within which nonfunctional osseous structures forms.

The group includes developmental and reactive or dysplastic lesions as well as neoplasm.

DEFINITION

Fibrous dysplasia of craniofacial bones is a benign non-neoplastic intermedullary cellular proliferation of fibroblasts with formation of irregular trabeculae of bone or ovoid calcification with indistinct encapsulated borders.

CLASSIFICATION

According to World Health Organization (WHO) classification the concept of a spectrum of clinicopathological entities in which the diagnosis can only be made on the basis of a full consideration of clinical, histological, and radiological features

WHO 2005 classification of these lesions are as follows:

Fibrous dysplasias
Monostotic fibrous dysplasia
Polyostotic fibrous dysplasia
Craniofacial fibrous dysplasia
Osseous dysplasias
Periapical osseous dysplasia
Focal osseous dysplasia
Florid osseous dysplasia
Familial gigantiform cementoma
Ossifying fibroma
Conventional ossifying fibroma
Juvenile trabecular ossifying fibroma
Juvenile psammomatoid ossifying fibroma

FIBROUS DYSPLASIA

An asymptomatic regional alteration of bone in which the normal architecture is replaced by fibrous tissues and non-functional trabeculae like osseous structures; lesions may be monostotic or polyostotic, with or without associated endocrine disturbances.

Authorities have suggested five main clinical subtypes.
1. Monostotic
2. Polyostotic
3. Polyostotic with pigmentation (Jaffe)

4. Polyostotic with pigmentation and endocrine dysfunctions (McCune -Albright)
5. Craniofacial fibrous dysplasia.

Etiology

- Fibrous dysplasia represent a non-neoplastic hamartomatous growth resulting from deranged mesenchymal activity due to osseous maturation arrest, osseous metaplasia and trauma
- Fibrous dysplasia is considered to be a developmental hamartomatous fibro-osseous disease of unknown etiology
- It may represent developmental arrest in a benign fibro-osseous proliferation that lacks the ability to fully differentiate
- Clinical severity depends upon point in time during fetal or postnatal life that the mutation of gene occurs.
  - Undifferentiated stem cells (embryologic life)—Jaffe-Lichtenstein or McCune Albright syndrome
  - Skeletal progenitor cells—polyostotic fibrous dysplasia
  - Post-natal life—monostotic fibrous dysplasia.

Clinical Features

Monostotic Fibrous Dysplasia of Jaws
- Limited to single bone (Figs 29.1 and 29.2)

- 80 – 85% of cases
- Any bone of skeleton may be involved, but, lower limbs are most commonly affected, than ribs and cranial bones
- Jaws are also commonly affected
- Maxilla > mandible. Almost always buccal cortical plate is expanded
- Patient unable to call when lesion 1st noticed
- Most of times diagnosed in 2nd decade of life
- Sex : M = F
- Mandibular lesions are truly monostotic
- Maxillary lesions often involve adjacent bones such as zygoma, sphenoid, occiput so better called as craniofacial fibrous dysplasia
- Teeth involved remains firm, but displaced by bony mass
- Painless swelling in affected area, slow growth
- Swelling is non tender on palpation
- Seldom there is disturbance of function, teeth may be displaced, occlusion interfered with or failure of eruption
- The optic canal can be narrowed by fibrous dysplasia, although it seems unlikely that any associated vision loss can be relieved by orbital decompression
- Typically lesions undergo periods of activity and periods of quiescence

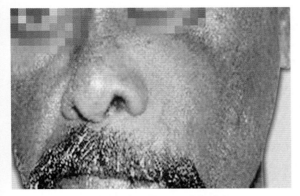

Fig. 29.1: Swelling on left side of face

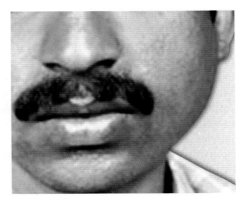

Fig. 29.2: Clinical photograph showing swelling in left molar region

- When they are active, they are often symptomatic in that the patient may perceive a throbbing or discomfort, the swelling increases, and the lesions appear hot on a bone scan and can, in fact, mimic osteomyelitis. In a quiescent phase they may be totally asymptomatic.

Polyostotic Fibrous Dysplasia

- Involvement of two or more bones
- Relatively uncommon
- Bone involved varies from few to 75% of skeleton
- It is recognized earlier than monovariant
- Lesion occurs in bone of one limb (particularly lower)
- When upper limbs are affected, there may be one or more skull lesions as well
- Disease manifests by bowing, thickening of long bones
- Symptoms related to long bone lesions are pathologic fracture and leg length discrepancy as a result of involvement of upper portion of femur causing hockey stick deformity
- Facial asymmetry
- Polyostotic fibrous dysplasia and café au lait pigmentation is seen in Jaffe-Lichtenstein syndrome
- Polyostotic fibrous dysplasia, café au lait pigmentation and multiple endocrinopathies are characteristic features of McCune Albright syndrome (sexual precocity, pituitary adenomas or hypothyroidism)
- Café au lait pigmentation are well defined, generally unilateral tan macule on trunk and thighs. These may be congenital, and margins are typically irregular like a coast line
- Sexual precocity most common manifestation and manifest as menstrual bleeding during first few months of life. Others being accelerated skeltal growth, hyperthyroidism, hyper- parathyroidism, diabetes mellitus, gynecomastia
- It should be noted that fibrous dysplasia affecting the jaws and craniofacial bones may differ in two important ways from lesions affecting the axial skeleton
- First, head and neck lesions are diffuse and poorly demarcated, while axial lesions may be

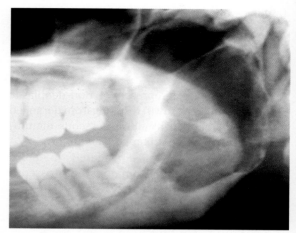

Fig. 29.3: OPG showing unilocular radiolucency involving ramus

more radiolucent and well circumscribed with a corticated outline
- Secondly, head and neck lesions, particularly when mature, may contain lamellar bone, but this is not described in other bones.

Radiological Features

- In earlier stages radiolucent/mottled appearance is seen (Fig. 29.3)
- Fine ground glass opacification, resulting from super imposition of a myriad of poorly calcified trabeculae, in a disorganized pattern
- Lesions not well demarcated
- A very characteristic pattern resembling orange peel is seen in the intra oral films of those areas that show the ground glass appearance in ordinary extra oral radiographs
- Narrowing of periodontal ligament spaces.
- In maxilla sinus floor is displaced superiorly, increased density of skull involving the occiput, sphenoid, roof of orbit and frontal bone.

Histopathologic Features

- No distinguishing histological features between the three types of fibrous dysplasia
- The normal bone is replaced by cellular fibrous tissue composed of spindled fibroblasts in a moderate amount of collagen

- This contains fine branching, irregularly shaped, curvilinear trabeculae of woven bone (immature), not connected to each other with little evidence of osteoblasts rimming, which have been linked to Chinese script writing
- The fibrous tissue has a monotonous cellularity and the fine pattern of bony trabeculae is repeated throughout the entire lesion. Rather than being a haphazard mixture of woven bone lamellar bone and spheroid particles
- Spherical, cementicle or psammomatoid calcifications may be seen in a minority of lesions, but they are never prominent
- In older or mature lesions there may be lamellar bone with mature trabeculae arranged in elongated parallel arrays
- A characteristic feature of fibrous dysplasia that may help distinguish it from ossifying fibroma is that the lesional bone merges imperceptibly with adjacent cancellous bone or with the overlying cortex
- Most often, however, the pathologist is faced with curetted fragments making distinction from other fibro-osseous lesions impossible. Only correlation with clinical and radiographic information can lead to a final diagnosis
- Some of the earlier literature dealing with this disease suggested that it represents a permanent maturation arrest in the woven bone stage and proposed that lesions demonstrating lamellar bone transformation should not be diagnosed as fibrous dysplasia
- However it is generally well accepted now, that lesions of fibrous dysplasia of the jaws, especially the craniofacial type will mature over a period of time and lesional tissue may show lamellar bone
- The presence of lamellar bone and osteoblastic rimming does not exclude the diagnosis of fibrous dysplasia, as would be the case for lesion occurring outside maxillofacial bone
- In an ideal biopsy the margins of the lesion and the overall pattern may be clearly apparent, allowing some confidence in a histological diagnosis.

Differential Diagnosis

- Primarily from ossifying fibroma
- Paget's disease share some features but occurs in much older age group, has bilateral distribution and alkaline phosphatse levels are elevated
- Chronic osteomyelitis may mimic mottled radiographic appearance of fibrous dysplasia. But along with it, inflammation, pain and purulent discharge are also seen.

Treatment and Prognosis

- Treatment is pursued only when lesions are cosmetically unacceptable or interfere with sight, breathing, mastication or speech
- Following growth, fibrous dysplasia slows after onset of puberty. So for smaller lesions no treatment is needed
- For larger disfiguring ones cosmetic and functional correction and osseous recontouring.
- About 25–50% of patients after surgery may experience regrowth
- Some clinicians believe, cosmetic surgical osteoplasty will accelerate it from an indolent to an aggressive course
- It is of utmost important to biopsy the lesion, as other more serious disease may have similar pictures
- Most lesions of monostotic type do not require treatment untill the patient has reached early adulthood
- Lesions should not be treated by radiotherapy in an attempt to halt growth, because the risk of malignancy in later life is greatly enhanced
- In case of polyostotic fibrous dysplasia, it is impossible to treat all lesions and remove all pigmentation in patients with McCune Albright syndrome
- Surgical management is directed towards alleviating functional disturbances
- Malignant transformation is rare in less than 1% of cases.

OSSEOUS DYSPLASIAS (OD)

- Benign fibro-osseous lesions of the jaws closely associated with the apices of teeth and containing amorphous spherical calcifications thought to resemble an aberrant form of cementum: lesions are usually without signs and symptoms
- Most commonly encountered fibro-osseous lesions
- Represent a spectrum of lesions, probably reactive in nature, which only differ by their clinical presentation and radiological appearances
- All types affect the tooth-bearing areas of the jaws and appear to arise from the periodontal ligament and form cementum, or cementum-like tissue
- Shares many pathologic features similarity with fibrous dysplasia and ossifying fibroma
- For unknown reasons they all have a predilection for black females
- In the third to fifth decades, where the prevalence may be as high as 6%
- It is likely that these categories may represent variants/spectrum of same pathologic processes.

Based on clinical and radiologic features types of osseous dysplasia are
Periapical cemento-osseous dysplasia
Focal cemento-osseous dysplasia
Florid cemento-osseous dysplasia
Familial gigantiform cementoma

Periapical Osseous Dysplasia

- Also known as cementoma, fibrocementoma, sclerosing cementoma, periapical osteofibrosis, or periapical fibro-osteoma
- A non-neoplastic lesion affecting the periapical tissues of one or more teeth and with histologic features similar to those of cementossifying fibroma group but with out a sharply defined margin

- Believed to be a reactive fibro-osseous lesion derived from odontogenic cells in the periodontal ligament
- Periapical region
- In the anterior mandible asymptomatic condition
- Solitary or as multiple radiolucent lesions at the apices of the lower incisor teeth, which remain vital.

Clinical Features

- Correlate with the maturity of the lesion
- Three stage process—osteolytic, cementoblastic and maturation
- Early in a lesion's course, an enlarging mass of fibrous tissue replaces periapical bone
- The fibrous tissue usually retains continuity with the periodontal ligament tissue
- Later, small round or ovoid calcifications form within the fibrous mass near the involved root surface. These depositions are composed of bone, cementum, or a nondescript "cementum-like bone."

> The radiographic features are diagnostic hence biopsy of these lesions are not done.

Focal Osseous Dysplasia

- A solitary lesion in the posterior jaws, most often the mandible
- Usually at the site of a previous tooth extraction
- Occasionally they may be found at the apices of a molar tooth
- Asymptomatic, painless, well-circumscribed lesions that may be radiolucent or have variable amounts of opacity
- Rarely exceed 2 cm in diameter and they are most probably reactive in nature
- Radiographically completely radiolucent to dense radio opaque with a thin rim of peripheral radiolucency
- Lesions tend to be well defined, but borders are slightly irregular.

Florid Osseous Dysplasia

- Usually affects both sides of the jaw in a symmetrical manner, usually the mandible but all four quadrants may be affected
- Patients may complain of dull pain, alveolar sinus tract may be present, exposing yellowish avascular bone to oral cavity.

Histopathologic Features (Fig. 29.4)

- All three patterns exhibit similar histopathologic features
- Pictures correlate well with radio appearances
- Tissue consists of fragments of cellular mesenchymal tissues composed of spindle shaped fibroblasts and collagen fibers with numerous small blood vessels
- Free hemorrhage is typically noted interspread throughout
- Within fibrous connective tissue background, mixture of woven bone, lamellar bone and cementum like particles are seen
- The proportion of each mineralized material varies from lesion to lesion, and from area to area
- As the lesion matures, it becomes more sclerotic. The ratio of fibrous connective tissue to mineralized material decreases
- With maturation, the bone trabeculae become thick curvilinear structures, said to resemble shape of ginger roots
- With progression to final radio opaque stage, individual trabeculae fuses and forms large lobular masses composed of sheets or fused globules of relatively acellular and disorganized cemento-osseous matter
- Slootweg considered a sharply defined margin, the only distinguishing feature between conventional ossifying fibroma and focal cemento-osseous dysplasia
- The areas of dense bone have reduced vascularity and so are less able to cope with the usual transient infections
- On occasion after patients become edentulous some of dense sclerotic bone nodules break

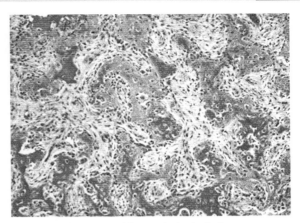

Fig. 29.4: Histopathological view

through the surface, because they do not resorb at the same rate as normal vascularized alveolar bone.

Treatment and Prognosis

A correct diagnosis after radio clinical examination, establishing the diagnosis will exclude any treatment and surgical intervention.

- Regular follow up is only required
- Complication may arise in later stages owing to avascularity, so proper oral health care must be maintained to avoid any pocket formation, extraction.

Familial Gigantiform Cementoma

- Similar in presentation to florid osseous dysplasia but it has a familial basis
- Disorder of gnathic bone that ultimately leads to the formation of massive sclerotic masses of disorganized mineralized material
- An autosomal dominant disorder, with variable expressivity
- Few genuine cases have been recorded, it appears not to have any gender or racial predilections, and it presents at a younger age, often becoming apparent in childhood
- Patients begin to develop radiographic alterations during 1st decade

- Lesions may grow rapidly and result in facial deformity, a feature that is rare in florid osseous dysplasia
- Osseous pathoses is limited to jaws, with multifocal involvement of both jaws
- If not treated osseous enlargement ceases by 5th decade
- Radiologically, initial features resemble those seen in cemento-osseous dysplasias appearing as multiple radiolucencies in periapical areas with progression affected sites expand to involve much of normal bone, developing a mixed radio pattern
- Affected bones are very sensitive to inflammatory stimuli and become necrotic with slightest provocation.

OSSIFYING FIBROMA (FIGS 29.5 TO 29.8)

- The most widely used term was cemento-ossifying fibroma
- This was coined on the basis that most lesions may be associated with the teeth or may contain cementum-like spherical calcifications
- A benign osteogenic, well demarcated neoplasm composed of calcified material and a fibroblastic stroma, which may be very cellular
- Various terms have been used from time-to-time like when bone predominates in a particular lesion, it is ossifying fibroma. Curved/linear trabeculae or spheroidal like calcifications are seen in cementifying fibroma
- However, lesions not associated with the jaws, particularly in the sinonasal regions frequently contain these types of calcifications and it is now recognized that cementum and bone are essentially the same tissue
- Ossifying fibroma is a true neoplasm with significant growth potential
- Can resemble focal COD histologically
- True lesions relatively rare, previous reported examples actually being focal COD
- Composed of fibrous tissues that contain variable mixture of bony trabeculae, cementum-like spherules or both
- Origin has been suggested to be odontogenic or from PDL but identical lesions have been reported in orbital, frontal, ethmoid, temporal bones, so making it still a debatable question
- In many respects it may be regarded as a type of osteoblastoma and in some cases the histological distinction from osteoblastoma may be difficult
- However, within the spectrum of these lesions, a variant was recognized that most often occurs in young people and may be rapidly growing and aggressive
- In 1992 WHO classification this was called 'juvenile (aggressive) ossifying fibroma'.

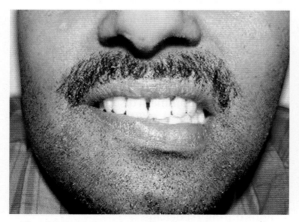

Fig. 29.5: Extraoral swelling in right molar region

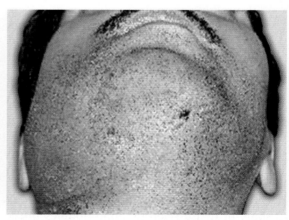

Fig. 29.6: Previous surgical mark and marked swelling

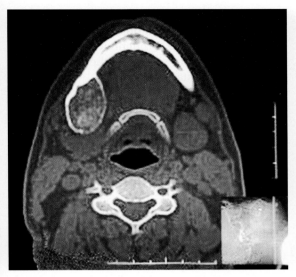

Fig. 29.7: Expansion of cortex and thinned margins

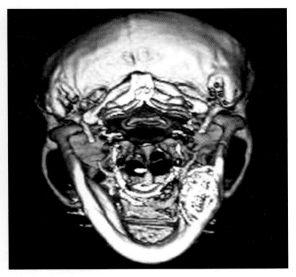

Fig. 29.8: 3-D CT showing expansion of lingual cortex

Subsequently, two histologically distinct lesions have become known under this term.
- The original 'WHO-type' lesion with trabecular calcifications and
- A lesion most often associated with the sinonasal regions with spherical or psammomatoid calcifications
- Both lesions are recognized as being aggressive in their behaviour in that they may grow to large sizes, permeate the bones and recur
- It should be noted that extraosseous or peripheral lesions known as peripheral ossifying fibroma (soft fibroma, peripheral fibroma with calcifications or peripheral odontogenic fibroma) is reactive in natur
- It is not the extraosseous counterpart of central ossifying fibroma.

Clinical Features
- Ossifying fibroma is found in the tooth-bearing areas of the jaws and has a slight predilection for the posterior mandible
- Small lesions are asymptomatic, detected coincidentaly

- Large lesions present as painless swelling with facial asymmetry
- Pain and paresthesia are rare.

Radiographic Features
- Because the lesion is usually slow growing, the bony cortices and covering mucosa remain intact
- Lesions continue to enlarge after cessation of normal skeletal growth, unlike monostotic fibrous dysplasia
- Occurs most often in the canine fossa and zygomatic arch area. When ossifying fibroma involves the maxillary sinus, it may completely fill the sinus cavity and expand the sinus walls
- In the mandible, ossifying fibroma frequently develops inferior to the premolars and molars
- The radiographic density of the ossifying fibroma is dependent on its stage of development
- Bone destruction that occurs early in lesion formation causes a unilocular radiolucent defect within the bone. Subsequent calcification that takes place within the lesion results in the appearance of radiopaque foci

- The radiopaque calcified areas tend to coalesce, and the lesion may become very radiopaque after several years
- The radiographic appearance may be radiolucent, radiopaque, or a mixture. Growth tends to be concentric within the medullary part of the bone, with outward expansion approximately equal in all directions. This expansion may result in osseous deformity. In such cases, the margins become thinned but remain intact
- The borders of the ossifying fibroma are usually well defined. A thin radiolucent line representing a fibrous capsule separates the mixed-density lesion from surrounding bone
- Sometimes the bone next to the lesion may develop a hyperostotic border. A thin shell of bone usually forms along the lesion
- When it grows beyond the confines of the jaw, it maintains a thin capsule of new subperiosteal cortical bone, an important feature that distinguishes it from the more destructive growth pattern of intraosseous osteosarcoma.

Histopathological Features

- At surgical exploration well demarcated from surrounding bone, permitting easy separation from bony bed
- Similar to that of fibrous dysplasia. A large number of fibroblast with flat, elongated nuclei are present within a network of interlacing collagen fibers
- The calcified component is usually a combination of bony trabeculae and strongly basophilic cementum like structures with variable osteoblastic rimming
- Osteoclast like giant cells and occasional aneurysm bone cavity components characterized by sinusoid blood space may be present
- The lesion is composed of cellular fibrous tissues containing spindled fibroblasts, often with a storiform appearance
- The bone is deposited in a variable pattern. There may be irregular thin trabeculae of woven bone, sometimes rimmed by osteoblasts but often apparently emerging directly from the fibrous tissue

- A common feature is the presence of "Chinese character" shaped islands of bone or calcification distributed throughout the connective tissue, somewhat similar to the trabeculae in fibrous dysplasia
- Histologic appearance may be indistinguishable from fibrous dysplasia, the lesion itself is encapsulated and behaves as a neoplasm
- Peripheral osteoblastic rimming is usually present
- The spherules of cementum-like material often demonstrate peripheral brush border that blend into adjacent connective tissues
- Intralesional hemorrhage is unusual
- Microscopically, the ossifying fibroma and cementifying fibroma are very similar. However, the cementifying fibroma has a greater tendency to form more cementum-like material that is more ovoid and more heavily calcified than that produced by the ossifying fibroma
- In the ossifying fibroma, the calcified material is more spiculated and reminiscent of woven bone, with that at the periphery being more lamellar in appearance.

A key feature of ossifying fibroma that distinguishes it from fibrous dysplasia is the pattern of mineralization, in ossifying fibroma it varies from place to place within the lesion, whereas in fibrous dysplasia, the pattern tends to be uniform throughout the lesion.

JUVENILE OSSIFYING FIBROMA

- An actively growing lesion consisting of a cell rich fibrous stroma, containing bands of cellular osteoid without osteoblastic rimming together with trabeculae of more typical woven bone
- Controversial lesion, distinguished on basis of age of the patient, common sites of involvement, and clinical behavior
- Two different neoplasms under this term are trabecular and psammomatoid
- Malignant change in ossifying fibromas has not been reported

- Conventional ossifying fibroma occurs in the tooth-bearing areas of the jaws and may be odontogenic in origin in that it arises from tissues of the periodontal membrane
- The juvenile variants arise outside of the tooth-bearing areas, either in the jaws or the craniofacial bones in younger people and have a tendency towards aggressive behavior.

Important Feature

- Well circumscribed, slow growth, lacks continuity with adjacent bones
- The lesion can be noted even at the age of 6 months
- Both pattern with similar radiographic features and growth patterns, but trabecular pattern diagnosed initially in younger patients (Fig. 29.9A)
- Trabecular...mean age...11 years
- Psammomatoid...mean age...22 years (Fig. 29.9B)
- Both pattern in either jaw with maxillary predominance
- Discovered upon routine radiological examination but cortical expansion may result in noticeable facial enlargement
- Complications arise due to impingement on neighboring structures
- With persistent growth, sinus lesions may penetrate orbital, nasal, cranial cavities resulting in nasal blockage, proptosis, exophthalmos

- Lesions are circumscribed radiolucencies that in some cases may contain central radiopacities
- When it grows beyond the confines of the jaw, it maintains a thin capsule of new subperiosteal cortical bone, an important feature that distinguishes it from the more destructive growth pattern of intraosseous osteosarcoma
- Ossifying fibromas rarely erode or displace teeth and are generally slow growing and expansile.

Histopathological Features

- Both patterns typically non-encapsulated, but like ossifying fibroma (and unlike FD) it is well demarcated from the surrounding bone
- In both types of juvenile ossifying fibroma the appearances can vary from area to area with regard to the relative proportion of mineralized tissue or fibrous stroma
- Tumor consists of cellular fibrous connective tissue that exhibits areas that are loose and other zones that are so cellular that the cytoplasm of individual cells is hard to discern because of nuclear crowding
- Mitotic figures may be found but not numerous
- Mineralized components in both pattern is different
- Areas of hemorrhage and small clusters of multinucleated giant cells are usually seen

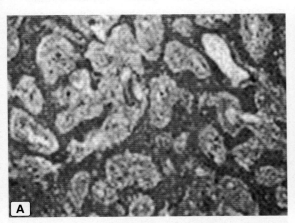 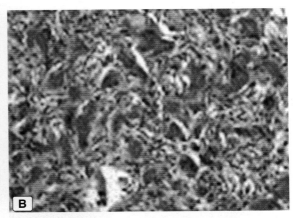

Fig. 29.9: Two ossifying fibromas of the mandible showing (A) cellular stromas with trabecular and droplet or (B) psammomatoid bone

- The trabecular variant is composed of densely cellular fibrous tissue with little collagen, containing thin strand-like trabeculae of osteoid and woven bone (Fig. 29.9)
- Osteoblasts are prominent and may be incorporated into the osteoid material. It is sometimes difficult to distinguish the cellular osteoid from the fibrous stroma
- The psammomatoid variant is also densely cellular but the calcifications are spherical or lamellated like typical psammoma bodies
- They may have a 'feathered' or 'fluffy' margin where the osteoid merges or projects into the cellular stroma—sometimes in a thorn-like pattern.

Treatment and Prognosis

- Small lesion is treated well by surgical curettage/enucleation
- In absence of a reliable diagnostic/ prognostic predictor to indicate the potential of COF for aggressive behavior or the likelihood of recurrence regular radiographic follow up shall be pursued
- Large tumors/sudden growth spurt en bloc resection is secondary definitive therapy
- If tumor is only partially removed, continued growth necessarily do not follow.

CASE NUMBER 1

A case of asymptomatic non-progressive swelling of the mandible (Figs 29.10 to 29.16).

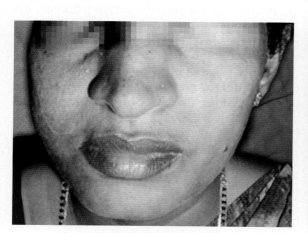

Fig. 29.10: Facial swelling: Right side

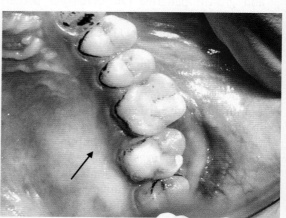

Fig. 29.11: Intraoral picture showing diffuse expansion in maxilla

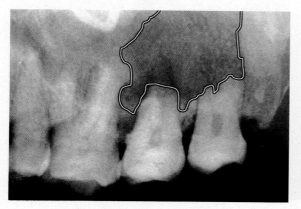

Fig. 29.12: IOPA radiograph

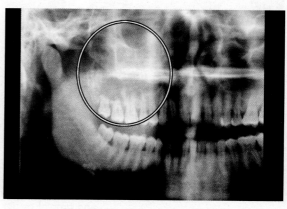

Fig. 29.13: Orthopantomogram

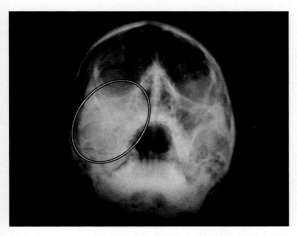

Fig. 29.14: PNS view

Forty years old female complains of swelling over the right cheek area of 7 months duration.

History of Present Illness

- Insidious onset
- Asymptomatic and nonprogressive.
- Associated with intra oral swelling over right maxillary posterior region of 4 months duration
- No history of trauma
- No history of bleeding, pus, pain or any other associated secondary or systemic changes
- No nasal complaints in the form of nasal stuffiness or bleeding from the nose.

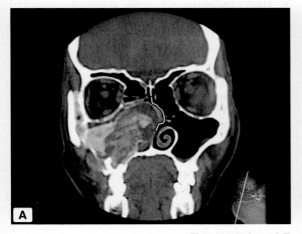
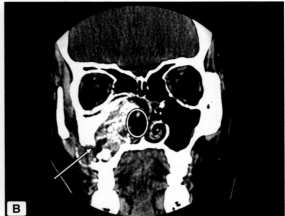

Figs 29.15A and B: CT imaging (coronal)

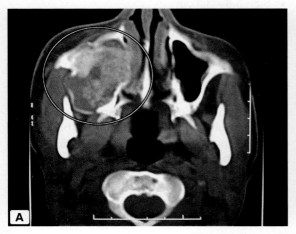
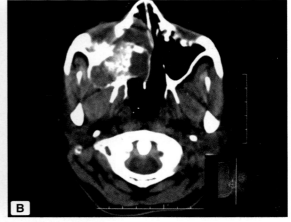

Figs 29.16A and B: CT imaging (axial)

Past Medical History

Non-contributory.

General Physical Examination

Moderately built and moderately nourished
- No signs of pallor, icterus, cyanosis, clubbing, edema
- Vital signs—within normal limits.

Head and Neck Examination

- TMJ—no clinically detectable abnormalities
- No palpable lymph nodes.

Examination of Lesion

Inspection
- Facial asymmetry—right side of lower 2/3rd the face
- Approximate size—1 × 1 inch
  Diffuse borders
  Overlying skin—normal

Palpation
Inspector finding are confirmed.

Intraoral Examination

Inspection (Fig. 29.11)
- Mouth opening—normal
- Diffuse expansion of jaw—right maxillary posterior area
- *Extensions*: Anteroposteriorly—distal of 15 to tuberosity region
- Approximate size—2.5 cm
- Buccal basal bone expansion—partial obliteration of the buccal vestibule
- Mucosa—normal
- Palatal expansion—minimal
- Mild blanching.

Palpation
- Ill defined enlargement involving the basal bone only
- Tender
- Consistency—bony hard except at buccal aspect of 17 - soft
- Grade II mobility—17.

Chairside Investigations
- Vitality test: 16,17,18 nonvital
- Aspiration of lesion: Negative.

Impression
A benign neoplasm arising from maxillary basal bone which has windowed the bone irt 17 and extended superiorly.

Differential Diagnosis

- Benign odontogenic tumors
- Benign non-odontogenic tumors
- Maxillary antral tumors.

Investigations

- Hazy radiolucency with multiple, calcified specks above the apices of roots of teeth (Fig. 29.12)
- Size: About 2.5 cm
- Periphery: Well defined
- Shape: Ill defined
- Loss of lamina dura at 17,18 and resorption of roots of 16, 17, 18 (Fig. 29.13)
- Ill defined hazy radiopacity
- Resorption of the roots of 17,18
- Haziness of the right maxillary sinus
- Non-uniform opacification
- Ill defined border
- Well defined, expansile mass lesion occluding the right maxillary sinus extending inferiorly upto the right maxillary alveolus
- *Size*: 5.6 × 3.3 cm
- Destruction of the lateral wall of the right maxillary sinus
- Evidence of specks of calcification and cystic spaces
- *Size of the lesion*: 5.2 × 4.2 cm
- Evidence of destruction of medial, anterior, lateral wall of the right maxillary sinus, (R) maxillary alveolus, middle and inferior turbinates
- Cystic spaces and calcific specks noted
- Part of the lesion shows ground glass appearance.

Impression
Ill defined expansile mass lesion in the right maxillary sinus with cystic areas and calcific specks within it.

Diagnosis

Aggressive ossifying/cementifying fibroma.

CASE NUMBER 2

Twenty-third year old female patient with a complaint of painless swelling in the left lower third of the face (Fig. 39.17 and 29.18).

History of Present Illness

- Duration of 20 years
- Mother noticed nodular swellings in the gum pads at 2 years of birth
- Painless, gradual enlargement by age 10— unilateral enlargement of left side of lower jaw
- Surgically treated at age 10 for asymmetry with moderate esthetic improvement
- Developed a painless, slow growing enlargement on the left buccal aspect of the lower jaw
- Gradually enlarged in size causing facial asymmetry—finally attaining its present proportions
- No history of discharge, ulcerations, paresthesia, interference with swallowing, jaw movements, tongue movements.

Medical, Drug, Personal History

Noncontributory.

General Physical Examination
- Moderately nourished and built
- Normal vital signs
- No other lumps and swellings in any other part of the body.

Extraoral Examination

- Facial asymmetry present
- Diffuse, swelling in left lower third of the face approximately 8 × 5 cm in size
- Borders
- Normal skin
- Non-tender
- Bony hard
- Overlying skin is pinchable. Lower border, lateral aspect expanded.

Intraoral Examination

- Partial increase of left buccal vestibular depth
- Normal mucosa
- Midline shift
- Bicortical expansion
- Non-tender
- Bony hard.

Provisional Diagnosis

Benign odontogenic tumor/cyst/bone tumor of the mandible.

Differential Diagnosis

- Ameloblastoma
- Odontogenic keratocyst
- Central giant cell granuloma
- Dentigerous cyst
- Fibrous dysplasia
- Cemento-ossifying fibroma.

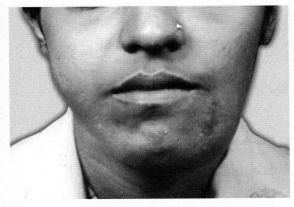

Fig. 29.17: Facial swelling and surgical scar

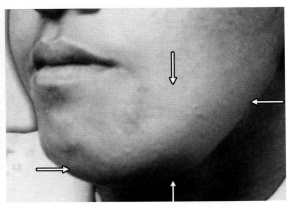

Fig. 29.18: Facial asymmetry and expansion

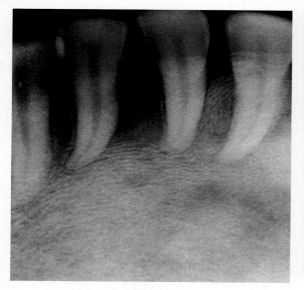

Fig. 29.19: IOPA   **Fig. 29.20:** Occlusal

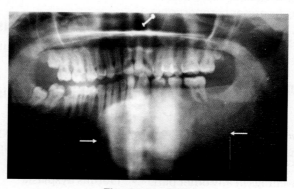

Fig. 29.21: OPG

Investigations

Radiographs

- Intraoral radiographs showing loss of normal bony architecture (Fig. 29.19)
- Occlusal showing bony expansion (Fig. 29.20).
- Panoramic showing expansion in the left para symphysis and body area (Fig. 29.21)

Differential Diagnosis

- Fibrous dysplasia
- Paget's Disease
- Hyperparathyroidism
- Diffuse sclerosing osteomyelitis
- Cemento-ossifying fibromas.

Serum Chemistry

- Serum calcium
- Serum phosphorous
- Alkaline phosphatase.

Final Diagnosis

Fibrous dysplasia.

30

Vascular Anomalies

INTRODUCTION

The term vascular lesions is used to define a variety of neoplasms or malformations originating from blood vessels or vascular structures. Although, this term is generally sufficient to describe the nature of the lesion, vascular lesions can be divided into two groups; hemangiomas and vascular malformations.

Hemangiomas are the most common vascular lesions occurring in infancy and childhood. Hemangiomas must be differentiated from vascular malformations because of the different treatment approaches and different clinical course. Hemangiomas involute over time, under the influence of hormones and angiogenesis factors. Vascular malformations are composed of mature blood vessels and do not involute over time.

More than 60 percent of vascular malformation occurs in head and neck region. Vascular malformation in head and neck region are divided into venular malformation, venous malformation, lymphatic malformation, arteriovenous malformation and mixed malformation which includes mixed venous-lymphatic malformation and mixed venous-venular malformation.

HEMANGIOMAS OF THE MAXILLOFACIAL REGION

Introduction

- Vascular tumor growing by cellular proliferation
- Most common—tumor of infancy

- Synonymous with:
  - Capillary hemangioma
  - Hypertrophic hemangioma
  - Juvenile hemangioma
  - Benign hemangioendothelioma
- Vascular anomalies have existed as a clinical entity for over 100 years
- Most common congenital deformity (Fig. 30.1)
- Tend to be most overdiagnosed but grossly undertreated conditions in the head and neck
- Endothelial cells show:
  - Very few (if any) mitotic figures
  - Very long doubling times
- Thymidine incorporation studies of hemangioma documented increased endothelial cell turnover.

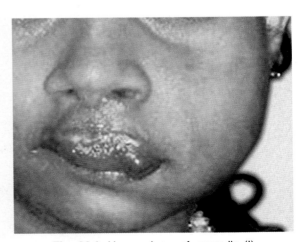

Fig. 30.1: Hemangioma of upper lip (l)

Embryology

Woolard-embryonic Vascular Development

- *Stage 1*: Primitive capillary network is formed of interlacing blood spaces differentiated from primitive mesenchyme
- *Stage 2*: Primitive capillaries coalesce into large plexiform structures
- *Stage 3*: Primitive elements then disappear and mature vascular stems appear with the capillary beds
- *Stage 4*: Focal failure of this developmental sequence with persistence of primitive vascular structures result in arteriovenous malformation.

Classification

- Clinical appearance
- Histopathological basis (Virchow and Wagner)
- Endothelial characteristics (Mulliken and Glowacki classification)
- International Society for the Study of Vascular Anomalies Classification.

Virchow (1863)

Anatomicopathological classification—based on channel architecture
- Angioma simplex—capillaries
- Angioma cavernosum—larger channels
- Angioma racemosum—markedly dilated interconnected vessels.

Mulliken and Coworkers (1982)

Biological classification (Flowchart 30.1)
- Hemangiomas: Lesions demonstrating endothelial hyperplasia
- Malformations: Normal endothelial turnover

Hemangiomas

- Superficial (capillary hemangioma)
- Deep (cavernous hemangioma)
- Compound (capillary cavernous hemangioma).

Vascular malformations
Simple lesions
• Low flow lesions
• Capillary malformation
• Venous malformation
• Lymphatic malformation
• High flow lesions
• Arterial malformation
Combined lesions
• Arteriovenous malformations
• Lymphovenous malformations
• Other combinations
Lymphatic malformations
Lymphangioma circumscriptum
Cavernous lymphangioma
Cystic hygroma

HEMANGIOMA

Clinical Presentation (Figs 30.2 to 30.6)

- Nearly 1/3 present as small macular spot
- Most appear 1-4 weeks
- Female:Male = 3:1
- Eighty percent solitary, head/face most common site
- Rapid postnatal growth and very slow involution

Flowchart 30.1: Biological classification of endothelial hyperplasia

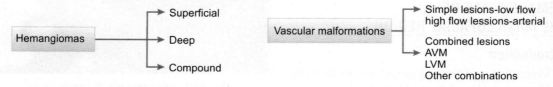

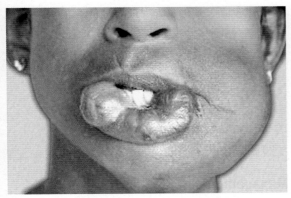

Fig. 30.2: Hemangioma of lower lip

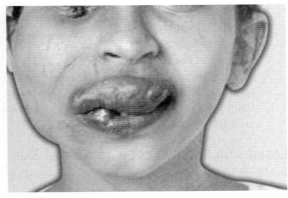

Fig. 30.3: Hemangioma of upper lip (II)
(*Courtesy:* Dr Vikram Shetty)

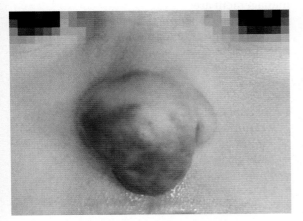

Fig. 30.4: Hemangioma at nose tip
(*Courtesy:* Dr Vikram Shetty)

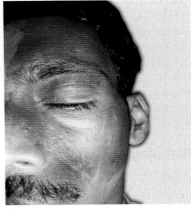

Fig. 30.5: Note the facial staining/pigmentation

- Proliferating hemangioma rarely causes bony or cartilaginous distortion or hypertrophy
- Macrotia or jaw enlargement may also occur secondary to increased blood flow (Fig. 30.2)
- May produce mass effect, i.e. depression of calvaria, shift of nasal skeleton, secondary enlargement of orbit.

Phases

- Proliferation: 1–10 months
  - Most rapid 1–4 months
  - Complications occur in this phase
  - Plump rapidly dividing endothelial cells
  - Increased mast cells—neoangiogenesis

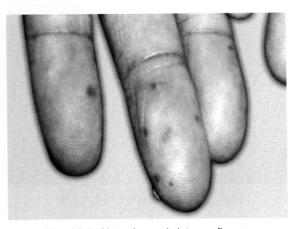

Fig. 30.6: Note tiny red dots on fingers

- Involution: After 6–10 months
  - Soften, gray surface
  - 50 percent gone by age 5
  - 90 percent gone by age 9
  - Multilamination of basement membrane
  - Interaction between mast cells and local macrophages, fibroblasts and multinucleated giant cells.

Lesions Do Not Always Leave Normal Skin

Residual atrophy, wrinkling, telangiectasias, pallor and redundant tissue are common.

Diagnosis

- Present at birth
  Yes—VM
  No—Hemangioma
- Rapid proliferation
  Yes—Hemangioma
  No—VM
- Involution
  Yes—Hemangioma
  No—VM.

Differential Diagnosis

Port-wine Stains

Present since birth and stay flat (Fig. 30.5).

Spider Angiomas

Tiny on face and hands (Fig. 30.6).

Investigations
Ultrasonography
Doppler analysis
Magnetic resonance imaging
Computerized tomography
Angiography (Figs 30.7 and 30.8).

Management

Wait and watch recommendation of the past is not always in the patient's best interest. Goals of management are:
- Preventing function threatening complications
- Preventing/reducing permanent disfigurement
- Minimizing psychosocial stress for the patient and family.

Surgical Treatment

- Surgical excision
  - Lenticular excision
  - Circular excision and purse string closure
- Embolization
- Compression therapy
- Cryosurgery
- Radiation.

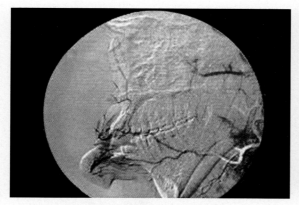

Fig. 30.7: Hemangioma of lower lip angiography

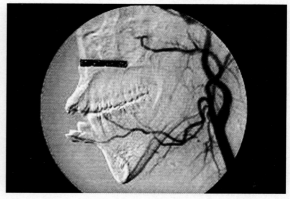

Fig. 30.8: Angiography of hemangioma of lower lip showing large tongle of vessels over the angle of mandible

Medical treatment
Steroids
Interferon 2α
Vincristine
Sclerosing agents—foam sclerotherapy
Becaplermin gel
Lasers
Beta-blockers

ROLE OF β-BLOCKERS IN MANAGEMENT OF HEMANGIOMAS

During the growth phase, two major proangiogenic factors are involved: basic fibroblast growth factor (bFGF) and vascular endothelial growth factor (VEGF). Histologic studies have shown that both endothelial and interstitial cells are actively dividing in this phase.

During the involution phase, apoptosis has been shown.

Potential explanations for the therapeutic effect of propranolol—a nonselective beta-blocker—on infantile capillary hemangiomas include vasoconstriction, which is immediately visible as a change in color, associated with a palpable softening of the hemangioma; decreased expression of VEGF and bFGF genes through the down-regulation of the RAF–mitogen-activated protein kinase pathway (which explains the progressive improvement of the hemangioma); and the triggering of apoptosis of capillary endothelial cells

Approach in Management of Hemangioma

Williams et al proposed a new treatment strategy based on
Stage of lesion
Type of lesion
Size and site of lesion
Management of residual deformity.

Proliferative Phase

Aim
- To eradicate the lesion completely
- To stunt its growth, so that by the time proliferation is complete, a small less disfiguring lesion is left.

Early proliferation
- Pulsed dye laser
- High potency topical corticosteroids (clobetasol propionate).

Late proliferation
- Potassium titanyl phosphate laser
- Nd:YAG laser
- Intralesional steroids
- Oral corticosteroids.

Involutive Phase

Aim
- To improve appearance and esthetics
- Treatment should never give a worse result than after normal involution.
  Rapid involuters—60 percent no treatment
  Slow involuters—80 percent need treatment.

Early involution
- Superficial lesions—pulsed dye laser (Fig. 30.9)
- Deep lesions—copper bromide and Nd:YAG laser (Fig. 30.10)
- Compound lesions—lasers and surgical excision.

Late involution: Management of residual deformity.

Telangiectasia
- Pulsed dye laser
- Copper bromide and Nd:YAG laser.

Fibrofatty Tissue
- Best treated by surgical excision.
- Thermoscalpel and lasers should also be considered.

Epidermal Atrophy
CO_2 laser and Er:YAG laser for skin resurfacing.

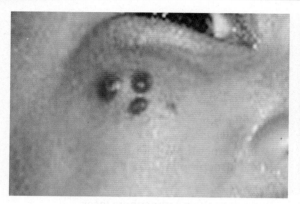

Fig. 30.9: Superficial hemangioma

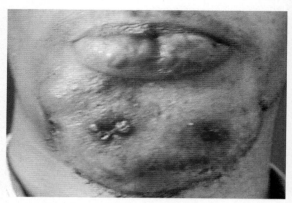

Fig. 30.10: Deep hemangioma

Complications
Ulceration (Fig. 30.11)
Infection
Visual impairment
Airway obstruction
Congestive heart failure
Kasabach-Merritt syndrome
Posterior fossa defects

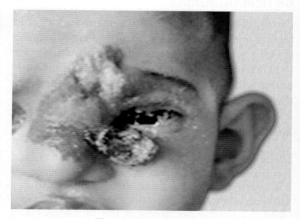

Fig. 30.11: Ulceration

- Topical antibiotics
- Barriers +/– occlusive dressings
- Oral antibiotics; analgesics
- Pulsed dye laser
- Oral prednisone (2 mg/kg).

Visual Impairment

- Oral prednisone
- Intralesional steroids
- Pulsed dye laser if early
- Elliptical surgical excision
- Referral to ophthalmology.

Airway Obstruction

- Direct laryngoscopy for stridor

- Oral prednisone and CO_2 laser
- Surgical excision.

Kasabach-Merritt Syndrome

- Severe thrombocytopenia and hemorrhage because of platelet trapping within the tumor
- Not associated with the common hemangioma of infancy
- The overlying skin is deep red-purple in colour, tense and shiny
- Ecchymosis appears over and around the tumor, and there are generalized petechiae
- Fibrinogen markedly low, fibrin split products increased, PT elevated.

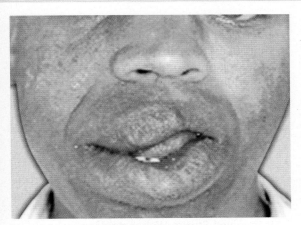

Fig. 30.12: Hemangioma of lip

Posterior Fossa Defects

PHACE
- Posterior fossa malformation
- Hemangioma (segmental) (Fig. 30.12)
- Arterial anomalies
- Cardiac anomalies
- Eye defects.

Discussion
- Natural history and appearance can distinguish vascular lesions
- Not all hemangiomas are benign
- Psychological impact should be considered
- Treatment is conservative in majority
- Future therapies will likely be directed at restoring the balance of factors of angiogenesis through the administration of angiogenesis modulators.

VASCULAR MALFORMATIONS

Introduction

The term "vascular malformation" is used to describe a group of lesions, present at birth formed by an anomaly of angiovascular or, lymphovascular structures. Vascular lesions are among the most common congenital and neonatal abnormalities with a reported 60 percent of them occur in maxillofacial region. The understanding of vascular malformation greatly facilitated by the work of Mulliken and Glowacki, who developed a biological classification of vascular anomalies encompassing clinical findings and thier behavior. Vascular malformations never involute, their early treatment is not controversial. Clinically variety of different treatment options have been proposed.

In most cases, they might require sclerotherapy, laser pharmacologic, and surgical treatment depending on their topography, type and depth. Rare extensive conditions do require multimodality. Vascular malformations are also classified according to hemodynamic features during angiography. Venous and lymphatic malformation are classified as "low-flow" lesions. Arterial, arteriovenous malformations and arteriovenous fistulas are categorized as "high-flow lesions", because the best care involves determination of slow-flow or fast-flow. Total removal is not possible in many clinical conditions, hence recurrence.
- Different and unique clinical identity
- Abnormal embryonic and fetal morphogenesis
- Vascular malformations are present at birth but may not be clinically or cosmetically significant until later in life when the abnormal vessels progressively dilate, resulting in increased vascular pigmentation, surface textural irregularities, soft tissue bulk, and/or functional problems
- Principal cell type, degree of blood flow or lymph flow important.

Pathogenesis

Thoma's Law
- Caliber of blood vessel is determined by velocity of blood flow
- Vessel length is determined by pull on vessel walls of blood flow
- Vessel thickness is determined by the blood pressure within it
- New capillaries will form in response to terminal blood pressure in regions whereas capillary size is reduced in presence of reduced pressure.

Clinical Presentation

- Present at birth and grow with the child
- Male: female ratio = 1:1
- Diagnosis not at birth usually
- Infection, hormonal changes, trauma
- Secondary effects on bone
- Color of lesion—filling nature
- Low flow lesions—nonpulsatile, no palpable thrill—capillary, lymphatic, venous, mixed
- High flow—warm, tender swelling & asymmetry present; bruit detected—arterial, arteriovenous.

Treatment

- Some superficial malformations are highly responsive to laser photocoagulation, whereas others persist despite repeated treatments
- Well-circumscribed lesions may be cured by surgical excision or sclerotherapy, but large lesions with transmural extension may be unresectable and resistant to repeated sclerosis
- High-flow lesions such as AVMs may be palliated with repeated embolization or completely cured by a combination of embolization and radical resection
- Treatment and prognosis are heavily dependent upon the type and extent of each malformation
- Extensive malformations are best evaluated by a magnetic resonance imaging (MRI) scan with contrast
- If a high-flow lesion is suspected, a simultaneous magnetic resonance angiogram (MRA) will assist the interventional radiologist in planning a diagnostic or therapeutic arteriogram.

Capillary Vascular Malformations

- Capillary vascular malformations (port-wine stains) are comprised of dilated capillaries and venules in the dermis layer, which impart a pink or purple hue to the involved skin
- Capillary hemangioma is a benign rapidly growing usually solitary lesion which occurs in the skin and mucous membrane
- It was first described as human botryomycosis by Poncet and Dor in 1897
- It is also known as pyogenic granuloma

- It is a benign capillary proliferation with a microscopically distinctive lobular structure that affects the skin and mucous membrane of nasal region or oral cavity, sometimes occurs as pedunculated or broad based and can vary in size from few mm to several cm
- Mean depth—0.46 mm
- Infancy—macular
- Capillary—angel's kiss or stork's bite
- Portwine stains—flat, pink macular—birth; raised, nodular, darken to deep red—0.3 percent
- The pigmentation often follows a dermatomal distribution, and if the V1 distribution of the face is involved Sturge-Weber syndrome should be ruled out with periodic ophthalmologic testing for glaucoma (Figs 30.13 and 30.14)
- A history of seizures is also suggestive of this syndrome, secondary to leptomeningeal involvement
- Although port-wine stains can be located anywhere on the body, facial involvement is obviously the most cosmetically and psychologically significant
- Most pediatric port-wine stains are flat and pink, but over time they may become darker and raised as the individual dermal vessels continue to dilate and engorge
- Laser is considered to be the treatment of choice, the first clinically useful laser being the continuous-wave argon laser. Its blue-green wavelength (488, 515 nm) was semiselectively absorbed by oxyhemoglobin, causing photocoagulation and blanching of the dermal vessels
- The argon laser was particularly useful for hypertrophic adult port-wine stains which are darker and thicker than pediatric stains
- Children tend to have much lighter capillary vascular malformations, and nonspecific epidermal and dermal absorption of argon light caused hypertrophic scarring
- Other continuous-wave lasers that have been useful in the treatment of adult port-wine stains include the copper vapor laser, but most of these lasers have been replaced by newer laser technology

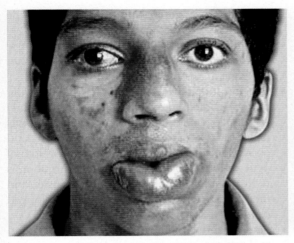

Fig. 30.13: Skin color and lip swelling

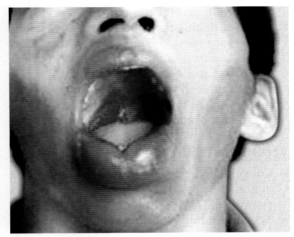

Fig. 30.14: Intraoral redness on right side of palate

- The KTP laser remains one of the last clinically useful continuous-wave lasers for the treatment of vascular lesions, but pulsed laser technology is well accepted as the delivery system of choice for superficial vascular lesions because of its efficacy, speed, and extremely low risk of scarring
- Using the principle of selective photothermolysis, the pulsed yellow dye laser delivers a very high energy but short duration pulse to the involved skin. Yellow light (585 nm) is selectively absorbed by oxyhemoglobin, which causes the dermal vessels to rupture rather than coagulate. There is significantly less heat transfer to the surrounding dermis compared with continuous-wave lasers, thereby decreasing the risk of thermal injury to the skin. Each pulse leaves a very obvious purpuric spot that lasts for about 2 weeks. It may take at least 2–3 months to determine the benefit of a laser session, and patients should be advised that multiple treatments 3–5 are routinely needed to achieve maximum benefit. It should also be emphasized that very few port-wine stains are ever completely obliterated because yellow laser light cannot reach vessels in the deep dermis. Treatment sessions are concluded when no additional lightening is observed

- Lasers that may have additional benefit for persistent port-wine stains include the 595-nm lasers: V-beam (Candela) and the Photogenica V-Star (Cynosure, originally designed for deeper and larger leg spider veins). Theoretically the longer wavelength penetrates more deeply into the dermis
- The 595-nm laser has been marketed as the first pulsed laser that does not cause purpura, specifically targeting adult patients who are reluctant to walk around for 2 weeks with dark spots on their faces
- Very deeply penetrating lasers such as the 800 nm diode laser, designed for spider veins and hair removal, are theoretically ineffective in the treatment of superficial capillary malformations but may be useful in treating thick hypertrophic stains and possibly in treating persistent stains that have reached maximum benefit with the pulsed yellow dye laser
- Capillary vascular malformations involving the maxillary and mandibular dermatomes commonly result in hypertrophy of the involved vermilion that is resistant to laser photocoagulation. Localized unilateral hypertrophy can often be addressed by excision of a tranverse mucosal ellipse, hiding the scar just inside the red line that separates dry from

wet vermilion. More significant hypertrophy requires debulking in both a transverse and vertical direction, and multiple vertical wedges can be excised in addition to the transverse ellipse. If the skin of the upper lip is also hypertrophic and ptotic, a combination skin and vermilion debulking may be necessary to decrease the amount of asymmetry.

VENOUS MALFORMATIONS

- Congenital localized or ecstatic veins with abnormal collections of irregular venous channels
- Acquired adult venous malformations of the head are most commonly seen as small venous lakes in the lower vermilion
- They are soft and easily compressible and fill slowly when pressure is released (Fig. 30.15)
- These are readily treatable by a variety of modalities that include laser photocoagulation and direct surgical excision
- Unlike cutaneous capillary vascular malformations, venous malformations are usually unresponsive to the 585 nm pulsed yellow dye laser because the depth of penetration is too shallow and the duration of energy delivery is too brief (450 microseconds)
- Pulsed lasers designed for treating leg spider veins (595 nm dye lasers) have deeper penetration and longer pulse widths (up to

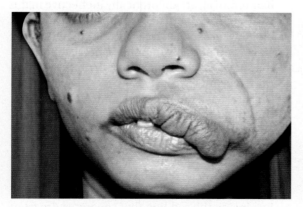

Fig. 30.15: Swelling of upper lip on left side

1500 microseconds) and therefore may be efficacious for small venous malformations
- The diode laser (800 nm wavelength, pulse duration of up to 100 milliseconds) is another example of a potentially useful laser
- The continuous-wave lasers (KTP and the older and less-available argon and copper vapor lasers) rapidly coagulate small venous malformations using 1 to 2 W of power, a defocused beam, and glass slide compression to improve the depth of penetration. Unlike intact skin, the vermilion is more tolerant of nonspecific heat transfer and therefore is less likely to scar with prolonged exposure to laser energy
- Larger venous malformations of the vermilion and mucosa can be treated with prolonged exposure to KTP laser photocoagulation (on the order of seconds), with visible blanching and shrinkage of the malformation as the heat penetrates into the deeper tissues
- Alternatively, the bare fiber of the KTP laser can be passed transmucosally into the heart of the malformation for deep photocoagulation. The fiber can be passed through a hypodermic needle or the fiber tip can be placed against the mucosa and a brief burst of energy is applied to vaporize a small opening. It is advisable to insert the fiber through normal mucosa 1–2 cm away from the actual malformation to avoid bleeding and the need to oversew the puncture site. The fiber can be palpated and repositioned within the malformation to insure correct placement. 5–10 W of continuous power usually produces visible transillumination of the laser light, audible popping, and sometimes visible tissue contraction. It is important to avoid fiber placement too close to the skin as skin perforation and sternation
- Initial attempts at localized sclerotherapy may result in acceptable improvement.

Lymphatic and Venolymphatic Malformations

- Lymphatic and venolymphatic malformations are among the most challenging and the most frustrating malformations to treat (Figs 3.16 to 30.20)

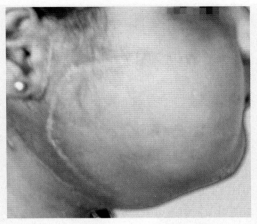

Fig. 30.16: Note old surgical scar

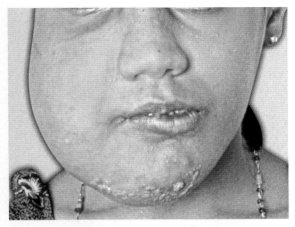

Fig. 30.17: Facial presentation

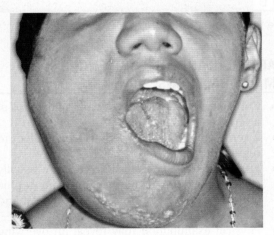

Fig. 30.18: Note gross facial asymmetry

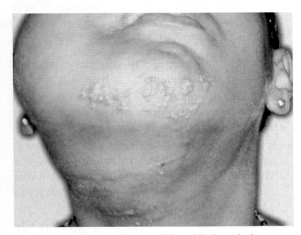

Fig. 30.19: Lesion on right: side basal view

- Even small, apparently localized lesions may have microscopic extension into normal-appearing tissue, making complete excision difficult and recurrence or persistence common
- Lymphatic malformations may be characterized by a large cystic component (still called a cystic hygroma in the pediatric literature), but more often they are composed of a myriad of small cysts and abnormal lymphatics with associated venous abnormalities
- Patients may present with periodic bouts of cellulitis best treated by oral or systemic antibiotics
- More commonly they are plagued by periodic bleeding and drainage from superficial lymphatics, particularly when the tongue is involved

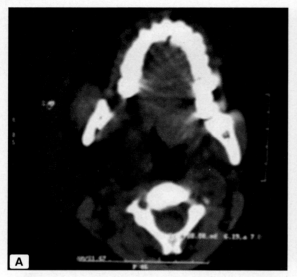 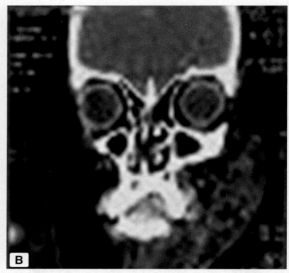

Figs 30.20A and B: Note the extent of lesion

- Although, it is possible to surgically debulk a large tongue, it is palliative at best
- Another option is to vaporize the many lymphatic vesicles with a carbon dioxide laser, but again the treatment is at best palliative
- Sclerotherapy is only an option for large cystic spaces, and an MRI scan helps to determine whether or not these exist in sufficient size to attempt sclerosis by an interventional radiologist
- Surgical debulking is difficult because of the fibrotic consistency that obliterates natural tissue planes
- Dissection of facial nerves and muscles is tedious and often futile, with high rates of facial nerve injury. Hours of meticulous dissection followed by postoperative edema and persistent soft tissue hypertrophy result in a disappointing degree of improvement. Bony hypertrophy may result in malocclusion requiring extensive orthognathic surgery
- Still, surgical debulking may represent the best chance for improvement.

ARTERIAL AND ARTERIOVENOUS MALFORMATIONS

- Congenital vascular lesions varying degrees of arteriovenous shunting
- Arteriovenous channels that have failed to regress during birth
- True AVMs of the head and neck are usually evident in childhood, may become hypertrophic during puberty, and usually slowly expand during adult life
- Physical examination may reveal an overlying capillary vascular malformation (Parkes-Weber syndrome), increased skin temperature, visible and palpable pulsations, a palpable thrill, and/or an audible bruit
- An MRI/MRA scan is the study of choice and should precede an arteriogram
- Treatment should be tailored to the individual patient
- Simple ligation of the feeding artery is contraindicated as it results in the rapid formation of a collateral arterial supply and makes interventional radiologic maneuvers difficult

- Other treatment options include conservative observation, highly selective embolization of the smallest feeding arteries (sometimes combined with direct sclerosis of the draining veins), and complete surgical excision (often preceded by arterial embolization of the major feeding vessels)
- Unlike ligation of the main feeding artery, selective embolization seeks to obliterate the tiny end-arteries and arterioles of the malformation, theoretically reducing the tendency to develop a collateral circulation. Simultaneous sclerosis of the large draining veins may cause a desirable shutdown in blood flow to and from the malformation
- This may be a lifesaving maneuver in the face of massive hemorrhage following dental extraction when an AVM involves the maxilla or mandible
- Interventional embolization alone is rarely curative, but it is an option that can be used periodically as a palliative maneuver in patients with extensive, unresectable AVMs
- Surgical excision of the entire AVM is the treatment goal whenever possible, but the timing of such radical surgery depends greatly upon the location, the age of the patient, the reconstructive plan, and the current morbidity and risk of the untreated AVM
- The hormonal changes of puberty seem to stimulate the development of additional arteriovenous shunts in many patients, causing significant hypertrophy and deformity at an age when appearance is particularly important
- Complete excision and reconstruction can achieve both a cure and an improvement in appearance in selected patients
- Partial excision is an option in patients with extensive malformations, in whom complete excision would risk significant bleeding or result in unacceptable deformity
- Large resections may require sophisticated flap reconstruction, often in the form of a microsurgical free flap transfer.

CASE NUMBER 1

Sturge-Weber Syndrome (Figs 30.21 to 30.29)

A 26-year-old male reported to the department of oral and maxillofacial surgery with a chief complaint of enlarged lower lip of 10 years duration.

History of Presenting Illness

- Progressively increased in size to attain its present size
- Difficulty in speech is associated with the lip enlargement
- Purplish red pigmentation on the face noticed since birth which reduced in severity on the right side but has remained persistent on the left side.
- Complete redness of the left eye since the age of 10 years
- Poor vision in the left eye which gradually resulted in complete loss of vision in the left eye past 6 years.

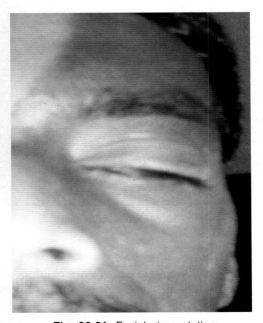

Fig. 30.21: Facial pigmentation

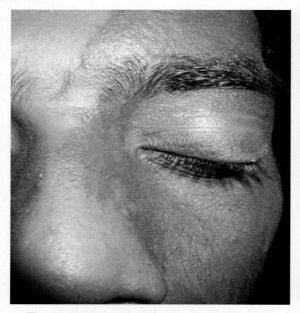

Fig. 30.22: Lesion showing involvement of face

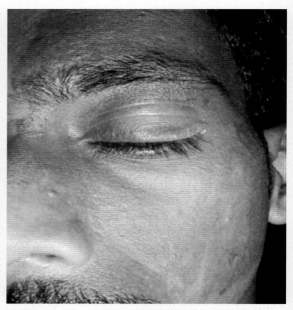

Fig. 30.23: Lesion involving forehead and face

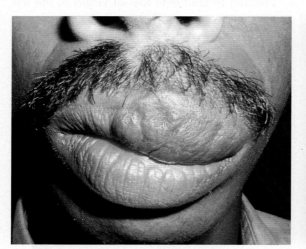

Fig. 30.24: Lip involvement

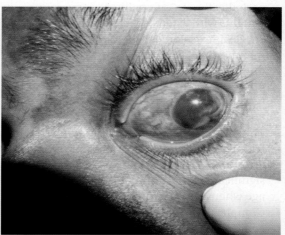

Fig. 30.25: Involvement of sclera

Medical History
- History of epileptic seizures since childhood
- Presently on carbamazepine 60 mg + 30 mg daily
- Last episode of epileptic seizure 2 months back.

Family History
No history of familial, contagious, hereditary disease

General Physical Examination
- Conscious and cooperative with average intelligence level

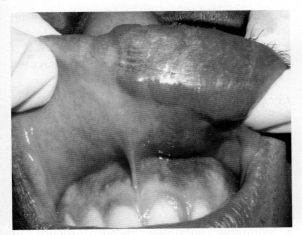

Fig. 30.26: Lesion involving lip

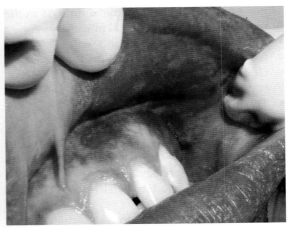

Fig. 30.27: Upper vestibular involvement

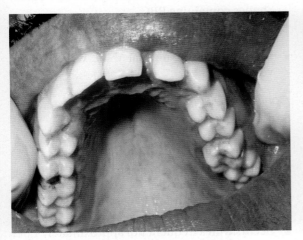

Fig. 30.28: Involvement of palate

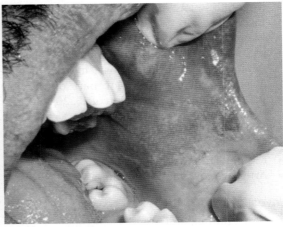

Fig. 30.29: Involving buccal mucosa

- Moderately built and nourished
- Normal gait and posture
- Normal vital signs.

Extraoral Examination Inspection

- Diffuse purplish red patch/ macular pigmentation seen on the left half of the face involving the upper lips
- Skin lesion was accurately demarcated in the midline and involved the upper lip, nose, forehead, scalp
- Normal skin texture.

- Right eye conjunctiva erythematous
- Sclera was affected.

Palpation

- Raised temperature noted in the lesion
- Left half of upper lip enlarged, soft in consistency
- Blanching of the macular area on application of digital pressure.

Intraoral Examination Soft Tissue

- Diffuse macular erythematous patches seen on the left buccal mucosa, alveolar mucosa,

posterior part of the left palatal mucosa in the region of 25,26,27 and labial mucosa
- Blanches on digital pressure
- No changes were noticed on the tongue
- Generalized erythematous marginal gingiva, soft and edematous with scalloped margins
- Texture was firm and resilient.

To Summarize
- Eighteen year-old male with complaint of enlarged lower lip of duration 10 years progressively increased in size associated with purplish pigmentation persistent on the left side of the face.
- A unilateral erythematous macular patch involving the entire left half of the face
- Skin lesion was accurately demarcated in the midline and involved the upper lip, nose, forehead, scalp
- Blanching on application of pressure.
- Intraorally diffuse erythematous macular patch of the buccal mucosa, labial mucosa, alveolar mucosa, posterior part of the left palatal mucosa in the region of 25, 26, and 27.

Differential Diagnosis
- Sturge-Weber syndrome
- Klippel-Trenauay syndrome
- Arteriovenous malformation.

Investigations
- Conventional radiographs
- Ultrasonography
- Computed tomography
- Ophthalmic consultations
- Biopsy.

Panoramic: Panoramic radiograph showed normal anatomic landmarks. No radiographic changes noticed.
Lateral skull view and PA view did not show any calcifications.

Ultrasonography
- Gray scale ultrasonography shows a well defined anechoic area with a posterior acoustic enhancement

- A feeding artery was seen in connection with the lesion
- No internal calcifications were seen
- Color Doppler study showed an increased vascularity.

Computed tomography
- Evidence of extensive cortical calcification along the left cerebral hemisphere predominantly in the temporoparietal and occipital regions
- Minimal calcifications seen in the right occipital lobe region.

Histopathology
- Submitted specimen shows presence of numerous endothelial lined spaces of irregular shapes containing RBC
- The surrounding stroma shows presence of muscle tissue and adipose tissue
- Several areas of normal thick walled blood vessels seen.

Confirmed Diagnosis
Sturge-Weber syndrome.

Sturge-Weber Syndrome

- *Synonym*: Encephalotrigeminal or leptomeningeal angiomatosis
- William Allen Sturge first described a syndrome in 1879 in a six and half-year-old girl
- Occurs with a frequency of approximately 1 per 50,000.

Definition
- Sturge-Weber syndrome is a neurocutaneous syndrome characterized by port-wine stain (facial nevus flammeus), congenital glaucoma, and underlying anomalous leptomeningeal venous plexus and the lack of normal cortical venous drainage
- It has been postulated that venous stasis results in hypoperfusion of the subjacent brain parenchyma, progressively insufficient to meet metabolic demands, particularly in the presence of seizures

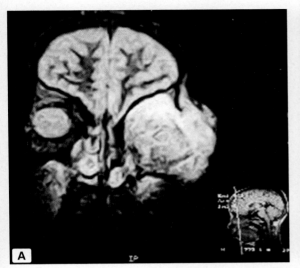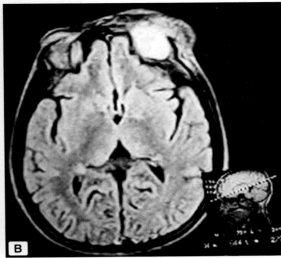

Figs 30.38A and B: MRI showing extent of lesion

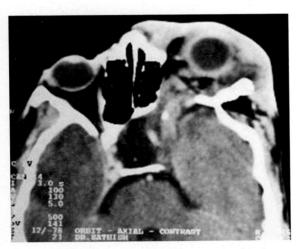

Fig. 30.39: CT contrast showing extent of lesion

6

Section

Examination of Temporomandibular Joint Disorders

Temporomandibular Joint Ankylosis

31

INTRODUCTION

Mastication, digestion, speech, appearance and oral hygiene are all affected in extremely disabling condition known as temporomandibular joint (TMJ) ankylosis.

This can also cause severe psychological stress because of facial disfigurement. TMJ ankylosis occurring in childhood can impair mandibular growth and function. Which may later on produce severe facial asymmetry and mandibular retrusion causing serious difficulties in breathing during sleep.

Ankylosis of the TMJ is a distressing structural condition that mainly occurs after trauma, or local or systemic infection. It is a challenge for oral and maxillofacial surgeons to prevent reankylosis after arthroplasty or reconstruction.

DEFINITION

Intracapsular adhesions or an actual ossification that tether the condyle to articular fossa or eminence is termed ankylosis.

- Hypomobility/ immobility of the joint
- Obliteration of the joint space with abnormal bony morphology
- Ankylosis is a Greek word, meaning, 'stiff joint'.

CLASSIFICATION

- By combination of location
- By type of tissue involved
- By extent of fusion.

General Classification

- True/false ankylosis
- Extra-articular/intraarticular ankylosis
- Fibrous/bony ankylosis
- Unilateral/bilateral ankylosis
- Partial/complete ankylosis.

Kazanzian's
True – intra-articular
False – extra-articular
Topazian's – true ankylosis
Type I – affects the condyle only
Type II – intermediate
Type III – entire condyle, coronoid, cranial base
Rowe's (according to tissue involved)
Fibrous ankylosis
Fibro-osseous ankylosis
Osseous ankylosis
Cartilaginous ankylosis
Osteocartilaginous ankylosis

Grading of TMJ Ankylosis by Sawhney (1986)

Type I: Condylar head is present without much distortion. Fibrous adhesions make movement impossible.

Type II: Flattening of condyle and bridging of bone on the lateral surface.

Type III: Bony block bridging across the ramus and zygomatic arch and elongation of coronoid process.

Type IV: Entire joint is replaced by bony mass, normal anatomy totally destroyed.

Etiology of TMJ Ankylosis

Trauma

- Congenital
- At birth (forceps delivery)
- Hemarthrosis
- Condylar fracture—intra- /extracapsular.

Infections

- Chronic suppurative otitis media
- Parotitis
- Tonsilitis
- Furuncle
- Abscess around the joint
- Osteomyelitis of the jaw
- Actinomycosis.

Inflammation

- Rheumatoid arthritis
- Osteoarthritis
- Septic arthritis.

Rare causes

- Polyarthritis
- Measles.

Systemic Diseases

- Smallpox
- Scarlet fever
- Typhoid
- Gonoccocal arthritis
- Marie Strumpell disease
- Scleroderma
- Beriberi
- Ankylosing spondylitis.

Other Causes

- Bifid condyle
- Prolonged trismus
- Prolonged immobilization
- Burns.

Pathophysiology

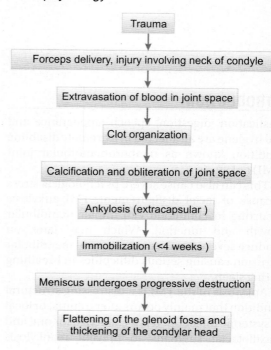

Factors Contributing to Ankylosis

- Age of patient
- Site and type of fractures
- Length of immobilization
- Damage to the meniscus.

Incidence of ankylosis following condylar fracture is more in children than in adults

- In children, the cortical bone is very thin and the condylar neck relatively broad
- There is interconnecting plexus of blood vessels penetrating the bone extending into the capsule
- An impact on chin during the first few years of life on the condyle breaks into small fragments

filling the hemarthrosis with highly osteogenic particles
- Due to immobilization (>4 wk) there is organization of fibrosseous mass converted into a bony ankylosis
- Due to histological difference between adult and child condyle which prevents many crushing injuries and potential for bony fusion.

Diagnosis
- History of trauma, infections, etc.
- Restricted or nil oral opening
- Difficulty in mastication
- Pain is usually absent
- Protrusive movements not possible on involved side
- Radiographic findings are important in arriving at final diagnosis.

Unilateral Ankylosis (Figs 31.1 to 31.3)
- Onset in childhood
- Facial asymmetry
- Deviation of chin on affected side
- Fullness of face on affected side
- Antegonial notch on affected side
- Flatness and elongation on unaffected side

- Oral opening minimal
- Cross bite may be seen.

Bilateral Ankylosis (Figs 31.4 to 31.7)
- Micrognathic mandible
- Bird-face deformity
- Neck chin angle reduced
- Bilateral antegonial notch
- Class II malocclusion

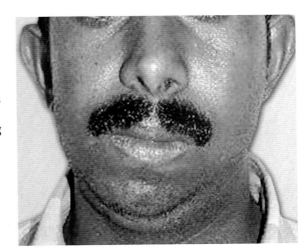

Fig. 31.1: Unilateral ankylosis left side: Frontal view. Note the facial asymmetry

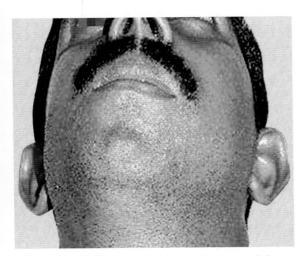

Fig. 31.2: Unilateral ankylosis. Note the deviation

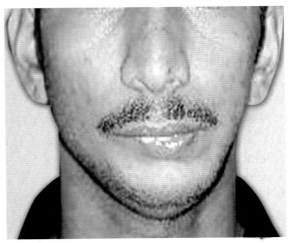

Fig. 31.3: Unilateral ankylosis left side. Frontal view

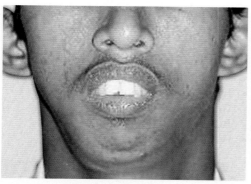

Fig. 31.4: Bilateral ankylosis

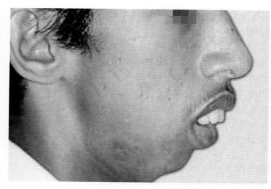

Fig. 31.5: Hypoplastic mandible

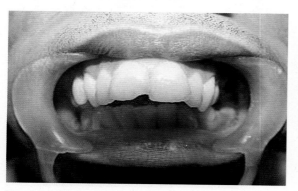

Fig. 31.6: Skeletal class II due to ill developed mandible

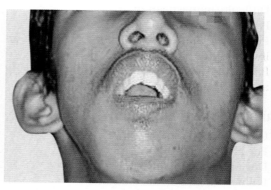

Fig. 31.7: Reduced mouth opening

- Oral opening less than 5 mm
- Anterior open bite
- Multiple carious tooth.

Radiographic Features

Orthopantomograph (Fig. 31.8)

- Antegonial notch can be seen
- Unilateral and bilateral ankylosis can be distinguished.

Lateral Oblique View (Fig. 31.9)

- Anteroposterior dimension of condyle
- Elongation of coronoid can also be seen.

PA View (Fig. 31.10)

- Mediolateral extent of condyle
- Highlights asymmetry in unilateral ankylosis.

CT Scan (Figs 31.11 and 31.12)

- Helpful guide for surgery
- Relation to medial cranial fossa, anteroposterior width, mediolateral depth
- Bony fusion can be seen.

Radiographic Findings in Fibrous Ankylosis

- Reduced joint space (Fig. 31.13)
- Hazy appearance
- Normal anatomy of TMJ.

Radiographic Findings in Bony Ankylosis

- Complete obliteration of joint space
- TMJ anatomy is distorted
- Condylar head is deformed
- Elongation of coronoid process can also be seen.

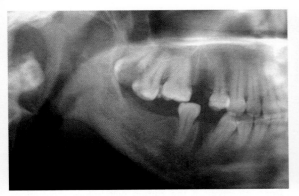

Fig. 31.8: Orthopantomograph

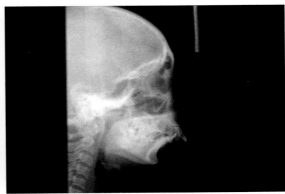

Fig. 31.9: Lateral cephalogram

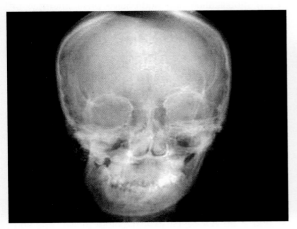

Fig. 31.10: PA skull view

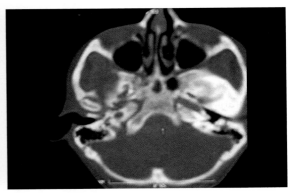

Fig. 31.11: CT showing fusion

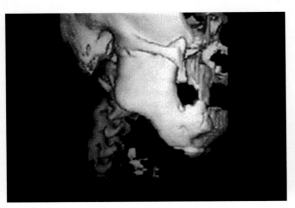

Fig. 31.12: 3-D CT showing fusion

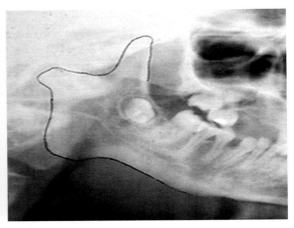

Fig. 31.13: OPG showing reduced joint space

Sequelae of Untreated Ankylosis
- Facial growth and development affected
- Speech impairment
- Nutrition impairment
- Respiratory distress (tongue fall in sleep)
- Malocclusion
- Poor oral hygiene
- Multiple carious and impacted teeth.

Management
- Always surgical
- Depends upon
  - Age of onset
  - Extent
  - Unilateral or bilateral involvement
  - Associated facial deformity.

Aims of Surgery
- Release of ankylosed mass
- Creation of functional joint
- Restoration of vertical height
- Restoration of normal facial growth pattern
- Prevention of recurrence
- Esthetics improvement.

Leeonard B Kaban's protocol for management of TMJ ankylosis
Early surgical intervention
Aggressive resection (gap = 1–1.5 cm) especially medial aspect of the ramus
Ipsilateral coronoidectomy and temporalis myotomy, the interincisal opening should be = 35 mm
Contralateral coronoidectomy and temporalis myotomy necessary if maximal incisal opening <35 mm
Lining of glenoid fossa with temporalis fascia
Reconstruction of the ramus with either dictraction osteogenesis or a costochondral graft
Early mobilization and aggressive physiotherapy for six months
Regular long-term follow-up
To carry out cosmetic surgery when the growth of the patient is completed

Sahwney classification according to the type of ankylosis
Type I and II: A discrete section of condyle is excised with a reciprocating saw and a gap of 3–5 mm is made, fibrous adhesion is removed. If meniscus is intact, no interpositional material is required and if meniscus is damaged/absent interpositional material is inserted
Type III: Extra-articular bony bridge extending from zygomatic arch to the ramus is removed
Type IV: New joint is fashioned to restore function in children (12–13 years of age). Intermaxillary fixation for 10–14 days followed by early mobilization and physiotherapy

The 7-step new protocol
Aggressive excision of the fibrous and/or bony ankylotic mass
Coronoidectomy on the affected side
Coronoidectomy on the contralateral side, if steps 1 and 2 do not result in a maximal incisal opening greater than 35 mm or to the point of dislocation of the unaffected TMJ
Lining of the TMJ with a temporalis myofascial flap or the native disc, if it can be salvaged
Reconstruction of the ramus condyle unit with either distraction osteogenesis or costochondral graft and rigid fixation
Early mobilization of the jaw. If distraction osteogenesis is used to reconstruct the ramus condyle unit, mobilization begins the day of the operation. In patients who undergo costochondral graft reconstruction, mobilization begins after 10 days of maxillomandibular fixation
All patients receive aggressive physiotherapy

Surgical Approaches to TMJ

- Submandibular (Risdon's) (Fig. 31.14)
- Postramal (Hind's)
- Postauricular
- Endural
- Rhytidectomy approach
- Preauricular (Fig. 31.15)
  - Dingman's
  - Blair's
  - Thoma's
  - Popowich's modification of Al-Kayat and Bramley's
- Hemicoronal and bicoronal (Obwegeser's).

Advantages of *Popowich* modification of *Al-Kayat and Bramley's* approach
Reduction in incidence of facial nerve palsy
- Provision for donor site for temporalis fascia
- Dissection through avascular zone
- Improved visibility (facial planes)
- Good cosmetic result
- Avoidance of auriculotemporal nerve anesthesia
- Reduction in total operating time.

Surgical Techniques

- Condylectomy
- Gap arthroplasty
- Interpositional arthroplasty.

Condylectomy (Fig. 31.16)

Indications: Fibrous ankylosis
- Horizontal osteotomy cut at the level of condylar neck
- Vital structures on medial aspect should be preserved
- Condylar head is separated and rest of stump is smoothened.

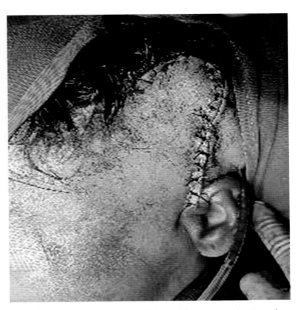

Fig. 31.15: Preauricular incision with temporal extension

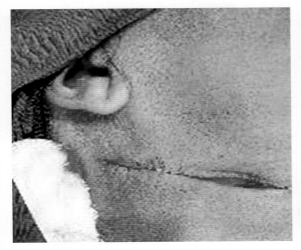

Fig. 31.14: Submandibular incision

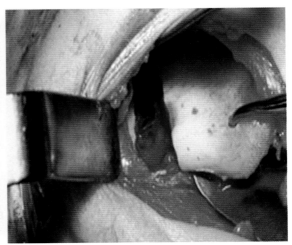

Fig. 31.16: Condylectomy intraoperative

Gap Arthroplasty (Figs 31.17A and B)

Indications: Extensive bony ankylosis

- Identification of previous joint structure and roof of glenoid fossa is impossible
- Level of section below the previous joint space
- Two horizontal osteotomy cuts and removal of bony wedge
- Gap of at least 1 cm to prevent reankylosis
- No substance is interposed between the two cut bony surfaces.

Interpositional Arthroplasty
(Figs 31.18 to 31.23)

- Creation of a gap
- Addition of a barrier material to prevent reankylosis and to restore vertical ramus height
- Replacement of the mandibular condyle and ramus
- Reconstruction of the glenoid fossa
- Replacement of the meniscus

- Interpositional materials may be autogenous, heterogenous, or alloplastic.

Interpositional Materials
Autogenous
• Temporal fascia
• Temporal fascia and pericranium
• Fascia lata
• Dermal graft
• Auricular cartilage
• Costochondral cartilage and bone composites
Allogenic
• Freeze dried dura
• Cryopreserved cartilage
• Allogenic bone
Alloplastic
• Metals—stainless steel alloy
• Cobalt chromium alloy
• Titanium
• Ceramics—aluminum oxide
• Hydroxyapatite
• Polymers—dimethylsiloxane
• Composites—teflon, silastic, proplast

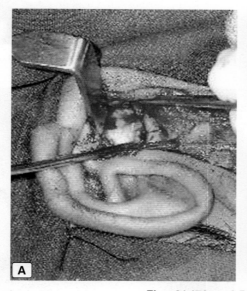 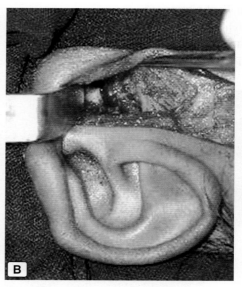

Figs 31.17A and B: Gap arthroplasty

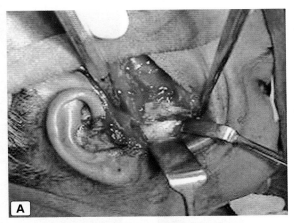

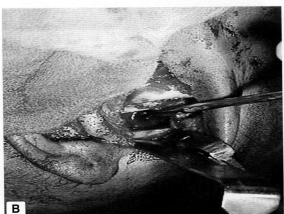
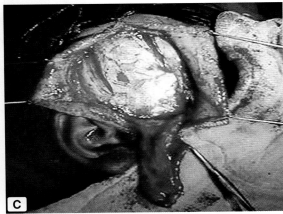

Figs 31.18A to C: With temporal fascia-interpositional arthroplasty

Role of temporalis fascia and muscle flap in TMJ surgery described by MA Pogrel and LB Kaban
Temporal muscle has dual origin from the inner temporal line of the temporal fossa and deep temporal fascia
Temporal muscle has dual origin from the inner temporal line of the temporal fossa and deep temporal fascia
Middle
Middle temporal artery, a branch, the superficial tempral artery provides blood supply to temporalis fascia
Primary blood supply is from anterior and posterior deep temporal artery
Temporalis fascia and temporalis muscle individual blood supply and may be dissected as separate unit
Temporalis muscle is innervated by anterior and posterior and occationally middle temporal nerve
Vascular supply and nerve supply enter the muscle and fasciafrom inferior middle and posterior direction for this reason both andteriorly and posteriorly based flaps are possible

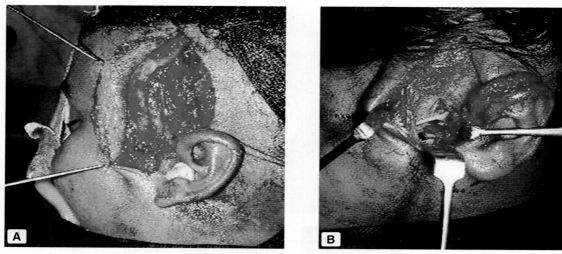

Figs 31.19A and B: Interpositional arthroplasty

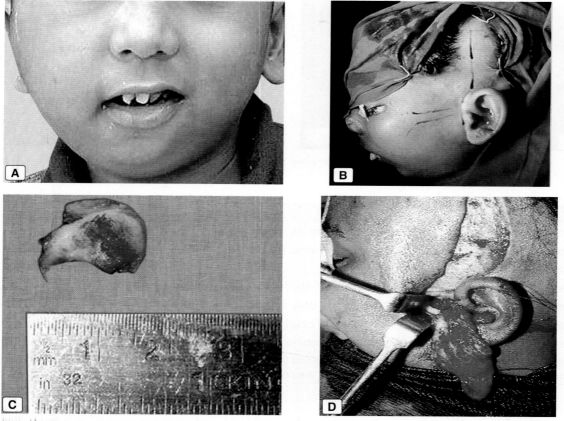

Figs 31.20A to D: (A) Preoperative, (B) Incision marking, (C) Removed ankylosed mass, (D) Interposition material placement,

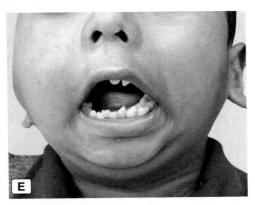

Figs 31.20 E: Postoperative mouth opening

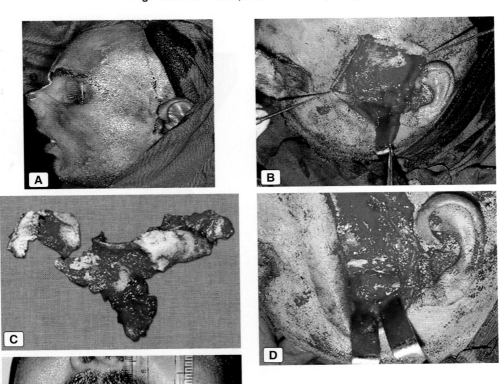

Figs 31.21A to E: (A) Incision marking, (B) Surgical dissection, (C) Excised ankylosed mass, (D) Interposition material, (E) Postoperative mouth opening (*Courtesy:* R Prasad)

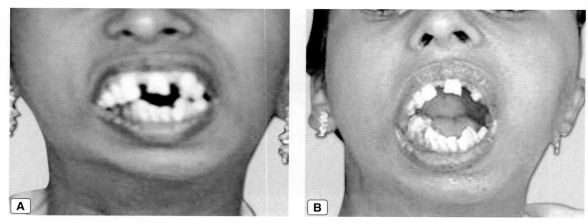

Figs 31.22A and B: (A) Ankylosis bilateral before treatment, (B) Ankylosis bilateral after treatment

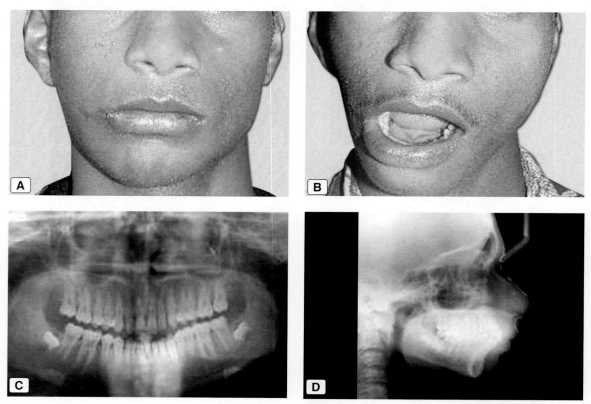

Figs 31.23A to D: (A) Ankylosis unilateral, (B) Ankylosis unilateral with mouthopening, (C) OPG showing ankylosis; (D) Lateral cephalogram showing ankylosis feature

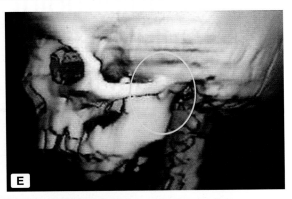

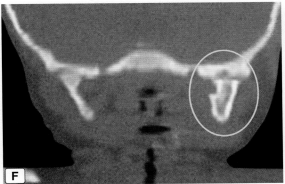

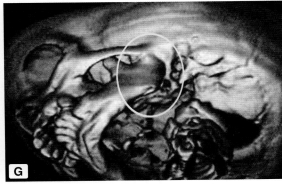

Figs 31.23E to G: (E) 3D CT showing ankylosis; (F) 3D CT showing ankylosis; (G) CT showing ankylosis

Alloplastic reconstruction
Advantages
• Lack of a donor site
• Immediate return to function
Complication
• Foreirgn body reaction to some materials
• Erosion of metal condylar prostesis into the glenoid fossa
• Suboptimal postoperative range of motion
• Loosening of the screw and loss of stability

Autogenous costochondral Grafts
Advantages
• Biologic acceptability
• Remodeling by appositional growth
Disadvantages
• Increased operating time
• Additional surgical site
Complications
• Donor site morbidity
• Potential overgrowth of graft
• Suboptimal postoperative range of motion

Temporomandibular Joint Dislocation, Subluxation, and Hypermobility

32

INTRODUCTION

Temporomandibular joint (TMJ) dislocation is a fairly common finding. The types of dislocation can be according to location or duration. TMJ becomes dislocated when the condyle moves too far and gets stuck in front of the articular eminence.

- Dislocation is a complete separation of the articular surfaces with fixation in an abnormal position. Luxation and dislocation are synonymous. The key terms used include hypormobility, acute dislocation, long standing dislocation, recurrent dislocation and habitual dislocation. Subluxation is substituted for the term dislocation when dislocation is incomplete
- Anterior acute dislocation of the condyle occurs, in which the normal anatomic relationships within the joint have been completely disrupted, with the condyle displaced and fixed anterior to the articular eminence
- A dislocation that remains locked anteriorly for several days and years is an old or *long-standing* dislocation
- Condylar recurrent or Habitual dislocation or subluxation is called when there are abnormal anterior excursions of the condyles beyond the articular eminence, but the patient is able to manipulate it back into normal position. The articular surfaces maintain partial contact and the condyle is able to return to the glenoid fossa voluntarily or aided by self manipulation.

ETIOLOGY

- Acute anterior dislocation is precipitated by either intrinsic or extrinsic trauma
- A wide yawn is a frequent cause of spontaneous (intrinsic) dislocation
- Other forms of intrinsic events such as vomiting, singing laughing, screaming, wide biting, and seizures can also bring about episode of acute dislocation.

Extrinsic Causes

- Traumatic reasons which forces the condyle out of the fossa
- External force such as a blow to the mandible, usually with the mouth in an open position, can result in mandibular dislocation
- Acute dislocation found the most common cause to be a blow on the chin with the mouth open in males and dental extractions in females
- Manipulation of the jaw during intubation for general anesthesia, endoscopy and dental extraction is another extrinsic cause
- Laxity of ligaments and capsule and abnormalities of skeletal form are predisposing factors in both acute and chronic forms of dislocation
- Inadequate healing after injuries, occlusal disharmonies and long-standing degenerative joint disease can cause looseness of the capsule and ligaments.

Systemic Hypermobility

Familial hypermobility syndromes loose-jointed individuals with articular symptoms comprise a very heterogeneous group.

> In the Ehlers-Danlos syndrome, the degree of hypermobility and the incidence of dislocation are closely related.
> Here dislocations of the temporomandibular joint are often recurrent

Occlusal Factors

- Long-term overclosure and loss of physiologic vertical dimension secondary to loss of dentition can contribute to subluxation and dislocation
- Overclosure produces stretching and loosening of joint ligaments and joint laxity
- Asymmetry of the condylar position due to mandibular malposition may be caused by occlusal interferences (Fig. 32.1).

Drug-associated Dislocation

- Spontaneous dislocation of the mandible can occur due to extrapyramidal reactions caused by antipsychotic drugs
- Prochlorperazine causes left facial weakness and wild facial contortions, followed by a unilateral mandibular dislocation.

Psychogenic Dislocation

- Hysteria can be the cause of habitual dislocation of the mandible
- Ligaments lax and subluxation or dislocation can easily occur
- It is important to recognize early that habitual dislocation may be the presenting feature of an underlying psychiatric disturbance.

DIAGNOSIS

- A thorough history and physical examination is important to evaluate properly all categories of dislocation

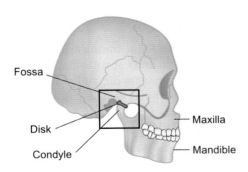
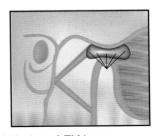
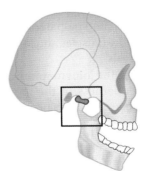
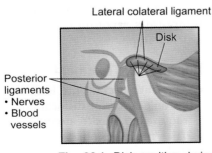

Fig. 32.1: Disk position during opening and closing of TMJ

- It is important to determine the cause and onset of the dislocation
- A spontaneous intrinsic dislocation only occurs in an anterior direction
- Acute, initial spontaneous and extrinsic traumatic anterior dislocations are treated differently from chronic repetitive dislocation
- A prior history of local joint laxity, internal derangements, and other temporomandibular joint disorders will influence the outcome of treatment
- Neurological and musculoskeletal disorders such as Parkinson's disease and epilepsy and other systemic disorder of hypermobility are important to recognize.

Clinical Examination

- Spontaneous dislocation from a wide yawn is often bilateral, but a blow to the chin with the mouth open usually creates a unilateral dislocation
- The lateral pole of the condyle produces a characteristic protuberance anterior to and below the articular eminence which can usually be seen and palpated
- Palpation of the muscles and joints is a valuable aid to diagnosis
- Tenderness in the joint may indicate a fracture; where as tenderness in the temporal fossa is more characteristic of dislocation.

Unilateral Acute Dislocation

- Mouth is partly open
- Difficulty in mastication and speech
- Profuse drooling of saliva
- A deviation of chin toward contralateral side
- Lateral cross bite and open bite on the contralateral side
- Affected condyle is not palpable.

Bilateral Acute Dislocation

- Pain, inability to close the mouth
- Tense masticatory muscles
- Difficulty in speech

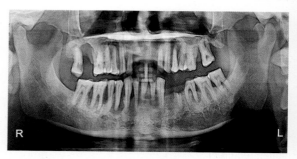

Fig. 32.2: Recurrent dislocation resulting from bifid condyle

- Excessive salivation
- Protruding chin
- Gagging of molar teeth
- Anterior open bite
- Difficulty in swallowing and drooling of saliva.

Radiographic Examination

- Plains flims, such as transcranial radiograph and lateral tomograms, OPG, etc.
- Arthrographic studies with recurrent dislocation have enabled a differentiation to be made between meniscotemporal and meniscocondylar types
- MRI and CT scanning are useful in identifying ligament and capsular tears and stretching
- Electromyographic studies also provide valuable information (Fig. 32.2).

TREATMENT

Numerous treatments have been used for dislocation of the mandible. They include injection of sclerosing solutions, physical therapy, eminectomies, joint placation, pterygoid and temporalis myotomies, condylectomies and articular implants.

Nonsurgical Treatment

- The initial acute, the long standing and the chronic recurring dislocations of the mandible require different treatments
- The major problem to overcome in all dislocation is muscle contraction

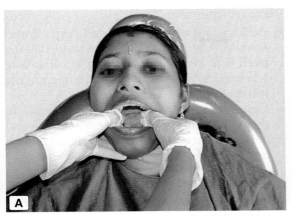
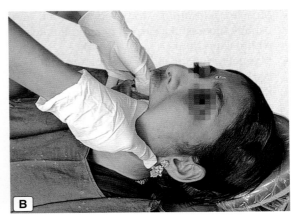

Figs 32.3A and B: Hippocrates method

- The acute dislocation needs immediate attention for relief of pain and anxiety and to minimize damage to the joint structure
- Reduction and immobilization for 4 weeks will allow damage ligaments, capsule, and disk to heal.

Acute Dislocation

- Initial treatment is aimed at reducing tension, anxiety, and muscle spasm by using the simplest methods
- A tranquilizer or sedative drug provides necessary relaxation
- Also pressure and message over coronoid processes can benefit
- An impressive simple technique is injecting local anesthetic into the depression in the glenoid fossa left by the dislocated condyle
- Manipulation is the next step
- Hippocrates remains an effective way to manipulate and reduce the dislocated mandible (Figs 32.3A and B)
- Operator stand in front of the patient who is sitting with the head supported
- Thumbs are wrapped in gauze and placed on the occlusal surfaces of the mandibular molars or alveolar ridges
- The lower border of the mandible is grasped with the fingers and the patient is encouraged to relax

- By pressing firmly on the molars and elevating anteriorly with simultaneous backward pressure the condyle is relocated.

Yurino's Method

- Places the patient in a supine position without a pillow
- The patient is encouraged to relax completely while the operator stands near the patient's head and holds the body of the mandible from the opposite side
- The patient is asked to open and close the mouth and although it is difficult to do so, it is important for the patient to attempt this alone
- The operator moves the mandible up and down in phase with the patient's opening and closing movements
- The operator then locates the dislocated condyle with his thumb and simultaneously with the patient's closing motion pushes it completely downward while moving the body of the mandible upward
- By this procedure the condyle moves over the articular eminence and slips into the fossa.

Long-standing Dislocation

- The difficulty in reducing mandibular dislocation increases proportionately with time

- Muscle relaxation and manipulation are usually successful if carried out immediately or within a few hours
- Manual reduction either under LA or under GA is tried first
- If manual reduction fails, then open reduction can be done. It consists of opening the joint through preauricular incision and direct vision manipulation
- Condylectomy, eminectomy is last resort.

Recurrent Dislocation

Physical Therapy

- The use of isometric exercises to improve opening and closing patterns is most important.
- Synchronized isometric contraction exercises of masticatory opening muscles and their antagonists should be performed on a regular basis

> Isometric exercise similar to that described by Poswillo is very helpful

- This relatively simple exercise trains the suprahyoid muscles to stabilize the mandible and reduce forward movement of the condyle in the early opening phase
- The exercise should be carried out several times a day for 4 weeks until dislocations are no longer a problem
- Then the exercise should be done indefinitely once or twice a day to maintain the stability and to prevent a return to paranormal function.

Symptomatic Treatment

- Analgesics and nonsteroidal anti-inflammatory drugs will relieve locomotor system pain whether in the joint, bone, tendon, ligament, or muscle
- Muscle relaxants and tranquillizers are useful.

> An injection of a steroid such as methylprednisone gives excellent results in persistent synovitis in the hypermobility syndrome.
>
> Long-acting corticosteroids should be avoided as they may lead to connective tissue atrophy and weakening of collagenous tissue, which may contribute to increasing joint laxity

Occlusal Treatment

- Occlusal disturbances, such as cuspal interferences and non occlusion due to missing teeth with loss of vertical support, should be corrected to prevent their contributing to the instability of the joint
- However, appliances can be useful in those individuals with coexisting internal derangement of the disk, bruxism, and muscle hyperactivity.

Chemical Capsulorrhaphy

- Injection of sclerosing agents into the supporting ligaments or into the joint
- The objective is to produce fibrosis and tightening of the capsular ligaments, thus limiting motion of the mandible
- The use of sodium psylliate emulsion, sodium morrhuate, sodium tetradecyl sulfate has been advocated
- The disadvantange in their use is the inability to predict the amount of limitation that will be produced.

SURGERY FOR SUBLUXATION AND DISLOCATION

Indications

Disabling recurrent dislocation and long standing dislocation not responsive to closed manipulations and other nonsurgical treatment.

Contraindications

- Acute dislocation
- Habitual dislocation with significant psychologic influence.

  Three broad categories of procedures:
  - Designed to limit translation
  - To eliminate blocking factors in the condylar path of closure
  - Combination of both.
- Limiting translation are anchoring, blocking, and myotomy procedures
- Procedures that eliminate blocking factors in the condylar path of closure include diskectomy and eminectomy

- The combination procedures are condylotomy, condylectomy, high condylectomy, and lateral pterygoid myotomy with diskectomy.

Procedures to Limit Translation (Figs 32.4 to 32.7)

Anchoring Procedures

- Anchoring procedures reduce or eliminate the anterior or translational motion of the condyle
- The operations described in the literature include:

    – Capsulorrhaphy
    – Capsular plication
    – Ligamentopexy
    – Flap secured to the capsule
    – Autogenous and alloplastic slings between the condyle and zygomatic process.

Blocking Procedures

Designed to create an obstacle to the condyle in its opening path
Include both soft tissues and bony procedures

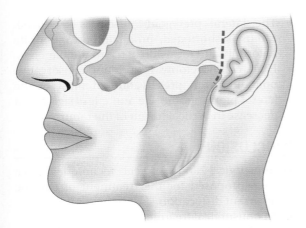

Fig. 32.4: Preauricular incision marking

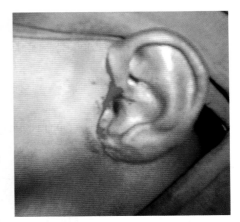

Fig. 32.5: Preauricular incision

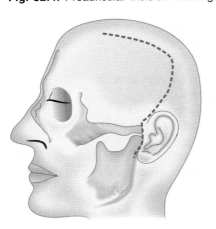

Fig. 32.6: Al-Kayat and Bramley's incision marking

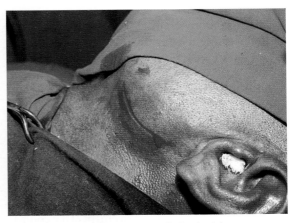

Fig. 32.7: Submandibular incision

Soft tissue procedures

- Konietzny surgically creates a closed lock by the disk
- The posterior ligament of the disk is released and the anterior attachment is preserved
- The disk is pulled anteriorly and inferiorly and is anchored vertically in front of the condyle by suturing it *to* the lateral pterygoid muscle inferiorly and *to* the capsule laterally.

Bony procedures: These procedures increase the height of the articular eminence by osteotomies, bone grafts, and metal implants.

Lindemann made an oblique osteotomy to increase the height of the articular tubercle. Bone of the tubercle and eminence was tilted inferiorly and anteriorly
Gossere and Dautry: The zygomatic arch is cut vertically in front of the joint and lowered

Eliminating Blocking Factors in the Condylar Path

Eliminating obstacles in the condylar path that prevent reduction of the condyle into the glenoid fossa
The two procedures, which accomplish this, are diskectomy and eminectomy

Diskectomy

Diskectomy has been advocated by Ashurst and Axhausen for recurrent dislocation.

Procedure
- Surgical approach to TMJ
- Eminectomy and eminoplasty are frequently used
- Techniques to correct recurrent dislocation.

Combined Procedures to Eliminate Blocking and Limit Translation

- Lateral pterygoid myotomy with diskectomy
- Condylotomy
- Condylectomy.

Lateral Pterygoid Myotomy with Diskectomy
- First described by Boman
- Restricts anterior gliding movement of the condyle and eliminates obstruction caused by the disk.

Condylotomy
- First described for treatment of painful joints with internal derangement
- Later advocated by Poswillo for treatment of recurrent dislocation
- Condylotomy is an osteotomy through the condylar neck which is performed through an extraoral or an intraoral approach.

Condylectomy
- The blocking effect of the condyle on the disk or eminence is removed in this procedure
- A complete condylectomy also has the disadvantage of producing facial and occlusal deformity
- The lateral pterygoid muscle is sacrificed; ramus is shortened, producing an open-bite deformity and retrusion of the mandible
- High condylectomy is a more conservative operation with preservation of most of the lateral pterygoid muscle and a less significant decrease in vertical height of the ramus.

CONCLUSION

- Nonsurgical and surgical techniques have been proposed for the treatment of chronic recurrent dislocation
- In nonsurgical treatment
- Bandages
- Splints
- Sclerosing agents
- Introduction of botulinum toxin in reducing dislocation.

Surgical techniques used were
- Myotomy
- Capsular placation
- Sacrification of the temoralis tendon
- Open condylotomy
- Insertion of implants into the articular eminence
- Down-fracturing of the zygomatic arches
- Augmentation of the eminence by allografts
- Eminectomy.

Of these procedures eminectomy and augmentation of the articular eminence by bone grafts are the most popular.

Internal Derangements of Temporomandibular Joint and Myofascial Pain Dysfunction Syndrome

33

INTRODUCTION

Temporomandibular disorders can be a wide range of clinical conditions involving the temporomandibular joint (TMJ). Chronic closed lock of the temporomandibular joint is the result of internal derangement of the joint subsequent to disk displacement without reduction. Clinically condylar hypomobility together with mouth opening restriction may be observed. Other entities are severe decrease in maximal interincisal opening, such as osteoarthritis, myofascial pain and disfunction, TMJ fibrous or bony ankylosis, and anchored disk phenomenon.

TMJ disorders are multifunctional disorders with variety of etiological factors involving physical, psychological, emotional, social, and local factors
Derangements of the condyle-disk complex
Structural incompatibility of the articular surfaces
Inflammatory disorders

DERANGEMENTS OF THE CONDYLE-DISK COMPLEX

- Result of abnormal biomechanical function between the condyle and the disk
- These disorders are a result of a derangement in the structure of the condyle-disk complex; they have been referred to internal derangements
- Internal derangements are defined as intra-articular tissue interfering with the normal smooth action of a joint

- Disk displacement is by far the most common cause of internal derangement of the TMJ
  - Disk displacement and disk dislocations with reduction
  - Disk dislocations without reduction.
- Disk is in a normal superior position when the posterior band of the disk is in the 12 o'clock position on top of the condyle in the closed mouth position
- Variations in the superior position occur when the posterior band is anterior to the 12 o'clock position
- The anterior prominence of the condyle and the inferior concavity of the central thin zone of the disk are in contact and the anterior prominence of the condyle is within the biconcave portion of the disk.
- If these two surfaces are separated by at least 2 mm then the disk is considered displaced.

Disk Displacements and Disk Dislocations with Reduction (Fig. 33.1)

Represent the early stages of disk derangement disorders.

Cause

- Elongation of the capsular and discal ligaments coupled with thinning of the articular disk
- Commonly result from macrotrauma or microtrauma
- Orthopedic instability and joint loading combine as causative factors

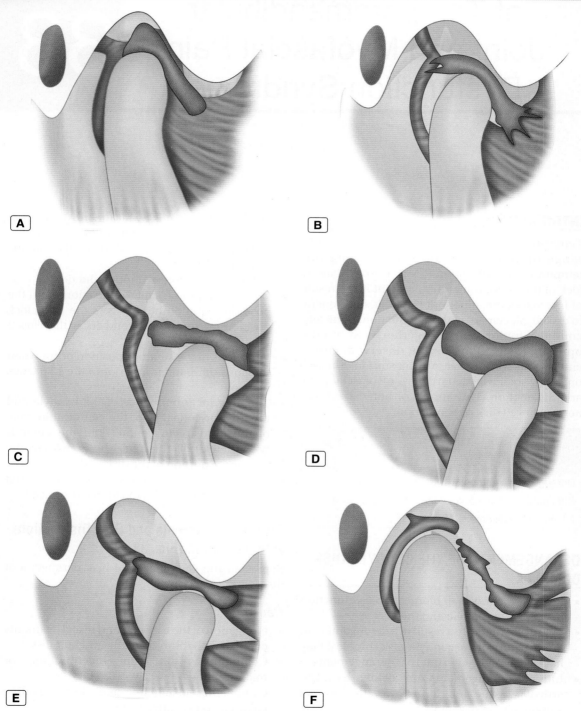

Figs 33.1A to F: Disk displacement with reduction

- Heavy and prolonged loading of the articular tissues exceeds the functional capacity of the articular tissues and breakdown begins (hypoxia reperfusion injuries)

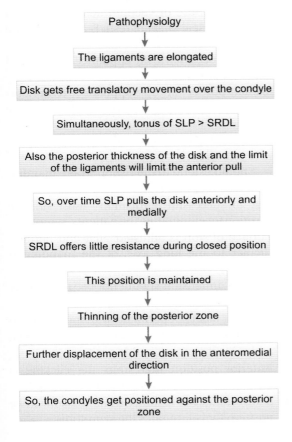

- With or without audible clicking, the displacement and reduction of the disk can be felt as jarring sensation or palpation posterior to the joint or with fingers towards the mandibular angle.

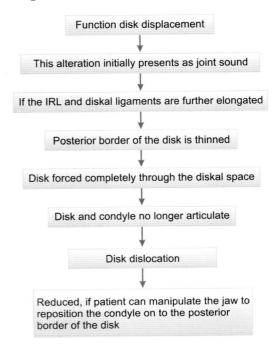

Definitive Treatment

Re-establish a normal condyle-disk assembly.

Anterior repositioning appliance
- In the early 1970s, Farrar introduced the anterior mandibular repositioning appliance
- Provides an occlusal relationship that requires the mandible to be maintained in a forward position
- Re-establish the normal condyle-disk relationship with the least protrusion of the mandible
- Achieved clinically by monitoring the clicking joint
- Idea behind the appliance is to reposition the disk back on the condyle (recapture the disk)
- Originally suggested to be worn 24 hours a day for as long as 3–6 months

Clinical Characteristics
- Normal range of movement with restriction only associated with pain
- Discal movement can be felt by palpation of the joints during opening and closing
- Deviations in the opening pathways are common
- Lateral movements: Laterotrusive to the affected side is normal and laterotrusive to the contralateral side impaired
- Clinically, the disk displacement can be associated with joint, muscle and facial pain

- In many patients advancing the mandible for a period of time prevents the condyle from articulating with the highly vascularized, well innervated retrodiscal tissues
- During forward repositioning, the retrodiscal tissues undergo adaptive and reparative change; tissues can become fibrotic and avascular
- However recent studies have shown that the disks generally are not recaptured by anterior repositioning appliances
- Instead as the condyle returns to the fossa, it articulates on the adapted retrodiscal tissues
- If these tissues have adequately adapted, loading occurs without pain even though the disk is anteriorly displaced
- Result is a painless joint that may continue to click with condylar movement
- Reconstruction of the dentition or orthodontic therapy should be reserved only for those patients who present with a significant orthopedic instability.

Disadvantage

- Some patients develop a posterior open bite (result of reversible, myostatic contracture of the lateral pterygoid muscle).

The philosophy now is to reduce the time the appliance is worn so as to limit the adverse effects on the occlusal condition.

Anterior positioning appliance

- Is an interocclusal device that encourages the mandible to assume a position more anterior than the intercuspal position
- Goal is to provide a better condyle-disc relationship in the fosse so that tissues have a better opportunity to repair or adapt
- Change the position temporarily to enhance adaptation of the retrodiscal tissues
- Once the tissue adaptation has occurred, appliance is eliminated and condyle to assume the musculostable position and function painlessly on the adaptive fibrous tissue.

Method of Fabrication

- Full arch hard acrylic device
- Can be used in either arch
- An alginate impression is first made
- With a pressure or vacuum adapter, a 2 mm thick hard clear sheet of resin is adapted to the cast
- Adapted occlusal resin appliance is removed from the stone cast
- Labial border of the appliance terminates between the incisal and middle thirds of the anterior teeth
- Anterior stop is constructed:
  - 4 mm wide
  - Should extend to the region where mandibular central incisor will contact
- Key to successful fabrication—most suitable position for eliminating the patients' symptoms
- Surface of stop is adjusted—flat and perpendicular to the long axes of the mandibular incisors
- Vertical dimension should not be significantly increased
- Posterior teeth not in contact with the appliance
- Protrude the mandible—slightly and to open and close the mouth in this position
- Anterior position that stops the clicking is located and marked with red marking paper
- Shortest anterior distance from musculostable position that eliminates the symptoms.
  1 mm groove in the contact area.
  Note: There should not be any joint sounds during opening and closing.
- Self curing acrylic is added to the remaining occlusal surface so that all occlusal contacts can be established
- Anterior guiding ramp on the anterior palatal area is constructed by an excess of acrylic located lingual to the mandibular anterior teeth when occluded
- Patient is asked to slowly close into the grooved area on the anterior stop

- Slightly more anterior position—once anterior stop contacted the mandible is slowly moved posteriorly until the groove is felt
- Occlusion—flat occlusal contacts
  - Anterior guiding ramp (mandible to assume a more forward position to ICP)
- RAMP—smooth sliding surface so as not to promote catching or locking of the teeth
- Repeated attempts to eliminate the appliance fail to control symptoms, orthopedic instability should be suspected
- For some patients—more traditional muscle relaxation appliance that opens the bite but does not anteriorly reposition the mandible can reduce symptoms
- Factors that determine the length of time an appliance has to be worn (retrodiscal tissues to adapt):
  - Acuteness of the injury
  - Extent of the injury
  - Age and health of the patient.

Stabilization appliance

- Provides an occlusal relationship considered optimal for the patient
- Condyles are in their most musculostable position when the teeth are contacting evenly and simultaneously
- Canine disocclusion of the posterior teeth during eccentric movement provided
- Goal is to eliminate any orthopedic instability between the occlusal position and the joint position
- Decreases the parafunctional activity that often accompanies periods of stress
- Maxillary device is more stable and covers more tissue -more retentive and less likely to break
- Final criteria
  - Accurately fit the maxillary teeth, with total stability and retention
  - In centric relation all posterior mandibular buccal cusps must contact on flat surfaces with even force

- Protrusive movement—mandibular canines must contact the appliance with even force
- Lateral movement—only mandibular canine should contact
- Mandibular posterior teeth must contact only in the centric relation closure
- Occlusal surface as flat as possible.

Supportive Therapy

- Patient education
- Encouraged to decrease loading of the joints
  - Softer foods
  - Slower chewing
  - Smaller bites
- If inflammation is suspected—NSAID prescribed
- Moist heat or ice can be used
- Distractive manipulation by a physical therapist may assist in healing
- PSR (physical self regulation) techniques should be provided to the patient
- Reduce loading to the joint and generally down regulate the CNS
- Help decrease pain and improve the patients coping skills.

Disk Dislocation without Reduction (Figs 33.2A and B)

Clinical condition in which the disk is dislocated most frequently anteromedially from the condyle and does not return to normal position with condylar movement.

Cause

Macrotrauma and microtrauma.

History

- Report the exact onset of this disorder
- Sudden change in range of mandibular movement that is very apparent to the patient
- Gradual increase in intracapsular symptoms before the dislocation
- Most often joint sounds are no longer present immediately after the dislocation.

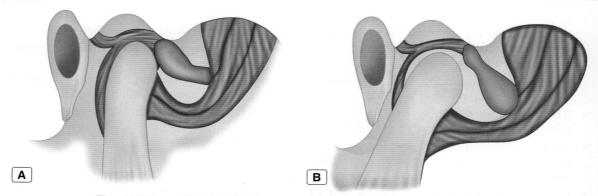

Figs 33.2A and B: Disk displacement without reduction: (A) Closed (B) Open

Types

Non-reducing disk displacement can be sub-divided into acute phase and chronic phase.

Clinical Characteristics

- Limited mandibular opening (25–30 mm)
- Affected joint does not show translatory movement. Only rotational whereas, unaffected shows both so when patient opens wide, midline shifts to the affected side, called as deflection
- Normal eccentric movement to the ipsilateral side and restricted eccentric movement to the contralateral side
- Joint pain on jaw function
- Tenderness over the affected joint
- History of clicking that disappears at the onset of a sudden limitation of mouth opening.

Definitive Treatment

> Murakami et al in 1995 suggested that the treatment goal should be to normalize masticatory function and to eliminate the associated pain.

> Primary conservative treatment consist of medication, physiotherapy and occlusal splint

> If conservative management fails surgical treatment fails surgical intervention is necessary

Technique for manual manipulation:
- Dependent on three factors:
  1. Level of activity in the superior lateral pterygoid muscle

2. The disk space must be increased so that the disk can be repositioned on the condyle
3. Condyle must be in maximum forward translatory position.

- First attempt to reduce the disk—patient attempt to reduce the dislocation without assistance
- Patient is asked to move the mandible to the contralateral side of the dislocation as far as possible-from this eccentric position, the mouth is opened maximally
- Clinician places the thumb intraorally over the mandibular second molar on the affected side
- Fingers are placed on the inferior border of the mandible anterior to the thumb position
- Firm but controlled downward force is then exerted on the molar at the same time upward force is applied by the fingers
- The opposite hand stabilizes the cranium above the joint that is being distracted
- The condyle is brought downward and forward which translates it out of the fossa
- Distractive force has been applied for 20–30 seconds, it is discontinued
- If the disk has been successfully reduced, patient opens the mouth to full range
- An *anterior positioning appliance* is immediately placed to prevent clenching on the posterior teeth which would likely displace the disk again.

Chronic Phase

- Normal condyle-disk relationship not established: Condition progresses to chronic, non-reducing disk displacement
- With the condyle functioning off the disk, capsule and disk attachments progressively elongate, allowing the disk to be pushed gradually further forwards before condylar translation is obstructed
- Minor deflection of the mandibular midline at mouth opening is best observed when looking at the facial midline from above
- Patients with permanent disk dislocation—stabilization appliance that will reduce the forces to the retrodiscal tissues.

Supportive Therapy

- Educating the patient
- Not to open the mouth too widely, especially immediately after dislocation
- Decrease hard biting, gum chewing
- NSAIDs for pain and inflammation
- Heat or ice application to reduce pain.

Surgical considerations
Arthrocentesis
Arthroscopy
Arthrotomy
Plication
Diskectomy
Disc implants like silastic and proplast teflon

Arthrocentesis

Temporomandibular joint arthrocentesis entails placing two needles into the joint space for purposes of lysis and lavage via hydraulic distension. For arthropathy patients unresponsive to nonsurgical care, arthrocentesis is a simplified alternative to the most common arthroscopic surgical procedure. It is minimally invasive and may be performed in the office with comparable success and diminished morbidity in this technique normal ringer lactate used as a hypotonic solution.

Arthroscopy

Arthroscopic procedure are strongly indicated for closed condylar lock which was first described by Onishi in 1975.

STRUCTURAL INCOMPATIBILITY OF THE ARTICULAR SURFACES

- Can originate from any problem that disrupts normal joint functioning like trauma, pathologic process and excessive mouth opening
- These disorders are characterized by deviating movement patterns that are repeatable and difficult to avoid
  - Deviation in form
  - Adhesions
  - Subluxation
  - Spontaneous dislocation.

Deviation in Form

- Includes a group of disorders that are created by changes in the smooth articular surface of the joint and the disk
- An alteration in the normal pathway of condylar movement.

Cause: Trauma

Clinical characteristics

- Repeated alteration in the pathway of the opening and closing movements
- Click or deviation in opening always occurs at the same position of opening and closing
- May or may not be painful.

Definitive Treatment

- Return the altered structure to normal form
- Bony incompatibilty—smoothed and rounded
- Disc is perforated or misshapen—discoplasty

Supportive Therapy

- Patient education is encouraged to learn a manner of opening and closing that avoids or minimizes the dysfunction

- The increased interarticular pressure associated with bruxism can accentuate-stabilization appliance to decrease the muscle hyperactivity
- Pain analgesics to prevent the development of secondary central excitatory factors.

Adherences and Adhesions

- Adherences—Temporary sticking of the articular surfaces during normal joint movements
- Adhesions—More permanent and is caused by fibrosis attachment of the articular surfaces
- May occur between the disk and the condyle or the disk and the fossa.

Cause

- Adherences prolonged static loading of the joint structures
- If the adherence is maintained the more permanent condition of adhesion may develop
- May also develop secondary to hemarthrosis caused by macrotrauma or surgery.

History

- Adherences that develop occasionally but are broken or released during function can be diagnosed only through history
- Patient will report a long period when the jaw was statically loaded, followed by a sensation of limited mouth opening
- As the patient tries to open a single click is felt and normal range of movement is immediately returned
- The click or catching sensation does not return during opening or closing unless the joint is again statically loaded for a prolonged time
- These patients typically report that in the morning the jaw appears stiff until they pop it once and normal movement is restored
- Patients with adhesion often report restriction in the opening range of movement
- Related to the location of the adhesion.

Clinical Characteristics

- Adherences produce temporary restrictions in the mouth opening until the click occurs
- Adhesions produce more permanent limitation in the mouth opening
- Degree of restriction is dependent upon the location of the adhesion
- If only one joint is affected, the opening movement deflect to the ipsilateral side
- When permanent the dysfunction can be great
- In the inferior joint cavity—sudden jerky movement during opening
- In the superior joint cavity—restrict movement to rotation and thus limit the patient to 25–30 mm of opening
- If adhesion between disk and fossa—during mouth opening – force the condyle across the anterior border of the disk
- As disk is thinned and the anterior capsular and collateral ligaments elongated, the condyle moves over the disk and onto the attachment of the superior lateral pterygoid muscle
- In these cases the disk becomes dislocated posteriorly
- Far less common than an anterior dislocation
- Symptoms are constant and repeatable.

Definitive Treatment

- Decreasing loading to the articular surfaces.
- Loading related to either diurnal or nocturnal clenching
- Diurnal clenching-patient awareness PSR techniques
- Nocturnal clenching-stabilization appliance
- When adhesions are present-breaking the fibrous attachment
- Arthroscopic surgery
- Adhesions that are painless and produce only minor dysfunction.

Supportive Therapy

- Passive stretching
- Ultrasound—loosen the fibrous attachments
- Distraction of the joint.

INFLAMMATORY DISORDERS OF THE TMJ

- Continuous joint area pain accentuated by function
- Secondary central excitatory effects—cyclic muscle pain, hyperalgesia, referred pain:
  - Synovitis
  - Capsulitis
  - Retrodiskitis
  - Arthritides.

Synovitis and Capsulitis

Cause

- Trauma
- Spreading infection—antibiotic medication.

History

Macrotrauma.

Clinical Characteristics

- Any movement that tends to elongate the capsular ligament will accentuate the pain
- Pain: Directly in front of the ear and the lateral aspect of the condyle is tender to palpation.

Definitive Treatment

- Condition is self limiting—trauma is no longer present
- Recurrence of trauma—athletic appliance
- Secondary to microtrauma associated with disk derangement should be treated.

Supportive Therapy

- Restrict all mandibular movement within painless limits
- Soft diet, small movements and small bites are necessary
- Constant pain—mild analgesics like NSAID
- Thermotherapy—moist heat for 10–15 minutes for 4 or 5 times
- Ultrasound therapy—2–4 times per week
- Acute traumatic injury—single injection of corticosteroid to the capsular tissues.

Retrodiskitis

Inflammatory condition of the retrodiscal tissues is known as retrodiskitis.

Cause: Trauma

History

- Extrinsic trauma—report the incidence
- Intrinsic trauma—a more subtle history
  - Gradual onset of the pain
  - Progressive onset of the condition (clicking, catching).

Clinical Characteristics

- Constant preauricular pain accentuated with jaw movement
- Clenching the teeth, increases the pain
- If tissues swell: Loss of posterior occlusal contact on the ipsilateral side.

Definitive Treatment for Retrodiskitis from Extrinsic Trauma

Cause of macrotrauma is not present—no definitive treatment is indicated.

Supportive therapy
- Analgesics for pain
- Restrict movement within painless limits
- Soft diet
- Ultrasound and thermotherapy
- Single intracapsular injection of corticosteroids.

Definitive Treatment for Retrodiskitis from Intrinsic Trauma

- Intrinsic trauma often remains and continues to cause injury to the tissues
- Eliminating the traumatic condition.

Supportive therapy
- Volutarily restricting use of the mandible to within painless limits
- Analgesics when pain not resolved with the positioning appliance
- Thermotherapy and ultrasound.

Arthritis

- Arthritis: Inflammation of the articular surfaces of the joint
- Osteoarthritis is the most common arthrides affecting the TMJ
- Referred to as degenerative joint disease.

Cause

- Overloading of the articular structures of the joint
- Joint surfaces are compromised by disk dislocation and retrodiskitis
- Not a true inflammatory response
- Non-inflammatory condition—articular surfaces and their underlying bone deteriorate
- When bony changes are active, the condition is active and often painful osteoarthritis
- Cause can be identified—secondary osteoarthritis
- Cause cannot be identified—primary osteoarthritis.

History

- Unilateral joint pain that is aggravated by mandibular movement
- Pain constant but worsens in the late afternoon or evening
- Secondary central excitatory effects are present.

Clinical Characteristics

- Limited mandibular opening
- Crepitation
- Lateral palpation of the condyle increases the pain
- Manual loading of the joint
- TMJ radiographs—structural changes in the subarticular bone of the condyle or the fossa (flattening, osteophytes, and erosions).

Definitive Treatment

- Decrease mechanical overloading of the joint structures
- Attempt to correct the condyle—disc relationship (anterior positioning appliance)

- Muscle hyperactivity—stabilization appliance
- PSR techniques

Supportive therapy

- Self limiting disorder
- Conservative treatment is indicated for most patients—reduce symptoms and hasten the adaptive process
- Pain medication and anti-inflammatory agents
- Restrict the movement to within painless limits
- Soft diet
- Thermotherapy
- Passive muscle exercises
- Single injection of corticosteroids.

Osteoarthrosis

- Bony changes are active—osteoarthritis
- Remodeling occurs the condition can become stable, bony morphology remains altered-osteoarthrosis.

Cause

Overloading.

History

Does not report symptoms, the history may reveal a time when symptoms were present.

Clinical Characteristics

- Osteoarthrosis confirmed—structural changes in the subarticular bone are seen on the radiographs
- No clinical symptoms of pain
- Crepitation is common.

Definitive treatment

- No therapy indicated
- If orthopedic instability—dental therapy.

MYOFASCIAL PAIN DYSFUNCTION SYNDROME

Introduction

Myofascial pain dysfunction is a major cause of musculoskeletal pain. It is a frequent cause of neck

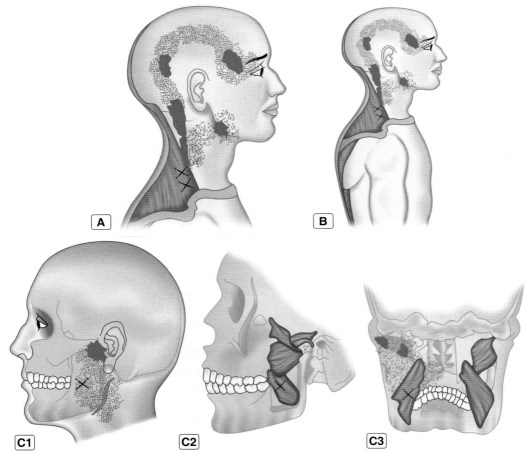

Figs 33.3A to C: Trigger points location over different muscles: (A) Head region, (B) Trapezius, (C) Medial pterygoid

pain and back pain. The traditional and narrow definition of myofascial pain is that it is pain that arises from trigger points (TRPs) in a muscle. TRPs are small and sensitive areas in a muscle that spontaneously or upon compression cause pain to distant region, known as the referred pain zone. Myofascial pain can vary from localized pain to a diffuse headache with neck pain. It is an extremely common and frustrating problem. Trigger points can cause intence spreading pain as a result of neural feedback (Figs 33.3A to C). It may present as regional musculoskeletal pain, as neck or back pain and may also present as shoulder pain.

Myofascial pain (MFP) which is treatable is often underdiagnosed and hence undertreated. With rehabilitation many patients do not have to continue to suffer unnecessary pain that affects their daily activities and quality of life. If left undiagnosed, untreated, it may lead to chronic pain with overlying psychosocial and functional problems, which leads to further distress, anxiety and even depression. This major source of musculoskeletal dysfunction requires more focused clinical attention which bears great impact on the quality of patients life.

Precipitating factor of MFP may cause the release of acetylecholine at motor end plates, sustained muscle fiber contraction and local ischemia with release of vascular and neuroactive substances, and muscle pain. More acetylcholine may then be released, thus perpetuating the facial spasm and muscle pain .

History

- 1956 Schwartz: TMJ pain dysfunction syndrome-spasm of masticatory and perimasticatory musculature
- 1969 Laskin: Myofascial pain dysfunction syndrome-psychophysiologic theory.

Definition

Myofascial pain dysfunction syndrome (MPDS) is a pain disorder in which unilateral pain is referred from the trigger points in myofascial structures to the muscles of the head and neck (Figs 33.3A to C).

Pathophysiology Psychological Occlusal Intrinsic Joint Disorder

- Muscular hyperfunction
- Physical disorders
- Injuries to tissues
- Parafunctional habits
- Disuse
- Nutritional problems
- Physiological stress
- Sleep disturbances.

Signs and Symptoms

- Pain—head and neck
- Limitation of motion of jaw
- Joint noises
- Tenderness to palpation of muscles of mastication
- Associated symptoms of MPDS: Neurologic, otologic-ear pain, GIT disturbance, musculosketal.

Examination

- Physical examinaton:
- Muscular examination
- Dental/occlusal examination
- Cervical examination
- Psychological evaluation
- Internal derangement.

Treatment

Education and Self Care

- Reassurance of the patient
- Elimination of self injurious oral habits like jaw clenching, chewing gums
- Provide information on jaw care associated with daily activities.

Pharmacotherapeutic Modalities

- NSAIDs
- Muscle relaxants
- Ethylchloride spray or intramuscular injections of LA in the affected muscles.

Physiotherapeutic Modalities

- Heat application
- Ultrasound
- Cryotherapy
- Massage with counter irritants and vibrators
- Use of vapocoolent sprays like ethyl chloride spray
- TENS
- Electrogalvanic stimulation.

Intra-articular Injections
Auriculotemporal Nerve Block
Behavioral/Relaxation Therapy

- Biofeedback
- Hypnosis
- Cognitive behavioral therapy
- Occlusal splints.

Clinical Cases of Temporomandibular Joint Pathology

34

CASE NUMBER 1

A 16-year-old female patient reported to the department of oral and maxillofacial surgery with complaints of pain and deviation of the jaw towards right side since last 2 days.

History of Presenting Illness

- An unintentional blow to the left side of face 2 days back
- Deviation to the right side (Fig. 34.1)
- Unable to bring back into position
- Associated with mild pain.

Past History

- Similar incident 5 years back
- Blow to left side of face
- Jaw deviation to right
- Sought medical advice after a week

- Diagnosed: dislocation of temporomandibular joint (TMJ) (left side)
- Dislocation reduced and IMF done for 1 week.
- *Medical history*: Nothing relevant reported
  Personal history: Mixed diet
  – No parafunctional habits.

General Physical Examination

- Conscious, cooperative and well oriented
- Vitals – stable
- No signs of pallor, icterus, cyanosis, clubbing, edema and lymphadenopathy.

Extraoral Examination

Inspection flatness on the left side of face and protrusion of the mandible (Fig. 34.2).
Palpation: Tenderness over the left preauricular region

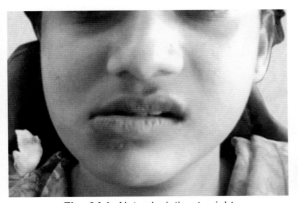

Fig. 34.1: Note deviation to right

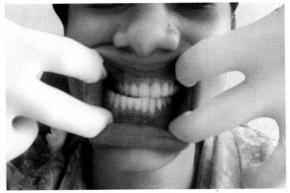

Fig. 34.2: Note cross bite on right side

Intraoral Examination

Provisional Diagnosis

TMJ dislocation – left side.

Investigations

- OPG (Fig. 34.3)
- Transcranial view (Fig. 34.4).

Final Diagnosis

Left TMJ recurrent dislocation.

Treatment

Reduction of dislocation (Figs 34.5 to 34.10)

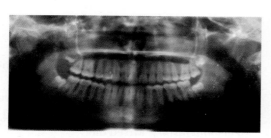

Fig. 34.3: Dislocated condyle

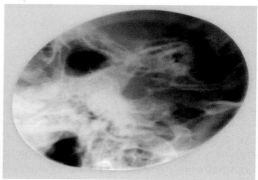

Fig. 34.4: Condylar dislocation

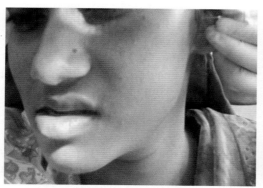

Fig. 34.5: Step I in reduction

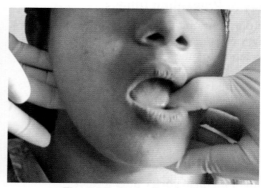

Fig. 34.6: Reduction in progress

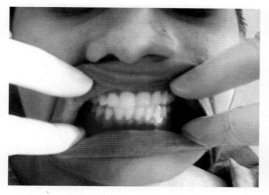

Fig. 34.7: Occlusion after reduction

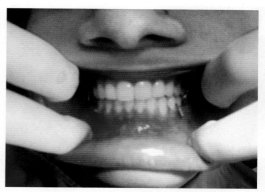

Fig. 34.8: Intermaxillary fixation

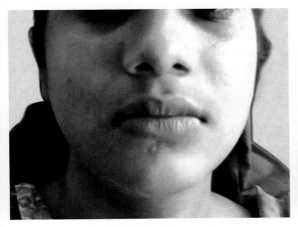

Fig. 34.9: Post-treatment

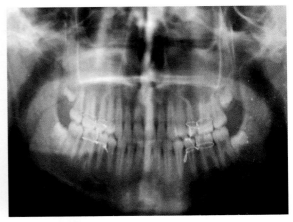

Fig. 34.10: OPG

CASE NUMBER 2

A 37-year-old gentleman reported to our department with the chief complaint of inability to open mouth widely (Figs 34.11).

History of Present Illness

He had history of trauma 10 years back with restricted mouth opening since 6 years.

Medical History

No relevant history.

Drug History

Nothing contributory.

Dental History

Patient underwent conservative treatment for the same at a local dentist.

Family History

No contributing factors.

General Physical Examination

- Patient is moderately built and nourished
- Cooperative
- Vitals
  - BP: 150/90 mm of Hg
  - Pulse: 88/min
  - CVS, CNS, RS – NAD

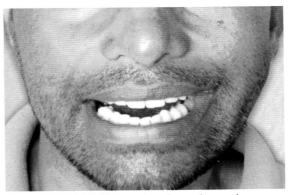

Fig. 34.11: Note reduced mouth opening

Extraoral Examination

- No gross facial asymmetry detected
- Deviation of mandible and chin to the left on opening
- Mouth opening was 18 mm
- Slight deviation of the mandible to the left on closing.

Radiographs

OPG shows no clear joint space (Fig. 34.12)

Clinical Diagnosis

Fibrous ankylosis left side.

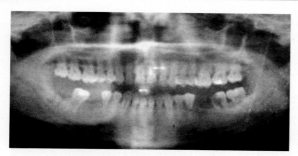

Fig. 34.12: Joint space not clear

CASE NUMBER 3

A 26-year-old male patient reported to our department complaining of lower jaw being deviated to one side and sharp pain in the right TMJ while chewing food.

History of Presenting Illness

- Patient noticed the lower jaw getting progressively deviated to the left side since 4 years.
- Associated with the pain in the right TMJ.
- Pain is nonradiating and is relieved on taking medication.

Medical History

No relevant medical history.

Past Dental History

- History of visit to a local dentist 10 months back for the same complain.
- He was informed about the need of surgery for right TMJ.
- But due to time constraints was unable to undergo treatment.

General Physical Examination

- Conscious and cooperative
- Well built and nourished
- No signs of pallor, icterus, cyanosis, clubbing, edema
- Vital signs - normal

Extra Oral Examination

- Gross facial asymmetry detected
- Reduced fullness of face on left side
- Midline shifted to left in the lower 3rd of the face
- Chin and mandible deviated to left side

Inspection

- Reduced range of movement
- Deviation to left side on closing the mouth
- Mouth opening – 40 mm

Palpation

- Bulge of condyle felt 2.5 cm anterior to the tragus on right side
- No clicking
- No tenderness
- No crepitation

Intraoral Examination

- Teeth present
  87654321   12345678
  8765432   12345678
- FPD with 41
- Cross bite present
- Calculus and stains present

Provisional Diagnosis

- Osteochondroma of right condyle
- Chondroma of right condyle
- Osteoma of right condyle

Investigations

See Figures 34.13 to 34.21.

Treatment

Intentional fracture of condyle +
- Excision of bony lesion +
- Recontouring of condylar head +
- Reimplantation of condyle (Figs 34.22 to 34.29).

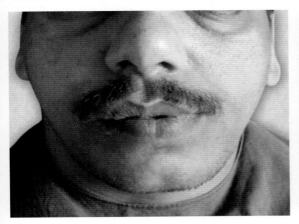

Fig. 34.13: Note deviation

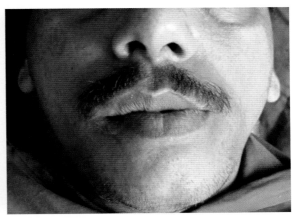

Fig. 34.14: Marked facial asymmetry

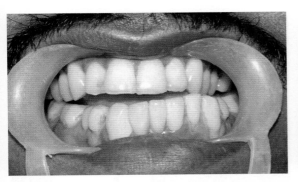

Fig. 34.15: Preoperative occlusion

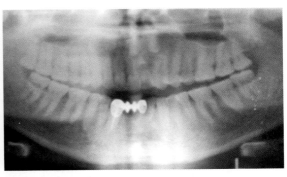

Fig. 34.16: OPG: Note distorted right condylar head

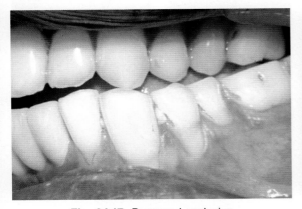

Fig. 34.17: Deranged occlusion

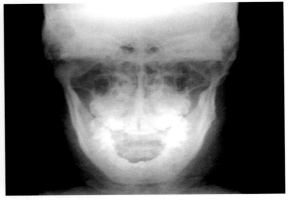

Fig. 34.18: Transcranial view: Note distorted right condylar head

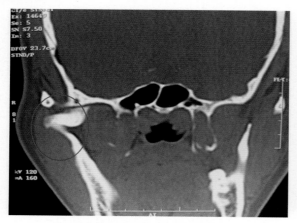

Fig. 34.19: Note right condylar head

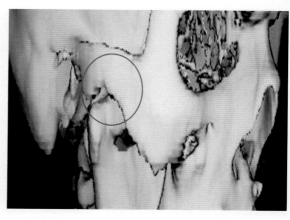

Fig. 34.20: Note distorted right condylar head

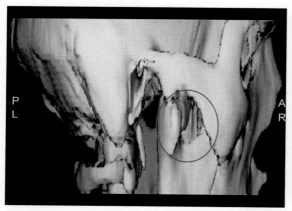

Fig. 34.21: Note distorted right condylar head anatomy

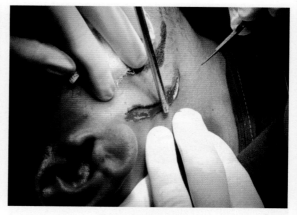

Fig. 34.22: Incision

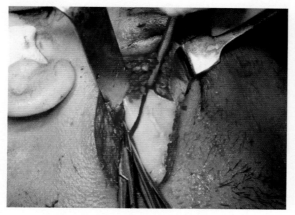

Fig. 34.23: Intentional fracturing condyle

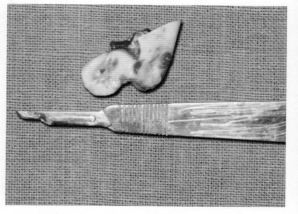

Fig. 34.24: Bony lesion attached to condylar head

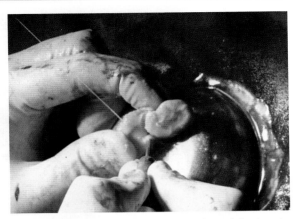

Fig. 34.25: Surgical recontouring of condylar head

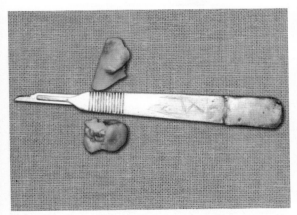

Fig. 34.26: Condylar head seperated from lesion

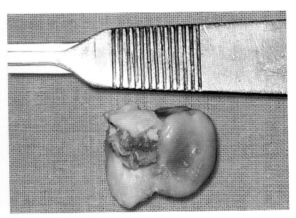

Fig. 34.27: Bony lesion

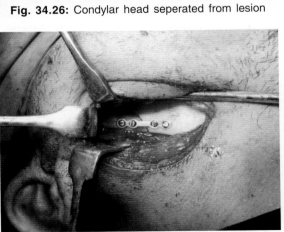

Fig. 34.28: Replated condylar head

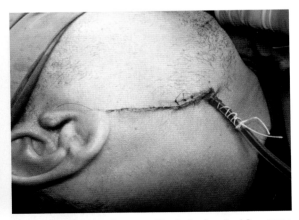

Fig. 34.29: Skin closure with drain *in situ* (*Courtesy* of Figures 34.22 to 34.29: Dr Murlee Mohan)

OSTEOCHONDROMA OF THE CORONOID PROCESS (FIGS 34.30 TO 34.34)

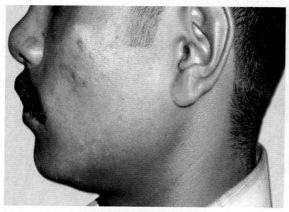

Fig. 34.30: Zygomatic prominence

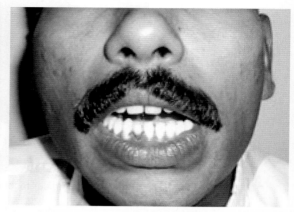

Fig. 34.31: Reduced mouth opening

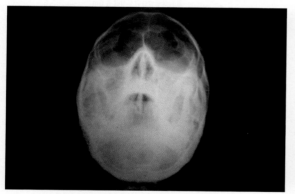

Fig. 34.32: Note coronoid process

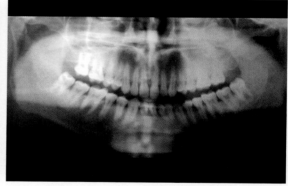

Fig. 34.33: Note left coronoids distorted anatomy

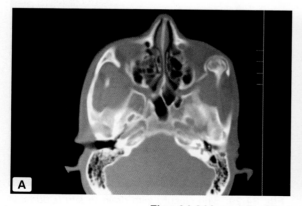

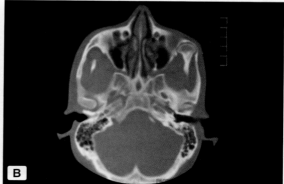

Figs 34.34A and B: CT showing coronoids enlargement

Section

7

Maxillofacial Infections

Fascial Spaces and Odontogenic Infections

35

INTRODUCTION

Infections in the oral and maxillofacial areas are frequently originated as odontogenic infections, even though majority of odontogenic infection are easily controlled with antibiotics and specific treatments (incision and drainage and extraction), fulminant infection and severe complication are possible. Spread of infections through deep fascial spaces is determined by the presence and pattern of loss of connective tissue.

Airway obstruction, necrotizing fasciitis, cavernous sinus thrombosis, extension to other areas and death are considered major complications.

Infection

- The lodgement and multiplication of an organism in or on the tissue of a host constitutes infection
- It does not invariably result in disease, but is a rare consequence of infection, which is a common natural event
- Establishing an infection involves three factors:
  - The host
  - The agent
  - Environment.

Inoculation

It is characterized by the entry of pathogenic microbes into the body without disease occurring.

Inflammation

It is the localized reaction of vascular and connective tissue of the body to an irritant, resulting in the development of an exudate rich in proteins and cells. This reaction is protective and aims at limiting or eliminating the irritant with various procedures while the mechanism of tissue repair is triggered. Depending on the duration and severity, inflammation is distinguished as acute, subacute or chronic.

Acute Inflammation

This is characterized by rapid progression and is associated with typical signs and symptoms. If it does not regress completely, it may become subacute or chronic.

Subacute Inflammation

This is considered a transition phase between acute and chronic inflammation.

Chronic Inflammation

- This procedure presents a prolonged time frame with slight clinical symptoms and is characterized mainly by the development of connective tissue
- Inflammation may be caused by, among other things, microbes, physical and chemical factors, heat, and irradiation
- Regardless of the type of irritant and the location of the defect, the manifestation of inflammation is typical and is characterized by

the following clinical signs and symptoms—rubor (redness), calor (heat), tumor (swelling or edema), dolor (pain), and functio laesa (loss of function)

- The natural progression of inflammation is distinguished into various phases. Initially vascular reactions with exudate are observed (serous phase), and then the cellular factors are triggered (exudative or cellular phase). The inflammation finally resolves and the destroyed tissues are repaired. On the other hand, chronic inflammation is characterized by factors of reparation and healing. Therefore, while acute inflammation is exudative, chronic inflammation is productive (exudative and reparative). Understanding the differences between these types of inflammation is important for therapeutic treatment.

Serous phase: This is a procedure that lasts approximately 36 hours and is characterized by local inflammatory edema, hyperemia, or redness with elevated temperature, and pain. Serous exudate is observed at this stage, which contains proteins and rarely polymorphonuclear leukocytes.

Cellular phase: This is the progression of the serous phase. It is characterized by massive accumulation of polymorphonuclear leukocytes, especially neutrophil granulocytes, leading to pus formation. If pus forms in a newly developed cavity, it is called an abscess. If it develops in a cavity that already exists, e.g. the maxillary sinus, it is called an empyema.

Reparative phase

- During inflammation, the reparative phenomena begin almost immediately after inoculation
- With the reparative mechanism of inflammation, the products of the acute inflammatory reaction are removed and reparation of the destroyed tissues follows. Repair is achieved with development of granulation tissue, which is converted to fibrous connective tissue, whose development ensures the return of the region to normal.

INFECTIONS OF THE OROFACIAL REGION

- Majority (i.e. 90–95%) of infections, which manifest in the orofacial region are odontogenic
- Of these, approximately 70% present as periapical inflammation, principally the acute dentoalveolar abscess, with the periodontal abscess following, etc.

Objectives

- Understand the microbiology of odontogenic infections
- Understand the signs symptoms and findings in patients with odontogenic infections
- Review the various pathways of spread with odontogenic infections
- Understand the medical and surgical management of odontogenic infections
- Infections of orofacial and neck region, particularly those of odontogenic origin, have been one of the most common diseases in human beings
- Most of these infections can be managed successfully without any complications but if unattended can produce serious complications and can prove fatal
- Early recognition of orofacial infection and prompt, appropriate therapy is absolutely essential
- A thorough knowledge of anatomy of the face and neck is necessary to predict pathways of spread of these infections and to drain these spaces adequately.

Etiology

Based on the Origin of Infection

- Odontogenic
  - Pulp disease
  - Periodontal disease
  - Secondarily infected cysts or odontomes
  - Remaining root fragment
  - Residual infection
  - Pericoronal infection
- Traumatic
- Implant surgery
- Reconstructive surgery

- Infections arising from contaminated needle punctures
- Secondary to oral malignancies
- Salivary gland infections

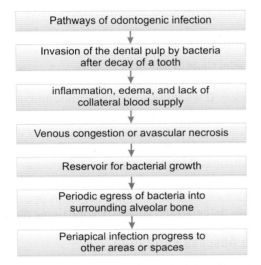

- Serious dental infection spreading beyond the tooth socket is more common due to the pulpal infection than the periodontal infection. The principal infection progress can vary according to the following:
  – The number and virulence of the organism
  – Host resistance
  – Anatomy of the involved area.

Microbiological Factors

- Odontogenic infections are multimicrobial
- Gram (+) cocci, aerobic and anaerobic:
  – Streptococci and their anaerobic counterpart, peptostreptococci
  – Staphylococci, and their anaerobic counterpart, peptococci
- Gram (+) rods:
  Lactobacillus, Diphtheroids, Actinomyces
- Gram (–) rods:
  Fusobacterium, Bacteroids, Eikenella, Pseudomonas (occasional).

Host Factors

Immunity against intraoral infection is composed of three sets of mechanisms:

- Humoral factors
- Cellular factors
- Local factors.

Decrease in one of these mechanisms and it increases the potential for infection.

Humoral Factors

- Circulating immunoglobulins, along with complement, combine with microbes to form opsonins that promote phagocytosis by macrophages
- IgA prevents colonization of microbes on oral mucosal surfaces
- In presence of infection, histamine, serotonin, prostaglandins support inflammation → vasodilation and increased vascular permeability.

Cellular Factors

- Phagocytes engulf and kill microbes, removing them, preventing replication
- Lymphocytes produce lymphokines and immunoglobulines (aids humoral)
- Lymphokines stimulate reproduction of other lymphocytes, and kills antigens.

Local Factors

Specific factors leading to resistance:
- Abundant vascular supply allowing humoral and cellular response
- Mechanical cleansing by salivary flow
- Secretory IgA contained within saliva
- High epithelial turnover and sloughing, taking with it adherent bacteria
- A variety of microflora normally preventing selection for a single organism by competing for nutrients or release of by-products.

Historical Features

- Slowly enlarging swelling with a dull ache or recurrent draining abscess that swells and drains spontaneously is not likely to require aggressive treatment within the hour—the patient's immune response is effectively containing the spread of infection
- However, 24-hour painful swelling causing pain during swallowing or severe trismus needs aggressive and prompt treatment

- Immediate treatment or referral is critical when patient's immune system has not been able to contain the infection.
- Specific warning signs include:
  - Dyspnea (difficulty breathing)
  - Dysphagia (difficulty/pain with swallowing)
  - Severe trismus
  - Rapidly progressive swelling.

TYPES OF INFECTION

- Acute:
  - Acute periapical abscess
  - Acute periodontal abscess
  - Cellulitis.
- Chronic:
  - Chronic abscess leading to fistulous tract or sinus formation.
- If untreated or improperly treated, infections can lead to:
  - Focal osteomyelitis
  - Widespread osteomyelitis
  - Fistulous tract
  - Intraoral or cutaneous soft tissue abscess
  - Cellulitis
  - Bacteremia—septicemia
  - Deep fascial space infection
  - Ascending facial cerebral infection.

Basis of Causative Organisms

- Bacterial infection:
  - Odontogenic infections in orofascial region
  - Nonodontogenic infection like tonsillar, nasal and furuncle of overlying skin.
- Fungal infection
- Viral infection.

Clinical Features

- Inflammation is tissue response to injury or invasion by microorganisms that involve vaso-dilation, capillary permeability, mobilization of leukocytes, and phagocytosis.

Cardinal Signs of Inflammation

- Red, hot, swelling, pain, with loss of function
- Other findings: regional lymphadenopathy, fever, elevated white blood cell count, tachy-cardia, tachypnea, dehydration, malaise.

Cellulitis

- Initial stage of infection
- Is spreading infection of loose connective tissue. It is a diffuse, erythematous, mucosal or cutaneous infection
- Diffuse, reddened, soft or hard swelling that is tender to palpation
- Inflammatory response not yet forming a true abscess
- Microorganisms have just begun to overcome host defenses and spread beyond tissue planes.

True Abscess Formation

- As inflammatory response matures, may develop a focal accumulation of pus (Fig. 35.1)
- Is a circumscribed collection of pus in a pathological tissue space. A true abscess is a thick walled cavity containing pus
- May have spontaneous drainage intraorally or extraorally.

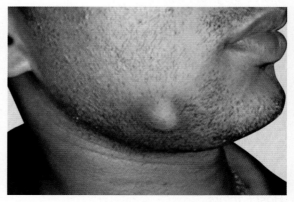

Fig. 35.1: Extraoral swelling

Oral Tissue Examination

Examine Quality and Consistency

- Soft to fluctuant (fluid filled) to hard (indurated)
- Color and temperature determine the presence and extent of infection.

Normal versus Abnormal Tissue Architecture

- Distortion of mucobuccal fold
- Soft palate symmetric with uvula in midline (deviation indicates involvement of lateral pharyngeal space)
- Nasal tip, nasolabial fold, circumorbital areas

Identify Causative Factors

- Tooth, root tip, foreign body, etc.
- Vital signs should be taken.
- Temperature >101–102°F accompanied by an elevated heart rate indicate systemic involvement of the infection and increased urgency of treatment.

Periodontal Abscess

- This is an acute or chronic purulent inflammation, which develops in an existing periodontal pocket
- Clinically, it is characterized by edema located at the middle of the tooth, pain and redness of the gingiva. These symptoms are not as severe as those observed in the acute dentoalveolar abscess
- Treatment of the periodontal abscess is usually simple and entails incision, through the gingival sulcus with a probe or scalpel, of the periodontal pocket that has become obstructed.

Acute Dentoalveolar Abscess

This is an acute purulent inflammation of the periapical tissues, presenting at nonvital teeth, especially when microbes exit the infected root canals into periapical tissues.

Local Symptoms

Pain

- The severity of the pain depends on the stage of development of the inflammation. In the initial phase, the pain is dull and continuous and worsens during percussion of the responsible tooth or when it comes into contact with antagonist teeth. If the pain is very severe and pulsates, it means that the accumulation of pus is still within the bone or underneath the periosteum
- Relief of pain begins as soon as the pus perforates the periosteum and exits into the soft tissues.

Edema

- Edema appears intraorally or extraorally and it usually has a buccal localization and more rarely palatal or lingual. In the initial phase soft swelling of the soft tissues of the affected side is observed, due to the reflex neuroregulating reaction of the tissues, especially of the periosteum. This swelling presents before suppuration, particularly in areas with loose tissue, such as the sublingual region, lips, or eyelids. Usually the edema is soft with redness of the skin
- During the final stages, the swelling fluctuates, especially at the mucosa of the oral cavity. This stage is considered the most suitable for incision and drainage of the abscess.

Other Symptoms

There is a sense of elongation of the responsible tooth and slight mobility; the tooth feels extremely sensitive to touch, while difficulty in swallowing is also observed.

Systemic Symptoms

The systemic symptoms usually observed are: Fever, which may rise to 39–40°C, chills, malaise with pain in muscles and joints, anorexia, insomnia, nausea, and vomiting. The laboratory tests show leukocytosis or rarely leukopenia, an increased erythrocyte sedimentation rate, and a raised C-reactive protein (CRP) level.

Complications

If the inflammation is not treated promptly, the following complications may occur—trismus, lymphadenitis at the respective lymph nodes, osteomyelitis, bacteremia and septicemia.

Diagnosis

- Diagnosis is usually based upon clinical examination and the patient's history
- Localization of the responsible tooth
- In the initial phase of inflammation, there is soft swelling of the soft tissues. The tooth is also sensitive during palpation of the apical area and during percussion with an instrument, while the tooth is hypermobile and there is a sense of elongation
- In more advanced stages, the pain is exceptionally severe, even after the slightest contact with the tooth surface. Tooth reaction during a test with an electric vitalometer is negative; however, sometimes it appears positive, which is due to conductivity of the fluid inside the root canal
- Radiographically, in the acute phase, no signs are observed at the bone (which may be observed 8–10 days later), unless there is recurrence of a chronic abscess, where upon osteolysis is observed
- Differential diagnosis of the acute dentoalveolar abscess includes the periodontal abscess.

Spread of Pus inside Tissues

- Inflammation may spread in three ways:
  - By continuity through tissue spaces and planes
  - By way of the lymphatic system
  - By way of blood circulation.
- The most common route of spread of inflammation is by continuity through tissue spaces and planes. First of all, pus is formed in the cancellous bone, and spreads in various directions by way of the tissues presenting the least resistance. Whether the pus spreads buccally, palatally or lingually depends mainly on the position of the tooth in the dental arch, the thickness of the bone, and the distance it must travel
- Purulent inflammation that is associated with apices near the buccal or labial alveolar bone usually spreads buccally, while that associated with apices near the palatal or lingual alveolar bone spreads palatally or lingually respectively. For example, the palatal roots of the posterior teeth and the maxillary lateral incisor are considered responsible for the palatal spread of pus, while the mandibular third molar and sometimes the mandibular second molar are considered responsible for the lingual spread of infection
- Inflammation may even spread into the maxillary sinus when the apices of posterior teeth are found inside or close to the floor of the antrum
- The length of the root and the relationship between the apex and the proximal and distal attachments of various muscles also play a significant role in the spread of pus. Depending on these relationships, in the mandible pus originates from the apices found above the mylohyoid muscle, and usually spreads intraorally, mainly towards the floor of the mouth (sublingual space). When the apices are found beneath the mylohyoid muscle (second and third molar), the pus spreads towards the submandibular space resulting in extraoral localization
- Infection originating from incisors and canines of the mandible spreads buccally or lingually, due to the thin alveolar bone of the area. It is usually localized buccally if the apices are found above the attachment of the mentalis muscle
- In the maxilla, the attachment of the buccinator muscle is significant. When the apices of the maxillary premolars and molars are found beneath the attachment of the buccinator muscle, the pus spreads intraorally; however, if the apices are found above its attachment, infection spreads upwards and extraorally. Exactly the same phenomenon is observed in the mandible as in the maxilla if the apices are found above or below the attachment of the buccinator muscle
- The initial stage of the cellular phase is characterized by accumulation of pus in the alveolar bone and is termed an intra-alveolar abscess

In the cellular stage, depending on the pathway and inoculation site of the pus, the acute dentoalveolar abscess may have various clinical presentations, such as:
Intra-alveolar
Subperiosteal
Submucosal
Subcutaneous, and
Fascial or migratory—cervicofacial

- The pus spreads outwards from this site and, after perforating the bone, spreads to the subperiosteal space, from which the subperiosteal abscess originates, where a limited amount of pus accumulates between the bone and periosteum
- After perforation of the periosteum, the pus continues to spread through the soft tissues in various directions. It usually spreads intraorally, spreading underneath the mucosa forming the submucosal abscess
- Sometimes, it spreads through the loose connective tissue and, after its pathway underneath the skin, forms a subcutaneous abscess
- While other times it spreads towards the fascial spaces, forming fascial space abscesses. The fascial spaces are bounded by the fascia, which may stretch or be perforated by the purulent exudate, facilitating the spread of infection. These spaces are potential areas and do not exist in healthy individuals, developing only in cases of spread of infection that have not been treated promptly
- Acute diffuse infection, which spreads into the loose connective tissue to a great extent underneath the skin with or without suppuration, is termed cellulitis (phlegmon).

Principles in Treatment of Oral and Paraoral Infections

- Remove the cause
- Establish drainage
- Institute antibiotic therapy
- Supportive care, including proper rest and nutrition.

FASCIAL SPACE INFECTIONS

- These infections involve fascial spaces and are usually of odontogenic origin
- Each of these pathologic conditions is described below, including discussion of their anatomic location, etiology, clinical presentation, and therapeutic treatment.

Classification of fascial spaces

Based on Mode of Involvement

- Direct involvement:
  - Primary spaces—maxillary and mandibular spaces
- Indirect invovlement:
  - Secondary spaces.

Spaces Involved in Odontogenic Infections

- Primary maxillary spaces—canine, buccal and infratemporal spaces
- Primary mandibular spaces—submental, buccal, submandibular and sublingual spaces
- Secondary fascial spaces—masseteric, pterygomandibular, superficial and deep temporal, lateral pharyngeal, retropharyngeal, prevertebral spaces, parotid space.

Spaces of Clinical Significance

Face:
- Buccal
- Canine
- Masticator
- Masseteric compartment
- Pterygoid compartment
- Zygomaticotemporal compartment.

Suprahyoid:
- Sublingual
- Submandibular
- Lateral pharyngeal
- Peritonsillar.

Infrahyoid:
- Anterovisceral (pretracheal).

Space of total neck:
- Retropharyngeal
- Danger space
- Space of carotid sheath.

Numbered Spaces of Grodensky and Holyoke

Space 1: Superficial to superficial fascia hence synonymous with subcutaneous space.

Space 2: Group of spaces surrounding strap muscles lying superficial to sternothyroid-thyrohyoid or between sternothyroid-thyrohyoid and sternohyoid-omohyoid.

Space 3: Superficial to visceral division of middle layer of deep cervical fascia. It contains pretracheal, retropharyngeal and lateral pharyngeal spaces.

Space 3A: Carotid sheath.

Space 4: Potential space between the alar and prevertebral division of posterior layer of deep cervical fascia. Also called "Danger space".

Space 4A: Posterior triangle of the neck, posterior to carotid sheath.

Space 5: Prevertebral space.

Space 5A: Enclosed by prevertebral fascia, posterior to the transverse process of the vertebrae as it surrounds scalene and spinal posture muscles.

Abscess of Base of Upper Lip

This abscess develops at the loose connective tissue of the base of the upper lip at the anterior region of the maxilla, beneath the pear-shaped aperture (Figs 35.2 and 35.3).

Etiology

It is usually caused by infected root canals of maxillary anterior teeth.

Clinical Presentation

- Swelling and protrusion of the upper lip
- Obliteration of the depth of the mucolabial fold.

Treatment

- The incision for drainage is made at the mucolabial fold parallel to the alveolar process
- A hemostat is then inserted inside the cavity, which reaches bone, aiming for the apex of the responsible tooth, facilitating the evacuation of pus
- After drainage of the abscess, a rubber drain is placed until the clinical symptoms of the infection subside.

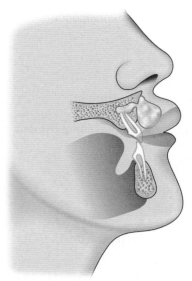

Fig. 35.2: Spread of infection upper to lower anterior

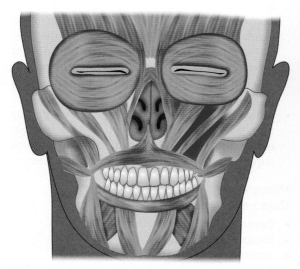

Fig. 35.3: Cannine space infection

Canine Fossa Space/Infraorbital Space

The canine fossa is a small space between the levator labii superioris and the levator anguli oris muscles.

Involvement

- Odontogenic infections arising from maxillary canine and premolars and sometimes from mesiobuccal root of first molar
- Nasal infections; less frequent.

Boundaries

- Inferiorly—caninus muscle
- Anteriorly—orbicularis oris
- Posteriorly—buccinator muscle
- Medially—anterolateral surface of maxilla.

Clinical Features

- Swelling of cheek and upper lip
- Obliteration of nasolabial fold (Fig. 35.4 and 35.5)
- Drooping of angle of the mouth
- Edema of lower eyelid
- Offending tooth may be mobile and tender to percussion.

Treatment

- The incision for drainage is performed intraorally at the mucobuccal fold (parallel to the alveolar bone), in the canine region
- A hemostat is then inserted, which is placed at the depth of the purulent accumulation until it comes into contact with bone, while the index finger of the nondominant hand palpates the infraorbital margin
- Finally, a rubber drain is placed, which is stabilized with a suture on the mucosa.

Palatal Abscess

- Intraorally a well-defined circumscribed fluctuant swelling is seen, which is confined to one side of the palate, adjacent to the offending tooth
- Incision and drainage (I and D).

Buccal Space

- The space in which this abscess develops is between the buccinator and masseter muscles
- Superiorly, it communicates with the pterygopalatine space; inferiorly with the pterygomandibular space. The spread of pus in the buccal space depends on the position of the apices of the responsible teeth relative to the attachment of the buccinator muscle. Location of root tip to the level of origin of buccinator muscle determines the spread of infection either intraorally into the vestibule or deep into the buccal space.

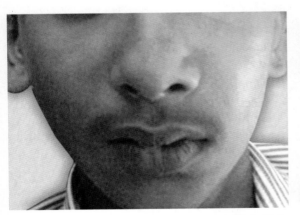 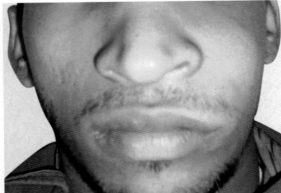

Figs 35.4 and 35.5: Notice obliterated nasolabial angle

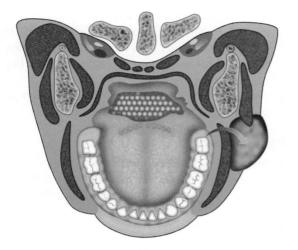

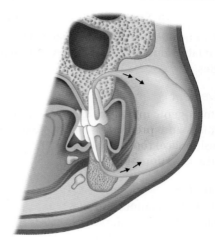

Figs 35.6 and 35.7: Buccal space infection (internal view)

Boundaries (Figs 35.6 to 35.8)

- Anteromedially—buccinator musle
- Posteromedially—masseter overlying the anterior border of the ramus of the mandible
- Laterally by forward extension of deep fascia from the capsule of parotid gland and by platysma muscle
- Inferiorly limited by the attachment of the deep fascia to the mandible and by depressor anguli oris
- Superiorly the zygomatic process of the maxilla and zygomaticus major and minor muscles.

Teeth Commonly Involved

- Maxillary and mandibular premolars and molar
- Pericoronitis in lower third molar.

Clinical Features

- Fluctuant swelling of cheek with an obvious swelling of the face
- Infection from the buccal space may extend upwards into temporal space or gravitate down into the submandibular space.

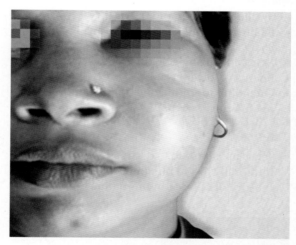

Fig. 35.8: Buccal space infection (external view)

Treatment

- Access to the buccal space is usually intraoral for three main reasons:
  - Because the abscess fluctuates intraorally in the majority of cases
  - To avoid injuring the facial nerve
  - For esthetic reasons.

- The intraoral incision is made at the posterior region of the mouth, in an anteroposterior direction and very carefully in order to avoid injury of the parotid duct
- A hemostat is then used to explore the space thoroughly
- An extraoral incision is made when intraoral access would not ensure adequate drainage, or when the pus is deep inside the space. The incision is made approximately 2 cm below and parallel to the inferior border of the mandible.

Submental Space

Boundaries

- *Laterally*: Lower border of the mandible, anterior belly of digastric
- *Superiorly*: Mylohyoid muscle
- *Inferiorly*: Suprahyoid portion of the investing layer of deep cervical fascia which is covered by platysma superficial fascia and skin.

Contents

Submental lymph nodes and anterior jugular vein.

Etiology

Infection of the submental space usually originates in the mandibular anterior teeth or is the result of spread of infection from other anatomic spaces (mental, sublingual, submandibular).

Clinical Features

- Extaorally distinct firm swelling in the midline beneath the chin skin overlying may be boardlike and taut (Figs 35.9 to 35.11). Fluctuation may be present
- Intraorally the offending tooth may exhibit tenderness to percussion and may show mobility.

Treatment

- After local anesthesia is performed around the abscess, an incision on the skin is made beneath the chin, in a horizontal direction and parallel to the anterior border of the chin (Fig. 35.12).

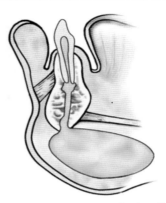

Fig. 35.9: Submental space infection (internal view)

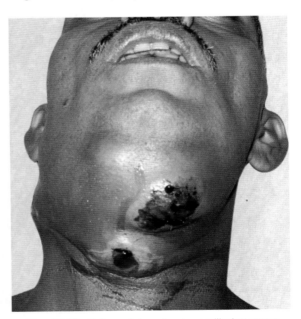

Fig. 35.10: Submental and submandibular space infection with fasciitis

- The pus is then drained in the same way as in the other cases (Fig. 35.13).

Submandibular Space

Boundaries

- Anteromedially: Floor is formed by mylohyoid muscle, covered by loose areolar tissue and fat

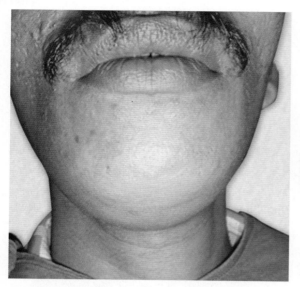

Fig. 35.11: Submental space infection (external view)

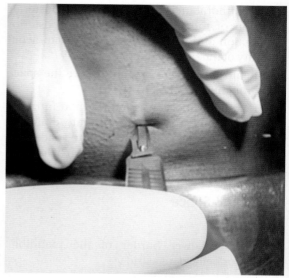

Fig. 35.12: Stab incision with number 11 blade

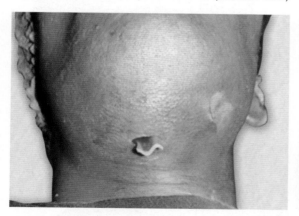

Fig. 35.13: Incision and drain *in situ* (in patient of Figures 35.11)

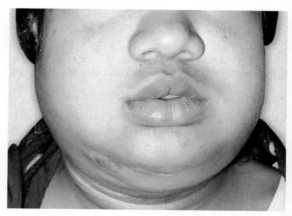

Fig. 35.14: Note facial swelling (front view)

- Posteromedially: Floor is formed by hyoglossus muscle
- Superolaterally: Medial surface of the mandible below mylohyoid ridge
- Anterosuperiorly: Anterior belly of digatric
- Posterosuperiorly: Posterior belly of digastric, stylohyoid and stylopharyngeus muscles
- Laterally: Platysma and skin.

Contents

Superficial lobe of submandibular gland and lymph nodes, facial art and vein, marginal mandibular nerve.

Clinical Features

- Extraorally firm swelling in the submandibular region, generalized constitutional symptoms, tenderness and redness over the skin (Figs 35.14 to 35.17)

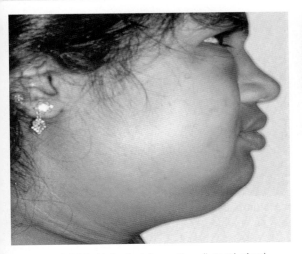

Fig. 35.15: Note facial swelling (lateral view)

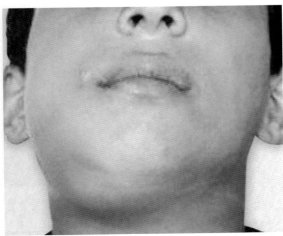

Fig. 35.16: Submandibular swelling

- Intraorally moderate trismus, teeth affected is sensitive to percussion and are mobile, dysphagia.

Treatment

- The incision for drainage is performed on the skin, approximately 1 cm beneath and parallel to the inferior border of the mandible
- During the incision, the course of the facial artery and vein (the incision should be made posterior to these) and the respective branch of the facial nerve should be taken into consideration. A hemostat is inserted into the cavity of the abscess to explore the space and an attempt is made to communicate with the infected spaces (Fig. 35.18)
- Blunt dissection must be performed along the medial surface of the mandibular bone also, because pus is often located in this area as well
- After drainage, a rubber drain is placed (Fig. 35.19 and 35.20).

Sublingual Space

- This is a V shaped trough lying lateral to muscles of tongue, including hyoglossus, genioglossus and geniohyoid
- There are two sublingual spaces above the mylohyoid muscle, to the right and left of the

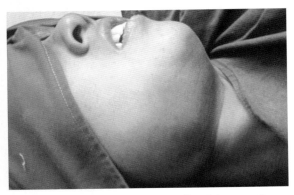

Fig. 35.17: Submandibular swelling intraoperative

midline. These spaces are divided by dense fascia (Fig. 35.21).

Boundaries

- *Superiorly*: By the mucosa of the floor of the mouth
- *Inferiorly*: Mylohyoid muscle
- *Medially*: Hyoglossus, genioglossus, and geniohyoid muscle
- *Laterally*: Medial side of the mandible above the mylohyoid muscle
- *Posteriorly*: Hyoid bone.

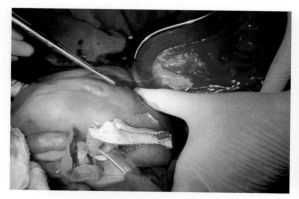

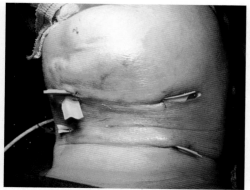

Fig. 35.18 and 35.19: Incision and drain *in situ* (in patients of Figure 35.15)

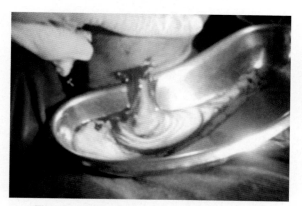

Fig. 35.20: Incision and drain intraoperative (in patient of Figures 35.17)

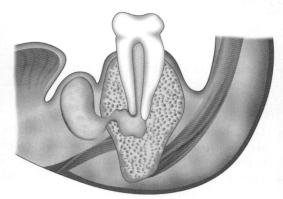

Fig. 35.21: Sublingual space infection

Clinical Features

- Extraorally little/no swelling, pain and discomfort during swallowing. speech may be affected
- Intraorally firm painful swelling in floor of the mouth, tongue may be pushed superiorly—causing airway obstruction. Inability to protrude tongue beyond vermillion border of upper lip.

Treatment

- The incision for drainage is performed intraorally, laterally and along Wharton's duct and the lingual nerve
- In order to locate the pus, a hemostat is used to explore the space inferiorly, in an anteroposterior direction and beneath the gland

- After drainage is complete, a rubber drain is placed.

Infratemporal space (Figs 35.22 to 35.26)

Clinical Features

- Trismus
- Bulging of temporalis muscle
- Marked swelling of the face on the affected side in front of ear, overlying TMJ, behind the zygomatic process.

Complications

Cavernous sinus thrombosis—through pterygoid plexus and inferior opthalmic vein via superior orbital fissure.

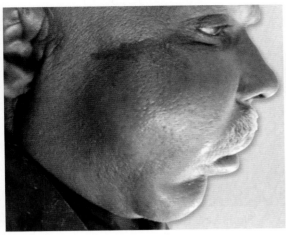

Fig. 35.22: Note swelling extension to temporal region

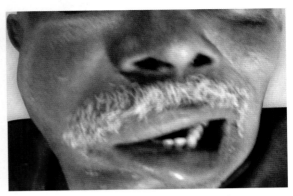

Fig. 35.23: Reduced mouth opening

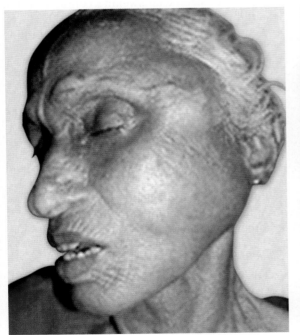

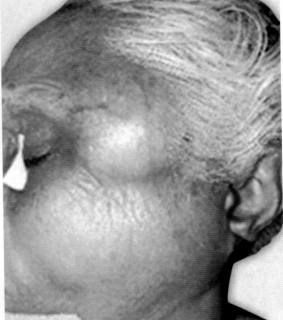

Fig. 35.24 and 35.25: Swelling at temporal region

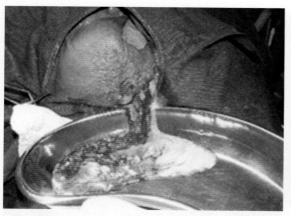

Fig. 35.26: Incision and drain *in situ* in patients of Figure 35.26

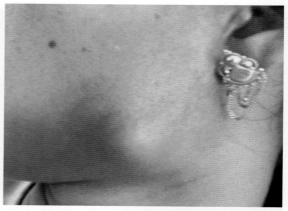

Fig. 35.27: Submasseteric space infection

Secondary Fascial Spaces

Masseteric

- Pterygomandibular
- Superficial and deep temporal
- Lateral pharyngeal
- Retropharyngeal
- Prevertebral spaces
- Parotid space.

Submassetric Space

Boundaries

- *Anteriorly*: Anterior border of masster muscle and buccinator
- *Posteriorly*: Parotid gland and posterior part of masseter
- *Inferiorly*: Attachment of the masseter to the lower border of the mandible
- *Medially*: Lateral surface of the ramus of the mandible
- *Laterally*: Medial surface of the masseter muscle.

Contents

Masseteric nerve, superficial temporal artery and transverse facial artery.

Clinical Features

- Moderate size facial swelling confined to the outline of masseter muscle (Fig. 35.27)
- Tenderness over the angle of the mandible (Fig. 35.28)
- Trismus
- Pyrexia and malaise.

Pterygomandibular Space

Boundaries

- Laterally: Ascending ramus of mandible
- Medially: Lateral surface of medial pterygoid muscle
- Posteriorly: Parotid gland
- Anteriorly: Pterygomandibular raphae
- Superiorly: Lateral pterygoid muscle.

Clinical Features

- Trismus
- Dysphagia
- Medial displacement of the lateral wall of pharynx
- Redness and edema of area around third molar
- Difficulty in breathing
- Spread of infection from 3rd molar.

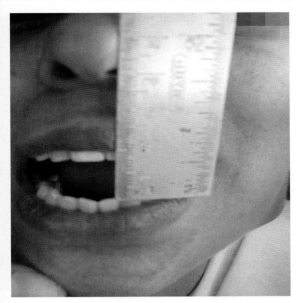

Fig. 35.28: Reduced mouth opening

Temporal Space Superficial Temporal Space

Boundaries
- Laterally: Temporal fascia
- Medially: Temporalis muscle.

Clinical Features
- Swelling limited superiorly and laterally by temporal fascia and inferiorly by zygomatic arch
- 'Dumbell shape' swelling if associated with buccal space due to lack of swelling over zygomatic arch
- Severe pain and trismus.

Deep Temporal Space

Boundaries
- *Laterally*: Medial surface of temporalis muscle
- *Medially*: Temporal bone and greater wing of sphenoid

Clinical Features
- Less swelling than superficial temporal space
- Difficult to diagnose

- Considerable pain and trismus
- Difficult to elicit fluctuation because of depth.

Parotid Space

- Rare from extension of odontogenic infection
- Blood borne/retrograde infection through parotid duct.

Boundaries
- *Superiorly*: Zygomatic arch
- *Inferiorly*: Lower border of mandible
- *Anteriorly*: Anterior border of mandibular ramus
- *Posteriorly*: Retromandibular area.

Clinical Features
- Severe pain radiating to ear and accentuated by eating
- Dehydration—due to insufficient consumption of fluids.

Differential Diagnosis
Submasseteric infection
Distinguished by
- Lack of trismus
- Eversion of ear lobe
- Escape of pus from parotid duct on milking.

Pharyngeal Space

- Lateral/parapharyngeal space
- Retropharyngeal space.

Lateral Pharyngeal Space

An inverted pyramid with its base at the base of the skull and apex at the hyoid bone.

Boundaries
- *Medially*: Superior pharyngeal constrictor muscle (lateral wall of pharynx)
- *Laterally*: Fascia of medial pterygoid, deep capsule of parotid gland
- *Anteriorly*: Palatal muscle superiorly, buccinator, superior constrictor, stylohyoid and posterior belly of digastric inferiorly

- *Posteriorly*: Carotid sheath posterolaterally and retropharyngeal space posteromedially
- *Inferiorly*: Hyoid bone.

Contents

- Carotid artery, internal jugular vein, vagus nerve, cervical sympathetic chain.
- *Aponeurosis of Zuckerkandl and Testut* divides this space into anterior (prestyloid) and posterior (poststyloid).

Clinical Features

- Anterior compartment—pain, fever, chills, medial bulging of lateral pharyngeal wall with deviation of palatal uvula from midline, dysphagia, swelling below angle of mandible and trismus.
- Posterior compartment—absence of visible swelling and trismus but respiratory obustruction, septic thrombosis of internal jugular vein and carotid artery hemorrhage may occur.

Peritonsillar Abscess

Enlarged and Inflamed Tonsil

Origin of infection:
- *Direct*: Sublingual space, submandibular space, lateral pharyngeal space.
- *Indirect*: Pterygomandibular space lateral pharyngeal space.

Spread of Infection

- Upwards through various foramina at base of skull causing cavernous sinus thrombosis, meningitis and brain abscess
- Posteriorly to retropharyngeal space or carotid sheath.

Investigation

CT scan more useful in diagnosis.

Route of Spread

- Submandibular (one side) sublingual
- Submental space contralat submandibular

or

- Sublingual space opp sublingual extend posterior over edge of mylohyoid submandibular submental space

or

- Submandibular pterygomandibular space pharyngeal space mediastinum.

Investigation

Cervical soft tissue films and CT before attempting tracheostomy.

Management

- General principle
- Establishment of drainage
  - Extraoral
  - Intraoral
- Removal of source of infection
  - Immediate
  - Delayed.

Surgical Therapy

Surgical technique for incision and drainage of an abscess helps:
- To get rid of toxic purulent material
- To decompress the edematous tissues
- To allow better perfusion of blood, containing antibiotic and defensive elements
- To increase oxygenation of the infected area.

Hilton's Method of Incision and Drainage

This method of opening an abscess ensures that no blood vessel or nerve in the vicinity is damaged.

Steps

- Topical anesthesia
- Stab incision made over a point of maximum fluctuation in most dependant area along skin creases through skin and subcutaneous tissue
- If pus is not encountered further deepening of surgical site is achieved with sinus forceps (to avoid damage to vital structures)
- Closed forceps are pushed through the tough deep fascia and advanced towards pus collection

- Abscess cavity is entered and forceps opened in a direction parallel to vital structures
- Pus flows along the sides of beaks
- Explore the entire cavity for additional loculi
- Placement of drains—corrugated rubber drain is inserted into the depths of abscess cavity and external part is secured to wound margin with help of suture
- Drain is left for at least 48 hours until complete drainage of abscess
- Dressing is applied over the site of incision taken extraorally without pressure.

Medical Therapy

Supportive care
- Aids in patients own body defenses on combating infection
- Administration of antibiotics
- Hydration of patient
- Analgesics for pain
- Bed rest
- Application of heat in the form of moist packs and/or mouth rinses
- Opening tooth for drainage.

These treatments will result in resolution of periapical osteitis/cellulitis, sometimes will progress from one stage to another until an abscess develops and surgical intervention becomes necessary.

Antibiotic Therapy

Decided based on patients systemic condition and type of infection, organism.

Noncompromised patients
- Well localized abcess, surgical drainage and therapy will resolve infection without antibiotic cover.
- In case of poorly localized, extensive abscess antibiotic is must.
- *In compromised patients* and patients with trismus, airway compromise and fever antibiotic cover is must.

- In patients with diminished host defense like uncontrolled diabetics, immunocompromised patients, chronic alcoholics, IV drug abusers, also requires antibiotic cover.

Principles of antibotic administration
- Proper dosage
- Proper route of administration
- Consistent route of administration
- Proper time interval
- Combination drug therapy.

Selection of antibiotics
- Narrow spectrum
- Based on identification of causative organism and sensitivity
- Compatible with patient's drug history
- Initially always empirical selection is done based on knowledge of the flora of oral infection, later after lab results specific antibiotics is instituted.
- Bactericidal antibiotics are preferable to bacteriostatic antibiotics because they can independently destroy invading organisms.
- Penicillin is an empirical drug of choice. β-lactamase producing organisms such as bacteroids are insensitive to penicillin.
- Oral clindamycin, amoxicilin-clavulanic acid (augmentin), first or second-generation cephalosporins are also useful in orofacial infections.

CASE OF A SUBMANDIBULAR SPACE INFECTION

A 38-year-old female patient complaint of pain and swelling in the right side of the face (Figs 35.29 to 35.33).

History of Present Illness

- Patient had pain in the lower right posterior tooth associated with swelling since 5 days
- Visited a local dentist—*antibiotics and analgesics*
- Pain and swelling increased

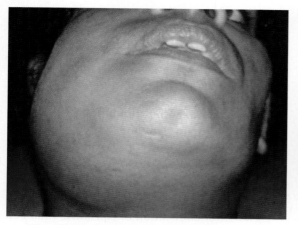

Fig. 35.29: Swelling at submandibular region

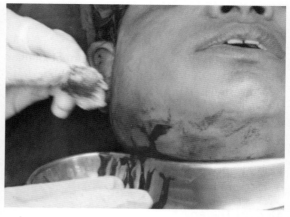

Fig. 35.30: Incision and drain

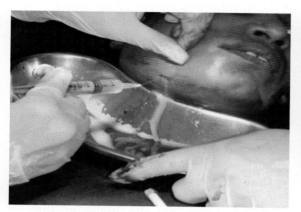

Fig. 35.31: I and D and irrigation of wound

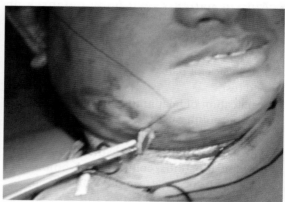

Fig. 35.32: Placement of drain

Past Medical History

No history of diabetes mellitus, hypertension and drug allergy.

Personal History

No habits, brushes once daily.

Physical Examination

Vital Signs

- Temperature—101°F
- Blood Pressure—mild elevation
- Pulse >100
- Increased respiratory rate—18.

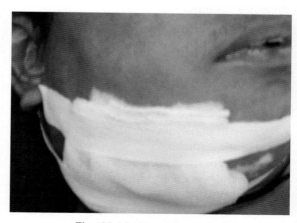

Fig. 35.33: Dressing applied

Extraoral Examination

Inspection

- Facial asymmetry noticed due to a diffuse swelling involving submandibular region
- A firm, hard, diffuse, tender swelling present in the submandibular region measuring 8 × 6 cm (approx)
- Trismus present
- Erythema present.

Palpation

- Local rise of temperature over the swelling area
- Overlying skin is taut and non-pinchable.

Intraoral Examination

Decayed lower right mandibular molar.

Provisional Diagnosis

Submandibular space infection.

Differential Diagnosis

- Lymphoma arising in the lymph nodes of upper neck
- Secondary deposits of a malignant neoplasm.

Radiological Examination

OPG shows grossly decayed 47.

Principles in Treatment of Oral and Paraoral Infections

- Remove the cause
- Establish drainage
- Institute antibiotic therapy
- Supportive care, including proper rest, and nutrition.

Removal of the Cause

- Extraction of 47 under L.A.

Incision and Drainage

- Hilton's method of drainage
- Approximately 5 mL of pus is drained
- Irrigation of the wound
- Corrugated rubber drain placed and sutured with 3.0 silk
- Sterile, thick gauze dressing is then placed and held in place with adhesive straping.

Drug Therapy

- Inj crystalline penicillin 20 lakh units IV 6 hourly
- Inj metrogyl 500 mg IV 8 hourly
- Inj diclo 50 mg IM 12 hourly
- Inj rantac 150 mg IV 12 hourly
- Chlorhexidine mouthwash 6 hourly
- IV fluid ringers lactate/DNS 80 mL hourly
- Hot fomentation.

Re-evaluated the Next Day

- Oral diet
- Improved mouth opening
- IV stopped
- Mouth opening exercises.

The Day After

- No fresh complaints
- Mouth opening approximately 22 mm
- Mouth opening exercises with mouth gag
- Minimal discharge (serosanguinous) about 2 mL
- Patient feeling fit and fine.

CASE REPORTS

- Buccal space infection (Fig. 35.34)
- Submandibular space infection (Figs 35.35 to 35.38)
- Temporal infection (Figs 35.39 to 35.42).

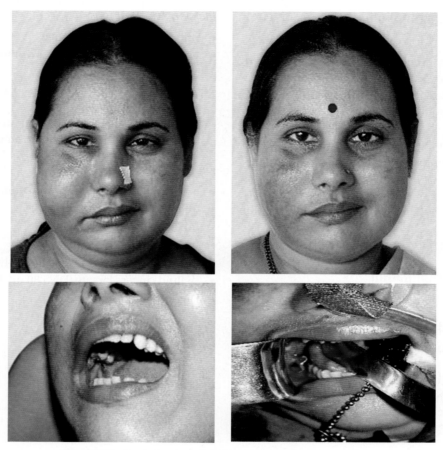

Fig. 35.34: Buccal space infection: Pre- and postoperative

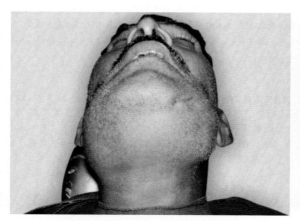

Fig. 35.35: Submandibular space infection

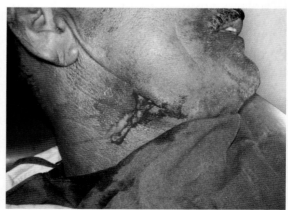

Fig. 35.36: Incision and drainage

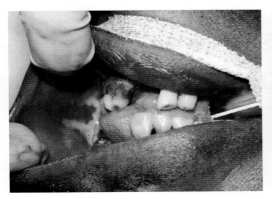

Fig. 35.37: Intra oral pus drainage

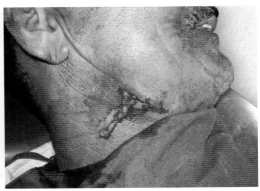

Fig. 35.38: Incision and drainage

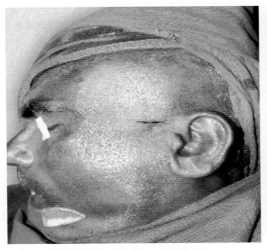

Fig. 35.39: Temporal swelling

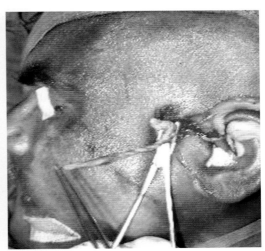

Fig. 35.40: Postoperative

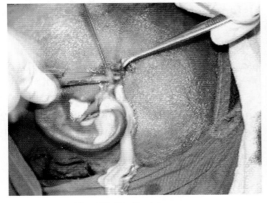

Fig. 35.41: Draining pus

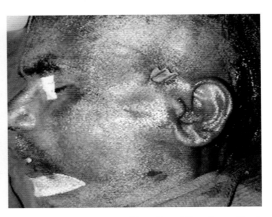

Fig. 35.42: Breaking of locules: Hilton's method

Osteomyelitis and Osteonecrosis

36

INTRODUCTION

The word "osteomyelitis" originates from the ancient Greek words osteon (bone) and muelinos (marrow) and means infection of medullary portion of the bone.

Osteomyelitis usually encompasses the cortical bone and periosteum as well. It can therefore be considered as an inflammatory condition of the bone, beginning in the medullar cavity and haversian systems and extending to involve the periosteum of the affected area. The infection becomes established in calcified portion of the bone when pus and edema in the medullary cavity and beneath the periosteum compromises or obstructs the local blood supply. Following ischemia, the infected bone becomes necrotic and leads to sequester formation, which is considered a classical sign of osteomyelitis (Topazian 1994, 2002).

Definition
Osteomyelitis can be defined as the inflammation of bone and bone marrow along with surrounding periosteum
Inflammatory condition involves all the structure of bone, e.g. bone marrow, Haversian system, periosteum and epiphysis

CLASSIFICATION

Classification Based on Pathogenesis (From Vibhagool 1993)

I. Hematogenous osteomyelitis (common in pediatrics)
II. Osteomyelitis secondary to a contiguous focus of infection (periapical pathology or failed implants and bone grafts or transition from acute condition)
III. Osteomyelitis associated with or without peripheral vascular disease (because of emergence of resistant microorganisms)

Dual Classification Based on Pathological Anatomy and Pathophysiology (From Vibhagool 1993 and Cierny 1985, and Cierny-Mader Staging System of Osteomyelitis)

I. Anatomic types

Stage I: Medullary osteomyelitis—involved medullary bone without cortical involvement; usually hematogenous.

Stage II: Superficial osteomyelitis—less than 2 cm bony defect without cancellous bone.

Stage III: Localized osteomyelitis—less than 2 cm bony defect on radiograph, defect does not appear to involve both cortices.

Stage IV: Diffuse osteomyelitis—defect greater than 2 cm. Pathologic fracture, infection, nonunion.

II. Physiological class

A host: Normal host

B host: Systemic compromised host, local compromised host

C host: Treatment worse than disease.

Classification based on clinical picture, radiology, pathology and etiology

Acute suppurative osteomyelitis (rarefactional osteomyelitis)

Chronic suppurative osteomyelitis (sclerosing osteomyelitis

Chronic focal sclerosing osteomyelitis (pseudo-Paget, condensing osteomyetitis)

Chronic diffuse sclerosing osteomyelitis

Chronic osteomyelitis with proliferativeperiostitis (Garrè's chronic nonsuppurative sclerosing osteitis, ossifying periostitis)

Specific osteomyelitis
- Tuberculous osteomyelitis
- Syphilitic osteomyelitis
- Actinomycotic osteomyelitis

Classification Based on Clinical Picture and Radiology

I. Acute/subacute osteomyelitis

II. Secondary chronic osteomyelitis

III. Primary chronic osteomyelitis.

Classification Based on Clinical Picture and Radiology, Etiology, and Pathophysiology.

The arbitrary time limit of one month is used to differ acute from chronic osteomyelitis but the moment sign of discharging sinus appears that stage onwards is considered chronic osteomyelitis.

I. Acute forms of osteomyelitis (suppurative or nonsuppurative)
- Contagious focus
  - Trauma
  - Surgery
  - Odontogenic Infection
- Progressive
  - Burns
  - Sinusitis
  - Vascular insufficiency
- Hematogenous (metastatic)
  - Developing skeleton (children)

II. Chronic forms of osteomyelitis
- Recurrent multifocal
  - Developing skeleton (children)
  - Escalated osteogenic (activity < age 25 years)
- Garrè's
  - Unique proliferative
  - subperiosteal reaction
  - Developing skeleton (children and young adults)
- Suppurative or nonsuppurative
  - Inadequately treated forms
  - Systemically compromised forms
  - Refractory forms (chronic recurrent multifocal osteomyelitis CROM)
- Diffuse sclerosing
  - Fastidious microorganisms
  - Compromised host/pathogen interface.

Classification Based on Clinical Picture and Radiology

Classification of chronic osteomyelitis forms only.

I. Primarily chronic jaw inflammation
- Osteomyelitis sicca (synonymous osteomyelitis of Garrè, chronic sclerosing nonsuppurative osteomyelitis of Garrè, periostitis ossificans)
- Chronic sclerosing osteomyelitis with fine-meshed trabecular structure
- Local and more extensive very dense sclerosing osteomyelitis

II. Secondary chronic jaw inflammation

Hierarchic order of classification criteria	Classification criteria	Classification groups
First	Clinical appearance and course of disease Radiology	Major groups Acute osteomyelitis (AO) Secondary chronic osteomyelitis (SCO) Primary chronic osteomyelitis (PCO)
Second	Pathology (gross pathology and histology)	Differentiation of cases that cannot clearly be distinguished solely on clinical appearance and course of disease; important for exclusion of differential diagnosis in borderline cases
Third	Etiology Pathogenesis	Subgroups of AO, SCO, and PCO

III. Chronic specific jaw inflammations
- Tuberculosis
- Syphilis
- Actinomycosis.

Classification Based on Clinical Picture, Radiology and Etiology
Topazian RG

I. Suppurative osteomyelitis
- Acute suppurative osteomyelitis
- Chronic suppurative osteomyelitis
  - Primary chronic suppurative osteomyelitis
  - Secondary chronic suppurative osteomyelitis
- Infantile osteomyelitis

II. Nonsuppurative osteomyelitis
- Chronic sclerosing osteomyelitis
  - Focal sclerosing osteomyelitis
  - Diffuse sclerosing osteomyelitis
- Garrè's sclerosing osteomyelitis
- Actinomycotic osteomyelitis
- Radiation osteomyelitis and necrosis

Classification Based on Clinical Picture and Radiology (J Can Dent Assoc. 1995 Classification)

I. Suppurative osteomyelitis
- Acute suppurative osteomyelitis
- Chronic suppurative osteomyelitis

II. Nonsuppurative osteomyelitis
- Chronic focal sclerosing osteomyelitis
- Chronic diffuse sclerosing osteomyelitis
- Garrè's chronic sclerosing osteomyelitis (proliferative osteomyelitis).

III. Osteoradionecrosis

Osteomyelitis of the Jaws (The Zurich Classification System)

- At the Department of Cranio-Maxillofacial Surgery at the University of Zurich, the classification system for osteomyelitis of the jaws uses a hierarchical order of classification criteria
- It is primarily based on clinical appearance and course of the disease, as well as on radiological features. Based on these criteria, three major groups of osteomyelitis can be distinguished:
  - Acute osteomyelitis (AO)
  - Secondary chronic osteomyelitis (SCO)
  - Primary chronic osteomyelitis (PCO).

ETIOLOGY

- Odontogenic infections
- Trauma
- Infections of orofacial region
- Infections derived by hematogenous routes.

   Other etiological factors, such as radiation, and certain chemical substances, among others, may also produce inflammation of the medullar space, the term "osteomyelitis" is mostly used to describe a true infection of the bone induced by pyogenic microorganisms (Marx 1991).

Acute Osteomyelitis ⇒ Secondary Chronic Osteomyelitis

- Neonatal, tooth germ associated
- Trauma/fracture related
- Odontogenic
- Foreign body, transplant/implant induced
- Associated with bone pathology and/or systemic disease
- Other (not further classifiable) cases.

Primary Chronic Osteomyelitis

- Early onset (juvenile chronic osteomyelitis)
- Adult onset
- Syndrome associated.

Predisposing Factors

- Conditions that alter host defences
- Conditions that alter vascularity of bone
- Virulence of organisms.

Conditions that Alter Host Defences

- Diabetes
- Leukemia
- Anemia
- Malnutrition
- Agranulocytosis
- Chronic alcoholism
- Sickle cell disease.

Conditions that Alter Vascularity of Bone

- Osteoporosis
- Therapeutic irradiation
- Paget's disease
- Fibrous dysplasia
- Bone malignancy.

Microbiology

- *Staphylococcus epidermidis*
- *Staphylococcus aureus*
- *Pseudomonas aeruginosa*
- *E. coli*
- *M. tuberculosis*
- *Actinomyces*
- *T. pallidum.*

Disease Mechanism Facilitating Bone Infection

Diabetes—Diminished leukocyte chemotaxis, phagocytosis and lifespan; diminished vascularity of tissue due to vasculopathy, thus reducing perfusion and the ability for an effective inflammatory response; slower healing rate due to reduced tissue perfusion and defective glucose utilization.

Leukemia—Deficient leukocyte function and associated anemia.

Malnutrition—Reduced wound healing and reduction of immunological response.

Cancer—Reduced wound healing and reduction of immunological response.

Osteopetrosis (Albers–Schonberg disease)—Reduction of bone vascularization due to enhanced mineralization, replacement of hematopoietic marrow causing anemia and leukopenia.

Severe anemia (particularly sickle-cell anemia)—Systemic debilitation, reduced tissue oxygenation, bone infarction (sickle cell anemia), especially in patients with a homozygous anemia trait.

IV drug abuse—Repeated septic injections, spreading of septic emboli (especially with harboring septic vegetation on heart valves, in skin or within veins).

AIDS—Impaired immune response.

Immunosuppression (steroids, cytostatic drugs)—Impaired immune response.

Cloaca—Hole formed in the bone during the formation of draining sinus.

Sequestrum—Fragments of necrotic bone embedded in pus.

Brodie's abscess—Reactive (woven) bone and granulation tissue at the metaphysis of long bone (especially upper end of tibia) formed from the periosteum and endosteum which surrounds the infection.

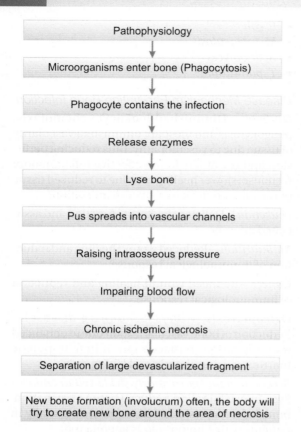

Pathophysiology

↓

Microorganisms enter bone (Phagocytosis)

↓

Phagocyte contains the infection

↓

Release enzymes

↓

Lyse bone

↓

Pus spreads into vascular channels

↓

Raising intraosseous pressure

↓

Impairing blood flow

↓

Chronic ischemic necrosis

↓

Separation of large devascularized fragment

↓

New bone formation (involucrum) often, the body will try to create new bone around the area of necrosis

Involucrum—Perisoteal reactive new (woven) bone formation around necrotic sequestrum.

Osteomyelitis in maxilla—is rare due to:
- Extensive blood supply
- Porous nature of membranous bone
- Thin cortical plates
- Abundant medullary spaces.

CLINICAL FEATURES

- The clinical appearance of acute osteomyelitis of the jaws may show a great variety, depending on the intensity of the disease and the magnitude of imbalance between the host and the microbiological aggressors
- Three principal types of clinical courses of acute osteomyelitis can be distinguished:
  - Acute suppurative
  - Subacute suppurative
  - Clinically silent with or without suppuration.

Acute Suppurative Osteomyelitis

- Generalised constitutional symptoms—The patient experiences a general malaise caused by high intermittent fever with temperatures reaching up to 39–40°C, often accompanied by regional lymphadenopathy
- Deep seated boring, continuous intense pain in the affected area
- Intermittent paresthesia or anesthesia of the lower lip (Vincent's symptom), indicating involvement of the inferior alveolar nerve
- Facial cellulitis
- Trismus—Local swelling and edema due to abscess formation causing limitation of jaw function
- Teeth become sensitive to percussion
- Foetid odour—caused by anaerobic pyogenic bacteria often is present
- In cases of a subacute or silent course, with or without suppuration, the clinical presentation is by definition less impressive. This can make an early diagnosis increasingly difficult, and in many instances these cases are not detected until they have become secondary chronic.

Chronic Osteomyelitis

- Pain and tenderness—pain is minimal
- The deep and intense pain frequently observed in the acute stage is replaced by a more dull pain
- Painful swelling caused by local edema and abscess formation in the acute stage is subsided by a harder palpable tenderness caused by periosteal reaction
- Nonhealing bone
- Induration of soft tissues
- Intraoral or extraoral draining fistulae
- Thickened or wooden character of bone
- Enlargement of mandible (Fig. 36.1)
- Pathological fractures may occur
- Sterile abscess
- Teeth become loose and sensitive to palpation and percussion.

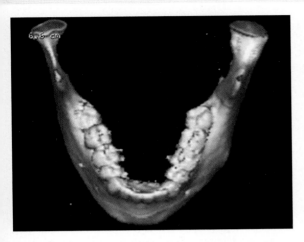

Fig. 36.1: The 3D reconstruction of the mandible clearly shows the enlarged angle, ascending ramus, and condyle of the left mandible

Actinomycotic and Other Rare Secondary Chronic Osteomyelitis of the Jaws

- Specific clinical findings can be found in acute and especially in secondary chronic osteomyelitis caused by *Actinomyces*, *Nocardia*, and *Mycobacteria*
- While *Actinomyces* is infrequently observed, the other pathogens are rarely associated with osteomyelitis of the jaws; however, if they are the causative pathogen, the clinical picture is somewhat atypical and hence deserves special recognition.

Secondary Chronic Osteomyelitis Associated with Bone Pathology

- There are several conditions which facilitate bone infection in the jaw
- Theoretically every pathological condition which alters bone physiology and/or vascularization of bone tissue may jeopardize host tissue defense mechanisms and hence may promote secondary infection. The unique location of the jawbones with their proximity to the heavily contaminated oral cavity makes them particularly vulnerable

- Depending on the nature of the underlying bone pathology, the clinical picture of succeeding secondary chronic osteomyelitis may differ from the average osteomyelitis infection established in "healthy bone"
- The initiation of infection is, like in regular acute and secondary chronic osteomyelitis, often a trauma such as extraction of a tooth or a dental infection leading to breakdown of the periodontal and/or mucosal barrier and promoting contamination and deep bone invasion of the jawbone. The further course of the disease is, however, strongly dependent on the reactive mechanisms of the host tissue (e.g. bone)
- In general, underlying bone pathology will reduce the defensive abilities of the host tissue and infection may spread faster than in healthy bone
- Clinical and radiological signs reflecting suppurative infection, such as abscess and fistula formation, are similar to osteomyelitis cases without associated bone pathology. Bone reaction to infection, like osteolysis, sclerosis, sequester formation, and periosteal reaction, however, may strongly differ, making correct diagnosis and determining the extent of the infection more challenging. In cases where necrotic bone is exposed to the oral cavity, secondary colonization of the bone and eventual deep bone invasion may occur.

Primary Chronic Osteomyelitis

- The term "primary chronic osteomyelitis," refers to a rare inflammatory disease of unknown etiology
- It is characterized as a strictly nonsuppurative chronic inflammation of the jawbone with the absence of pus formation, extra- or intraoral fistula, or sequestration
- The term "primary chronic osteomyelitis" also implies that the patient has never undergone an appreciable acute phase and lacks a definitive initiating event

- The disease tends to a rise de novo without an actual acute phase and follows an insidious course. In most cases of primary chronic osteomyelitis, periodic episodes of onset with varying intensity last from a few days to several weeks and are intersected by periods of silence where the patient may experience little to no clinical symptoms. In active periods dull to severe pain, limitation of jaw opening and/or myofacial pain, as well as variable swelling, may be observed. In certain cases regional lymphadenopathy and reduced sensation of the inferior alveolar nerve (Vincent's symptom) are also accompanying symptoms
- Primary chronic osteomyelitis of the jaws almost always targets the mandible.

Subclassification of Primary Chronic Osteomyelitis of the Jaws

Adult-onset primary chronic osteomyelitis
- Onset of symptoms in the adult patient after age 20 years
- The clinical symptoms of this disease are, as mentioned above, those of a chronic inflammation of the jawbone, excluding signs of suppuration
- Principally, the clinically observed symptoms in the adult patient are the same as in the child or adolescent patient with primary chronic osteomyelitis of the jaws, with swelling and pain (ranging from dull to sharp) being the most often observed. Intensity of these symptoms was less prominent in adult-onset cases. Furthermore, symptoms tended to be less intense as the disease progressed
- These results showed some correlation with radiological findings, which demonstrated more osteolytic findings and a greater periosteal reaction in cases of primary chronic osteomyelitis in children and adolescents compared with cases with onset in adult patients. Furthermore, a clear shift toward a more sclerotic pattern with normalization of the cortical architecture
- These findings may be explained by the fact that radiological remission takes longer with

extensive disease and patient age due to the general metabolic activity which decreases with age. In elderly patients residual sclerosis is more likely to persist
- An infection arising predominantly from a dental focus is the known etiology in cases of acute and secondary chronic osteomyelitis of the jaws. While an infectious etiology is also being discussed in primary chronic osteomyelitis, a chronic infection remains a readily discussed but still unproved hypothesis for this disease entity
- Currently favored hypothesis is that of a microorganism of low virulence functioning as a trigger that causes an exaggerated immune response in a genetically predisposed individual
- The genetic predisposition may also be an explanation for wide variety and intensity of possible extragnathic manifestations seen in some patients with primary chronic osteomyelitis of the jaws, which is discussed later
- Basic immunological parameters in patients with primary chronic osteomyelitis of the jaws demonstrate a mild elevation of the erythrocyte sedimentation rate and the C-reactive protein level. These findings are usually accompanied by a normal leukocyte count. During onset and active periods of the disease, subfebrile body temperatures may be noted. In less active or silent periods of primary chronic osteomyelitis the body temperature was found to be normal.

Early-onset primary chronic osteomyelitis (juvenile chronic osteomyelitis)
- Early-onset primary chronic osteomyelitis of the jaws describes cases with an onset in childhood or adolescence
- The clinical symptoms of early-onset primary chronic osteomyelitis are generally the same in younger patients as in adults but usually of stronger intensity
- In active periods of the disease, the swelling and tenderness of the jaw is more prominent, due to a more extensive periosteal reaction

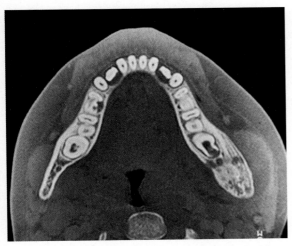

Fig. 36.2: Onion-like pattern of the periosteal reaction (ossifying periostitis)

- The swelling can create a voluminous expansion of the mandible with a pseudotumor-like appearance
- The radiological correlation of this pseudotumor is often a mixed pattern of small regions of osteolysis embedded in pronounced sclerotic bone
- The periosteal reaction may lead to destruction of the cortical-marrow architecture and/or form an onion-like picture (ossifying periostitis), resembling osteosarcoma or other bone malignancies (Fig. 36.2).

   In such instances a biopsy is the only possibility to rule out a malignancy.

Syndrome-associated Primary Chronic Osteomyelitis

SAPHO syndrome

- The term SAPHO syndrome describes a chronic disorder that involves the skin, bones, and joints
- SAPHO is an acronym that stands for morbid alteration of the dermatoskeletal system: synovitis; acne and pustulosis; hyperostosis; and osteitis

- The clinical picture is determined by chronic inflammation of one tissue or a combination of any of these tissues. According to Kahn, et al. (1994) three diagnostic criteria characterize SAPHO syndrome:
    - Multifocal osteomyelitis with or without skin manifestations
    - Sterile acute or chronic joint inflammation associated with either pustular psoriasis or palmoplantar pustulosis, acne, or hidradenitis
    - Sterile osteitis in the presence of one of the skin manifestations.

Chronic recurrent multifocal osteomyelitis

- CRMO is an inflammatory disorder that mainly affects the metaphyses of the long bones, in addition to the spine, pelvis, and shoulder girdle; however, bone lesions are described at any site of the skeleton including the jaws. Because the lesions in CRMO patients affecting the mandible radiologically resemble cases of primary chronic osteomyelitis in the same age group, Suei, et al. concluded that the latter may be considered the mandibular manifestation of CRMO (1995)
- Chronic recurrent multifocal osteomyelitis is usually characterized by periods of exacerbations and remissions over many years. Clinical diagnosis may be challenging because the clinical picture and course of the disease may vary significantly. Histological analysis of bone lesions in CRMO patients may help to differentiate them from other bone pathology, especially those which are malignant; however, they may resemble acute and secondary chronic osteomyelitis caused by microbiological infection. Therefore, an extensive microbiological work-up of the tissue biopsy, including PCR techniques, is essential in order to establish the diagnosis and hence decide on the treatment. It is of the utmost importance to avoid contamination when harvesting a bone biopsy from a lesion

for microbiological analysis. While lesions of CRMO in the mandible may be easier to access, an oral approach should be avoided for reasons mentioned previously. A biopsy from another part of the skeleton may therefore be of more diagnostic value, despite a possibly more invasive procedure to harvest the specimen

- Chronic recurrent multifocal osteomyelitis is an extremely rare disease
- The incidence might be around 1:1,000,000
- The disease has been predominantly described in children, but cases in adults have also been noted but seem to be significantly less frequent than in the former group.

INVESTIGATIONS PRIOR TO MANAGEMENT

- Bacterial culture or sensitivity testing
- Radiograph
  - Till at least 30–60% destruction of mineralized portion of bone takes place—this destruction is not visible on radiograph.
  - Acute osteomyelitis—not visible on radiograph
  - Chronic osteomyelitis—moth eaten appearance
- CT scan
  - More accurate as compared to radiograph
- MRI
  - More accurate as compared to CT scan.
  - Bone marrow changes and soft tissue changes are seen more accurately in MRI when compared to a CT scan
- Scintigraphy/bone scanning/radionuclide scanning
  - Measures physiological changes in bone.

GOALS OF MANAGEMENT

- Attenuate and eradicate proliferating pathological organisms
- Promote healing
- Re-establish vascular permeability
- The final common pathway in all treatment of acute and secondary chronic osteomyelitis of the jaws is to achieve a shift in the disturbed balance between the responsible pathogen(s)

and host defenses to the latter, allowing the body to overcome the infection

- Reduction of pathogens is achieved by surgical removal of infected and necrotic tissue as well as by antibiotic therapy
- Improvement of local vascularization is further accomplished by surgical decortication, exceeding conventional surgical debridement, which not only removes the poorly vascularized (infected) bone but also brings well-vascularized tissue to the affected bone, thus facilitating the healing process and allowing antibiotics to reach the target area; therefore, surgery and antibiotics are to be considered the major columns in treating osteomyelitis of the jaws
- Hyperbaric oxygen (HBO), which can be recognized as an adjunctive therapeutic modality in treatment of acute and secondary chronic osteomyelitis, supports host-defensive mechanisms and promotes tissue vascularization as well as has direct toxic effects on microorganisms causing the infection. Although never as dominating as surgery and antibiotic therapy, HBO is to be considered the third column in the armentarium for acute and secondary chronic osteomyelitis treatment
- A sufficient surgical debridement is as the most important factor in successful treatment of advanced acute and secondary chronic osteomyelitis of the jaws. The extent of the surgical debridement is dictated mainly by the extent of the infected bone. The most important surgical procedure to achieve a sufficient debridement and in addition bring well-perfused tissue in contact with the surgical site is the decortication procedure, which is considered the workhorse in surgical treatment of acute and secondary chronic osteomyelitis of the jaws
- The main goal in treatment of primary chronic osteomyelitis of the jawbone is cessation or amelioration of symptoms
- In addition, bone deformity may or must be surgically addressed. Dealing with symptoms, aside from surgery, several conservative treatment options are available. Even though the disease may not been cured, change of course and severity should be considered a sign of success.

Treatment Guidelines

- Disrupt infectious foci
- Debride any foreign bodies, necrotic tissues or sequestra
- Culture and identify specific pathogens for definitive antibiotic treatment
- Drain and irrigate the region
- Consider adjunctive treatment to enhance microvascular reperfusion
  - Trephination
  - Decortication
  - Vascular flaps
  - Hyperbaric oxygen therapy
- Reconstruction

Successful treatment is based on following fundamental principles
Early diagnosis
Bacterial culture and sensitivity testing
Adequate, appropriate and prompt antibiotic therapy.
Adequate pain control
Proper surgical intervention
Reconstruction

Principles of Therapy of Acute and Secondary Chronic Osteomyelitis

- The final common pathway in all treatment of acute and secondary chronic osteomyelitis of the jaws is to achieve a shift in the disturbed balance between the responsible pathogen(s) and host defenses to the latter, allowing the body to overcome the infection. This is primarily achieved by reduction of the pathogens by number and, on the other hand, by increasing host defense mechanisms and local tissue perfusion
- These goals are mainly achieved by surgery and antibiotics which are considered the major pillars in treatment of osteomyelitis of the jaws
- Reduction of the number of pathogens is the main effect of antibiotic therapy. Besides reducing the number of pathogens by removal of infected and necrotic tissue, surgical therapy furthermore brings well-perfused tissue to the affected area

- Despite the above mentioned limitations, HBO may be seen as a third pillar in treatment of acute and secondary chronic osteomyelitis. Its mechanisms in osteomyelitis therapy are to reverse the hypoxic state of the infected bone, enhancing leukocyte killing potential as well as its direct toxic effect on strict anaerobes and facultative anaerobes. Furthermore, HBO promotes angiogenesis in the tissue and hence increasing local tissue perfusion (Marx 1991).

Therapeutic Goals in Treatment of Acute and Secondary Chronic Osteomyelitis of the Jaws

- Eradication of infection and removal of infectious focus
- Pain management
- Limitation of further spreading of the disease
- Fracture prophylaxis, and stabilization of infected fractures
- Preservation of anatomic structures when possible
- Prevention of relapse of disease
- Prevention of (further) chronification of the infection
- Re-establishment of anatomy and function.

Principles of Treatment of Acute Osteomyelitis of the Jaws

- Establish correct diagnosis, based on history, clinical evaluation, and imaging studies
- Biopsy in unclear cases to rule out other pathology (e.g. malignancy)
- Determine extent of infected bone and soft tissue
- Evaluation and correction of host defense deficiencies when possible
- Removal of source of infection, usually a dental focus, foreign bodies/implants
- Local incision and drainage of pus
- Local curettage with removal of superficial sequestra and saucerization if necessary
- Collection of specimens for Gram stain, culture and sensitivity, histopathology
- Begin with empiric broad-spectrum antibiotic therapy and change to culture-guided antibiotics as soon as possible

- More extensive surgical debridement if necessary (e.g., decortication, resection)
- Possible adjunctive hyperbaric oxygen therapy.

Principles of Treatment of Secondary Chronic Osteomyelitis of the Jaws

- Establish correct diagnosis, based on history, clinical evaluation, and imaging studies
- Biopsy in unclear cases to rule out other pathology (e.g. malignancy)
- Determine extent of infected bone and soft tissue
- Evaluation and correction of host defense deficiencies when possible
- Surgical debridement of infected tissue dictated by extent of the lesion (removal of affected teeth and foreign bodies/implants, sequestrectomy, local curettage, saucerization, decortication, resection)
- Collection of specimens for Gram stain, culture and sensitivity, histopathology
- Begin with empiric broad-spectrum antibiotic therapy and change to culture-guided antibiotics as soon as possible
- Possible adjunctive hyperbaric oxygen therapy More extensive surgical debridement if necessary (e.g. repeated decortication, resection).

Conservative management
- Complete bed rest
- Supportive therapy
  - Nutritional support:
  - High protein diet
  - High caloric diet
  - Adequate multivitamins.
- Rehydration
  - Hydration orally
  - Administration of IV fluids.
- Blood transfusion
- Control of pain
- Antibiotic therapy
  - Systemic antibiotics
    - Penicillin—Antibiotic of choice for osteomyelitis of jaw
    - Metronidazole

- Cephalosporin
- Ciprofixacin
- Clindamycin, etc.

Note: Use antibiotics for 2–4 months.

- Local antibiotics –
  - Gentamicicn + polymethylmethacrylate delivery system – non resorbable
  - Gentamicin + collagen sponge – resorbable
  - Recent introduction of oxazoledinone— non synthetic antibiotic which has a strong action against gram positive pathogens
  - Tigecycline—first commercially available new class of antimicrobial agent. It is a glycycline derivative of tetracycline and can de administered parenterally and has bacteriostatic action, useful for antibiotic resistant organism.

- Closed wound irrigation – suction:
  - To achieve the desired effect locally it may be required to give very high doses of antibiotic systematically which on other hand will produce unwanted side effects
  - To overcome this problem, local application of the antibiotic may be effective
- Antibiotic impregnated beads:
  - PMMA (Polymethyl methacrylate) beads impregnated with antibiotics may be placed into the disease bone.
- Hyperbaric oxygen therapy: Hyperbaric oxygen is effective in treatment of osteomyelitis because:
  - Hyperbaric oxygen enhances lysosomal degradation.
  - The oxygen free radicals are formed which are toxic to anaerobic pathogens.
  - The elevated partial pressure of oxygen created which inactivate the exotoxins released by the pathogens.
  - The tissue oxygen level is elevated which enhances the healing.
  - It helps in neoangiogenesis by encouraging endothelial proliferation.
  - Increased vascularity

Surgical management
Extraction of offending teeth
Incision and drainage
Sequestrectomy
Saucerization
Decortication
Resection and reconstruction

Sequestrectomy

- Removal of sequestrum (dead necrotic bone)
- Once the sequestrum is formed in bone, it can undergo many changes—
  - It may get infected and form a chronic infective focus
  - May remain dormant with no changes in it.
  - May get revascularized and healing takes place
  - May get resorbed completely.

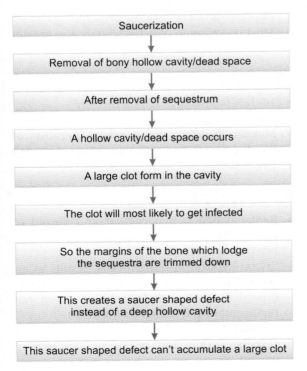

Saucerization of the Mandible (Step-by-step Procedure Modified After Topazian 2002)

- Access to the bone by creating a mucoperosteal flap, usually using a gingival crest incision
- Reflection of flap should be as limited as possible to preserve local bood supply
- Affected teeth (loosened and other dental foci within the affected area) are extracted
- The lateral cortex of the mandible is reduced using burs or rongeurs until the sufficient bleeding bone is encountered at all margins, approximately to the level of the unattached mucosa, thus producing a saucerlike defect
- Local debridement is performed by removing granulation tissue and loose bone fragments from the bone bed using curettes
- The debrided area is thoroughly irrigated with sterile saline solution with or without additional antibiotic, such as neomycin
- If there is substantial local bleeding due to hyperemia caused by the inflammatory process, a medicated pack may be placed and serve as local compression device
- The buccal flap is trimmed and a medicated pack (such as iodoform gauze lightly covered with antibiotic and local steroid ointment is placed for hemostasis and to maintain the flap in a retracted position. The pack is placed firmly without pressure and retained by several nonresorbable sutures, extending over the pack from the lingual to the buccal flap
- The pack is remained in situ for several days up to 2 weeks or even more in some instances and may be replaced serveral times until the surface of the bed of granulation tissue is epithelialized and the margins have healed.

Decortication (Mowlem's Decorticectomy)

- Surgical procedure in which the lateral and inferior cortical bone is removed (then underlying cancellous bone can be irrigated and debrided effectively)
- Cancellous bone is removed till the uninvolved area. This can be differentiated by the presence of bleeding point in vital bone compared to the necrotic bone which shows no bleeding when it is cut.

Resection and Reconstruction

- All the above procedures are not effective completely eliminating the infective process. It may be necessary to resect the infected part of jaw
- Once the part of the jaw is resected, it may be reconstructed using autologous bone graft or reconstruction plates.

Postoperative Care

- Continued use of antibiotics
- Warm saline mouth rinses
- Adequate hydration
- Complete bed rest.

Principles of Treatment of Primary Chronic Osteomyelitis

- Because primary chronic osteomyelitis responds to treatment inconsistently, all treatment options should be considered and applied on an individual basis
- As described previously, the course of early onset of primary chronic osteomyelitis (juvenile chronic osteomyelitis) may differ from the adult type
- In addition, the stage of disease may be different in an earlier period compared with a later stage. In the decision making process, the frequency of onset with pain, swelling, and limitation of mouth opening should be taken in to account as well; therefore, extent and aggressiveness of treatment may also differ. The large volume and extent of affected bone in most cases may suggest that complete surgical removal would be the best option
- Because involvement of reconstructed bone is frequently observed, resection and second-stage reconstruction should be considered carefully in late stage of disease (Eyrich et al. 1999)
- Especially in the early-onset cases of disease full-thickness resection of bone, such as continuity resection or hemimandiblectomy should not be carried out since some of the juvenile patients have shown remission at the end of bony growth

- Conservative therapy involves HBO, nonsteroidal anti-inflammatory drugs (NSAIDs), antibiotics
- HBO (twice daily sessions at 1.4 atmospheres for 45 min cycles) is applied, it seems to be important that the treatment period consist of a minimum of 20 or more sessions and that antibiotics be administered along with the HBO treatment.

OSTEONECROSIS AND HYPERBARIC OXYGEN THERAPY

DEFINITION

Osteoradionecrosis (ORN) is defined as exposed bone in the field of radiation that has failed to heal either spontaneously or with treatment for at least six months.

ETIOLOGY

- High dose radiation therapy
- ORN is a result of nonhealing, dead bone; Infection is not necessarily present.
- Most prevalent in patients who receive greater than 60 Gy radiation.

INCIDENCE

- 10–15% following radiation therapy
- Most commonly occurs in posterior mandible
- Maxilla is often not involved because of its decreased bone density and increased vascularity.

PATHOGENESIS

- Radiated bed is hypocellular and devoid of fibroblasts, osteoblasts, and undifferentiated osteocompetent cells
- Tissue hypoxia in normal cells, results in an imbalance where cell death and collagen lysis exceed the homeostatic mechanisms of cell replacement and collagen synthesis
- Metabolic demands exceed the oxygen and vascular supply and results in non healing wound.

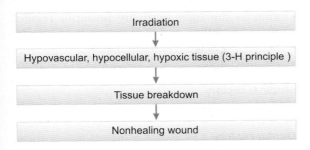

HISTOLOGIC FEATURES

- Osteoradionecrotic mandibles show several characteristic histologic changes
- The inferior alveolar artery (the predominant arterial blood supply to the body of the mandible) and periosteal arteries show significant intimal fibrosis and thrombosis
- Normal marrow will be replaced by dense fibrous tissue with loss of osteocytes
- Buccal cortical necrosis with sequestrum formation and periosteal fibrosis with a tendency to detach from the cortex.

Clinical manifestations
Pain
Orocutaneous fistula
Exposed necrotic bone
Pathologic fracture
Suppuration
Trismus
Fetid breath

CLINICAL CLASSIFICATION OF ORN

Type I: Trauma-induced ORN which occurs when radiation or surgical wounding are coupled closely together.

Type II: Also trauma-induced ORN, which occurs years after radiation therapy. Most common type.

Type III: Spontaneous ORN. Can occur anytime after radiotherapy but commonly occurs 6 months to 2 years following radiotherapy, without any obvious preceding surgical or traumatic event.

CLASSIFICATION OF ORN

Grade I: Most common presentation. Exposed alveolar bone is observed.

Grade II: Designates ORN that does not respond to hyperbaric oxygen therapy and sequestrectomy/saucerization.

Grade III: Full thickness involvement and/or pathologic fracture.

Schwartz and Robert Kagan

Stage 1: Exposed cortical bone necrotic

Stage 2: Cortical bone and underlying medullary bone necrotic
- Soft tissue ulceration is minimal
- Soft tissue necrosis (Fig. 36.3)
- Orocutaneous fisttulation

Stage 3: Full thickness of a segment of bone is involved
- Soft tissue Ulceration is minimal
- Soft tissue necrosis
- Orocutaneous fistulation.

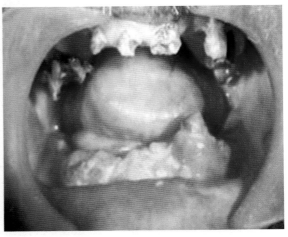

Fig. 36.3: Exposed cortical and medullary bone with soft tissue necrosis

Complications of ORN
Intractable pain
Drug dependency
Trismus
Nutritional deficiencies
Pathologic fractures
Oral and cutaneous fistulas
Loss of large areas of soft tissue and bone

DIFFERENTIAL DIAGNOSIS

- Persistent cancer
- Chronic osteomyelitis.

CASE PRESENTATION 1

A 35-year-old female patient with complaint of pain in the upper right back tooth region for a period of 3 months.

History of Presenting Illness

- Vesicle formation on the right middle third of the face 9 months ago
- Associated with severe pain and burning sensation

- Pain in the right maxillary posterior region since 3 months
- Loosening of teeth and exfoliation
- Pus discharge.

Medical History

Noncontributory.

Dental History

h/o extraction 2 weeks previously
- No known drug allergies
- No relevant personal history.

General Examination

- Moderately built and nourished
- No signs of icterus, pallor, associated systemic symptoms
- Right submandibular Lymphadenopathy

Extraoral Examination

- Extensive Scarring and hypopigmented areas over the middle third of the face (Figs 36.4 and 36.5)
- Unilateral
- Diffuse swelling over the right malar region
- Skin over swelling is erythematous
- Tender, soft in consistency
- Mild increase in temperature.

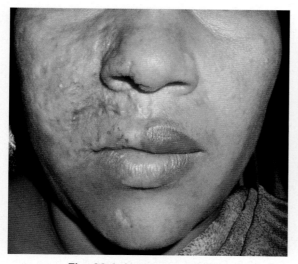

Fig. 36.4: Note extra-oral scar

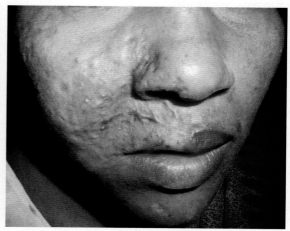

Fig. 36.5: Note hypopigmentation

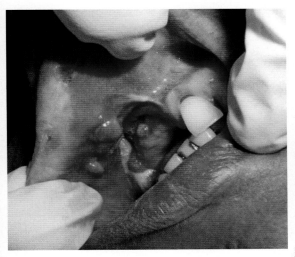

Fig. 36.6: Intraoral ulcer

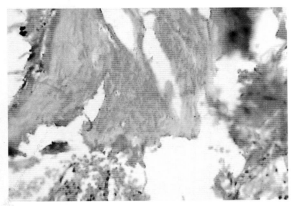

Fig. 36.7: Histopathology showing bone sequestra with necrosis

Intraoral Examination
- Ulcerated area (Fig. 36.6)
- Necrotic slough
- Exposed buccal cortical bone
- Pus Discharge
- Missing 11,12,13,14.
- Palatal Gingiva edematous, soft, tender
- Mobility of 15,16,17,18.

To Summarize

A 35-year-old female patient with a history of unilateral vesicular lesions on the right side of the face and currently presenting with exposed cortical bone in the right maxillary segment with pus discharge and tooth exfoliation.

Histopathological impression was suggestive of an infection of the bone (Fig. 36.7).

Provisional Diagnosis
- Postherpetic osteonecrosis
- Osteomyelitis
- Carcinoma.

Investigations
- Blood investigations
- Radiographs
- Exfoliative cytology.

Radiographs (Figs 36.8 to 36.10)
- Maxillary occlusal
- Panoramic
- Waters view
- Missing 11,12,13,14
- Missing 26
- Extensive right palatal bone loss
- Necrotic bone
- Granulation tissue.

ELISA

HIV positive.

Final Diagnosis

Postherpetic osteonecrosis.

Radiographic Findings
- Radiographic picture varies so greatly and hence the diagnosis of ORN is a clinical one
- Plain radiography of the mandible, such as panorex depicts areas of local decalcification or sclerosis (Fig. 36.11)
- Typical moth eaten appearance can be seen
- CT scanning and MRI may allow early diagnosis of ORN and better delineate the extent of disease
- MRI depicts ORN with reduced bone marrow signal intensity on T1-weighted images and increased signal intensity on T2-weighted images

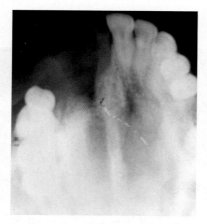

Fig. 36.8: Maxillary occlusal

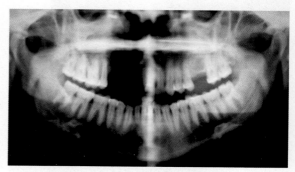

Fig. 36.9: Panoramic radiograph

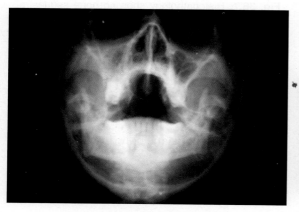

Fig. 36.10: Paranasal sinus view

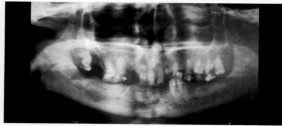

Fig. 36.11: Areas of local decalcification and typical moth-eaten appearance can be seen

- Absence of marrow signal on MRI can be used to identify significant radiation injury in the mandible
- Panoramic radiography and CT scan images can be used to determine sites of significant bone injury. Alteration in trabeculation, cortical thinning, and sclerosis are common findings in sites of injury
- Single-photon emission computed tomography (SPECT) imaging may have a role in the future as more experience is gained with this.

Treatment

- Medical therapy
- Surgical therapy

Medical Therapy

- Patient's motivation
- Oral prophylaxis
- Periodontal scaling
- Caries control
- Fabrication of fluoride trays
- Prior to radiotherapy prognosis for each tooth should be outlined
- Ideally, extractions should be performed 3 weeks (21 days) prior to beginning radiation therapy
- Extraction of teeth during radiation therapy should be discouraged and delayed until the completion of treatment with resolution of the oral mucositis

- Post-radiation dental extractions should be avoided. Surgery performed during the first 4 months after radiation therapy is usually associated with normal healing (Golden period)
- To prevent radiation caries, patients should begin daily fluoride treatment with 1% neutral sodium fluoride gel in prefabricated trays for 5 minutes each day. This practice should continue for life
- Medical therapy in treatment of ORN is primarily supportive, involving
  - Nutritional support
  - Superficial debridement
  - Oral saline irrigation
  - Antibiotics are indicated only for definite secondary infection.

Surgical therapy

In 1983, Marx demonstrated successful resolution of mandibular ORN in 58 patients using a staged protocol with HBO and surgery.

Marx University of Miami Protocol

Stage I

- Perform 30 HBO dives (1 dive per day, Monday to Friday) to 2.4 atmospheres for 90 minutes
- Reassess the patient to evaluate decreased bone exposure, granulation tissue covering exposed bone, resorption of nonviable bone, and absence of inflammation
- For patients who respond favorably, continue treatment to a total of 40 dives. For patients who are not responsive, advance to stage II.

Stage II

- Perform transoral sequestrectomy with primary wound closure followed by continued HBO to a total of 40 dives.
- If wound dehiscence occurs, advance patients to stage III.
- Patients who present with orocutaneous fistula, pathologic fracture, or resorption to the inferior border of the mandible advance to stage III immediately after the initial 30 dives.

Stage III

Perform transcutaneous mandibular resection, wound closure, and mandibular fixation with an external fixator or maxillomandibular fixation, followed by an additional 10 postoperative HBO dives.

Stage IIIR

- Perform mandibular reconstruction 10 weeks after successful resolution of mandibular ORN
- Marx advocates the use of autogenous cancellous bone within a freeze-dried allogeneic bone carrier
- Complete 10 additional postoperative HBO dives.

HYPERBARIC OXYGEN THERAPY

Definition

Short-term-100% oxygen inhalation therapy at a pressure greater than that of sea level. The pressure is usually about 2.4 absolute atmospheres or ATA.

Indications of HBO

Currently underseas and Hyperbaric Medical Society approves only the following indications for HBO:

- Air or gas embolism
- Carbon monoxide poisioning
- Clostridial myonecrosis
- Crush injury
- Decompression sickness
- Exceptional blood loss (anemia)
- Necrotizing soft tissue infections
- Osteomyelitis
- Osteoradionecrosis
- Skin grafts and flaps (compromised)
- Thermal burn.

Indications in OMFS

- Chronic refractory osteomyelitis of the jaws
- Chronic suppurative osteomyelitis
- Chronic diffuse sclerozing osteomyelitis

- Osteoradionecrosis
  - Stage I ORN
  - Stage II ORN
  - Stage III ORN
- Prevention of ORN
- Elective surgery in irradiated tissues
- Bony reconstruction of jaws
- Soft tissue reconstruction of oral cavity and neck.

Absolute Contraindications

- Untreated pneumothorax
- History of optic neuritis
- Fulminant viral infections
- Congenital spherocytosis.

Mechanism of Action of HBO

- HBO improves tissue healing by increasing the oxygen gradient in irradiated tissues
- Nonirradiated wounds, there is a central area of tissue injury surrounded by tissue with normal perfusion, setting up a steep oxygen gradient across the wound
- In wounds with radiation tissue injury, only shallow oxygen gradients are created
- Gradients have been shown to be the physical–chemotactic factor attracting macrophages to a wound
- Lactate, iron and steep oxygen gradients stimulate macrophage-derived angiogenesis factor and macrophage-derived growth factor, which in turn promote capillary budding and collagen synthesis
- Stimulus for fibroplasia and angiogenesis is therefore lacking in irradiated tissues
- HBO restores the steep oxygen gradient needed for wound healing.

Effects of Hyperbaric Oxygen (Tables 36.1 and 36.2)

- Primary effects
- Secondary effects.

Table 36.1: Primary effects

Mechanism	Effect	Clinical application
Hyperoxygenation	Greater oxygen carrying capacity Increased oxygen diffusion in tissue fluids	• Severe blood loss anemia • Crush injury • Graft and flap salvage
Decrease gas bubble size		• Decompression sickness • Air embolus syndrome

Table 36.2: Secondary effects

Mechanism	Effect	Clinical application
Vasoconsriction	• Decreased inflow into tissues • Decreased edema	• Crush injuries • Acute burns • Compartment syndrome
Angiogenesis	• Increased oxygen gradient • Increased fibroblast proliferation	• Graft and flap salvage • Osteoradionecrosis • Chronic wounds
Leucocytre oxidative killing	• Increased oxygen free radicals • Anaerobes lack • Superoxide dismutase to control oxygen free redicals	• Necrotizing soft-tissue infections • Chronic osteomyelitis

Types of Hyperbaric Oxygen Therapy Chambers

- Monoplace chambers
- Multiplace chambers.

Monoplace Chambers

100% oxygen, 2.0 ATA for 120 treatment minutes exclusive of pressurization and depressurization times used.

Advantages and disadvantages
- Claustrophobic environment
- Limited access to patient
- Whole chamber contains hyperbaric oxygen, increasing fire risk
- Lower cost
- Portable.

Multiplace Chambers

100% oxygen at 2.4 ATA for 90 treatment minutes exclusive of pressurization and depressurization times used.

Advantages and disadvantages
- More room
- Assistant can enter to deal with acute problems such as pneumothorax
- Hyperbaric oxygen is delivered via tight fitting mask, the rest of chamber gas can be air (reduced fire risk)
- Risk of cross infection when used for ulcers, etc.

Risks of Hyperbaric Oxygen

- Fire hazard
- Claustrophobia
- Reversible myopia
- Fatigue
- Headache
- Vomiting
- Barotrauma
  - Ear damage
  - Sinus damage
  - Ruptured middle ear
  - Lung damage

- Oxygen toxicity
  - Convulsions
- Decompression sickness
- Pneumothorax
- Gas emboli.

CASE PRESENTATION 2

A 65-year-old male patient complains of pain and pus discharge from lower right molar region for 1 year.

History of Presenting Illness

- Extraction of lower right back teeth was done 1 year back as they were mobile. It was followed by pain with pus discharge from the alveolus on right lower molar region (Fig. 36.12).
- Pain was continuous, severe pricking type radiating to right mandibular angle region. Pain is not relieved on taking medication and associated with mild fever and difficulty in eating
- Patient has consulted many dentists but no relief was found. Records of previous treatment not available
- Underwent radiotherapy for the treatment of a non healing ulcer present on palate, which was diagnosed as squamous cell carcinoma 1 year 10 months back
- Radiotherapy was done for a period of 1 month; 5 days/week. Lesion has healed.

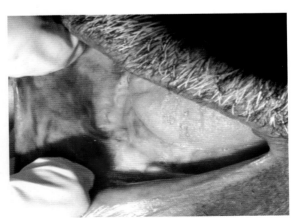

Fig. 36.12: Note pus in right molar region

Past Medical and Drug History

- Patient was hospitalized for eye surgery for decreased vision 5 months back
- No history of drug allergy.

Personal History

- Cleans mouth twice daily
- Mixed diet
- Habituated to beedi smoking for 35 yrs, 20–25 bidis/day. Occasional alcohol consumption present.

General Physical Examination

- Patient was conscious and cooperative. Poorly built and nourished
- Pallor present, sclera is pigmented, no cyanosis, clubbing, edema noted
- Eyes are sunken and skin is wrinkled
- Neck muscles are accentuated with prominent supraclavicular and suprasternal notch
- TMJ is normal on palpation
- No palpable lymph nodes present
- Hoarseness of voice noted.

Extraoral Examination

- No gross extraoral asymmetry

- Tenderness present over right mandibular angle region on palpation
- Lips are pigmented.

Intraoral Examination (Figs 36.13 and 36.14)

Inspection
- Completely edentulous
- A linear furrow is present on edentulous alveolar ridge measuring about 2.5 cm in length extending from 46 to 48
- Furrow is filled with pus and margins are raised with normal mucosal color.

Palpation
- Tender
- No alveolar bone expansion noted.
- Pus exudates from furrow on palpation.
- Dryness of mucosa felt on palpation.
- Labial mucosa, hard palate is pale and pigmented (Fig. 36.13).

To Summarize

- A 65-year-male reported with complains of pain and pus discharge from the lower right molar region of 1 year duration
- History of radiotherapy for the treatment of squamous cell carcinoma on palate, 1 year 10 months back

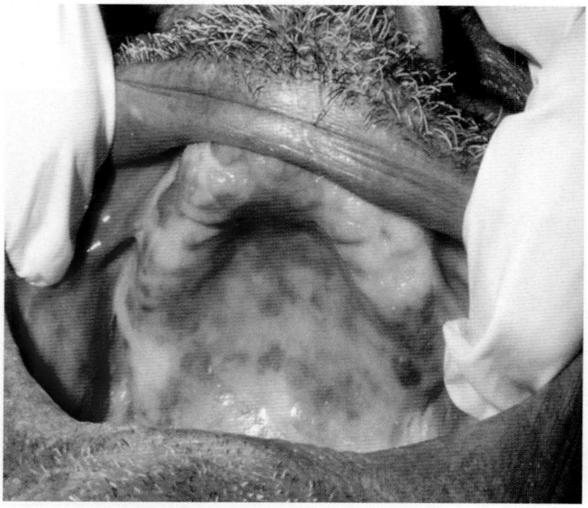

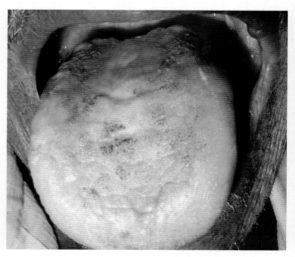

Fig. 36.13: Pigmentation at hard palate

Fig. 36.14: Tongue—depapillated

- Pus discharge noted after extraction of teeth in that region
- Intraorally a linear furrow was noted on right alveolar ridge with raised margins. Pus exudation noted from the furrow. No signs of inflammation present except for tenderness.

Provisional Diagnosis

Post-radiation therapy necrosis of mandible

Differential Diagnosis

- Chronic osteomyelitis
- Residual infection.

Investigations

OPG (Fig. 36.15)
- Reduced height of body of mandible on right side
- Superior border on right side shows loss of contour with irregular bony saucerizations
- Multiple irregular radiolucent areas found with necrotic bony spicules and no reactive bone is noted
- Obliteration of mandibular canal on right side
- Features are suggestive of post-radiotherapy osteomyelitic changes.

Fine Needle Aspiration Cytology

H&E and PAP stained smear shows normal superficial epithelial cells seen in singly or in clumps with numerous acute and chronic inflammatory cells. No evidence of malignancy or dysplasia or malignancy is seen in smears.

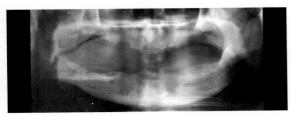

Fig. 36.15: OPG loss of contour with irregular bony saucerization with mandibular canal obliteration

Impression: Suggestive of acute inflammation.
Microbiology: Negative for acid fast-bacilli .
Diagnosis: Osteoradionecrosis.

CASE PRESENTATION 3

A 55-year-old male patient complains of pain and burning sensation of mouth for 3 months duration.

History of Presenting Illness

- Treated for carcinoma of larynx 10 months back and had received 20 fractions of radiation in 1 month duration
- Patient underwent dental extractions 3 months after radiotherapy and has not revealed about radiotherapy at that time
- Moderate and persistent pain through out the day for 10 months.

Medical History

- No history of diabetes or hypertension
- Radiotherapy 10 months for carcinoma of larynx.

Personal History

- Beedi smoker for 30 years, 30 beedis per day
- Alcoholic since 30 years.

General Physical Examination

- Moderately built
- Hoarseness of voice
- Vital signs:BP:130/80 mm Hg
- PR: 72/min
- RR: 22/min

Extraoral Examination

- Face: Alopecia present over the beard (Figs 36.16 and 36.17)
- Neck: Skin is fixed to the underlying connective tissue
- Lymph nodes : Not palpable.

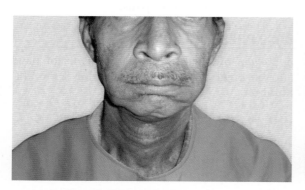

Fig. 36.16: Extraoral presentation

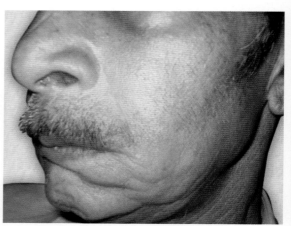

Fig. 36.17: Reduced beard growth

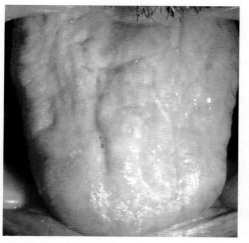

Fig. 36.18: Tongue: Smooth appearance, depapillated

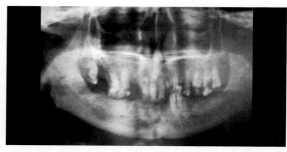

Fig. 36.19: Areas of local decalcification and typical moth eaten appearance can be seen

Intraoral Examination

- Mucosa: Pale, dry, edematous, tender on palpation
- Indirect laryngoscopy
  - Edema of epiglottis
  - Bilateral vocal cords not visible due to edema
- Tongue—smooth appearance (Fig. 36.18)
- Teeth present

$$\frac{86521 \quad 135678}{34}$$

- Generalized cervical caries
- Exposed bone in the region of

$$\overline{654321 \;|\; 1257}$$

Investigations

Orthopantomogram (Fig. 36.19).

Provisional Diagnosis

- Osteoradionecrosis, radiation caries
- Stage 2 Division B.

CASE 4 (FIGS 36.20 TO 36.23 A AND B)

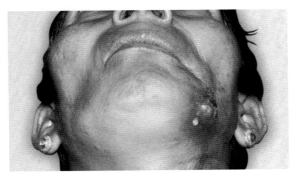

Fig. 36.20: Extraoral sinus

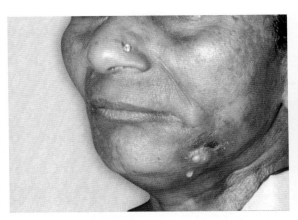

Fig. 36.21: Pus discharge can be seen

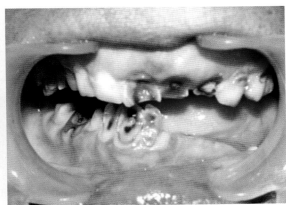

Fig. 36.22: Radiation carries

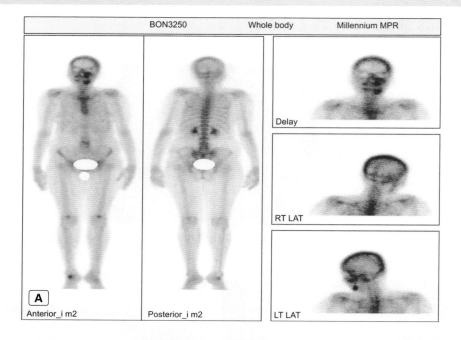

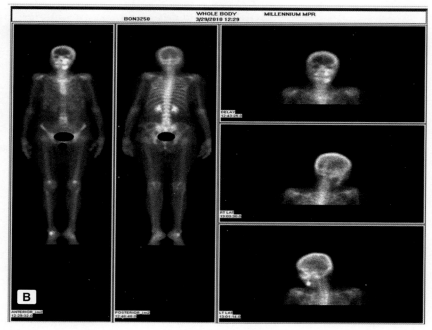

Figs 36.23A and B: Bone scan notice the hot spots at region of fistula in mandible

Section

8

Examination of Jaw Deformities

Diagnosis and Evaluation of Jaw Deformity

37

INTRODUCTION

Diagnosis and evaluation of jaw deformity involve good clinical evaluation, photograph, freehand surgical simulation based on cephalometric tracing and then transferred to study model surgery and computerized prediction software. Model surgery planning on dental casts is used for the final correction of facial deformity and malocclusion. Analysis of model surgery allows the transfer of planned three-dimensional movements for the surgical correction of complex dentofacial deformity.

One of the accuracy of the errors in orthognathic model surgery occurs in mounting the models on the articulator. The accuracy of the face bow transfer may differ from one type of face bow to another. When using a conventional articulator for orthognathic surgery, it is essential that the angle between the occlsial plane and Frankfort horizontal for the patient is the same as theangle between the occlsial plane and the upper member of the articulator on the maxillary model.

DEFINITION

Orthognathic surgery is the art and science of diagnosis, treatment planning and execution of treatment by combining orthodontic and OMFS to correct musculoskeletal, dento-osseous and soft tissue deformities of the jaws and associated structures.

- Dentofacial deformities affects 20% of population
- They demonstrate functional and esthetic compromise
- Occur unilaterally or bilaterally or may be expressed in vertical, horizontal and transverse facial planes.

DENTOFACIAL DEFORMITY (TABLE 37.1)

- Dental malocclusion
- Skeletal malocclusion.

Table 37.1: Various dentofacial deformity and their treatment options

Maxillary deformities
- Maxillary AP excess
- Maxillary AP deficiency
- Vertical maxillay excess
- Vertical maxillary deficiency
- Transverse maxillary deficiency
- Alveolar clefts

Mandibular deformities
- Mandibular AP excess
- Mandibular AP deficiency
- Mandibular AP asymmetry
- Chin deformities
- Macrogenia
- Microgenia

Combination deformities
- Short face syndrome
- Long face syndrome

Treatment options for dentofacial deformities
- Growth modification
- Orthodontic camouflage
- Orthognathic surgery

- These procedures are done by combination of teeth movement (orthodontics) and repositioning of jaw structures (orthognathic surgery)
- Orthodontist can align and decompensate the teeth in relation to upper and lower jaws
- Oral and maxillofacial surgeon can move facial skeleton, but can also provide detailed alignment and precise interdigitation of the teeth.

Common Diagnostic and Risk Factors

- Type of congenital or development deformity
- Type of acquired deformity
- Type of dento-osseous deformity
- Type of musculoskeletal deformity
- Respiratory problems
- Sinus or nasal airway disease
- Speech problems
- TMJ dysfunction
- Masticatory and swallowing difficulties
- Bone or soft tissue pathosis
- Severity of esthetic facial deformity
- Poor patient compliance and psychosocial impairment.

Basic Therapeutic Goals

1. *Function*
   - Normal masticaiton
   - Speech
   - Occular function
   - Respiratory function.
2. *Esthetic:* Establish facial harmony and balance.
3. *Stability:* Avoid short and long-term relapses.
   - Variations in facial proportions within normal limits make a human face interesting. It is the harmony and symmetry of each segment which contributes towards the total beauty of the face
   - Any deviation from the normal facial development brings about an unpleasant facial appearance with a disturbance in both aesthetics as well as function.

Treatment Plan

Personal, medical and dental testing:
- Analysis of facial aesthetics
- Lateral cephalometric analysis
- Occlusal analysis
- Final treatment plan
  - Presurgical orthodontics
  - Surgery plan
  - Postsurgical orthodontics
  - Maintenance.

Patient Evaluation

Evaluation of patient for orthognathic surgery is divided into four main areas:
- Patient concerns
- Clinical examination
- Radiographic imaging analysis
- Dental model analysis.

Patient Concerns

- Attention should be paid to chief complaint of patient, since ultimate aim of orthognathic surgery is to satisfy patient
- A surgeon should understand patient concern, expectation and motivation. This also gives idea to surgeon regarding psychological health of the patient
- Asking specific simple questions to patient prepare a preliminary problem list. This will help to identify the patient with unrealistic expectations
- The patient should understand his problem, all treatment options, anticipated outcomes and potential risk and complications.

System-oriented Physical Examination

Medical and dental history, physical examination, appropriate laboratory studies which may gives any positive findings, affecting the treatment plan. The proper history may help the surgery to prevent potentially life-threatening complications.

Patient Preparation

- The patient should sit upright in a straight backed chair with the examiner seated directly opposite at eye level

- The Frankfort horizontal plane should be parallel to the floor
- Once the head oriented properly, the mandibular condyles should be seated in glenoid fossae with the teeth lightly touching
- Evaluate centric occlusion and centric relation.
- Patient's lips should be relaxed and not forced together help to evaluate vertical facial height and the morphologic features, tooth-to-lip measurements, possible lip incompetence and evaluation of midlines and chin position, etc

Facial Evaluation
- The face is derived into equal thirds
- The upper facial third extends from the hairline to the glabella
- The middle third extends-from glabella to the subnasale to soft tissue menton
- Lower third extends from subnasale to soft tissue menton.
  Evaluation from frontal view should include the following 14 anatomic relationships.
- Forehead, eyes, orbits and nose are evaluated for symmetry, size and deformity
- Normal intercanthal distances 32 ± 3 mm for which 35 ± 3 mm blacks
- Normal interpupillary distances 65 ± 3 mm
- The intercanthal distance, alar base width and palpebral fissure width should all be equal
- Width of nasal dorsum should be one half the intercanthal distances and width of the nasal lobules should be 2/3rd the intercanthal distance
- A vertical line through the medial canthus and perpendicular to the pupillary plane should fall on the alar bases ± 2 mm
- The upper lip length is measured from subnasale to upper lip stomion (22 ± 2 mm for males and 20 ± 2 mm for females)
- A normal upper tooth—to lip relationship exposes 2.5 ± 1.5 mm of incisal edge to lips
- The facial midline, nasal midline, lip midline dental midline all should be in line and face should be reasonably symmetric, vertical and transversely

- During smiling the vermilion of the upper lip should fall at the cervicogingival margin with no more than 1 to 2 mm of exposed gingival
- The lower eyelid should be level/slightly above the most inferior aspect of the iris
- The distance from glabella to subnasale and subnasali to menton should be approximately in a 1:1 ration, providing that the upper tip length is normal
- The length of the upper lip should be 1/3rd the length of the lower facial third.

Lateral View Evaluation

Most valuable in assessing vertical and AP problems of the jaws:
- The distance form glabella to subnasale and from subnasale to soft tissue menton should be in a 1:1 ratio if the upper lip length is normal
- With the maxilla in normal AP position and the upper lip normal thickness, ideal chin projection is 3 ± 3 mm posterior to a line through subnasale that is perpendicular to a clinical Frankfort horizontal
- The morphologic characteristics and relationships of the nose, lips, cheeks and chin are evaluated
- The cervicomandibular angle is evaluated in reference to chin position
- Upper lip suprabasale should be 1 + 3 mm enterion to subnasale
- The length of the upper lip should be 1/3rd the length of lower facial height (third). Lower lip stomion to soft tissue menton should be twice the vertical dimension of the upper lip if the upper lip is normal in length
- A line perpendicular to Frankfort horizontal and tangist to the globe should fall on the infraorbital soft tissues J2 mm.

Oral Examination
- It helps to identify functional and esthetic deformities of dento-osseous and soft tissue structures

- Examine oral cavity for following features:
  - Dental arch form/length
  - Dental alignment/symmetry
  - Dental occlusion
  - Curve of Wilson and curve of Spee
  - Missing and carious teeth
  - Periodontal evaluation
  - Anatomic or functional tongue abnormalities.

TMJ Evaluation

TMJ provides foundation for orthognathic surgery. Presurgical TMJ pathology can result in unfavorable outcome such as condylar resorption, malocclusion, jaw dysfunction and facial deformity.

The Nose

History of nasal trauma since problems, mouth bleeding esthetic concerns, nasal airway obstruction and previous surgery is asked with the patient undergoing orthognathic surgery.

Radiographic evaluation
The imaging technique used in the diagnosis of dentofacial deformity can be devided broadly into 2 categories
• Routine radiograph: – Periapical—OPG are helpful in determining root angualtion, tooth alignment and existing pathology   – Lateral and PA cephalograms
• Other imaging modalities: TMJ tomograms, transcranial radiographs, water view, MRI and CT scan

Cephalometric Radiographs

- Lateral and PA cephalometric radiographs used to analyze skeletal, dentoalveolar and soft tissue relationships in the anterioposterior (AP), transverse and vertical dimensions
- Cephalometry is only an aid to clinical assessment and should not be used as sole diagnostic tool
- When a significant difference occurs, the clinical evaluation is for more important for treatment planning.

Cephalometric Analysis

- The cephalometric analysis helpful in diagnosing the problem helps in treatment planning and also allows clinician to evaluate changes after surgery
- These analyzes primarily designed to evaluate the position of the teeth with the existing skeletal pattern (Figs 37.1 to 37.4).

Cephalometric for Orthognathic Surgery (COGS) Analysis

- Chosen landmarks and measurements can be altered by various surgical procedures.
- The appraisal includes all facial bones and a cranial base reference.
- Rectilinear measurements can be readily transferred to a study cast for mock surgery.

Dental Model Analysis

- Arch length
- Tooth size analysis: Bolton's analysis
- Arch width analysis
- Cuspid-molar position
- Overbite overjet relation
- Tooth arch symmetry
- Model surgery.

Diagnostic List

The list includes:
- Functional
- Esthetic
- Dental problem.

Orthodontic Objectives

- Locate the teeth in optimal and decompensated position so that surgical correction is not hindered by the dentoalveolar component
- Presurgical phase takes 24–30 months, while the postsurgical detailing of occlusion requiring 4–6 months.

Orthodontic Teeth Movement for Surgical Patient

- Presurgical: Alignment, leveling, arch form compatibility, space for osteotomy

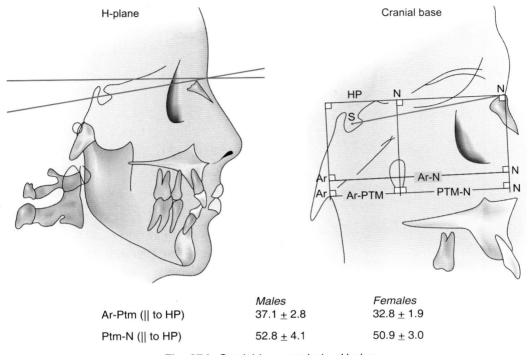

	Males	Females
Ar-Ptm (|| to HP)	37.1 ± 2.8	32.8 ± 1.9
Ptm-N (|| to HP)	52.8 ± 4.1	50.9 ± 3.0

Fig. 37.1: Cranial base analysis—H plane

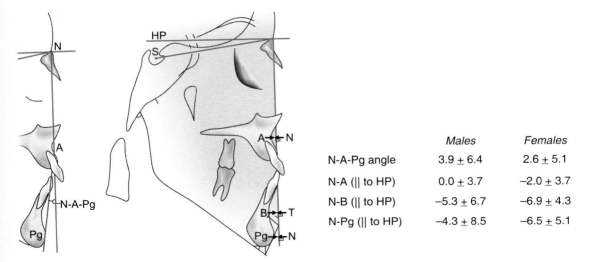

	Males	Females
N-A-Pg angle	3.9 ± 6.4	2.6 ± 5.1
N-A (|| to HP)	0.0 ± 3.7	−2.0 ± 3.7
N-B (|| to HP)	−5.3 ± 6.7	−6.9 ± 4.3
N-Pg (|| to HP)	−4.3 ± 8.5	−6.5 ± 5.1

Fig. 37.2: Cranian base analysis—horizontal measurement

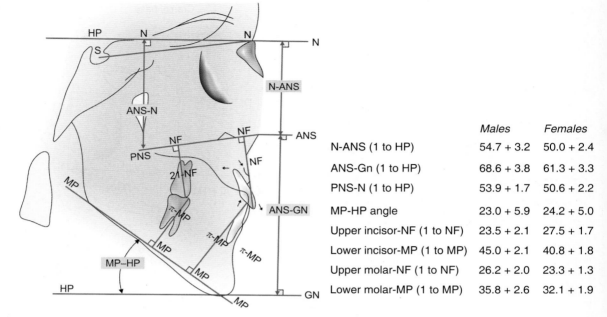

	Males	Females
N-ANS (1 to HP)	54.7 + 3.2	50.0 + 2.4
ANS-Gn (1 to HP)	68.6 + 3.8	61.3 + 3.3
PNS-N (1 to HP)	53.9 + 1.7	50.6 + 2.2
MP-HP angle	23.0 + 5.9	24.2 + 5.0
Upper incisor-NF (1 to NF)	23.5 + 2.1	27.5 + 1.7
Lower incisor-MP (1 to MP)	45.0 + 2.1	40.8 + 1.8
Upper molar-NF (1 to NF)	26.2 + 2.0	23.3 + 1.3
Lower molar-MP (1 to MP)	35.8 + 2.6	32.1 + 1.9

Fig. 37.3: Cranial base analysis—vertical measurement

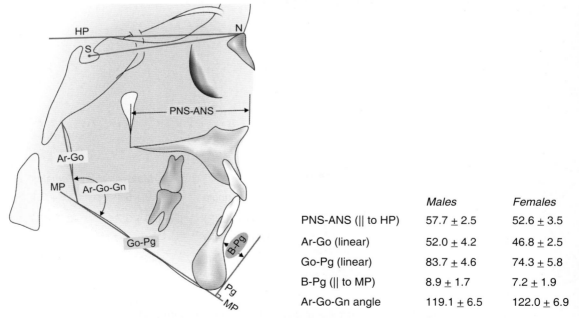

	Males	Females
PNS-ANS (‖ to HP)	57.7 ± 2.5	52.6 ± 3.5
Ar-Go (linear)	52.0 ± 4.2	46.8 ± 2.5
Go-Pg (linear)	83.7 ± 4.6	74.3 ± 5.8
B-Pg (‖ to MP)	8.9 ± 1.7	7.2 ± 1.9
Ar-Go-Gn angle	119.1 ± 6.5	122.0 ± 6.9

Fig. 37.4: Cranial base analysis—maxilla and mandible measurements

- Postsurgical: Posterior cross bite correction, extrusion for leveling and setting, detailing occlusion, root paralleling.

Diagnosis

- The jaws relation and facial proportion including the nose and the ears
- Orthodontics
- Periodontal condition
- Speech pattern
- Psychological condition.

Model Surgery

- Maxillary, mandibular, combined double jaw procedures
- Analytic model surgery allows the transfer of prescribed three dimensional movements
- For either maxillary or mandibular procedures make only one splint (final splint)
- For double jaw procedure
- Intermediate splint (wafer) to relate the osteotomized maxilla to the stable mandible
- Final splint to relate the osteotomized mandible to the fixated maxilla
- When the plan to operate the maxilla only or the mandible only, the use of semi-adjustable articulator and face bow transfer is not always required.
- Draw line in between the base and the cast to breakthrough to make the necessary movement.
- Hold U and L casts together in centric relation using bite registration
- Mount the two cast on articulator
- Separate the casts and make the vertical and horizontal reference lines
- Vertical reference lines at midline, canines, first molars and posterior to third molars regions
- Horizontal reference lines should be made parallel to each other and separated by 10–15 mm to allow you to reproduce the vertical movement within these two lines.

ESTHETIC SURGICAL PROCEDURES

Soft Tissue Procedures

- Fat augmentation
- Rhytidectomy
- Blepharoplasty
- Botox injections.

Hard Tissue Procedures

- Maxillary procedures
- Mandibular procedures.

Maxillary Procedures

Segmental osteotomy

- Single tooth osteotomy
- Corticotomy
- Anterior maxillary segmental osteotomy
  - Wassmund's technique
  - Wunderer's technique
  - Epker's anterior maxillary osteotomy
  - Cupar's technique
- Posterior subapical osteotomy of maxilla
  - Kufner
  - Schuchardt
  - Perko and Bell.

Total maxillary osteotomy

- LeFort I osteotomy
- LeFort II osteotomy
- LeFort III osteotomy.

Mandibular Procedures

Mandibular body osteotomies

- Anterior body
- Posterior body
- Mid symphysis.

Segmental subapical osteotomies

- Anterior subapical
- Posterior subapical
- Total subapical.

Genioplasties

- Horizontal osteotomy with AP reduction
- Tenon technique
- Double sliding horizontal osteotomy
- Alloplastic augmentation

- Vertical reduction
- Straightening
- Lengthening.

Mandibular ramus osteotomies
- Subcondylar ramus
- Vertical ramus osteotomy
- Sagittal split osteotomy.

CASE NUMBER 1

A 20-year male patient complains of irregular arrangement of teeth and bad smile (Figs 37.5 to 37.7).

Extraoral Examination

- Cephalic type — Brachycephalic
- Facial type — Leptoprosopic
- Facial profile — Convex
- Mandibular plane — Steep angle
- Lips — Consciously competent
- Everted lower lips
- Interlabial gap — 3–4 mm
- Incisal display
- On speech — 3–4 mm
- On smile — 1–2 mm of gingiva
- Mid face: Lower face – 65 : 75

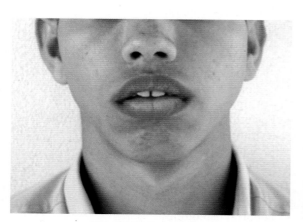

Fig. 37.5: Frontal view

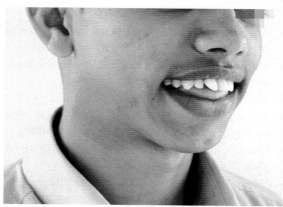

Fig. 37.6: Oblique view

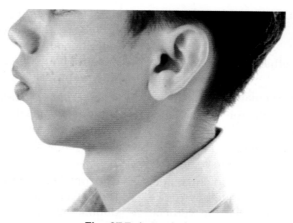

Fig. 37.7: Lateral view

Intraoral Examination

Maxillary Arch (Fig. 37.8)

- Symmetric
- Anterior spacing—7 mm.

Mandibular Arch (Fig. 37.9)

- Square shaped arch
- Anterior spacing—7 mm
- Posterior spacing—3 mm
- Missing first molars.

Tongue thrust present: Teeth in occlusion (Fig. 37.10)

- Overjet—15 mm
- Openbite—8 mm
- Midline deviation to left.

Cephalometric Analysis

See detail in Table 37.2 to 37.5.

Diagnosis

- Class II skeletal base (normal maxilla; retrognathic mandible with vertical growth pattern)

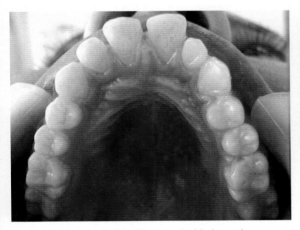

Fig. 37.8: Maxillary arch: V-shaped

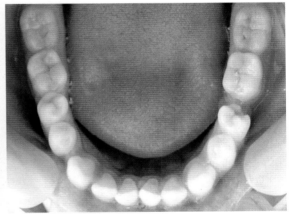

Fig. 37.9: Mandibular arch: square-shaped

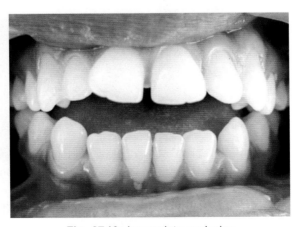

Fig. 37.10: Incomplete occlusion

Table 37.2: Downs analysis

Angles	Mean	Range	Actual
Facial angle	87.8	82 to 95	77
Angle of convexity	0	+10 to – 8	10
AB to N-Pg	– 4.8	0 to – 9	8
Mandibular plane	21.9	17 to 28	42
Y-axis	59.4	53 to 66	71
Cant of the occlusal plane	+ 9.3	+ 1.5 to + 14	15
Interincisal angle	135.4	130 to 150.5	97
Mandibular incisor to mandibular plane	91.4	– 8.5 to +7	+ 1
Mandibular incisor to occlusal plane	+ 14.5	+ 3.5 to + 20	28
Maxillary incisor to A-Pg line	+ 2.9 mm	– 1 to + 5 mm	17 mm

Table 37.3: Steiners analysis

Angles	Mean	Preorthopedic	Presurgery
SNA	82	82	
SNB	80	75	
ANB	2	7	
Gonion to gnathion	32	39	
Occlusal Pl to SN	14	16	
UI to N-A mm	4 mm	13 mm	
U1 to N-A angles	22	46	
L1 to N-B mm	4 mm	8 mm	
L1 to N-B angles	25	30	
U1 to L1 angles	131	97	

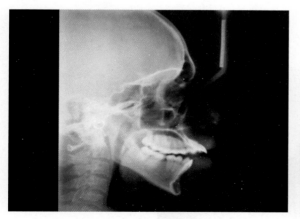

Fig. 37.11: Lateral cephalogram (Case 1)

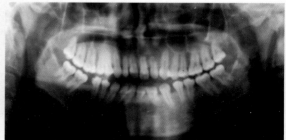

Fig. 37.12: Orthopantomogram (Case 1)

- Increased overjet (15 mm), anterior open bite (6 mm)
- Proclined incisors with spacing
- Convex facial profile with consciously competent lip.
- Cephalogram and OPG (Figs 37.11 and 37.12).

Landmarks	Mean female	Mean male	Pre-Rx	Inference	Presurgery	Postsurgery
Cranial base						
Ar-Ptm	32.8 ± 1.9	37.1 ± 2.8	37		37	
Ptm-N (ll to HP)	50.9 ± 3.0	52.8 ± 4.1	53		53	
Horizontal skeletal						
N-A-Pg (angle)	2.6 ± 5.1	3.8 ± 6.4	10		7	
N-A (ll to HP)	−2.0 ± 3.7	0.0 ± 3.7	−2		−1.5	
N-B (ll to HP)	−6.9 ± 4.3	-5.3 ± 6.7	−15		−12	
N-B (ll to HP)	−6.5 ± 4.3	-4.3 ± 8.5	−14		−11	
Vertical skeletal						
N-ANS (⊥ HP)	50.0 ± 2.4	54.7 ± 3.2	53		53	
ANS-Gn (⊥ HP)	61.3 ± 3.3	68.6 ± 3.8	77		77	
PNS-N (⊥ HP)	50.6 ± 2.2	53.9 ± 1.7	57		56	
MP-HP (angle)	24.2 ± 5.0	23.0 ± 5.9	32		32	
Vertical dental						
Upper incisor—NF	27.5 ± 1.7	30.5 ± 2.1	33		33	
Lower incisor to MP	40.8 ± 1.8	45.0 ± 2.1	39		41	
Upper molar to NF	23.3 ± 1.3	26.2 ± 2.0	29		29	
Lower molar to MP	32.1 ± 1.9	35.8 ± 2.6	30		33	
Vertical skeletal						
PNS-ANS	52.6 ± 3.5	57.7 ± 2.5	57		57	
Ar-Go	46.8 ± 2.5	52.0 ± 4.2	45		46	
Go-Pg	74.3 ± 5.8	83.7 ± 4.6	74		76	
B-Pg	7.2 ± 1.9	8.9 ± 1.7	5		5	
Ar-Go-Gn (angle)	122.0° ± 6.9	119.3° ± 6.5°	134		135	
Dental						
A-B (OP)	−0.4 ± 2.5	−1.1 ± 2.0	−5		−2	
Upper incisor-NF angle	112.5° ± 5.3°	111.0° ± 4.7°	133		130	
Lower incisor-MP angle	95.9° ± 5.7°	95.9° ± 5.2°	96		88	
OP upper-HP angle	7.1 ± 2.5	6.2 ± 5.1	3		6	
OP-HP angle			17		14	

Table 37.4: Cephalometrics for orthognathic surgery analysis (COGS)

Treatment Plan

- Presurgical orthodontics
  - Arch alignment
  - Closure of spaces
- LeFort I osteotomy (posterior maxillary impaction to reduce anterior open bite; set back to achieve class I canine relation)
- Advancement genioplasty (if required)?
- BSSO (if required)?
- Postsurgical orthodontics

- Contemporary surgical planning is concerned with designing an operation to meet individuals functional and esthetic needs
- A radiograph that delineates both soft and hard tissues is made with mandible in centric relation
- The maxilla is moved superiorly the amount necessary to achieve 2–3 mm of maxillary incisor exposure with upper lip at rest
- The magnitude of the superior movement of the posterior portion of the maxilla will usually be

Table 37.5: Holdaway's analysis		
Particulars	*Mean*	*Actual*
Facial angle	90	78
Upper lip curvature	2.5 mm	5 mm
Skeletal convexity @ pt A	−2 to + 2 mm	4 mm
H-line angle	7 to 15	24
Upper sulcus depth	5 mm	7 mm
Upper lip thickness	15 mm	15 mm
Upper lip strain	14–16	17 mm
Lower lip to H-line	−1 to +2 mm	13
Lower sulcus depth	5 mm	−6 mm
Soft tissue thickness	10 to 12 mm	3 mm

greater than the amount of superior movement of the anterior portion of the maxilla

- This is necessary to level to the maxillary occlusal plane and correct the anterior open bite
- Consequently there will be proportionally more autorotation of the mandible.

Closure of Open Bite

- It must be programmed before orthodontic treatment is initiated
- The selection of the sites for interdental osteotomy and transverse palatal bone incision is based on the location of the anterior open bite.

LeFort I Osteotomy

- Osteotome cuts are taken via horizontal buccal vestibular incision from canine to first premolar region
- Planned interdental osteotomy is etched into interproximal bone through retracted wound margins in canine first premolar interdental space posterior to the pterygomaxillary suture
- Parasagittal osteotomy is extended into the maxillary antrum below nasal floor and apices of maxilllary molar teeth
- The palatal mucosa is reflected minimally to maximize the attachment of mucoperiostium to the posterior maxilla
- The incompletely cut posterior portion of the palate is completely sectioned by malleting with an osteotome
- The posterior portion of the tuberosity is seperated from the pterygoid plate with an osteotome
- The repositioned segment is fixed with an arch wire ligated to the stable maxilla
- IMF is usually not necessary unless mandibular osteotomies are done.

CASE NUMBER 2

A 24-year old female complains of forwardly placed upper teeth and show of gums during smiling (Figs 37.13 and 37.14).

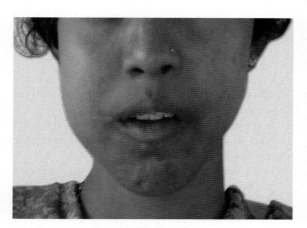

Fig. 37.13: Frontal view

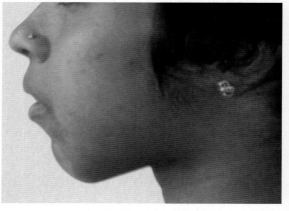

Fig. 37.14: Lateral view

History of Present Illness

- Known case of skeletal open bite (Fig. 37.15)
- Orthodontic treatment for past one and a half years (Fig. 37.16).

Medical History

No relevant past medical history.

Personal History

She had digit sucking until 15 years.

General Examination

Moderately built and nourished.

Intraoral Examination

- Anterior open bite with occlusion only at 2nd molar
- No canine relationship
- Lower dental midline shift to left
- Exposed implant screws on left buccal sulcus
- Poor periodontal support to lower anteriors
- COGS analysis (Table 37.6)

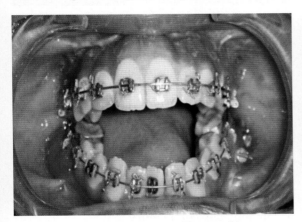

Fig. 37.15: Occlusion with open bite

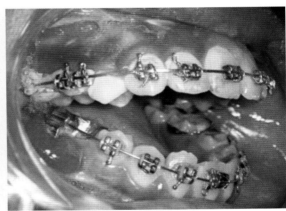

Fig. 37.16: Occlusion lateral view with anterior open bite

Table 37.6: COGS analysis				
Landmarks	Mean values	Pretreatment	Presurgical	Present status
AR-PTM	32.8	27	29	26 mm
PTM-N	50.9	54	53	56 mm
N-A-Pg	2.6+/–5.1	–5.5	–2	10
N-A	2.0+/–3.7	–5.5	–3.5	–3 mm
N-B	–6.9+/–4.3	–9	–15	–20 mm
N-Pg	6.5+/–5.1	–4.5	–10	–21 mm
N-ANS	50+/–2.4	59.5	56	61 mm
ANS-GN	61.3+/–3.3	81	78	81 mm
PNS-N	50.6+/–2.2	50.5	52	50 mm
MP-HP	24.2+/–5.0	35	40	55 mm
Upper incisor -NF	27.5+/–1.7	31	31	29 mm
Lower incisor -NF	40.8+/–1.8	36	39	41 mm
Upper molar -NF	23.3+/–1.3	28	30	28.5 mm
Lower incisor AR-MP	32.1+/–1.9	25	31	38 mm

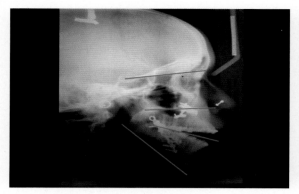

Fig. 37.17: Lateral cephalogram (Case 2)

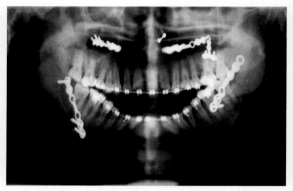

Fig. 37.18: Orthopantomogram (Case 2)

- Excessive granulation tissue in right buccal sulcus at the site of rigid fixation

Extraoral Examination
- Convex profile
- Long face with middle and lower third excess
- Incompetent lips
- Hyperactive mentalis
- Excessive exposure of anterior teeth on smiling
- Steep mandibular plane angle.

Provisional Diagnosis
Postsurgical relapse of skeletal open bite (Figs 37.17 and 37.18).

Problem List
Skeletal open bite 9 mm
- Increased skeletal anterior facial height

- Increased post dental height
- Absence of intercuspation in 1st molar and premolars
- No canine relationship
- Incompetent lips.

Treatment Objectives
- Reassurance of the patient
- Correction of anterior open bite
- Obtaining stable class I molar and canine relation
- Obtaining lip competency
- Prevention of surgical relapse.

Treatment Plan
- Revision LeFort I osteotomy and differential impaction
- BSSO and advancement +/– genioplasty
- Postsurgical orthodontics.

Principles and Protocols of Bimaxillary Surgery

38

INTRODUCTION

Surgical alterations in the position of the bony facial skeleton will inevitably affect the soft tissue–hard tissue relationships. The aesthetics nowadays the primary considerations, especially in maxillofacial surgery, and the orthognatic surgery. However, an aspect of orthognathic surgery that is seldom considered is the effect of the skeletal movements on the pharyngeal airway. Changes in airway dimensions have been demonstrated after surgical repositioning of the mandible or maxilla. All bimaxillary orthognathic patients are though candidate for surgical correction patients' assessment and selection remains main issues of diagnosis and treatment planning. Bimaxillary orthognathic cases require a decisive parameter both on their soft tissue profile and hard tissue consideration.

History
- 1960s, treatment of dentofacial deformity was changed from orthodontic treatment to orthodontic-surgical treatment
- Later single jaw surgical treatment was replaced by two jaw surgery
- In 1980s, two stage bimaxillary surgery was replaced by single stage procedure.

Indications
- Severe class III (>12 mm)
- Class III with vertical maxillary excess

CASE SERIES
- Class III with vertical maxillary deficiency
- Class III with transverse maxillary deficiency
- Class II with vertical maxillary excess
- Class II with vertical maxillary deficiency
- Class II with transverse maxillary deficiency
- Class I with vertical maxillary excess
- Class I with bimaxillary protrusion
- Asymmetric prognathism with deficient maxilla
- Asymmetry of maxilla and mandible
- Syndromic patients
- Sleep apnea.

Surgical Treatment Objectives

Initial Phase

Before orthodontic treatment and surgery (Figs 38.1 to 38.7).

Final Phase

Orthodontic treatment before and after surgery

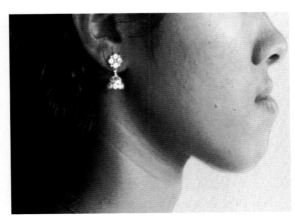

Fig. 38.1: Class III lateral view (patient 1)

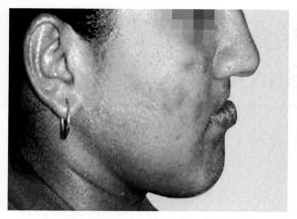

Fig. 38.2: Class III lateral view (patient 2)

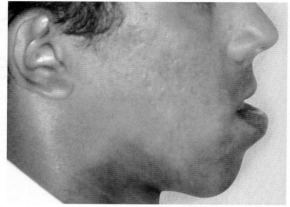

Fig. 38.3: Class III lateral view (patient 3)

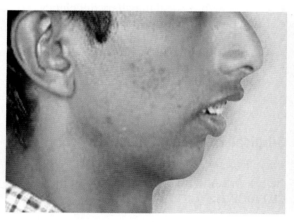

Fig. 38.4: Class II lateral view (patient 4)

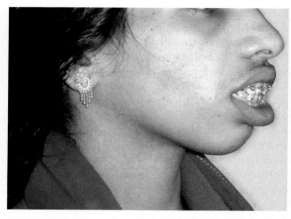

Fig. 38.5: Bimax protrusion: oblique view (patient 5)

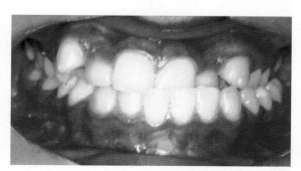

Fig. 38.6: Crossbite and asymmetric occlusion: intraoral (patient 6)

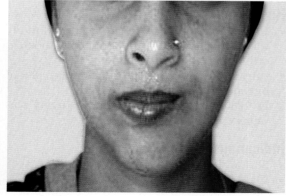

Fig. 38.7: Crossbite and asymmetric occlusion extraoral ((patient 7))

CEPHALOMETRIC TRACING AND OSTEOTOMY LINES (FIGS 38.8 TO 38.19)

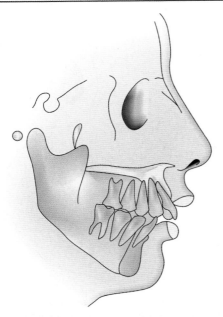

Fig. 38.8: Cephalometric tracing with stable landmarks

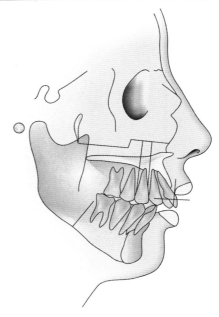

Fig. 38.9: Maxillary and mandibular osteotomy lines are marked

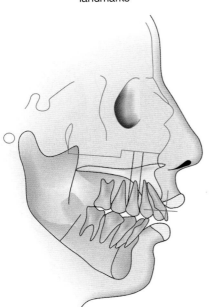

Fig. 38.10: Acetate sheet is placed. Stable landmarks and reference lines for upper central incisor are drawn

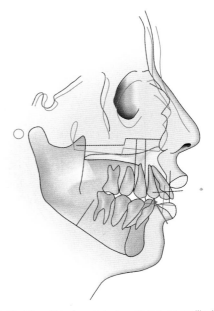

Fig. 38.11: Mandible is rotated until the unandibular central incisior is 2 mm above the horizontal line

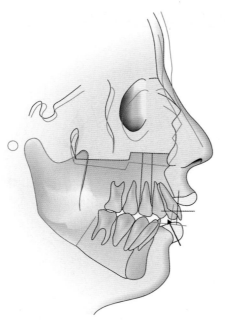

Fig. 38.12: Proximal segment of mandible is traced on acetate sheet

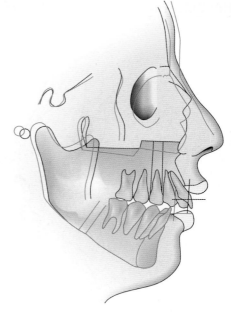

Fig. 38.13: Tracing is shifted to left so that mandibular central incisor is 1 mm behind the vertical line and trace the distal segment

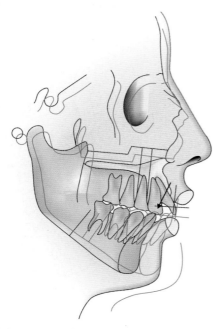

Fig. 38.14: Tracing is shifted such that the maxillary anterior teeth are in ideal relation with mandibular teeth

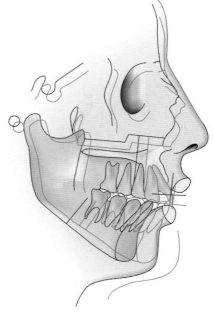

Fig. 38.15: Maxillary anterior segment is traced including horizontal and vertical osteotomy lines

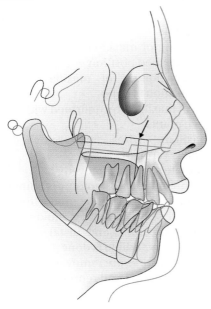

Fig. 38.16: Slide tracing to left side so that maxillary posterior teeth are in ideal occlusion with the mandibular teeth

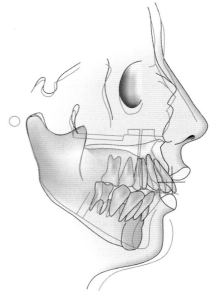

Fig. 38.17: Trace the skeletal structures and horizontal osteotomy line on posterior maxillary segment

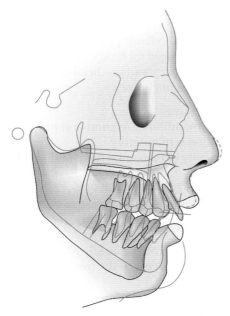

Fig. 38.18: Structures unaffected by surgery are superimposed and amount of hard and soft tissue changes are assessed

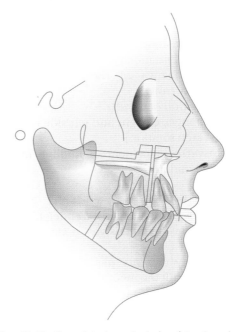

Fig. 38.19: Completed surgical visual treatment objectives

PLANNING

Model Surgery

- Maxillary cast is mounted on semi-adjustable articulator using face bow transfer
- Mandibular cast is mounted using occlusion as guide
- *Horizontal line*—used to plan vertical movements
- *Vertical line*—used to plan horizontal movements
- *Transverse changes* are recorded by measuring intercanine and intermolar distance measured across the palate
- Maxillary osteotomies are done and segments are stabilized
- Duplicate mandibular cast is articulated in final position
- Final splint is prepared
- Maxillary cast in desired position is articulated in articulator with mandibular cast
- Intermediate splint is fabricated with mandibular cast in initial position

Surgical Decision before Bimaxillary Surgery

- Vertical position of anterior maxilla (tooth-lip relation)
- Vertical position of posterior maxilla (vertical change of 2nd molar)
- Vertical change of right and left maxilla (maxillary cant)
- A–P position of maxilla
- A–P changes of right and left side of maxillary arch (arch rotation)
- Transverse placement of midline of maxilla (dental midline).

Surgical Procedure

- Patient position—reverse trendelenburg
- Anesthesia—hypotensive GA via nasotracheal tube
- Osteotomy cuts are placed on mandible on both sides till the medullary space
- Mandible is left intact and moistened packs are placed into the wounds
- External reference point (nasal pin) are placed and maxillary osteotomy is done

- Intermediate splint is placed between maxilla and mandible
- Repositioning of maxillomandibular complex is done to desired position
- After repositioning of maxilla to desired position fixation is done
- Position of maxilla is reconfirmed with external reference points
- Intermaxillary wires are removed and occlusion is verified
- Intermediate splint is removed
- Bilateral mandibular osteotomy is completed
- Final splint is placed and secured with wires
- Condyles are seated back to glenoid fossa
- Fixation of proximal and distal segment of osteotomized mandible is done
- Intermaxillary wires are removed
- Occlusion is verified and reproduced
- Final splint is secured back with wires or elastics.

Altered Orthognathic Surgical Sequencing

Mandibular surgery is done prior to maxillary surgery.

Advantages

- Simple and reliable procedure
- Eliminate need for final splint
- Better stability and predictability
- Less laboratory time.

Disadvantages

- Rigid mandibular fixation and proper condyle position is mandatory
- Difficulty in managing unfavorable split.

Postoperative Considerations

- Blood loss and postoperative edema is more in two jaw surgery as compared to single jaw surgery
- Chances of relapse are less as compared to single jaw surgery, if the treatment planning is accurate
- Other complications are similar to single jaw surgery, such as—nerve injury, infection, TMJ dysfunction, unfavorable occlusion and esthetic

Maxillomandibular Advancement for Obstructive Sleep Apnea

Goals of therapy:
- Maximize upper airway space and reduce upper airway resistance
- Advancement of maxilla—
  - Pulls soft tissue of palate forward and upward
  - Palatoglossus muscle forward
  - Open nasal valve
- Advancement of mandible—
  - More anterior position of tongue base
  - More favorable position of hyoid bone

Presurgical phase
- Two splints are prepared
- 1st registration of occlusion after 8–10 mm advancement of mandibular model.
- 2nd registration of final occlusion after the advancement of maxillary model to centric occlusion using the new mandibular position.

Surgical Procedure
- Mandible is advanced via bilateral sagittal split osteotomy placed into MMF using 1st splint

- Condyles are properly positioned and mandible is fixed
- MMF is released and advancement splint is removed
- Maxillary advancement is done using LeFort I osteotomy
- Maxillomandibular unit is then rotated up into bony contact
- Maxilla is fixed and bone graft is placed at lateral walls.

CONCLUSION

- If the discrepancy between the jaw is large then plan for two jaw surgery should be considered as it provides more favorable results and less chances of relapse
- Cephalometric prediction tracing and model surgery must be performed with meticulous attention as minor errors for two jaw surgery have magnified effect when compared with one jaw surgery.

Maxillary Orthognathic Procedures

39

INTRODUCTION

The elements of the facial skeleton can be repositioned, redefine the face through a variety of well stabilized osteotomies, including LeFort I type osteotomy, LeFort II type osteotomy, LeFort III type osteotomy, maxillary segmental osteotomies.

Various osteotomies are used to correct midfacial deformities, and the choice of procedure depends on the specific deformity. The LeFort osteotomies are named after the 3 classic lines of weakness of the facial skeleton described by Rene LeFort in 1901. The LeFort I ostetomy allows for correction primarily at the occlusal level affecting the upper lip position, nasal tip and alar base region, and the columella labial angle without altering the orbitozygomatic region. A modified high LeFort I osteotomy is often used when performing midfacial advancement for patients with cleft lip and palate. In addition to providing more malar projection a downward sloping osteotomy elongates the nasolabial region, which is frequently short in the patient with cleft. The LeFort II and III osteotomies generally are part of the treatment plan in the major craniofacial dysostosis syndromes. In some cases LeFort osteotomies are modified to address the specific clinical situation. For most maxillofacial deformities, the LeFort I osteotomy and its variations are adequate.

ANTERIOR MAXILLARY OSTEOTOMY

History

- 1921—Cohn-Stock were first to attempt to retract the anterior maxilla surgically

- A wedge shaped segment of bone was excised from the maxilla through a transverse palatal incision
- Relapse occurred in four weeks because the segment was mobilized by a greenstick fracture (inadequate mobilization).

Wound Healing

- 1965—Microangiographic studies performed by Bell on rhesus monkeys demonstrated that intraosseus and intrapulpal circulation to the segment was maintained when soft tissue was kept intact
- Osteonecrosis was minimal, and vascular ischemia was only transient when the anterior maxillary segment was pedicled to the labio-bucal or palatal mucoperiosteum
- Osseous union between most of the sectioned segments occurred within six weeks without immobilization of the mandible
- The possibility of rapid revascularization of the anterior maxillary bone segment was not supported by these studies
- With complete mucoperiosteal reflection, intra-osseoud necrosis, gross vascular ischemia, and nonunion resulted
- Nonpedicled, free anterior maxillary dental osseous segments did not revascularize
- Within one week, the segments became necrotic and did not heal with the proximal bone
- One stage and two stage procedures were devised to prevent impairment of vascular supply to anterior maxillary segment

- Stage one—palatal incision with palatal ostectomy and closure
- Stage two—vertical buccal incisions and completion of vertical cuts with mobilization and repositioning.

Indications

- Horizontal maxillary excess when posterior occlusion is correct
- Correction of anterior open bite
- Bimaxillary protrusion
- Correction of severe curve of Spee
- To correct protrusion of maxillary teeth with normal incisor inclination
- To retract anterior teeth in noncompliant patients for orthodontics
- Preexistent root pathology/resorption/ankylosis—contraindiction for orthodontics
- Inprovement in aesthetics by reducing prominence of upper lip relative to nose and lower face.

Sugrical Techniques

- Wunderer technique
- Downfracture/Cupar technique
- Wassmund technique.

Wunderer Technique (1963)

Surgical procedure (Fig. 39.1 to 39.3):

- Buccallabial vertical incision immediately anterior to the site of planned ostectomy
- Design incision so that line of wound closure is positioned over bone
- Posterior margin is elevated and reflected to expose the site of ostectomy
- Piriform aperture visualized by tunneling subperiosteally beneath anterosuperior margin
- Axial inclination of teeth are assessed by direct visualization, palpation of bone, and preoperative radiographs
- Extraction of necessary teeth
- Vertical osteotomies are made with a fissure bur or an oscillating saw

- Arching-incision is carried through tile palatal mucosa anterior to the site of ostectomy on one side to the contralateral interdental space
- Posterior margin is reflected a few millimeters beyond the ostectomy site
- Rounded tip bur should be used to prevent laceration to nasal mucosa
- Midline palatal osteotomy is carried deeper due to thicker nasal crest of maxilla
- Anterior maxillary segment is partially mobilized with posterior and inferior digital pressure
- Once superior movement is obtained, a large osteotome is manipulated to attain greater mobility and separation
- Remaining bony connections between segments are removed
- Midpalatal sagittal incision is made extending from the center of the transverse palatal mucosal incision anteriorly to the incisive canal
- Superior portion is sectioned midsagittaly with a fissure bur
- Segment is split by malletting a fine sharp osteotome
- With segment raised, the nasal mucoperiosteum can be carefully detached to facilitate:
  - Excision of nasal crest
  - Reduction of bony or cartilaginous nasal septum

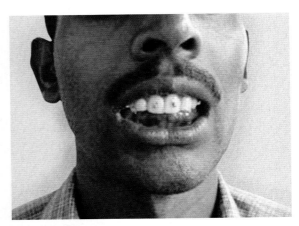

Fig. 39.1: Preoperative photograph (Front view)

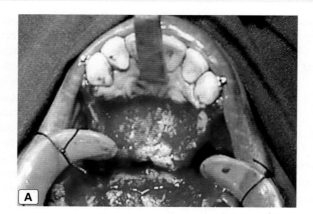

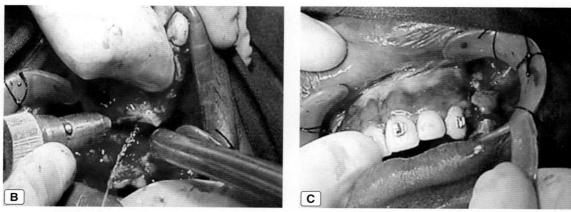

Figs 39.2A to C: Intraoperative (A) Anterior segmental osteotomy; (B) Recontouring of edges; (C) Segment in place

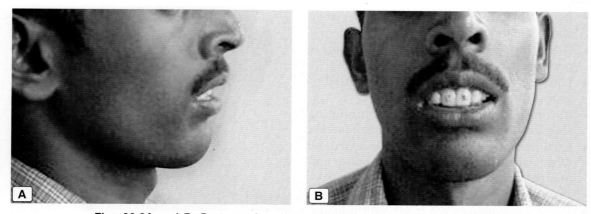

Figs 39.3A and B: Postoperative photograph: (A) Lateral view, (B) Front view

- The anterior maxillary segment may be stabilized with the use of an acrylic splint
- Intermaxillomandibular fixation
- Skeletal fixation—piriform aperture, zygomatic buttress, and infraorbital
- Excessive redundant palatal mucosa may be excised to facilitate closure of palatal mucosa.

Downfracture Technique (Cupar 1954)

- A circumvestibular incision is extended at least one tooth distal to the planned ostectomy site on one side to a similar area on the opposite side of the maxilla
- Superior margin is reflected to expose the lateral wall of maxilla and piriform aperture
- Extraction of necessary teeth
- The ostectomy site may be visualized by inferior retraction of the mucoperiosteal flap, or a vertical incision may be made immediately anterior to the site of the planned osteotomy
- Section of the lateral maxilia is excised from the extraction sites
- Vertical cuts are carried 4 or 5 mm above the canine apices and angled medially into the piriform aperture
- Transpalatal osteotomy is made through vertical osteotomy sites
- An osteotome is malleted into midpalatal and lateral osteotomy sites to facilitate downfracturing of anterior maxilla
- Anterior aspect of maxilla and nasal crest is reduced to prevent buckling of nasal septum
- Once downfractured, bone may be readily removed from transpalatal osteotomy sites
- A groove is made in the midline to accommodate the cartilaginous septum
- When superior movement of the maxilla exceeds the available bone, a portion of the cartilaginous nasal septum is removed
- The anterior maxillary segment, attached to the palatal soft tissue by a pedicle, is manipulated and any bony interference is removed.

Wassmund Technique

- A vertical incision is made in the interdental space immediately anterior to the distal bony margin of the planned ostectomy

- Incision is carried superiorly into the depth of the vestibule and directed slightly anteriorly so that the line of closure is positioned over the bone
- The lateroinferior portion of the bony anterior nasal aperture is visualized by subperiosteal tunneling
- A vertical incision overlying the anterior nasal spine is carried inferiorly 3–4 mm above the free gingival margin
- Extraction of necessary teeth
- A measured vertical section of alveolar bone is excised with a fissure bur or oscillating saw
- Buccal bone incision is carried 4 or 5 mm above the adjacent canine apex and then angled medially to the inferolateral part of the piriform rim
- Wound is packed for hemostasis and the opposite side is treated similarly
- Lateral palatal and transpalatal ostectomies are completed through the vertical ostectomy sites
- A palatal subperiosteal tunnel is developed and the palatal bone is sectioned transversely from the vertical ostectomv site of one side to the contralateral side
- Digital pressure on the palatal mucosa is essential to prevent trauma to the palatal and nasal mucosa during this relatively blind cut
- A midpalatal sagittal mucosal incision, immediately distal to incisive foramen, may be used to facilitate transverse palatal bone ostectomy
- Through the vertical midline incision, the Mucoperiosteum is elevated from the anterior nasal floor and nasal septum
- Septal osteotome is malleted between the anterior parts of the nasal septum and maxilia
- Anterior maxilla is mobilized with posterior and inferior digital pressure
- A prefabricated acrylic splint is used as an index for proper segment position
- If an anterior transverse maxillarv discrepancy exists. the segment is sectioned through the labial or palatal mucosal incisions
- Complete mobility and separation is obtained by manipulation with osteotome and removal of bone.

Conclusion

- Wunderer technique
  - Transpalatal incision
  - Two labial buccal incision.
- Downfracture technique
  - Circumvestibular incision.
- Wassmund technique
  - Two vertical buccal labial incisions.
  - Midpalatal sagittal incision.
- For posterior movement of anterior maxilla, a transverse palatal incision as described by Wunderer provides direct access and excellent visualization
- For superior repositioning of anterior maxilla, "downfracturing' technique provides excellent visualization as well as direct access to superior maxilla
- The Wassmund technique maintains excellent dual vascular supply of the anterior in maxillary segment by preserving both palatal and labial buccal soft tissue pedicles
- Technically, gaining access to the superior and palatal aspects of the anterior maxilla is more difficult
- The anterior maxilla must be mobile enough that it does not require any significant pressure to move it into the desired position.

LEFORT I OSTEOTOMY (FIG. 39.4)

Introduction

- First performed in 1927 by Dr Wassmund
- It has been used to correct skeletal open bite deformities related to maxillary deficiency or an anterior open bite
- LeFort I osteotomy has later been modified to LeFort II and even LeFort III osteotomies
- It permits simultaneous correction of vertical, anteroposterior, transverse deformities via appropriate repositioning and segmentalization of maxilla.

Revascularization Study of Bell

The study indicates that the maxilla can be mobilized and repositioned and healing continues as long as, mobilized maxilla is pedicled on broad soft tissue base.

Indications

- All instances of apertognathia
- Vertical maxillary excess
- Benefits of maxillary advancement, especially in cleft palate and post trauma patients
- In severe mandibular prognathism to reduce the amount of severe mandibular setback

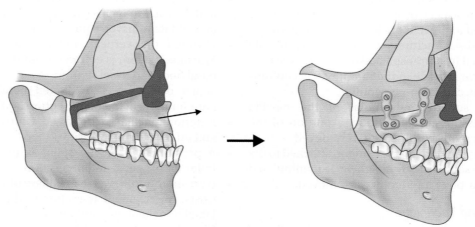

Fig. 39.4: LeFort I orthognathic surgery diagrammatic representation

- Nasomaxillary hypoplasia
- Inferior repositioning of maxilla—done in vertical maxillary deficiency
- Leveling of maxillary occlusal plane associated with hemifacial microsomia, Romberg's syndrome, unilateral condylar hyperplasia, etc.

Contraindications

- Whenever more than 5–6 mm of superior repositioning of the maxilla is required, the nasal cavity size will be reduced and flaring of the alar bases of nose will be seen with unaesthetic result
- And other systemic conditions which are contraindicated for surgeries.

Surgical Procedure

Position of the Patient

- Head should be elevated approximately 10 degree and modified hypotension should be maintained throughout the procedure [90 mm Hg of systolic blood pressure]
- It is critical to place an external reference pin and measure to the reproducible point on the maxillary incisors. This is done by placing the Kirschner wire through the skin and in to bone of the nasal bridge.

Incision

- Intraoral circumvestibular incision placed in the buccal vestibule, it extends from one zygomaticomaxillary buttress region to the other across the midline
- Subperiosteal dissection done
- Infraorbital nerve is exposed and protected
- Anterior nasal spine and piriform aperture are identified and septopremaxillary ligament is removed from the anterior nasal spine
- Nasal mucosa is dissected from the lateral nasal wall and floor
- Dissection of the posterior maxilla, which is tunneled to preserve a broad based intact mucosal pedicle

- Osteotomy should always be designed so that it terminates inferiorly in the piriform aperture region; this minimizes the risk to nasolacrimal system
- Vertical landmarks are placed on the maxilla at the piriform aperture, above canine and at the zygomaticomaxillary buttress using calipers
- Osteotomies initiate at the lateral wall of nose and proceeds to the zygomaticomaxillary buttress region
- Posteriorly osteotomy is directed inferiorly from the zygomaticomaxillary buttress to the junction of the maxilla and the pterygoid plates
- This minimizes the risk of damaging the maxillary artery and its terminal branches in the pterygopalatine fossa
- Spatula osteotome should be placed at the piriform rim and directed posteriorly and inferiorly along the lateral nasal wall towards the perpendicular plate of palatine bone.

Surgical Complication Related to This Step

- Incomplete sectioning of palatine bone can result in inadvertent fracture, which may extend to the orbit
- Several report suggest that inadequate sectioning of palatine bone resulted in vascular damage and even visual disturbances
- The maxilla and pterygoid plates are separated by malleting a curved osteotome from lateral to medial
- An index finger is used to palpate the inferior edge of the osteotome
- Similar procedure is repeated on the opposite side
- The maxilla is downfractured with hand presure or with maxillary mobilization forceps
- A rongeur reduces the nasal crest and lateral nasal walls.

Stabilization

Once the maxilla is repositioned, the distance between the vertical reference holes, external nasal pin and oral reference mark are measured to ensure correct vertical repositioning.

Wound Closure

- Upper lip closure is performed in layers
- The periostium and muscle layer are initially closed at four areas, both zygomaticomaxillary regions and nasal base regions
- Cinch suture is placed, it assist in controlling flare of the nasal base
- Mucosa of the lip closed with horizontal mattress suture in V–Y pattern.

Complications

- Relapse
- Nonunion
- Condylar retraction
- Bleeding
- Infraorbital nerve injury
- Infection

- Predictable soft tissue changes do occur after LeFort I osteotomy but it is difficult to control them due to there variable adabtability. A secondary soft tissue procedure is often needed to mask the soft tissue effect of procedure like reduction of anterior nasal spin, alar cinching and V-Y closure of the upper lip.

CASE SERIES

Case 1

Preoperative
See Figures 39.5 to 39.6.

Intraoperative
See Figures 39.7 to 39.13.

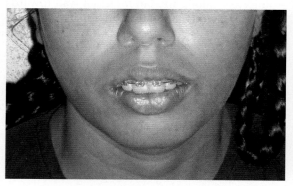

Fig. 39.5: Preoperative frontal view

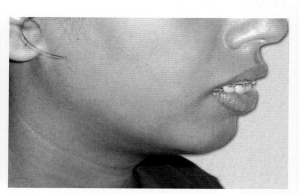

Fig. 39.6: Preoperative lateral view

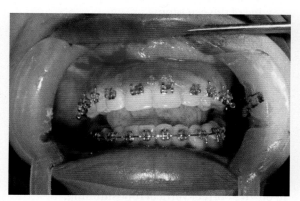

Fig. 39.7: Intraoperative incision

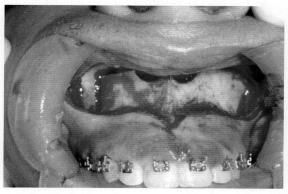

Fig. 39.8: Exposure and osteotomy cut given

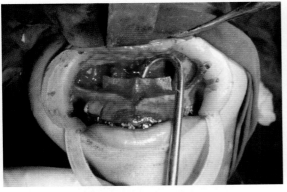

Fig. 39.9: Down fracture

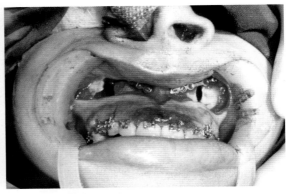

Fig. 39.10: Stabilized at new position

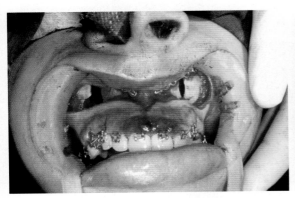

Fig. 39.11: Miniplate in use

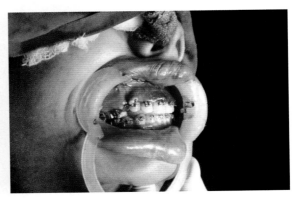

Fig. 39.12: Closure done

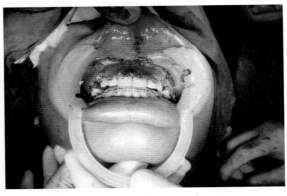

Fig. 39.13: After suturing

Case 2

Preoperative (Figs 39.14 to 39.16)

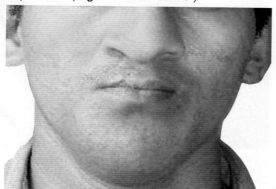

Fig. 39.14: Frontal view

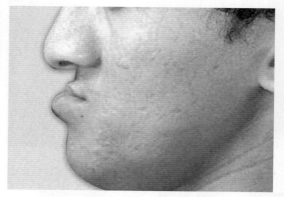

Fig. 39.15: Lateral view

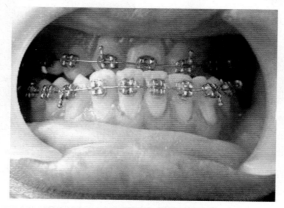

Fig. 39.16: Preoperative occlusion

Postoperative (Figs 39.17 to 39.19)

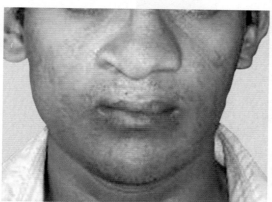

Fig. 39.17: Frontal view

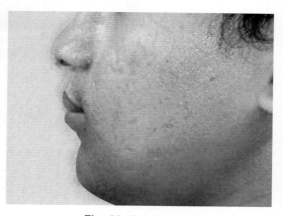

Fig. 39.18: Lateral view

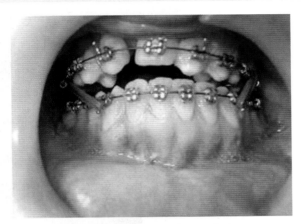

Fig. 39.19: Postoperative occlusion

Case 3

Preoperative (Figs 39.20 to 39.23)

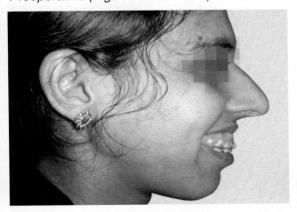

Fig. 39.20: Lateral view

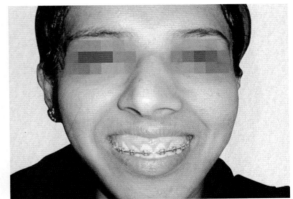

Fig. 39.21: Frontal view

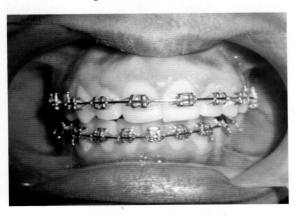

Fig. 39.22: Preoperative occlusion

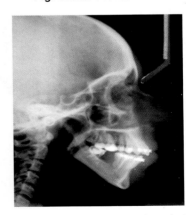

Fig. 39.23: Preoperative lateral cephologram

Postoperative (Figs 39.24 to 39. 27)

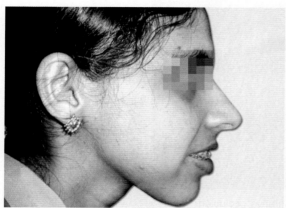

Fig. 39.24: Lateral view

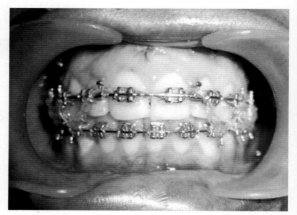

Fig. 39.26: Postoperative occlusion

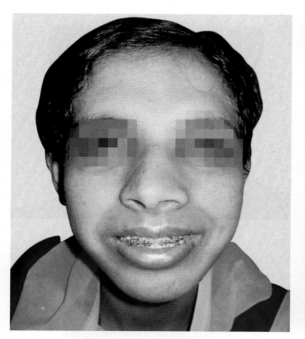

Fig. 39.25: Frontal view

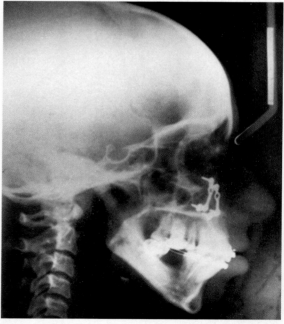

Fig. 39.27: Postoperative lateral cephologram

Case 4

Preoperative (Figs. 39.28 to 39. 30)

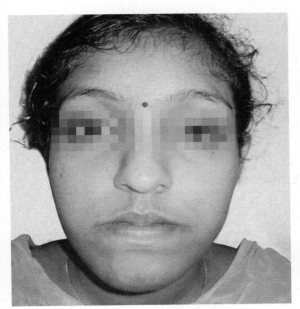

Fig. 39.28: Frontal view

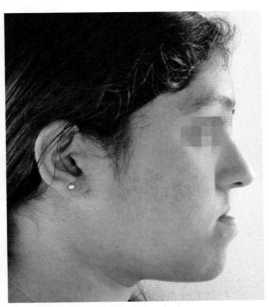

Fig. 39.29: Lateral view

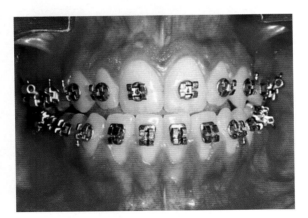

Fig. 39.30: Preoperative occlusion

Postoperative (Figs 39.31 to 39.33)

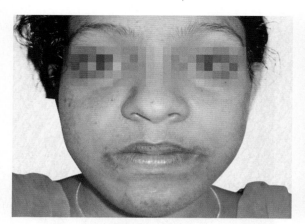

Fig. 39.31: Frontal view

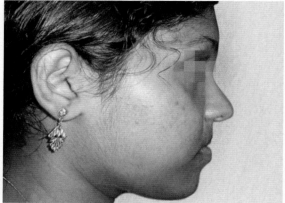

Fig. 39.32: Lateral view

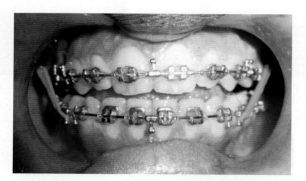

Fig. 39.33: Postoperative occlusion

Mandibular Orthognathic Procedures

40

INTRODUCTION

Mandible being the major constituent of facial skeleton and its prominent location of the facial bones any alteration can produce wide range of facial deformities. The entire mandible can be surgically altered by various type of osteotomies combined with displacement of bone, or the addition of bone by grafting. The mandible has been sectioned in practically every conceivable manner, and even in some cases combination of procedures is being done by a maxillofacial surgeon.

CLASSIFICATION OF OSTEOTOMIES OF THE MANDIBLE

Ramus osteotomies
The sagittal split and its modification
The vertical subsigmoid osteotomy through extraoral and intraoral approaches
The inverted L and C osteotomies of the ramus
Oblique subcondylar-condylotomy
Condylectomy

Osteotomies of the body and symphysis (Anterior to mental foramen)
Step osteotomy
Midline syphyseal
Posterior to mental foramen
Y-ostectomy
Rectangular ostectomy
Trapezoidal ostectomy
Inverted V ostectomy
Mandibuloplasty

Segmental procedures
Anterior
Kole procedure
Combined with midline symphyseal
Posterior and total

Genioplasties
Advancement
Reduction
Vertical reduction
Vertical augmentation
Asymmetric chin procedures
Alloplastic augmentation

Bilateral Sagittal Split Osteotomy: Advancement and Setback

History

- The bilateral sagittal split osteotomy (BSSO) is an indispensable surgical procedure for the correction of lower jaw deformities
- A surgical procedure resembling the sagittal split was described in 1942 in the German literature by Schuchardt
- Trauner and Obwegeser were the first to discuss its use in the English literature
- In 1961, Dal Pont changed the lower horizontal cut to a vertical cut on the buccal cortex between the first and the second molars, thereby obtaining broader contact surfaces and requiring minimal muscular displacement
- In 1968, Hunsuck modified the technique, advocating a shorter, horizontal medial cut,

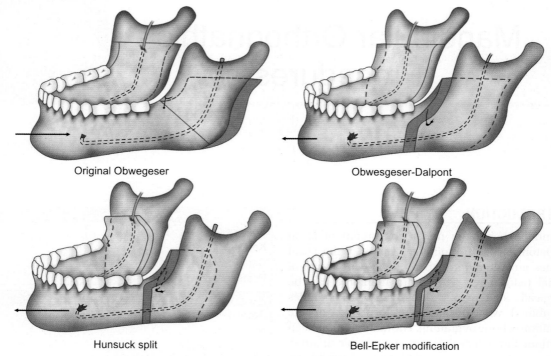

Original Obwegeser

Obwesgeser-Dalpont

Hunsuck split

Bell-Epker modification

Fig. 40.1: Modifications of bilateral sagittal spilt ramus osteotomy

just past the lingula, to minimize soft tissue dissection

- In 1977, Epker suggested several modifications. These included minimal stripping of the masseter muscle and limited medial dissection (Fig. 40.1)
- Bell and Schendel established the biologic basis for the BSSO, showing that with minimal detachment of the pterygomasseteric sling, intraosseous ischemia and necrosis of the proximal segment were significantly reduced
- In 1976, Spiessel advocated rigid internal fixation of the BSSO to promote healing, restore early function, and attenuate relapse
- Jeter and colleagues described a popular technique of placing three bicortical 2.0 mm position screws to fix the proximal and distal segments
- Blomqvist and others showed no significant differences in terms of relapse between mono-

cortical screws with miniplates and bicortical screws for mandibular advancements.

Indications

- Horizontal mandibular excess, deficiency, and asymmetry
- It is the procedure of choice for mandibular advancement
- Only when advancing the mandible beyond 10–12 mm should one give consideration to an extraoral procedure, because of minimal overlap between the proximal and the distal segments
- Excellent operation for a mandibular setback of small to moderate magnitude
- Minor asymmetries can easily be managed with a BSSO
- Minor anterior open bite
- For removal of impacted 3rd molar in ramus.

TECHNIQUE (FIGS 40.2 TO 40.14)

Soft Tissue

- Starting superiorly, two-thirds up the anterior border of the ramus, an incision is made through mucosa with a sharp scalpel or electrocautery
- The incision is carried inferiorly, lateral to the external oblique ridge to the area of the second molar, where the incision is made more lateral into the vestibule to the distal first molar
- Adequate attached tissue should be preserved medial to the incision to facilitate closure
- Hemostasis is obtained with electrocoagulation. The incision is continued through submucosa, muscle, and periosteum

- With a periosteal elevator, the periosteum is elevated, exposing the external oblique ridge. A notched coronoid retractor is inserted into the wound and used to retract the tissue superiorly until the tip of the coronoid is reached. This retraction is done gradually with gentle but firm force
- As the temporalis tendon is retracted superiorly, the sharp end of a periosteal elevator is used to release the remaining attachments of the tendon, especially on the medial side of the coronoid process
- A curved Kocher clamp is placed and secured with umbilical tape to the surgical drape with a Kelly forceps. It is important that the Kocher clamp be placed as close to the coronoid tip as

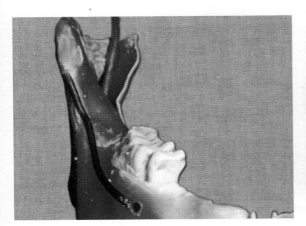

Fig. 40.2: Presentation of area anatomy

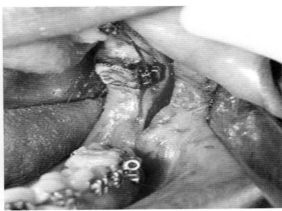

Fig. 40.3: Incision for BSSO

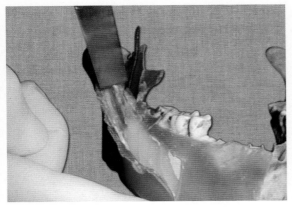

Fig. 40.4: Retraction of temporalis tendon

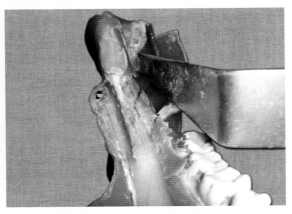

Fig. 40.5: Method to identify lingula

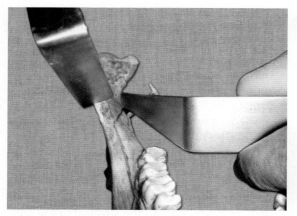

Fig. 40.6: Retraction to preserve neurovascular structure

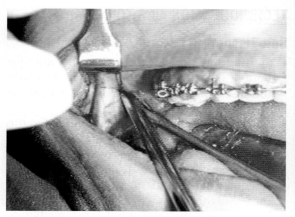

Fig. 40.7: Retraction of temporalis tendon

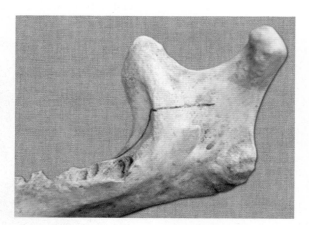

Fig. 40.8: Marking of medial cut on dry mandible

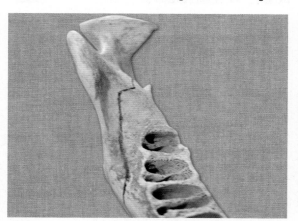

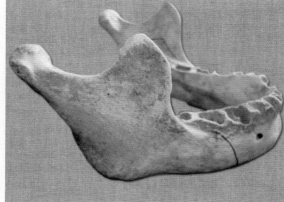

Figs 40.9 and 40.10: Marking of lateral cut on dry mandible

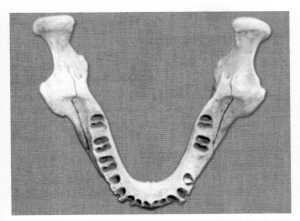

Fig. 40.11: Marking of cuts (superior view) on dry mandible

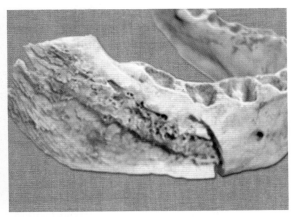

Fig. 40.12: Distal segment after BSSO osteotomy cut on dry mandible

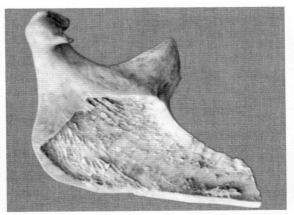

Fig. 40.13: Proximal segment after BSSO osteotomy cut on dry mandible

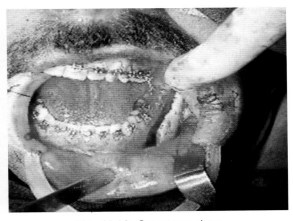

Fig. 40.14: Osteotomy done

- possible to allow access to the medial aspect of the ramus
- Subperiosteal dissection along the internal oblique ridge is carefully performed with the tip of the periosteal elevator
- Releasing tissue inferiorly to the level of the occlusal plane allows access and visualization of the medial aspect of the ramus
- Starting superiorly with the rounded edge of a periosteal elevator, the instrument is passed posteriorly and inferiorly until just superior and posterior to the lingula

- Once the lingula has been visualized and the medial osteotomy completed
- Reaching the inferior border, a periosteal stripper is inserted into the gonial notch and used to release the periosteum anteriorly until the first molar region is reached. The stripper is held flush with the inferior border of the mandible, and the superior aspect of the instrument should be perpendicular to the occlusal plane
- Inspection of the external oblique ridge will reveal the contour of the lateral cortex. As the

saw is brought down the ascending ramus, one must be cognizant of the contour of the lateral cortex, and the saw blade should parallel this lateral contour

- A fiberoptic retractor is inserted and turned at an angle to allow visualization of the external oblique ridge. A beveled cut is made through the inferior border perpendicular to the occlusal plane up to the external oblique ridge between the first and the second molar. The cut is stopped after extending 2 cm superior to the inferior border of the mandible
- A quarter-inch chisel is used, starting superiorly, to initiate the osteotomy. In progressive fashion, the chisel is malleted in place from superior to inferior, changing direction to match the contour of the ramus. As the bone is separated, it is important to observe whether it separates evenly. If it does not, one should recheck the osteotomy
- The cortices should be gently separated, looking for the neurovascular bundle
- For large advancements, beyond 7 mm, skeletal suspension wires may be helpful.

Fixation for Mandibular Advancement Bicortical Screws—Intraoral Approach

- If the gap between the proximal and the distal segments is small, then intraoral placement of bicortical screws is possible
- The screw placement will always be somewhat oblique when screws are placed from an intraoral approach
- If the gap between the segments is large, there may be limited overlap of the proximal and distal segments.

Bicortical Screws—Percutaneous Approach

- If the segments are flared at the anterior aspect of the osteotomy, it may not be possible to place a screw intraorally without a right-angled drill and screwdriver
- An alternative choice is a percutaneous approach.

Monocortical Screws and Plates

When asymmetry exists, it may be difficult to contour the proximal and distal segments to lie passively. In this case, a plate with monocortical screws may be used instead of bicortical screws.

Mandibular Setback

- The medial bone cut is identical to the cut used for advancement
- In the setback, a second bone cut is made distal to the first cut. The distance between the first and the second lateral cut is determined by the amount that the mandible is to be posteriorly repositioned
- The attachment of the medial pterygoid must be released from the medial aspect of the mandible
- Extensive contouring of the anterior ramus must be done to allow the segments to fit accurately. As the mandible is set back, there is greater contact at the anterior aspect of the proximal segment.

Complications
Condylar position
Malocclusion
Open bite
Lateral shift
Unfavorable splits
Proximal segment fractures
Small proximal fragment
Large proximal fragment
Distal segment fractures
Splits short of the lingula
Medial splits up the condyle
Distal segment splits (Behind the second molar)
Relapse
Nerve injury
TMJ dysfunction and hypomobility
Hemorrhage

CASES

Vertical Ramus Osteotomy and the Inverted-L Osteotomy (Fig. 40.15)

Indications for IVRO

- The primary indication for IVRO is treatment of patients with horizontal mandibular excess. The IVRO is a faster and simpler operation, rehabilitation time is shorter, and, most importantly, it has a much lower incidence of permanent inferior alveolar nerve injury when compared with SSRO

- Mandibular asymmetry often requires a largely rotational move of one or both mandibular rami to achieve correction. IVRO is indicated for the side or sides that move in a posterior direction.

Contraindications to IVRO

- The contraindication to IVRO is advancement of the distal, tooth-bearing mandibular segment
- Recent condylar fracture is a relative contraindication to IVRO
- Aesthetic assessment of the soft tissues of the neck is an integral factor in planning mandibular setback by ramus surgery (IVRO or SSRO).

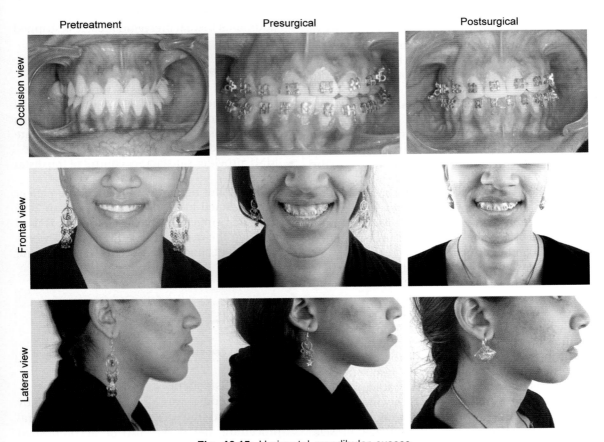

Fig. 40.15: Horizontal mandibular excess

Radiographic Evaluation before Surgery

Panoramic and lateral cephalometric radiographs are sufficient for the purpose of planning mandibular ramus osteotomy surgery.

IVRO Technique

- The incision is made over bone to minimize the risk of buccal fat pad herniation and to decrease the risk of food trap formation due to scar contracture
- The incision is carried forward 2–3 mm inferior and parallel to the mucogingival junction so that the buccinator muscle retracts with the lateral flap
- Blunt dissection of the soft tissues from the ascending ramus, with a blunt notched retractor or dual periosteal elevators, as high as the level of the sigmoid notch increases visualization of the osteotomy site and decreases the risk of injury to the long buccal and lingual nerves
- The periosteum is reflected from the lateral ramus to expose the sigmoid notch and posterior ramus
- The inferior border is stripped anterior to the antegonial notch
- The antilingula is a lateral prominence of the mid-ramus that generally corresponds to the entrance of the inferior alveolar nerve into the medial surface of the ramus
- The initial osteotomy cut should be a minimum of 6–8 mm in front of the posterior border
- Once the initial cut posterior to the foramen has been made, the osteotomy can be extended safely in either direction
- For setback of 4 mm or less, the inferior cut is carried parallel and about 9–10 mm anterior to the posterior border
- If a setback of 5 mm or greater is planned, the inferior osteotomy is angled progressively anterior, approximately parallel to the path of the inferior alveolar canal, to broaden the base of the proximal segment. If a 7 mm setback is planned, the inferior osteotomy should extend at least 12 mm forward of the mandibular angle. In this way, a residual sling of about 5 mm of masseter and medial pterygoid muscle and tendon would remain attached to the condylar segment following setback of the distal segment.

Muscle Stripping

- Once the cut is complete, the proximal segment is retracted laterally to expose the entire length of the medial pterygoid muscle
- The muscle and periosteum are stripped along the vertical length of the muscle an AP distance equivalent to the planned amount of setback
- The objective is to remove only enough muscle from the anterior and medial surface of the proximal segment to allow bony overlap
- Once preliminary medial pterygoid muscle reflection is completed, the same procedure is performed on the opposite side, and the patient is placed into MMF. The condylar segments are then rechecked. If necessary, additional medial pterygoid muscle is stripped to allow for passive overlap of the segments.

Fixation of the Segments

- Fixation of the segments is rarely necessary, because the combined effect of the medial pterygoid muscle and tendinous attachments of the masseter muscle provides adequate support and control of the proximal segment
- MMF provides satisfactory control of the distal segment
- Even without rigid or wire fixation, the patient is maintained in MMF for no more than 7–10 days after surgery. Light elastic traction is used to guide the occlusion for the next 4–5 weeks while initial bone healing occurs (Figs 40.16 and 40.17).

Complications of IVRO
Bleeding
Nerve injury
Unfavorable osteotomy

Inverted-L Osteotomy

- The procedure was originally described by Trauner and Obwegeser in 1957 as an intraoral procedure, but it can also be accomplished through a neck incision

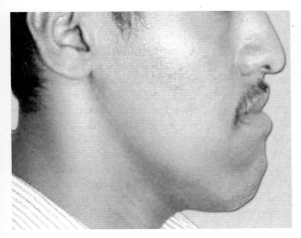

Fig. 40.16: Preoperative photograph

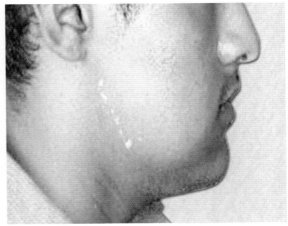

Fig. 40.17: Postoperative photograph

- The inverted-L osteotomy is a versatile procedure that can be adapted to treat a number of severe mandibular deformities
- For large (12 mm) advancements, concern over adequate bony interface between the proximal and distal segments and the concomitant problem of inability to place secure rigid fixation after SSRO are eliminated
- For mandibular setback of 10 mm or more, the inverted-L bypasses the need for coronoidotomy. There is less risk of condylar sag compared with IVRO, because the temporalis and pterygoid muscles remain attached to the condylar segment.

Anterior Mandibular Subapical Osteotomy

Indications

- When combined with an anterior maxillary subapical osteotomy, a nonskeletal open bite or bimaxillary protrusion can often be corrected, as long as there is not excessive lip incompetence or incisor exposure
- This procedure is often used to level the plane
- An anterior mandibular subapical osteotomy may be helpful in uprighting the anterior teeth to a more normal angulation, with positioning over basal bone, when orthodontic correction alone is not feasible

- This clinical situation may require the extraction of bicuspids to obtain space for posterior movements. When space constraints do not necessitate extractions, it is of paramount importance that the orthodontist diverge the roots of the teeth at the proposed osteotomy site to allow for the interdental cut without injury to adjacent teeth or the creation of periodontal problems
- This should be determined early during the planning phase and be part of the presurgical orthodontics. Failure to do this may result in delay of surgery or a compromised treatment plan.

Complications

- The direst complication is loss of bone and/or teeth in the osteotomized segment.
- A nonunion or malunion with resultant malocclusion.
- Neurosensory disturbances.

Mandibular Setback

- In gross mandibular prognathism in combination with a ramus procedure
- In mandibular prognathism where the body is long in relation to the ramus.

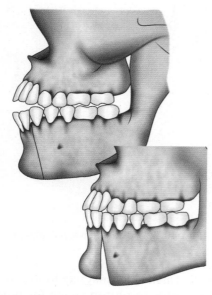

Fig. 40.18: Anterior body osteotomy to close an anterior open bite

Anterior Open Bite Closure and Curve of Spee Reduction (Fig. 40.18)

- Anterior open bite (AOB) closure does not usually lend itself to superior vertical movement of the anterior mandible because this may lead to excessive lower incisor show. If this movement is possible, then the result produces a stable closure of an AOB
- Surgical leveling of the curve of Spee using an anterior body osteotomy may be possible if the planned movements of chin advancement increase in anterior mandibular height, and setback of lower incisors coincide. There are often the advantages of a very pleasing increase in anterior mandibular height and no anterior stripping of the nutritive periosteum if the planning measurements are favorable.

Progenia Correction

In the class III situation, an anterior body osteotomy, with a planned wedge of bone removed to allow the setback, allows a measured correction to the progenia.

Genial Procedures

The chin is an element as important in facial profile as the nose and the forehead. It is subject to morphological anomalies in the sagittal, vertical, or transversal axes. Genioplasty used alone or in complement to other maxillomandibular osteotomies, allows for the correction of these malformations by modifying the position of the chin bones in three planes. Many types of genioplasty may be used to reach the desire goal, such as advancement, retraction, or adjustment of height or of symmetry. This genioplasty also has functional applications, notably in the treatment of obstructive sleep apnoea disorders.

Preoperative Evaluation

- Chin deformities can manifest in three dimensions, but the vast majority is in the horizontal plane (Fig. 40.19 and 40.20)
- Analysis of the deformity should involve careful scrutiny of the skeletal, dental, and soft tissue structures
- Vertical balance of the face can be judged by using relative size and proportions of the various structures
- Harmony is more important than absolute proportionality
- The face is considered balanced when the upper, middle, and lower thirds are of approximately similar size and the structures within each segment are When evaluating the chin, one must consider all structures
- Mentalis muscle activity must be closely evaluated and hyperactivity diagnosed
- When the chin is viewed in the horizontal plane, soft tissue contour is influenced by soft tissue thickness, as well as by the underlying bony chin contour
- The labiomental fold is influenced by the relative position of the maxilla; it is deepened in the presence of a deep bite or skeletal class II malocclusion, and flattened in a class III malocclusion.

Other Case of Genial Procedure

See Figures 40.21 to 40.29.

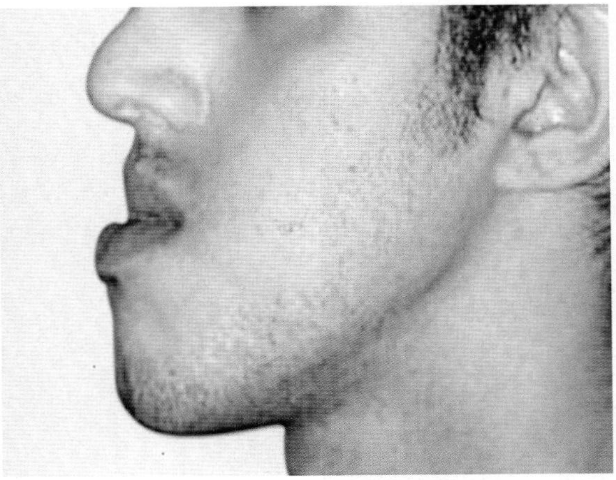

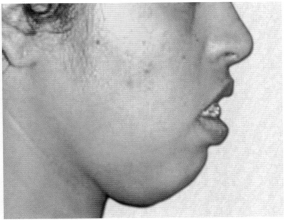

Fig. 40.19: Excess of chin

Fig. 40.20: Deficient chin (I)

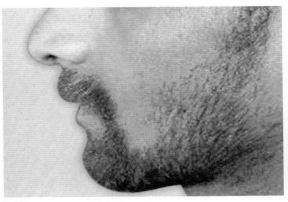

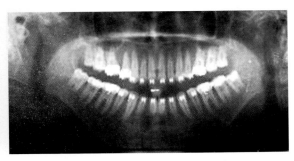

Fig. 40.21: Deficient chin (II)

Fig. 40.22: Preoperative OPG

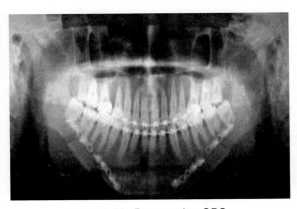

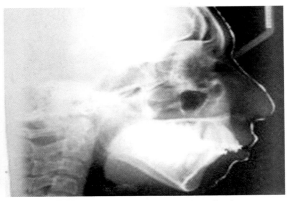

Fig. 40.23: Postopertive OPG

Fig. 40.24: Preoperative lateral ceph alogram

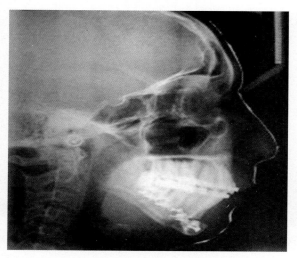

Fig. 40.25: Postoperative lateral cephalogram

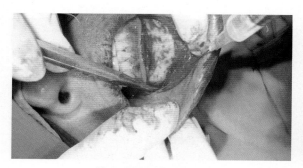

Fig. 40.26: Exposure

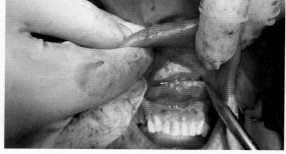

Fig. 40.27: Osteotomy cut given

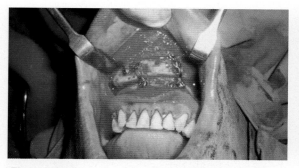

Fig. 40.28: Fixation and stabilization at new position

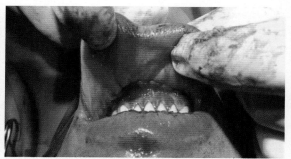

Fig. 40.29: Closure and suturing

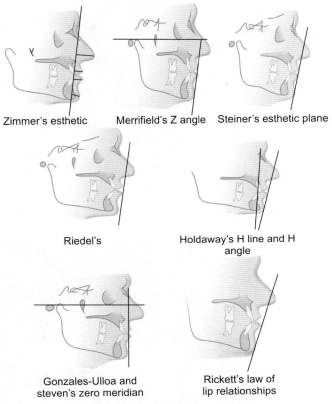

Zimmer's esthetic   Merrifield's Z angle   Steiner's esthetic plane

Riedel's

Holdaway's H line and H angle

Gonzales-Ulloa and steven's zero meridian

Rickett's law of lip relationships

Fig. 40.30: Soft tissue analysis

Soft Tissue Evaluation

- Soft tissue profile evaluation can be performed by any of several methods (Fig. 40.30)
- The upper lip should fall on the profile line, with the lower lip tangent to or slightly behind the profile line
- The aesthetic desires of the patient should be a priority and the clinical and radiographic assessment used to achieve that endpoint.

Horizontal Osteotomy with Advancement (Figs 40.31 to 40.33)

- Osseous genioplasties can be performed under general anesthesia or with IV sedation and local anesthesia

- The surgical approach to the anterior mandible consists of a bidirectional incision
- This incision should be initiated approximately halfway between the depth of the vestibule and the wet-dry line
- It should be marked at its midpoint and extended to approximately the canine region bilaterally
- Once mucosa has been incised, it is undermined, whereupon the mentalis muscle is divided on a bevel inferiorly toward bone. Sharp incision and reflection of periosteum from the anterior mandible can then be accomplished
- Periosteum should be left intact on the inferior border, and a minimum of 5 to 10 mm of perios-

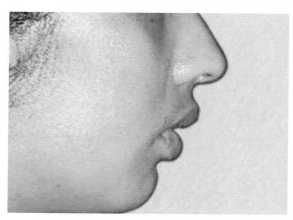

Fig. 40.31: Deficient chin (III)

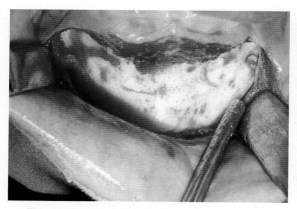

Fig. 40.32: Exposure and osteotomy cut given

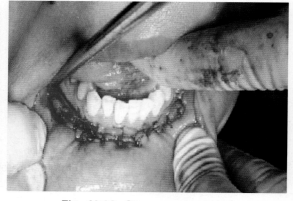

Fig. 40.33: Closure and suturing

teum should be maintained in the midpoint of the anterior mandible so that soft tissue support and blood supply are maintained.

- It is important that the bilateral mental nerves be identified
- Midline and paramidline orientation lines should be inscribed in the bone with a small bur to facilitate repositioning following any asymmetric or symmetric movements with anterior, posterior, or vertical changes
- The osteotomy can be completed with a reciprocating or oscillating saw

- Saw orientation must remain constant through-out the osteotomy to ensure a symmetric cut through the buccal and lingual cortices and to preclude bony interferences that might hamper the proposed movement. It is important that the buccal and lingual cortical cuts be complete where they join proximally
- Failure to adequately complete the lingual cortical cut in this area could result in mandibular fracture, which might require repair or compromise the inferior alveolar nerve or the esthetic result

- Upon completion of the osteotomy, the inferior fragment can be repositioned and stabilized using a variety of techniques, including unicortical or bicortical wires, bone plates, prebent chin plates, or lag screws
- One must keep in mind that when using transosseous wires, the degree of advancement available can be limited to the overall symphyseal thickness, and this must be determined before deciding on the method of stabilization.

Horizontal Osteotomy with Anteroposterior Reduction

- The surgical procedure is completed as described for advancement
- It is necessary, however, to reduce the proximal tips of the mobilized fragment to ensure a smooth transition along the inferior border and avoid palpable "wings"
- Additionally, the surgeon must be cognizant of potential changes in anterior vertical height of the mandible and take this into consideration when planning the orientation of the osteotomy.

Tenon Technique

- Michelet and associates originally described this technique in 1974
- The tenon technique allows for mortising of the tenon into the mobilized fragment when the chin is advanced. In the setback procedure, the tenon is reversed and the mobilized fragment is mortised into the mandible.

Double Sliding Horizontal Osteotomy

Occasionally, the chin is so deficient that a double sliding horizontal osteotomy must be used. The surgical technique involves creation of a stepped intermediate wafer of bone between the inferior fragment and mandible, which is also advanced to provide bony contact between the upper and lower fragments.

Vertical Reduction Genioplasty

- Vertical changes in chin height can be accomplished using a variety of techniques
- The magnitude is proportional to the amount and direction of horizontal movement. Approximately 3–5 mm of vertical change can be obtained.

Vertical Augmentation

- Vertical augmentation is indicated when it is desirable to increase the lower facial height, especially when the deficit is in the mandibular alveolus or symphysis
- Vertical augmentation is accomplished by interpositional grafting or alloplastic implant placement between the osteotomized segments following horizontal osteotomy of the mandible
- Barry Hendler, et al. described a modified technique for Mortised genioglossus advancement for treating obstructive sleep apnea and review the history of osteotomies in this region. This new osteotomy technique allows for greater soft tissue advancement of the hypopharyngeal region.

Horizontal-T Genioplasty

PD Grime described a technique in which a horizontal, single-slice of bone is sectioned from the inferior border of the chin, with preservation of the lingual soft tissue attachment, in the conventional manner. This is divided sagittally into three segments, which are not necessarily equal, and are then repositioned in the shape of a horizontal 'T'. To achieve this, the lateral segments are advanced and approximated in front of the central fragment which itself is also advanced. These are fixed in position and when desirable any voids may be filled with autogenous bone or hydroxyapatite.

Complications of genioplasty include
Prolonged neurosensory disturbance
Avascular necrosis of mobilized segments
Hemorrhage causing lingual hematoma
Possible airway compromise
Unesthetic soft tissue changes such as chin ptosis
Excessive lower tooth display
Bony resorption under alloplasts
Devitalization of teeth
Mandibular fracture
Creation of mucogingival problems
Asymmetry, and
An unesthetic end result

Alloplastic Augmentation

- The use of alloplasts affords the possibility of not only AP augmentation but also vertical and, more importantly, lateral augmentation
- The drawbacks of osseous genioplasty include the possibility of asymmetric advancement, inadvertent vertical changes, and narrowing of the anterior mandible with large advancements
- Implants should be stabilized with transosseous wires or position screws to ensure immobility.

Soft Tissue Changes

- Soft tissue changes associated with genioplasty are highly variable
- Vertical and horizontal reduction genioplasty appears to have the most variability in osseous-to-soft tissue change.

Section

Miscellaneous

Section 9

Miscellaneous

Imaging in Maxillofacial Pathology

41

INTRODUCTION

Imaging produces a picture of the internal layout which, the maxillofacial surgeon has inferred from the history and clinical examination of the patient. Radiology makes it possible to see what he suspects in his mind and also throws up new or unexpected information that is quite often complete. Technology has tried to keep up to the expectation of clinicians by providing many modes of imaging. All imaging modalities have their own place in pretreatment evaluation. It is for us to make use of them in the best possible way to benefit the patient.

Imaging helps:
- Develop a virtual operative environment
- Preview patients' anatomy in 2 and 3 dimensional formats
- To analyze and measure the patients' deviation from normal
- To have an accurate method of intraoperative navigation and measurements
- In an efficient and accurate transfer of information
- For accurate documentation and quantification of the pathology.

DIAGNOSTIC IMPORTANCE

- Key in evaluating the primary tumor
- Useful in defining the final extent
- Submucosal disease extension across tissue planes and nerves
- Especially invasion of tumors into the adjacent structures
- Nodal staging
- Guided biopsies.

IMAGING MODALITIES

- Plain conventional radiography
- CT scan
- MRI
- Scintigraphy
- Ultrasonography
- PET
- Optical coherence tomography
- Endoscopy
- Embolization
- Angiography
- Sialography

Plain Conventional Radiography

Versatile diagnostic tool projection radiographs, more commonly known as X-rays, are often used to determine the type and extent of a fracture as well as for detecting pathology in bone (Figs 41.1 to 41.13).

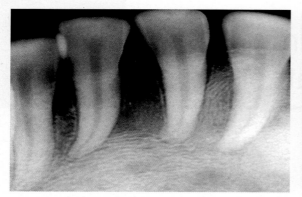

Fig. 41.1: IOPA showing loss of bony architecture

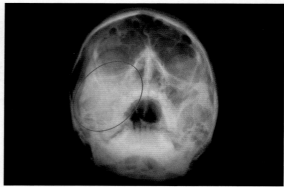

Fig. 41.2: PNS view haziness at right sinus

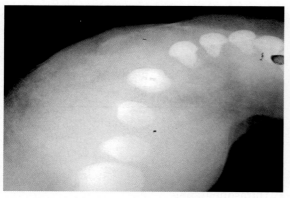

Fig. 41.3: Mandibular occlusal bicortical expansion

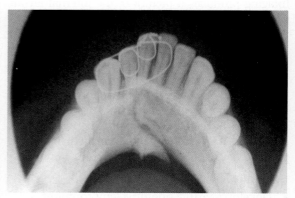

Fig. 41.4: Preoperative mandibular occlusal

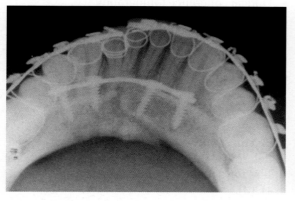

Fig. 41.5: Postoperative mandibular occlusal

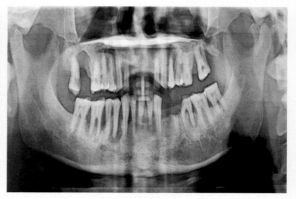

Fig. 41.6: OPG bifid condyle

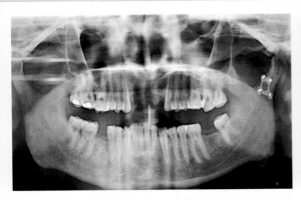

Fig. 41.7: OPG showing trapezoidal plate *in situ*

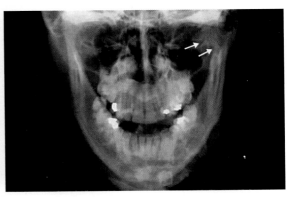

Fig. 41.8: PA mandible fracture and medially displaced condyle

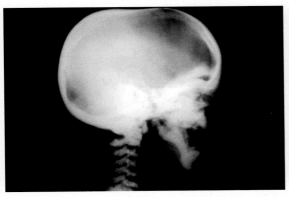

Fig. 41.9: Osteopetrosis (lateral skull): sclerosis of base of skull

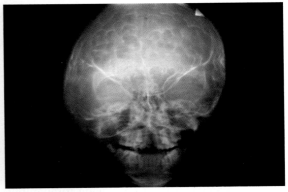

Fig. 41.10: Metal beaten appreance of PA skull (Crouzon's syndrome)

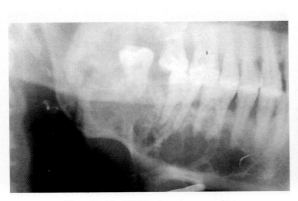

Fig. 41.11: OPG showing erosion

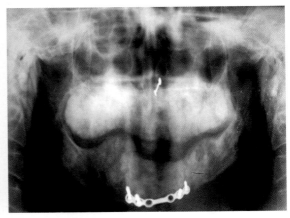

Fig. 41.12: OPG showing diffuse extensive radiopacity in maxilla

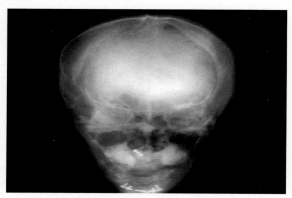

Fig. 41.13: Radiograph displayed diffuse, lobular, irregularly shaped radiopacities throughout the maxilla and mandible. Maxilla more radiopaque than mandible (florid cemento-osseous dysplasia)

Disadvantages

- Two-dimensional record of three-dimensional object
- Superimposition of various structures above and below the region of interest
- Requires multiple projections
- Poor understanding of structural relationships.

Computed Tomography

It is an imaging method employing tomography created by computer processing. Digital geometry processing is used to generate a three-dimensional image of the inside of an object from a large series of two-dimensional X-ray images taken around a single axis of rotation.

- Gold standard of imaging
- Gives cross-sectional information
- Allows evaluation of soft and hard tissues.

Techniques

- Plain studies without contrast
- Simple versus high resolution
- Contrast enhanced studies
- Reconstructions—coronal and sagittal view.

Advantages

- No special patient preparation

- Quick imaging decreases patient motion artifacts
- Exact contiguity of images
- Scan time <1 minute, transfer of information in seconds, display in 5 minutes
- Useful in emergencies, trauma and pediatric patients
- Evaluating necrosis of nodal metastases.

Disadvantages

- Requires a cooperative patient
- Respiratory motion or body motion affects imaging
- Medical radiation burden
- Allergic reaction to contrast medium.

Outstanding Features

- Useful to understand
- Complex anatomical relationships
  - Size of the stucture
  - Relative position
- Therefore, better surgical planning, decreased operating time
- Accurate documentation
- Postoperative evaluation and follow-up
- Excellent exchange of information
- Decreased radiation.

CT Plain (Figs 41.14 to 41.18)

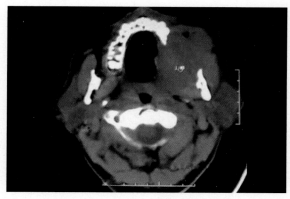

Fig. 41.14: CT plain showing tumor (I)

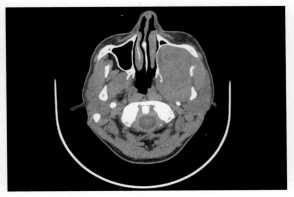

Fig. 41.15: CT plain showing tumor (II)

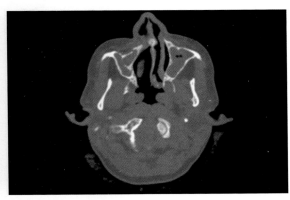

Fig. 41.16: CT plain showing fracture anterior wall of sinus

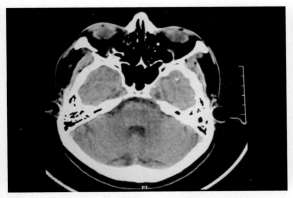

Fig. 41.17: CT plain showing fracture zygomatic process

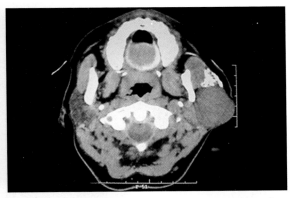

Fig. 41.18: CT plain showing lesion at parotid region

CT Contrast (Figs 41.19 to 41.22)

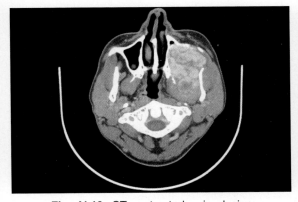

Fig. 41.19: CT contrast showing lesion

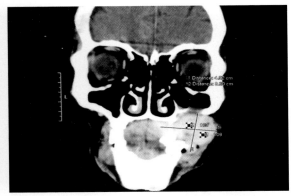

Fig. 41.20: CT axial view

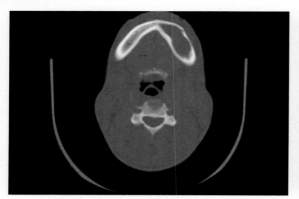

Fig. 41.21: CT radiolucency in anterior region

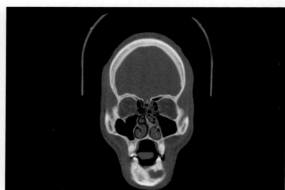

Fig. 41.22: CT radiolucency in anterior region axial cut

3D CT (Figs 41.23 to 41.28)

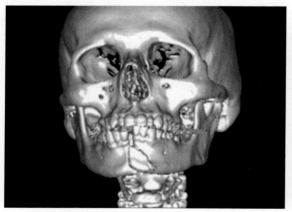

Fig. 41.23: 3D CT fracture mandible

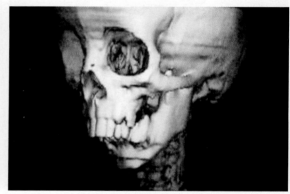

Fig. 41.24: TMJ ankylosis

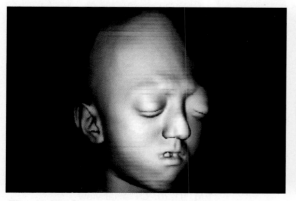

Fig. 41.25: Crouzon's syndrome facial reconstruction

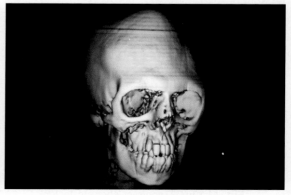

Fig. 41.26: Bony architecture

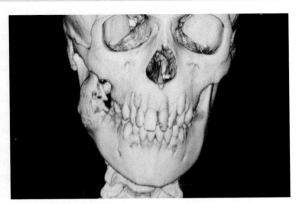

Fig. 41.27: Lesion at right angle region

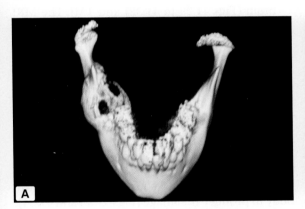 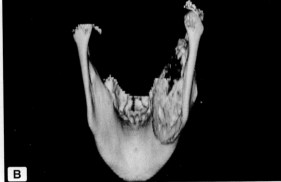

Figs 41.28A and B: (A) Anterior view, (B) Posterior view

Magnetic Resonance Imaging

MRI is based on magnetic property of nuclei with an odd number of protons, neutrons, or both. The hydrogen abundantly present in human body, as water is sensitive to magnetic field, can be easily evaluated using MRI.

Introduction

- Magnetic resonance imaging (MRI) has been used, extensively as a diagnostic tool in maxillofacial surgery.
- Nuclear magnetic resonance resulted due to the interaction of atomic nuclei within radiofrequency in a static magnetic field forms the basis for MRI.

History

- 1946 (Block and Purcell)
- 1972 (Lauterbeur—medical practice)
- Innovative and noninvasive technique
- Cornerstone of medical imaging
- Employs radiofrequency radiation in the presence of carefully controlled magnetic fields.

Advantages

- It is noninvasive and nonionizing.
- The images obtained are highly sensitive and specific
- Method of choice for the diagnosis of internal derangement in temporomandibular joint (TMJ) irrespective of displacements with or without reductions

- Provides a high degree of accuracy in detecting degenerative condylar conditions
- Simultaneous evaluation of soft and hard tissue relationship in both sagittal and coronal places.

Outstanding Features
- High quality cross-sectional images of body in any plane
- Superior soft tissue contrast
- Easier multiplanar imaging
- Perineural spread of disease and disease of skull base.

Limitations
- Inability to image bone due to lack of signal from cortical bone
- Motion artifacts
- Cardiac patients with pacemaker
- Presence of ferromagnetic materials in the patient such as respiratory assistance, and patients with surgically implanted metallic aneurysm clamp can restrict the performance of MRI
- In patients undergoing orthodontic treatment, appliances, arch wires palatal bars, lingual arches need to be removed before carrying out a MRI scan.

MRI in Temporomandibular Joint
- Diagnosis is a complex as well as a critical step in treatment of complications related to TMJ

- Jaw functions such as opening involves coordination between hard and soft tissues of the joint and muscles of mastication. Disruption in this coordination can lead to pain and dysfunction
- Degenerative arthritis and internal disk derangement are common complications related to this mechanism. These conditions require accurate diagnosis as mere clinical evaluation can lead to erroneous diagnosis
- Although artefacts are observed in MRI scans in patients with TMJ dysfunction, they are more concentrated at the face and mouth region and do not alter the quality of scans of brain (Figs 41.29 to 41.32) and TMJ. The MRI procedures are safe in patients with non- or weakly ferromagnetic objects. The procedure is also safe in patients who have devices with relatively strong ferromagnetic qualities. In such cases, the procedures should be carried out with the objects held in a way that prevents them from being disturbed by magnetic field interactions.

Ultrasonography

Based on reflection of sound waves within the body to produce the image (Figs 41.33 and 41.34).

Applications
- Widely used to detect lymph node metastases
- Examination of various masses in the neck

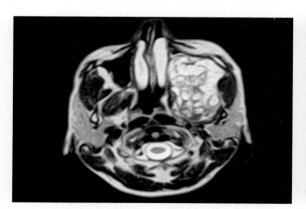

Fig. 41.29: MRI showing lesion

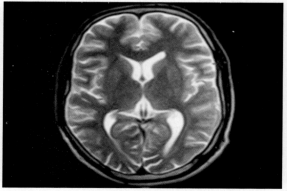

Fig. 41.30: MRI brain (I)

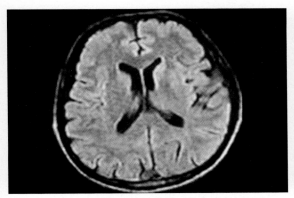

Fig. 41.31: MRI brain (II)

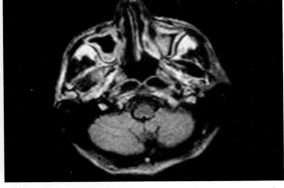

Fig. 41.32: MRI showing paranasal sinus mucosal thickening

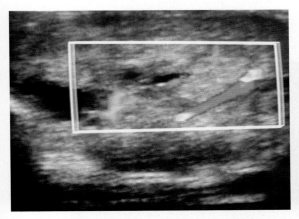

Fig. 41.33: Doppler of submandibular region

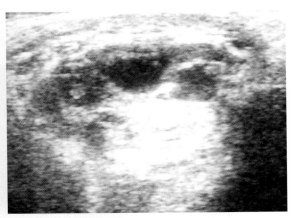

Fig. 41.34: USG of submandibular region

- Aids in differentiation of solid and cystic masses.
- Valuable for guided aspiration and biopsy.

Advantages

- Noninvasive
- Economical
- Quick
- No adverse reaction
- Mobile equipment.

Limitations

- High operator skill required
- Bone does not transmit sound.

Nuclear Medicine

Nuclear medicine encompasses both diagnostic imaging and treatment of disease, and may also be referred to as molecular medicine or molecular imaging and therapeutics.

- It has become an advanced diagnostic procedure in all fields of medicine
- Advanced procedures like single photon emission computed tomography (SPECT), positron emission tomography (PET), etc. hold lot of promise in all diagnostic areas
- The principle of nuclear medicine can be simplified into a procedure which detects

and produces an image of quantity as well as distribution of radioactivity of the injected isotope in a particular tissue studied.

Bone Scanning (Figs 41.35 and 41.36)

- Scintigraphy ("scint") is a form of diagnostic test where in radioisotopes are taken internally, either intravenously or orally, then gamma camera captures and forms two dimensional images from the radiation emitted by radio pharmaceuticals
- Bone scanning is a nuclear medicine technique, which is possibly one of the most commonly performed diagnostic procedures.
- It uses technetium 99m methylene diphosphonate, which is taken in bony areas of high metabolic osteoblastic activity or vascularity

- Bone scans are quite helpful in diagnosing and differentiating bony infections from soft tissue infections, e.g. dental osteomyelitis from cellulitis. While osteomyelitis shows more focal uptake in later phases, cellulitis shows a more diffuse uptake in early phases, followed by decreased uptake in later phases
- Both benign as well as metastatic bone tumors of oral regions show an increased uptake; however, this is nonspecific and increased uptake can be seen in other metabolic diseases like fibrous dysplasia and Paget's disease. Apart from that, increased uptake of isotopes is seen in inflammatory conditions of the temporomandibular (TMJ) joints
- However, the same is also seen in condylar hyperplasia, and clinically needs to be

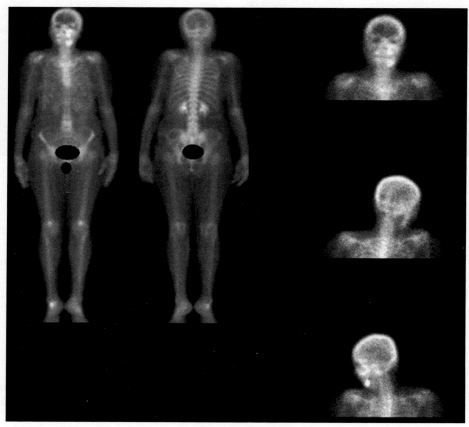

Fig. 41.35: Bone scan (I)

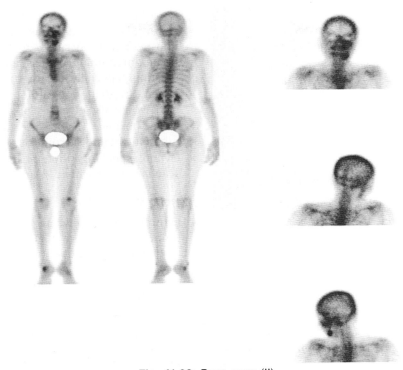

Fig. 41.36: Bone scan (II)

correlated with clinical assessment (including history and clinical examination) as well as other investigations, for correct diagnosis

- Decreased uptake of radioisotope in bone scan is seen in lesions resulting from radiation-treated tissues, vascularity compromised, and resulting necrosed tissue
- In oromaxillary regions, cases of dystrophic calcifications or chronic inflammatory changes should be considered in cases of decreased uptake seen
- Dynamic imaging in bone scans, with series of images with radioactive distribution use SPECT. These produce images in 3 planes and help in more accurate understanding and localizing specific target bone damage. SPECT images are used in pathologies of TMJ disease with MRI equivalent sensitivity.

Gallium Scan

- Gallium scan are used in detecting abscesses, osteomyelitis, and lymphomas
- Although not a favorite test, suspicion of osteomyelitis in dental and other areas can be confirmed and diagnosed effectively by Gallium scan
- Though triple phase bone scan test is the choice for osteomyelitis, it is nonspecific, and Gallium imaging increases the specificity of positive bone scan. Gallium scan is also used to monitor treatment response, with reduced gallium intake/accumulation indicating improvement in osteomyelitis.

Salivary Gland Studies

- Most salivary glands can be imaged and scintigraphy of glands is used for evaluation of normal functioning as well as lesions (Fig. 41.37)

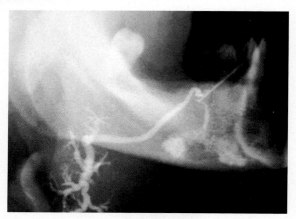

Fig. 41.37: Sialogram of submandibular salivary gland

- Radioactive substance with affinity for particular tissue is administered, with radioactivity measured by a scintillation camera
- Gland aplasia/agenesis, obstruction, trauma as well as fistulas in glands can be detected, and though study may not confirm the diagnosis but is definitely useful as an adjunct. Glandular mass lesions often present with lower uptake, though there are exceptions. Further, acute inflammation usually shows increase in uptake, while decrease intake is seen in chronic inflammatory states.

Positron Emission Tomography (PET) Scan

Advantages

- It is helpful in evaluating metabolic reactions in the body
- PET scans are usually useful in oral squamous cell carcinoma (OSCCA), and is able to detect pathology earlier than CT scan or a MRI
- PET scan can detect OSCCA at a stage when there are no palpable nodes in the neck, and is considered promising in this respect
- PET scan is also often helpful in localization of an occult primary tumor.

Disadvantages

- Accumulation and uptake may be seen in non-neoplastic tissue; e.g new granulation tissue, inflammatory areas, and postoperative scarring, especially in early stages
- Recent irradiation treatment in the OSCCA neck would also give false positive results
- False positive results are also seen with tuberculosis and sarcoidosis
- Overall speaking, though specificity in PET scan is high, sensitivity is an issue.

Lymphoscintigraphy

- Lymphoscintigraphy is showing excellent promise in oral malignancies and is an interesting scan modality. Already being used routinely in breast cancer and malignant melanoma, detecting oral malignancies seem to be effective with this technique
- The radioactive contrast is taken up through lymphatic channels to the first level of draining lymphatic area which is generally called the sentinel node. It is felt that the best prediction of spread of tumor can be done by evaluating sentinel node and lymphatic spread pattern. Metastases are usually evaluated in the sentinel node, and other nodes are considered free from disease if the sentinel node does not show any positive involvement. Sentinel node mapping has helped lot of breast cancer patients, by sparing many axillary nodal dissections/ persistent upper extremity lymphadema, and is considered promising for the same reasons in oral carcinomas. Many research studies are trying to evaluate the accuracy of sentinel node biopsy in management of oral carcinoma
- A lymph node which receives drainage from specific anatomic location in mouth, and is the first node draining the primary malignant site in oromaxillary areas can act as sentinel node, and is able to detect oral malignancies.

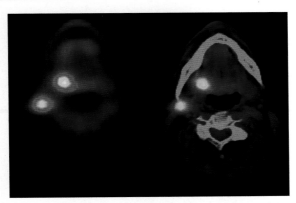

Fig. 41.38: A PET scan. (Left) Overlapped with a CT scan; (Right) PET-CT

SPECT

- The SPECT technology can be used in bone scans. With SPECT, the tomographic images are obtained in three planes (axial, coronal, and sagittal), which thereby facilitates more accurate interpretation and better localization of bone pathology
- In contrast to planar bone scanning, SPECT uses tomographic technology to provide three-dimensional images, which are more useful in localizing small lesions.

Applications

- Potential research tool in the future study of chronic idiopathic jaw pain.
- A negative bone SPECT rules out mandibular invasion of squamous cell carcinoma. And thereby, the inclusion of SPECT in the preoperative assessment would reduce unnecessary mandibular resections.
- In diagnosing and subsequently determining the therapeutic course in patients with asymmetrical mandibular condylar hyperplasia.
- In certain oncology patients treated with bisphosphonates, an increased uptake of 99 mTc-methylene diphosphonate in maxillary bones may suggest probable osteonecrosis of the jaw. Therefore in such cases, SPECT/CT is considered of diagnositic value in assessing the extent of the disease (Fig. 41.38).

Disadvantages

Cannot be routinely used for the detection of jaw pathoses.

Optical Coherence Tomography

- It is a recent development in optical engineering and biomedical imaging
- It is a new method of biomedical imaging that can generate high resolution, noninvasive imaging technique for biological tissues which can present even the cross–sectional images of micro structures
- It was first applied clinically to tomographic images of transparent tissues in the eyes for diagnosis of retinal macular diseases
- It has been applied even to accessible regions of the body such as sub surface imaging of skin, cancer lesions, oral vascular anomalies.

Management of Soft Tissue Facial Wound

42

INTRODUCTION

Principle objective of management of soft tissue facial wounds is minimization of scaring with its consequent long-term aesthetic and psychological impact. There are important differences between the orientation depth and regularity, character of surgical wound and soft tissue facial wound. All of these factors affect management and the healing process of soft tissue facial wound.

HEALING

Healing involves regeneration and repair:
- *Regeneration*: It refers to the replacement of lost cells by cells of same type. In human, regeneration of tissues is limited
- *Repair*: It involves the synthesis of connective tissue and its eventual maturation into scar tissue
- Wound healing is broadly divided into three stages:

Wound healing
Inflammation
Ingrowth of granulation tissue
Scar formation

- Regeneration depends upon two factors:
  - Replicative ability of surviving cells
  - Preservation of stroma.
- If basement membrane is damaged, epithelial cells proliferate in haphazard manner leading to formation of disarranged mass of cells (Fig. 42.1).

Proliferative Capacity of Tissues

Labile cells/intermitotic cells/continuously dividing cells
- Proliferate throughout the life
- Derived from stem cells
- Two groups
  - Hematopoietic cells of bone marrow
  - Covering epithelia.

Stable cells/quiescent cells
- Undergo few divisions
- Capable of division when activated
- Mesenchymal cells
- Liver cells
- Renal tubular cells
- Secretory epithelium of endocrine glands
- Smooth muscle.

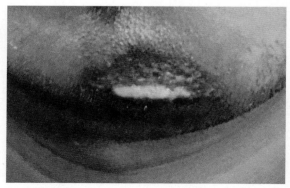

Fig. 42.1: Laceration at chin region healing

Permanent cells/static cells

- Highly specialized cells
- Do not replicate in postnatal life
- Neurons
- Cardiac myocytes
- Lens cells
- Skeletal muscle cells.

Healing of Soft Tissue Wounds

Process of healing of soft tissue wounds is elaborated in Flowchart 42.1.

Definition of Wound

- Loss of continuity of skin or mucous membrane due to injury. Soft tissue or bone may or may not be damaged.
  —Bailey and Love's Short Practice of Surgery
- An injury or damage, usually restricted to those caused by physical means with disruption of normal continuity of structures.
  —Dorland's Medical Dictionary
- Injury to any of the tissues of the body, especially that caused by physical means and with interruption of continuity.
  —Stedman's Medical Dictionary

Flowchart 42.1: Process of healing

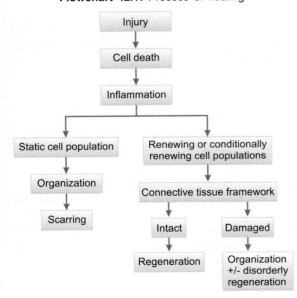

Classification of Wounds

WHO classification of physical and chemical Injuries relating to head and neck
Injury of Head and Neck (S00-S09)

- S00 : Superficial injury
- S01 : Open wound
- S02 : Fracture of skull and facial bones
- S03 : Dislocation, sprain and strain of joints & ligaments
- S04 : Injury of cranial nerves
- S05 : Injury of eye and orbit
- S06 : Intracranial injuries
- S07 : Crushing injury
- S08 : Traumatic amputation of a part of head
- S09 : Other and unspecified injuries (muscle, blood vessels, rupture of ear drum, etc.)

Centers for Disease Control and Prevention (CDC)

1. Classification of surgical wounds
   - Clean wounds
   - Clean contaminated wounds
   - Contaminated wounds
   - Dirty or infected wounds
2. Open and closed wounds
   - Open: Incisions, lacerations, abrasions, puncture wounds, penetration wounds and gun shot wounds.
   - Closed: Contusions, hematoma, crushing injuries.

Assessment of Wounds

Preparatory steps

- Prior to assessment of wound ensure adequate hemostasis
- Thorough irrigation with mild detergent agent (e.g. 1% Savlon)
- Povidone iodine spread over wound
- Blood clots to be removed
- Deep seated foreign material removed with fine curette or the point of No. 11 blade
- Lacerations in hairy area = hair shaven (essential landmarks, e.g. eyebrows and hairline preserved).

Phases of Wound Healing

Inflammatory phase

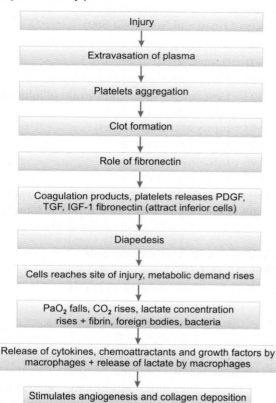

Proliferative phase

- Includes fibroplasia and matrix deposition, neovascularization and epithelization
- Characterized by the formation of granulation tissue.
- It has the appearance of pink granules protruding from the floor of the wound.

Proliferative phase
Fibroplasia and matrix deposition
Collagen synthesis
Angiogenesis
Epithelization

Maturational phase

Characterized by wound contraction and remodeling of scar.

Wound contraction

- Is the shrinkage of area of the wound by approximation of original edges
- Centripetal movement of the skin
- Believed to be brought by myofibroblasts
- Matrix metalloproteinases also appear to play a role.

Remodeling

- Breakdown and synthesis of collagen to achieve the preexisting organization
- Maximum tensile strength is approx. An 80% of original after 60 days.

Healing by Primary Intention

- Wounds sutured primarily with clips, sutures or adhesive materials, the wound healing occur with minimum scarring and it is known as healing by first/primary intention
- only focal disruption of epithelial basement membrane continuity
- Space rapidly fills with fibrin clotted blood
- Dehydration at the surface produces a scab to cover and protect the healing repair site.

The following reaction of wound healing can be divided into
Within 24 hours
By 3 days
By 5 days
During 2nd week
By the end of 1st month

Within 24 hours

- Acute inflammation quickly ensues
- At 8 hours: Incision is flanked by zone of necrotic tissue
- At 16 hours: Epidermis is thickened near line of demarcation between viable and necrotic

tissue. Tongue of epithelial cells is invading underlying dermis, separating necrotic from viable tissue

- At 24 hours: Advanced epithelial invasion, with two tongues moving towards each other
- At 40–48 hours: Tongues have met and severed the necrotic tissue (incorporated in scab) from underlying viable tissue.

Mechanism
- Increased mitotic activity by basal cells at the cut end of epidermis
- At both margins of incision, epidermis become thickened
- Migration of wound down into the upper part of the incisional gap and uniting the upper dermis
- Advancing epidermis cleaves the overlying necrotic epithelium and necrotic dermis from underlying viable dermis
- The scab over the migrated epidermis finally contains dry blood clot, dead epidermis, and fibers of collagen and elastin.

By day 3
- Neutrophils replaced largely by macrophages and granulation tissue progressively invade the incision space
- Collagen fibers are now evident and oriented vertically
- They do not bridge the incision
- Epithelial proliferation continues, yielding thickened epidermal layer.

By day 5
- Neovascularization reaches its peak as granulation tissue fills the incision space
- Collagen fibrils are abundant and begin to bridge the incision
- Epidermis recovers its normal thickness.

During second week
- Continued collagen accumulation and fibroblast proliferation
- Diminished leukocyte infiltrate, edema, and vascularity

- Long process of 'blanching' begins, increasing collagen deposition within incisional scar and regression of vascular channels.

By the end of first month
- Connective tissue largely devoid of inflammatory cells and covered by epidermis
- Dermal appendages destroyed in the line of incision are permanently damaged.

Response to sutures
- Healing by first intention of a wound more than minimal size requires wound to be sutured
- Insertion of suture itself entails incisional damage
- Granulomatous reaction evoked by both suture and downgrowing epithelium
- The earlier sutures are removed, the less will be granulomatous reaction
- Use of adhesive tape avoids even the lesser granulomatous response obtained by early removal of suture.

Healing by Secondary Intention
- Cell or tissue loss is more extensive, as in infarction, inflammatory ulceration, and abscess formation
- Regeneration of parenchymal cells alone cannot restore the original architecture in these situations
- Extensive in growth of granulation tissue from the wound margins, followed by accumulation of ECM and scarring
- Form of healing is known as secondary union or healing by second intention.

Events in healing by secondary intention
- Wound edges gape and open wound has a red base and margins that become swollen from inflammatory edema
- Floor of the wound exudes a yellowish pink fluid
- Pink fluid contains protein, including fibrinogen, and therefore coagulates over the wound
- Relatively wide separation of wound edges means that healing has to progress from base upward

- However, basic events in healing by second intention resemble those for first intention.
  - Acute inflammation and clearing of debris
  - Down growth of epidermis to form a layer of epithelium that separates viable pre-existing collagen of the dermis from injured necrotic collagen at the wound's margin.
- Meanwhile, the base of the coagulum becomes replaced by granulation tissue, produced by fibroblasts and vascular sprouts from adjacent viable dermis
- Concurrent with the development of granulation tissue, there is contraction of the wound induced by myofibroblasts
- The advancing sheets of epidermis finally cover the granulation tissue so that the scab is separated and cast off
- Progressive contraction decreases the size of the wound, and new epidermis is elevated by the increasing amount of granulation tissue.

Secondary healing differs from primary healing in several aspects
Large tissue defect intrinsically have a greater volume of necrotic debris, exudate and fibrin that must be removed
Much large amount of granulation tissue is formed
Wound contraction.

Wound contraction: Within 6 weeks, for example, large skin defects may be reduced to 5–10% of their original size, largely by contraction.

Wound strength
- Carefully sutured wounds have approx 70% of the strength of unwounded skin, largely because of placement of the sutures
- When sutures are removed usually at 1week, wound strength is approx 10% of that of unwounded skin, but this increases rapidly over the next 4 weeks
- Recovery of tensile strength results from collagen synthesis exceeding degradation during the first 2 months, and from structural modification of collagen (cross linking and increased fiber size) when synthesis declines at later times.

Healing by Tertiary Intention or Delayed Primary Closure
- Represented by contaminate wound
- Initially managed with repeated debridement and antibiotics
- Once ready for closure, surgical intervention is performed.

Nerve Injury
- Degeneration of entire neuron (including dendrites and synaptic nerve endings)
- Brain and spinal cord
  - Neuronal debris and myelin engulfed and phagocytosed by microglial cells
  - Neighboring astrocytes proliferate and replace neuron with scar tissue.
  - Nerve injuries (Seddon 1944).

Neuropraxia
- Transient block, incomplete paralysis, complete and rapid recovery
- No microscopic evidence of nerve degeneration
- Caused by pressure.

Axonotmesis
- Axons are damaged, surrounding connective tissue sheaths remain intact
- Wallerian degeneration occurs peripherally
- Caused by crush injuries and traction.

Neurotmesis
Complete section of nerve trunk also shows retrograde degeneration

Healing of Oral Mucosa
- Healing by primary intention is fairly similar to that of skin
- Absence of dry dermis and dry exudate (scab) formation over fibrin clot
- Epithelialization progresses more rapidly in the oral mucosa
- Oral cavity highly vascular

- Abundant amounts of various growth factors in saliva (PDGF, TGF–α, basic FGF and epidermal growth factor)
- EGF: Parotid gland major source, stimulates oral epithelial cell motility.

Characteristics of oral wounds

- Keratinized oral mucosa especially in areas of underlying bone heal with less/no scar formation
- Less scarring due to the presence of IL-10 which inhibits macrophage activity and prolongs monocyte activity.

Healing Muscles

Skeletal muscle

- Mostly composed of cells, with small volume of matrix
- Highly metabolic thus highly vascular
- Every muscle cell innervated
- Fibers → fascicle → perimysium → epimysium
- *Inflammation*: Stimulate regeneration of myofibers the dead muscle fibers are removed by macrophages. Satellite cells are activated within 18 hours of the injury, these cells are able to migrate, in response to a chemical stimulus
- Muscle may also heal with scar tissue instead of new muscle fibers
- This essentially means that the repaired muscle will not be as "strong" as it was before injury. Although it may be able to contract just as quickly.

Muscle injury
I – Damage to fibers without ECM disruption
II – Damage to nerves with intact ECM, vascularity
III – Necrosis of all components

Graft Healing

- Critical component of successful skin grafting is preparation of the recipient site
- Wound also must be free of necrotic tissue and relatively uncontaminated by bacteria.

Initial Adherence

- Initial adherence to the wound bed via a thin fibrin network that temporarily anchors the graft until definitive circulation and connective tissue connections are established
- Adherence begins immediately and is probably at its maximum by 8 hours postgrafting.

Plasmatic Imbibition

- The period of time between grafting and revascularization of the graft is referred to as the phase of plasmatic imbibition
- The graft imbibes wound exudate by capillary action through the sponge like structure of the graft dermis and through the dermal blood vessels
- This prevents graft desiccation, maintains graft vessel patency, and provides nourishment for the graft
- This process is entirely responsible for graft survival for 2–3 days until circulation is reestablished. During this time, the graft typically becomes edematous and increases in weight by 30–50%.

Revascularization

- Begins 2–3 days post grafting by a mechanism not completely understood
- Full circulation to the graft is restored by 6–7 days post grafting.

Theories
Establishment of direct anastomoses between graft and recipient blood vessels
Vascular in-growth of recipient bed vessels into the graft along the channels of previous graft vessels
New vascular in-growth of recipient bed vessels into the graft without regard for previous graft vessels

Wound Contraction

- Myofibroblast in the wound bed is believed to be responsible for this contraction
- In general, thicker grafts = lesser contraction
- Wounds covered with thin split-thickness skin grafts contract less than open wounds

- Ability of a skin graft to resist contraction is related to the thickness of deep dermal component included in the graft, not just the absolute thickness of the graft.

Regeneration

- Hair rarely grows from split-thickness grafts unless the grafts are quite thick. Hair is likely to grow from full-thickness grafts
- Sweat glands and sebaceous glands initially degenerate following grafting. Once again, they are more likely to regenerate in full-thickness grafts, because they are transferred as an entire functional unit. In split-thickness grafts, only a portion of the gland is transferred and the remaining portion may not regenerate.

Reinnervation

- Occurs from the recipient bed and the periphery along the empty neurolemmal sheaths of the graft
- Sensibility returns to the periphery of the graft and proceeds centrally. This process usually begins during the first month but is not complete for several years following grafting
- As reinnervation occurs, pain is usually the first perceived sensation followed later by touch, heat, and cold
- Usually the patient develops protective sensation but not normal perception.

Pigmentation

- Pigmentation returns gradually to full-thickness skin grafts, and they maintain a pigment similar to the donor site
- Split-thickness grafts may remain pale or white or may become hyperpigmented with exposure to sunlight
- It is generally recommended that the graft be protected from direct sunlight for at least 6 months after grafting or even longer.

Complications of wound healing
Infection
Bursting open of wounds (wound dehiscence)
Complications due to scarring
Hypertrophic scars and keloids
Implantation cysts
Contracture
Pigment changes

Biological Basis of Primary Wound Care

- Wound is said to be infected when it contains more than 10 organisms per gram of tissue
- Golden period does not apply to head and neck region
- Facial wound repair may be delayed up to 48 hours
- More important is surgical care delivered and tissue handling is of paramount importance.

Steps in wound managment
Anesthesia
Topical antiseptic and wound irrigant agents
Debridement
Wound closure
Hemostasis
Elimination of dead spaces
Skin closure
Topical medicaments

Wound Dressings

- Polyurethane films
- Hydrogels
- Foams
- Alginates.

Characteristics of ideal occlusive dressing

- Easy to apply and remove
- Transparent to visualize wound
- Semipermeable and absorption of exudate fluid

- Flexible and inexpensive
- Comfortable to the patient.

Interface dressing
- Most commonly used non-adherent composite dressings [TELFA] consist of mildly absorbent cellulose core covered on both sides by a perforated polyester film
- They are used as the sole-dressing for short term [24-48 hours] wound coverage in superficial, minimally exudative wounds or to support other dressings [e.g. Hydrogels]
- It has the tendency to become adherent in highly exudative wounds
- Recently, a non-adherent interpositional surface material [N-TERFACE] was evaluated for use in facial dermabrasion wounds.

Adjunct wound care
- The frequency of dressing change depends on the type of dressing used and the level of exudate
- If exudate breaks through the dressing or if the dressing becomes soiled, it should be removed.

Whether it is high energy ballistic and avulsion injury, a surgical incision, simple traumatic laceration, or complex blast injury, the same basic pattern of repair exists in all wounds. The differentiating factors are the length of time spent in the various phases of wound healing. The modifiying factors of foreign bodies, contamination, fragmentation, size of defect, associated thermal injury, and degree of functional impairment can alter the basic repair process of the body (Figs 42.2 and 42.3).

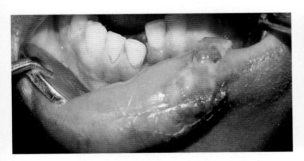

Fig. 42.2: Lip laceration

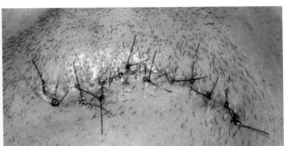

Fig. 42.3: Chin wound sutured

CASE SERIES

Case 1 (Figs 42.4A and B)

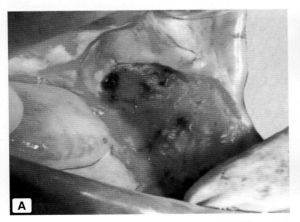
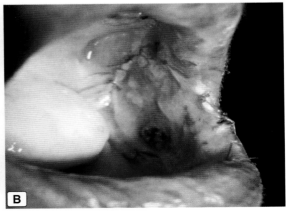

Figs 42.4A and B: Wound closure using collagen memberane

Case 2 (Figs 42.5A and B)

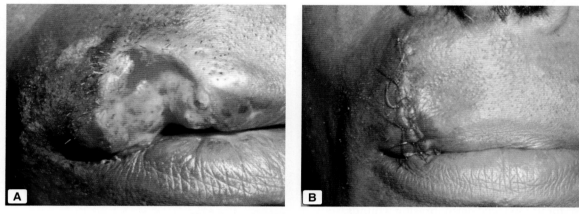

Figs 42.5A and B: Lip wound suturing

Case 3 (Figs 42.6A to C)

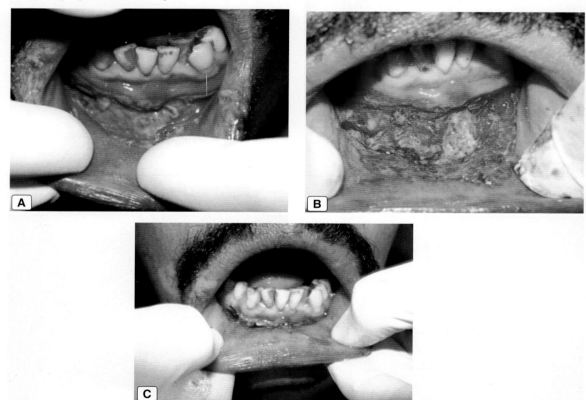

Figs 42.6A to C: Degloving injury. (A) Before debridement; (B) After debridement; (C) After suturing

Case 4 (Figs 42.7 and 42.8)

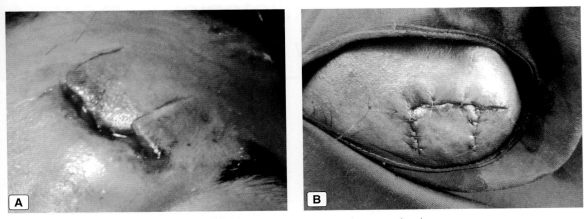

Figs 42.7A and B: Forehead injury and sutures in place

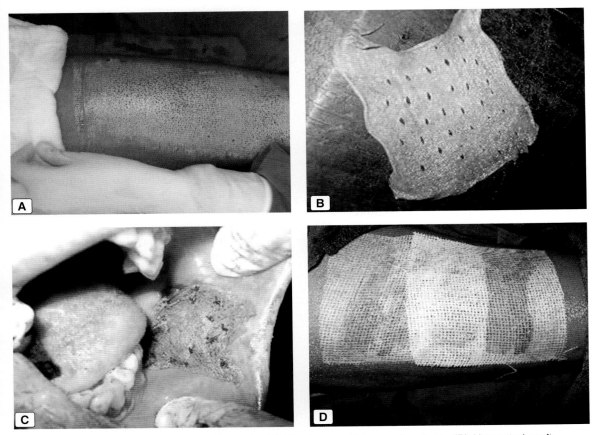

Figs 42.8A to D: Use of split skin graft. (A) Site from graft harvesting done; (B) Harvested graft; (C) Graft in place; (D) Donor site covered with dressing

43

Surgical Anatomy of Incisions in Maxillofacial Surgery

INTRODUCTION

Surgical incisions are always designed based upon certain anatomical landmarks. Applied anatomy and application of knowledge of basic of anatomy in maxillofacial clinical case is the most vital, without which surgery can not be attempted. Surgical incisions in maxillofacial region are as follows.

Maxillofacial Incisions

1. For mandible:
   - Submandibular incision
   - Risdon's incision
   - Retromandibular incision
   - Submental incision
2. For temporomandibular joint:
   - Preauricular incision with variation
   - Preauricular incision
   - Endaural incision
   - Intraoral incision
   - Temporal incision
   - Submandibular incision
3. For zygoma:
   - Gille's incision
   - Crow's foot incision
   - Lateral eyebrow incision
4. For orbit:
   - Transconjunctival
   - Infraorbital
   - Bicoronal

5. For nose:
   - Median vertical
   - H-shaped
   - Bilateral Z apporach
   - W shaped apporach
   - Coronal apporach.

Preoperative planning is required to achieve optimal cosmetic and functional results while making a skin incision. The healing process causes wound contraction and scarring, which can compromise function and appearance.

Obtaining accurate knowledge and assessment of nearby soft tissue and skeletal structures is crucial before making an incision. With planning incisions along relaxed skin-tension lines or at the border of facial aesthetic unit's adherence to techniques of tensionless wound closure, wound edge eversion and atraumatic handling of tissues optimizes scar appearance.

As restoration of facial appearance after incision being the most important area of concern for maxillofacial surgeon incisions for operation in the face must confirm to the basic requirements. But are fundamentally different to those of abdominal or thoracic surgery.

GENERAL GUIDELINES FOR INCISION PLACEMENT

Kruger (1989)

- Skin should be stretched in a way that the marked line rests on a solid bone, thereby providing a firm base or clean incision in one incising move

- Incision should be perpendicular to the skin and completely through it
- Cutting in an angle with an edge will decrease vascular supply and possibly result in a scar.

Norman and Bramley (1990)
Incision should be based on sound anatomical principles
Should have clear anatomical landmarks
Should be designed to give protection to important nerves in its vicinity
Should provide a relatively bloodless field
Should provide good visibility without skin tension
Should be rapidly and confidently executed
Should be uncomplicated in its repair
Should give good cosmetic result and minimal functional impairment
Should be easily teachable

David B Hom (2005)

- Incision should be placed along resting skin tension lines (RSTL). Avoid incisions perpendicular to RSTL
- Face can be considered in 6 major aesthetic units, i.e. forehead, eye and eyebrow, nose, lip, chin and cheek. Incision should be placed at the border of the facial units
- In hair bearing areas, blade should be parallel to hair follicles to prevent their transgression and damage
- Fusiform incisions' long axis should be parallel to RSTL, angle should be less than 300 to prevent dog ear deformity
- Bipolar cauterization must be used when close to nerve

Face has six major esthetic units comprising
Forehead
Eye and eyebrow
Nose
Lips
Chin
Cheek

Surgical incisions of the face are broadly divided into incisions for
Mandible
Temporomandibular joint
Zygoma
Orbit
Around the nose

INCISIONS FOR MANDIBULAR AREA

- Submandibular incision
- Risdon's incision
- Retromandibular incision
- Submental incision
- Modified submandibular incision.

Surgical Anatomy of Mandibular Area

Marginal mandibular branch of facial nerve: Supplies motor fibers to facial muscles in the lower lip and chin, it is the most important anatomic hazard in this incision.

It is important that while placing a submandibular incision it should be at least 1.5 cm below the inferior border of the mandible.

Facial artery: After its origin from the external carotid it runs upward, medial to the mandible and fairly close to the pharynx. It runs deep to the posterior belly of the digastric and stylohyoid muscles, then crosses above them to descend on the medial surface of the mandible grooving or passing through submandibular salivary gland as it rounds the lower border of the mandible. It appears on the external surface around the anterior border of the mandible and lies anterior to facial vein.

Facial vein: It is the primary venous drainage of the face, begins as angular vein, runs along the facial artery and lies posterior to it at the inferior border of the mandible.

Submandibular Incision (Figs 43.1 and 43.2)

Incision is made in two locations.
1. Parallel to the inferior border of the mandible

2. Parallel to or within the RSTL
- Used to approach the ramus of the mandible
- Used in mandibular ostotomies
- Used in submandibular gland surgeries
- Used to approach fractures of the angle or the body of the mandible.

Advantage: One of the most simple and useful incisions.

Disadvantage: Extraoral path and subsequent scar formation and possible damage to marginal mandibular nerve.

Risdon's Incision (Fig 43.3 to 43.6)

It is a modification of submandibular incision. Here the submandibular incision is extended posteriorly and curved in best cosmetic conformity with the angle of the mandible. It is taken 2 cm below the inferior border of the mandible.
- Used to expose the angle of the mandible
- Used access the TMJ and condylar fractures
- Used to access the ramus region
- Used to access the submandibular and the apex of the parotid gland.

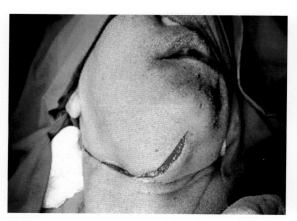

Fig. 43.1: Submandibular incision (I)

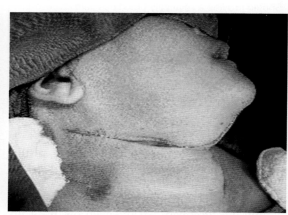

Fig. 43.2: Submandibular incision (II)

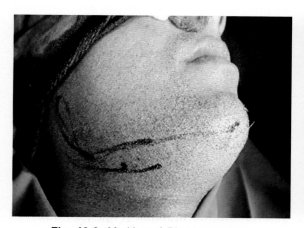

Fig. 43.3: Marking of Risdon's incision

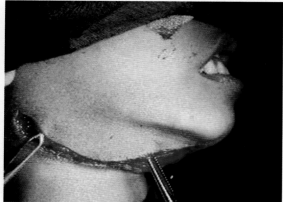

Fig. 43.4: Risdon's incision extended to mastoid region posteriorly

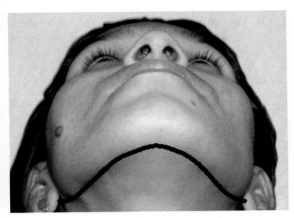

Fig. 43.5: Extended anteriorly for bilateral exposure of mandible

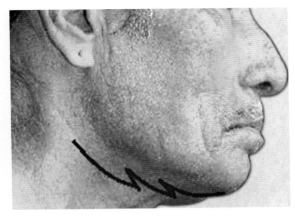

Fig. 43.6: Anterior extension or stepped manner

Advantage: Simple and versatile incision, can be extended and modified depending on the requirement.

Modifications

The incision begins approximately 1cm below the lobe of the ear and 1cm posterior to the ramus of the mandible. The parotid is retracted anteriorly and fibers of the masseter are separated bluntly along their vertical course, to reach the underlying ramus. This technique is also called HINDS technique.

Surgical Anatomy of Facial Nerve

The main trunk of the facial nerve emerges from the base of the skull at the stylomastoid foramen. It divides into temporofacial and cervicofacial divisions at the point inferior to the lowest part of the external auditory meatus.

Average distance from external auditory meatus to bifurcation is 2.3 cm.

Posterior to the parotid the nerve is at least 2 cm deep to the skin, then proceeds to the parotid gland and divide into their terminal branches.

The marginal mandibular nerve courses downward and anteriorly. It frequently arises from the main trunk well behind the posterior border in the lower 3rd of the ramus, thus leaves a void between buccal and marginal branches.

Retromandibular Vein (Figs 43.7A to D)

It is formed in the upper portion of the parotid gland, deep to the neck of the mandible, by the confluence of the superficial temporal vein and maxillary vein. It is lateral to external carotid artery. Both vessels are crossed by the facial nerve. Near the apex of the parotid gland the retromandibular vein gives of anterior communicating branch which joins facial vein just below the angle of the mandible.

- Used to expose the entire ramus of the mandible, from behind the posterior border.
- Useful in procedures involving the area on or near the condylar neck or head or ramus.
- Best suited to approach subcondylar fracture.

Advantage: Esthetically more pleasing, less conspicuous scar.

Alternate Approach

Modified BLAIR incision.

If added exposure is required, then preauricular and retromandibular incisions can be combined, which is known as modified Blair incision.

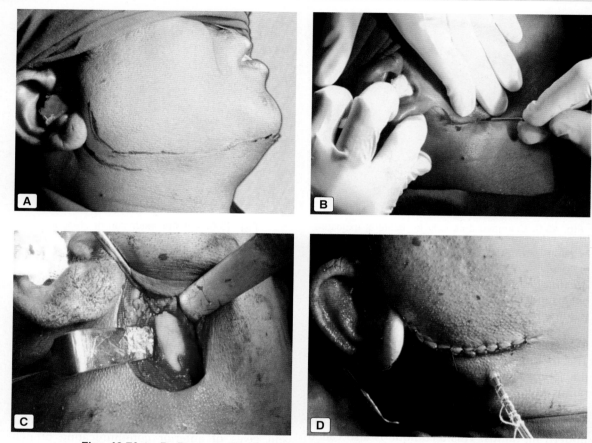

Figs 43.7A to D: Retromandibular incision. (A) Marking; (B) Incision; (C) Exposure; (D) Closure and suturing with drain *in situ*

Frequently used in TMJ ankylosis, surgery of the parotid and to get a wider access to the ramus of the mandible.

Submental Incision

The incision is given along the skin crease 1cm below the lower border of the mandible and parallel to it, provided it lies in the submental skin crease.

This approach is used for procedures, such as genioplasty and excision of the submental lymph node. But due to esthetic concerns extra oral incisions are avoided (Figs 43.8 and 43.9).

Surgical Anatomy
No major anatomical structures, but care should be taken not to strip the genial muscles.

Modified Submandibular Incision (Figs 43.10 to 43.12)

The submandibular incision for the temporomandibular region is the modified submandibular incision or the extended Risdon incision.

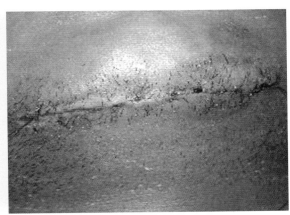

Fig. 43.8: Exposure and plating

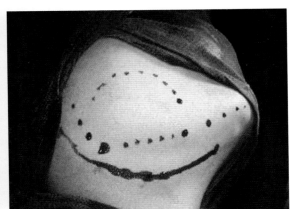

Fig. 43.9: Closure and subcuticular suturing

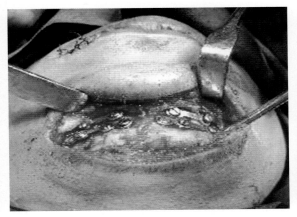

Fig. 43.10

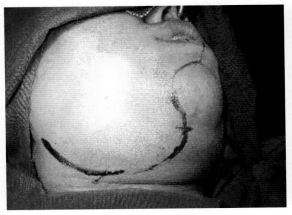

Fig. 43.11

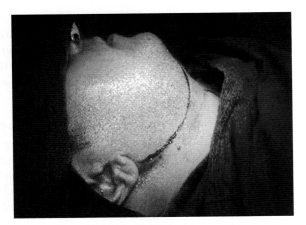

Figs 43.10 to 43.12: Incision marking

INCISIONS AROUND THE TEMPOROMANDIBULAR JOINT

Preauricular incision
• Al-Kayat and Bramley modification (1979)

Posterior auricular incision
• Circum meatal incision
• Endaural incision
• Face lift incision
• Extended Risdons incision
• Modified Blair incision.

Surgical Anatomy of the Temporomandibular Area

The important structure's in this region are:
• Parotid gland
• Superficial temporal vessels
• Auricotemporal nerve
• Facial nerve
• Temporomandibular joint.

Parotid Gland

It lies below the zygomatic arch, below and in front of the external acoustic meatus on the masseter muscle and behind the ramus of the mandible. The superficial pole lies on the TMJ capsule. The gland itself is enclosed in a capsule derived from the superficial layer of the cervical fascia.

Superficial Temporal Vessels

It emerges from the superior aspect of the gland and accompanies the auriculotemporal nerve. The superficial temporal vein lies superficial and usually posterior to the artery.

These vessels are a common source of bleeding.

Auriculotemporal Nerve

It is sensory to parts of the auricle, the external auditory meatus, tympanic membrane and the skin in the temporal area. It runs in the medial side posterior to the neck of the condyle and turns superiorly running over the zygomatic root of the temporal bone. Just anterior to the auricle it divides into its terminal branches.

Facial Nerve

After the nerve exits the stylomastoid foramen it enters the parotid gland. Here it divides into two main trunks and finally the terminal branch emerge out of parotid gland.

It is located 1.5–2.8 cm below the lowest concavity of the bony external auditory meatus.

Layers of the Temporoparietal Region

The temporoparietal fascia is the most superficial layer beneath the subcutaneous fat. This fascia is the lateral extension of the galea. The superficial temporal vessels run superficial to it and the temporal branch of the facial nerve runs deep to it.

The subgaleal fascia is well developed and is usually used as a plane of cleavage in standard preauricular approach.

Temporalis fascia arises from the superior temporal line and fuses with the pericranium. It split's into superficial and deep layers, between these layer a small amount of fat may be present.

A large vein frequently runs superficial to the temporal fascia which must be considered during incision.

Preauricular Incision (Figs 43.13 to 43.15)

This incision gives the easiest approach to the mandibular condyle. It is given just anterior to the pinna or alternately around the tragus and at the junction of the ear, and scalp superiorly. It is then directed obliquely forward and upward at an angle of 45. Usually posterior branch of superficial temporal artery requires ligation while its anterior branch and auricotemporal nerve are retracted anteriorly.

Al-Kayat and Bramley's Modification (1979)

This modification is done for wider exposure.

A question mark shaped incision is done, which avoids main vessels and nerves. About 2 cm above the malar arch, the temporalis fascia splits into 2 parts which can be easily identified by

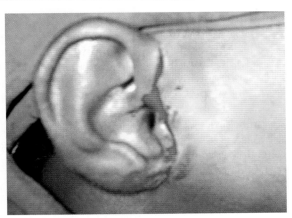

Fig. 43.13: Incision

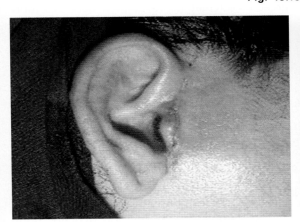

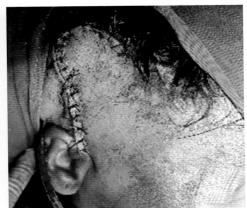

Figs 43.14 and 43.15: Closure and suturing

fat globules between the two layers, which form an important landmark.

In this technique, temporal fascia and superficial temporal artery are reflected with the skin flap. The incision should never be extended below the lobule of the ear as it increases the chances of damage to the main trunk of the facial nerve. It is particularly important in children where it may be quite superficial.

Posterior Auricular Incision

This incision was described by Alexander and James in 1975.

It is placed in the groove between the helix and posterior auricular skin so that the entire ear can be reflected anteriorly after completely dividing the cartilaginous external auditory canal. It gives a wide exposure to the joint with cosmetic advantage since the scar is completely hidden behind the auricle. But there may be partial stenosis of the auditory canal

Circum Meatal Incision

It is a modification of the preauricular incision. It incorporates elements of preauricular and postauricular incisions.

The preauricular incision commences at the upper border of the tragus & passes upward in preauricular crease to reach the most superior attachment of the helix to the scalp. From here incision is carried backward and downwards around the outer margin of funnel shaped bony auditory meatus to terminate just above the commencement of the mastoid process. The cosmetic results with this approach are excellent.

The only reported complication is transistent weakness of upper branch of facial nerve.

Endaural Incision (Fig. 43.16)

It was designed by Davidson in 1955.

It passes downward and backward in the cleft between the helix and tragus, and proceeds along the roof of the external auditory canal for approximately 1cm. It is then reversed and made at the anterior half of the meatal circumference at the junction of the cartilaginous and bony meati. A surgical cleft is thus created along almost in an avascular plane. Since the direction of the external auditory canal is downwards, forwards and medially directed, so the dissection should proceed in the same fashion otherwise the tympanic membrane can be injured.

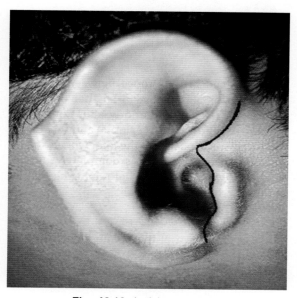

Fig. 43.16: Incision endaural

Face-lift Incision

It is also known as rhytidectomy incision.

It comprises of a preauricular component and a postauricular component, which may go into the hair line. It is a variant of the retromandibular incision with the difference being a more hidden location.

Advantage—decreased scar

Disadvantage—more time required for healing.

Surgical Anatomy

Greater auricular nerve: Most significant structure.

It begins in the neck as spinal roots of C2 and C3, which fuse on the scalene muscles to form the greater auricular nerve. It then becomes more superficial and crosses sterrnocleidomastoid muscle at an angel of 450 and splits into two.

It has a wide area of distribution.

Gilles Incision

It is also known as Gilles temporal approach. It was 1st introduced by Gilles, et al in 1927.

INCISIONS FOR THE ZYGOMA

- Gilles's temporal incision
- Crow's foot incision
- Lateral eyebrow incision.

The rational for the incision depends upon the fact that temporal fascia is attached to the outer aspect and superior border of the zygomatic arch and beneath this layer and is superficial to temporal muscles. There is a potential tissue plane into which a long flat and narrow instrument can be introduced to lift the depressed zygomatic bone or arch.

Surgical Anatomy

The superficial temporal artery crosses the posterior root of zygomatic process of temporal bone and bifurcates into anterior and posterior branch 5 cm above it. The anterior branch runs towards frontal tuberosity (William, et al 1999)

The incision 2.5 cm long is made above and parallel to anterior branch of superficial temporal artery and dissection is carried up to the temporal fascia. It is to be noted that if the incision is placed

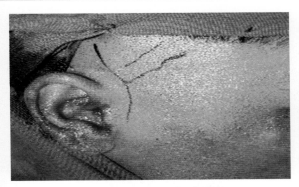

Fig. 43.17: Marking for incision

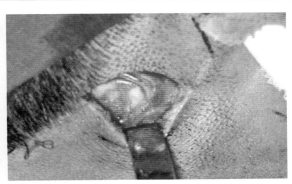

Fig. 43.18: Exposure of plane

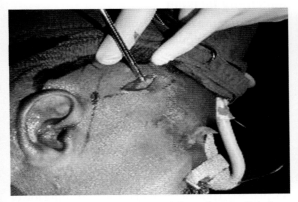

Fig. 43.19: Instrument advanced through potential plane

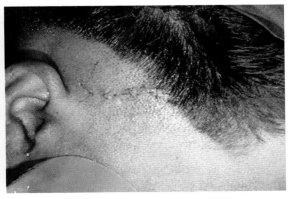

Fig. 43.20: Closure and suturing

too low then we may enter the lateral expansion of epicranial aponeurosis. If incision is placed too far posteriorly, the extrinsic muscle of the ear may be erroneously identified as temporal muscles (Figs 43.17 to 43.20).

Crow's Foot Incision

This incision is preferred in elderly patients in which there are well defined skin creases.

The incision is placed along skin crease in the lateral aspect about 1 cm above the outer cantus of the eye. It ensures an almost invisible postoperative scar (William 1994).

Lateral Eyebrow Incision

This is an ideal incision in young patients.

The incision is given through the outer end of the eyebrow. Here the incision should not be at right angel to the skin, but directed at an angel to the emerging hairs, so as to avoid transecting the hair follicles, which would impair their further growth (Converse 1974).

If the hairs are too thick, they may be trimmed slightly but not shaven off, since they provide a valuable guide to the alignment during skin closure. The periosteum should be incised and stripped away from outer and inner aspect of the zygomatic process of the frontal and zygomatic bones at a distance of 0.75 cm away from the bony margin. This decreases the risk of injury to branch of facial nerve (William 1994).

In this area there are no major neurovascular structures.

It gives simple and rapid access to the fronto-zygomatic area.

Occasionally, some hair loss may be present due to damage to the hair follicles

INCISIONS AROUND THE ORBIT

- Subcilliary incision
- Infraorbital incision
- Transconjuntival incision.

Surgical Anatomy

The orbital area in sagital section consists of four distinct layers.
- The skin along with subcutaneous tissue.
- The orbicularis oculi muscle surrounding the eye.
- The tarsus or orbital septum.
- The conjunctiva.

Skin

- Outermost layer
- Thinnest
- Has many elastic fibers
- Loosely attached to underlying muscle
- Blood supply from underlying muscle vessels.

Muscular Layer (Orbicularis Oculi)

- Subajdacent and adherent to skin
- Forms sphincter of eyelid
- Can be divided into palpebral and conjunctival
- Palpebral can be divided into pretarsal and preseptal.

    Nerve supply—branch of facial nerve that enter the muscle on the deep side.

    Blood supply—external facial artery tributaries that come from deep branch ophthalmic artery.

Orbital Septum/Tarsus

It forms a diaphragm between the contents of the orbit and superficial face. It is a facial extension of periostium of the bones of the face and orbit. The tarsal plate of the lower eyelid is a thin, pliable fibrocartilagenous structure that gives form and support to the lower eyelid. Laterally, it becomes a fibrous band and along with upper part becomes the lateral cantal tendon. Medially it also becomes fibrous and shelters the inferior lacriminal canaliculus behind it as it becomes the medial cantal tendon. Embedded within the tarsal plates are large sebaceous glands called the tarsal or meibomian glands, whose ducts may be seen along the lid margin.

A grayish line or a slight groove is visible between the lashes and the opening of the tarsal gland which represent the two fundamental portions of the eyelid, skin and muscle on one hand and tarsus and conjunctiva on the other. This indicates a plane along which the lid may be split into anterior and posterior portions with minimal scaring.

Subciliary Incision

It is given approximately 2 mm below the eyelashes and can be extended laterally as necessary (top line).

If natural skin crease line is used then the incision is located slightly inferiorly and should follow the crease line as it tails off (lower line).

Infraorbital Incision

The incision follows a line parallel to the margin of the lower eyelid, but not too close to the free edge. It is extended laterally and inferiorly at an angel 45, placed in one of the skin creases forming lower limit of crows foot wrinkles (Figs 43.21 to 43.23).

It gives an excellent exposure of the entire orbital floor and lower part of lateral and medial walls.

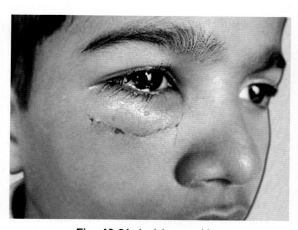

Fig. 43.21: Incision marking

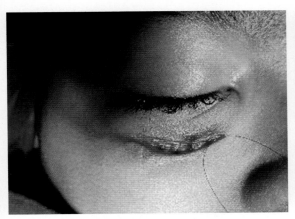

Fig. 43.22: Suturing procedure

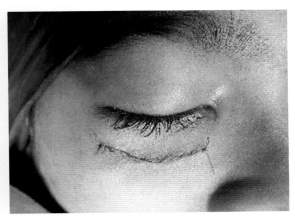

Fig. 43.23: Subcuticular suturing completed

Transconjuntival Incision

Also called as inferior fornix incision

Popular incision for exposure of orbital floor and infraorbital rim.

Advantage—produces excellent cosmetic result, because scar is hidden. Rapid and no skin or muscle dissection is required.

Disadvantage—medial extension is limited by lacrimal drainage.

Incision: Once the lower lid is everted and stabilized, the position of lower tarsal plate is noted through the conjunctiva. A small incision is made 3 mm below the tarsal plate on the medial aspect and in line with the punctum. The line of division is critical, if placed too low down near fornix, it will be below the fascia passing from the inferior rectus to tarsal plate, thus allowing the escape of periorbital fat. If placed too high, there may be distortion of lower eye lid (Williams 1994).

INCISIONS AROUND THE NASAL COMPLEX

- External nasal incision
- Endonasal/internal incision
- Median vertical incision of nose
- H-shaped incision
- Bilateral – Z incision
- W-shaped incision
- Bicoronal incision.

Surgical Anatomy

The nose has the form of a triangular pyramid, with its summit corresponding to the root of the nose and a base into which two nostrils open.

External nasal bony framework—consist of paired nasal bones, supported posteriorly by nasal process of frontal bone and laterally by nasal process by frontal process of maxilla. The inferior edge is continuous with the upper lateral triangular cartilage which extends underneath the nasal bone to 4–7 mm. This area is often called "keystone area."

External Nasal Cartilage Framework

The upper lateral cartilages are paired structures that form the greater part of the middle 3rd of the lateral nasal wall. Their medial border are fused with the lateral expansion of anterior border of the septal cartilage in its upper 2/3rds. The attachment between the alar and upper lateral cartilages is folded back by 2–3 mm and is frequently called the scroll area.

The alar (lower lateral) cartilage are paired structures that have medial and lateral crura. The two medial crura come together at the midline and take part in forming the columella

The posterio-inferior edges of the medial crura diverge and attach to the septal cartilage by fibrous tissue. The lateral crura are quadrilateral and usually convex.

Nasal Septum

It is made up of 6 structures, the septal crest of maxilla, perpendicular plate of palatine bone, perpendicular plate of ethamoid bone, the vomer, the cartilaginous septum, and the membranous septum.

External Nasal Incision

It is a bilateral marginal incision connected by a transcolumellar incision. The soft tissue is elevated off the cartilage and nasal bone exposing the entire tip and dorsum. Marginal incision follows the free caudal margin of the lower lateral cartilage and not the margin of the nostril. Incision should not be placed on the soft triangle. Next a stair step or inverted V incision in the skin across the columella connects the ends of these incisions.

Endonasal Incision

Involves marginal incision and an inter-cartilaginous incision to a partial or complete transfixion incision. Marginal incision for exposure of the dome and lateral crus should follow the free caudal margin of the lower lateral cartilage and not the margin of the nostril.

Intercartilaginous incision divides the junction of the U/L lateral cartilage. The incision traverses the aponeurotic like fibroareolar tissue that maintains the attachment between them (scroll area)

Transfixation Incision

It is made at the caudal end of the septal cartilage and connected to the intercartilaginous incision. It is important to extend the transfixation incision around the septal angle to permit the release of the alar cartilages from their septal attachments when complete exposure by a marginal incision is required.

Median Vertical Incision

A 2–3 mm vertical incision is made from the forehead down to the base of the nose (Fig. 43.24).

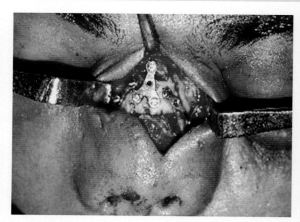

Fig. 43.24: Nasal fracture reduction and stabilization through vertical incision

This is used to access fractures of nasal skeleton and medial canthal ligament (Stanc 1970).

H-shaped Incision

It was 1st described by Converse and Smith in 1962. and then later modified by Mustarde in 1980

This incision is a curved lateral nasal incision made over anterior lacriminal crest to expose structures around the medial canthus (Fig. 43.25).

It gives excellent exposure of nasal bridge and canthal ligaments, but inadequate access to frontal bone.

Bilateral–Z incision

This incision is in shape of the letter Z. It is placed on either side of nose (Fig. 43.26).

It was described by Dingman, et al in 1969.

This incision is used to access the medial canthal area and the lateral aspect of the nose.

W-shaped Incision

It is a curved transverse incision made across the base of the nose within a skin crease with its convexity upwards (Fig. 43.27).

It was given by Bowerman in1975.

Care is taken to identify and preserve the supraorbital nerves and vessels.

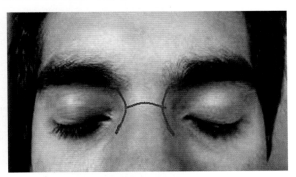

Fig. 43.25: H incision marking

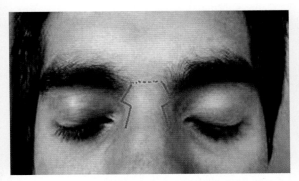

Fig. 43.26: Z incision marking

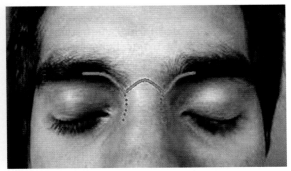

Fig. 43.27: W-shaped incision marking

This incision gives excellent visibility and access to various bone fragments for plating.

Bicoronal Incision

Here the preauricular incision is extended across the scalp within the hairline. The soft tissue is divided down to the subaponeurotic areolar tissue by dissecting along this plane, thus virtually degloving the forehead.

Advantage—very good cosmetic outcome and wide exposure

SUMMARY AND CONCLUSION

Surgical incisions of the face should be based on anatomical landmarks and underlying structures.

It is important to protect the underlying nerves and vessels. It is very important to keep in mind the cosmetic effect.

The amount of access required is also important in selecting the incision. Absorbable buried suture can be used to approximate deeper layers to avoid excessive tension on the skin. Non absorbable or absorbable sutures can be used on the skin surface with gentle eversion of skin edges. Generally 5-0 to 3-0 absorbable sutures for deeper layers and 6-0 to 5-0 sutures for skin. Differential undermining of wound edges in the subcutaneous plane may be needed to avoid distortion of nearby structures. This can be accompanied by creating subcutaneous plane on one side of the wound.

Fluid, Electrolyte, and Acid–Base Balance

44

INTRODUCTION

- The maintenance of normal volume and normal composition of the extracellular fluid is vital to life. Proper management of fluid and electrolytes in maxillofacial surgical patient is of extreme importance. Three types of homeostasis are involved in fluid and electrolyte maintenance: fluid balance, electrolyte balance, and acid-base balance.
- The ICF contains nearly 2/3rd of total body water; the ECF contains the rest. Exchange occurs between the ICF and ECF.

Definitions

Anion gap
A concept used to estimate anion and cation levels in serum and conditions that influence them
Extracellular fluid (ECF)
The compartment outside of cells that contains approximately one third of volume of the body water
Henderson-Hasselbach equation
An equation for stating the expression for the dissociation constant of an acid
pH = 6.1 + log HCO_3^-/($PaCO_2$)
Metabolic acidosis
Acidosis resulting from increase in acids other than carbonic acid
Metabolic alkalosis
Alkalosis in which plasma bicarbonate is increased and there is a rise in plasma concentration of CO_2

Oncotic pressure
The total influence of the protein on the osmotic activity of plasma water
Osmotic pressure
The pressure that develops when two solutions of different concentrations are separated by a semi permeable membrane
Respiratory acidosis
Acidosis secondary to pulmonary insufficiency resulting in retention of CO_2
Respiratory alkalosis
Alkalosis with an acute reduction of plasma with a proportionate reduction in plasma CO_2

Fluid Compartments

- Body fluids include water and solutes
- About 2/3rd of the body's fluid is located within cells and is called intracellular fluid (ICF)
- The other 1/3rd called extracellular fluid (ECF) includes interstitial fluid, plasma and lymph, GI tract fluids, synovial fluid, fluids of the eyes and ears, CSF, pleural, pericardial and peritoneal fluids and glomerular filtrate
- The term fluid balance means that various body compartments contain the normal amount of water
- An inorganic substance that dissociates into ions is called an electrolyte. Fluid balance and electrolyte balance are interrelated
- Water is the largest single constituent in the body 45–75% of total body mass

- Daily water gain and loss are about 2.5 litres.
- Sources of water gain are ingested liquids and foods, and water produced by cellular respiration and dehydration synthesis reactions
- Water is lost by the process of urination, evaporation from the skin surface, exhalation of water vapor, and defecation. In women also menstrual flow
- The main way to regulate body water gain is by adjusting the volume of water intake, mainly by drinking more or less fluid. The thirst center in the hypothalamus governs the urge to drink
- Although increased amounts of water and solutes are lost through sweating and exhalation during exercise, loss of excess water or excess solutes depends mainly on regulating excretion in the urine
- The extent of urinary NaCl loss is the main determinant of body fluid volume, whereas the extent of urinary water loss is the main determinant of body fluid osmolarity
- Angiotensin II and aldosterone reduce urinary loss of Na^+ and Cl^- and thereby increase the volume of body fluids
- ANP promotes natriuresis, elevated excretion of Na^+ (and Cl^-), which decreases blood volume
- The major hormone that regulates water loss and thus body fluid osmolarity is ADH
- An increase in the osmolarity of interstitial fluid draws water out of cells and they shrink slightly. A decrease in the osmolarity of interstitial fluid also causes cells to swell
- When a person consumes water faster than the kidneys excrete it or renal fn. Is poor-water intoxication, cells swell.

Ions: when inorganic salts are in solution, as in extracellular or intracellular fluids they dissociate into ions. There are two kinds of ions.
- *Cations*: electropositive—sodium potassium, calcium, magnesium
- *Anions*: electronegative—chlorides, phosphate, bicarbonate.

Collectively they are called electrolytes.

Chemical concentration, reactivity, and osmotic power of these ions is described in milimoles/liter

Osmolality: Measures the concentration of particles in the solution

Osmolarity: Is a measure of the osmoles of solute per liter of solution

Osmolality: Is a measure of the osmoles of solute per kilogram of solution

Plasma osmolality can be approximated by the following formula:

Plasma osmolality(mosm/l): 2(Na$^+$ + K$^+$) + (BUN ÷ 2.8) + (Glucose ÷18)

Serum Electrolytes

Cations

Sodium: A positively charged electrolyte that helps to balance the fluid levels in the body and facilitates neuromuscular function

Potassium: A main component of cellular fluid helps to regulate the neuromuscular function and osmotic pressure

Calcium: affects neuromuscular performance and contributes to skeletal growth and blood coagulation.

Magnesium: Influences the muscle contraction and intracellular activity.

Anions

Chloride: Regulates the blood pressure.

Phosphate: Impacts metabolism and regulates acid base balance and calcium levels.

Bicarbonate: Assists in the regulation of blood pH levels. Bicarbonate insufficiencies and elevations cause acid base disorders.

Body Fluid Spaces

Total body water: approximately 40L (60%) of the body weight in adult male (Table 44.1).

Intracellular: 2/3rds of the body water (30–40% of total body weight) 25–30 liters. Is measured by subtracting ECF fluid from total body water (Table 44.2).

It is a part of protoplasm of cells, largest portion within skeletal muscles.

Potassium and magnesium are principle cations, phosphates and proteins principal anions.

Extracellular: 1/3rds of body fluids (20% of body weight) (Table 44.3)
- Intravascular: 5% of body weight
- Interstitial: 15% of body weight

Table 44.1: Percentage of body weight in fluid

Age group	Percent of body weight is fluid
Embryo	97%
Newborn	77%
Adult	60%
elderly	54%

Table 44.2: Concentration of different ions in intracellular fluid

K$^+$	125 mEq/L
Mg^{++}	40 mEq/L
Na$^+$	10 mEq/L
Phosphates	150 mEq/L
Proteins	40 mEq/L

Table 44.3: Concentration of different ions in extracellular fluid

Na$^+$	135–145 mEq/L
K$^+$	3.5–5.5 mEq/L
Ca^{++}	3 mEq/L
Mg^{++}	2 mEq/L
Cl$^-$	114 mEq/L
HCO$_3^-$	30 mEq/L

Osmolality: (total particle concentration) is same in all fluid compartment and is 280–295 mmol/kg (Table 44.4).

Fluid intake: Exogenous—either drunk/ingested in solid food avg. 2–3 liters/day. Endogenous—released during oxidation of ingested food. Normal is <500 mL/day (Table 44.5).

SODIUM

About 44% of sodium is extracellular, 47% in the bone and 9% in intracellular fluid.

Total sodium content of blood is 90 gm (3900 mEq/L) total body requirement per day—app 5 gm or 1 mmol/kg NaCl or 500 mL of isotonic 0.9% saline.
- Plasma level 135–145 mEq/L
- Intracellular 5–10 mEq/L.

Sodium conversion following trauma: Following trauma of any kind there is a period of sodium conversion which varies with degree of tissue injury, in which there is almost no excretion of sodium. Output of sodium during this period not more than 10 mEq/L following surgery this period is of approx 48 hr, due to increased adrenocortical

Table 44.5: Average daily fluid balance in a70 kg adult

Intake	Output
Water from beverage – 1200ml	Urine – 1500 ml
Water from solid food – 1000ml	Insensible fluid loss – 500-900ml
Water from oxidation – 300ml	Faeces – 100 ml

Table 44.4: Concentration of different ions in body secretions

Secretion	Total per 24 hr	Na$^+$ mEq/L	K$^+$ mEq/L	Cl$^-$ mEq/L	HCO$_3^-$ mEq/L
Plasma		137–145	3.5–5.5	95–105	22–25
Saliva	1500 mL	15	40		
Gastric	2500 mL	50	10	80	
Intestinal	3000 mL	140	10	100	25
Biliary	500 mL	140	5	100	30
Pancreatic	800 mL	140	7	70	120

activity due to this it is not wise to administer large quantities of saline immediately after surgery (unless there is a continuing loss or patient is already in deficiency).

Hyponatremia: serum Na + <135 mEq/L

Sodium losses: sodium rich losses from GI tract-vomiting; severe diarrhea in cases of dysentery, ulcerative colitis, cholera; intestinal obstruction; intestinal fistulae.

Following Burns

Renal losses: Addison's disease. Prolonged diuretic use.

Water retention and dilutional hyponateremia: prolonged infusion of dextrose 5%, transurethral resection of prostrate (TRUP) syndrome, medical causes –CCF, cirrhosis of liver.

SIADH (syndrome of inappropriate ADH secretion).

Postoperative hyponatremia: with a normal or increased ECF volume as a result of prolonged administration of sodium free solutions.

C/F in its most usual mild form it is asymptomatic; symptomatic when it falls below.

120 mEq/L features of extracellular dehydration, wrinkled dry skin, subcutaneous tissue feels lax. Reduced BP, increased pulse rate, shrunken eyes, dry coated tongue, thrist is not particularly evident, urine is scanty and of high color, nausea and vomiting, drowsiness, weakness, convulsions, coma.

Packed cellvolume (hematocrit) provides an index of degree of hemoconcentration provided there is no preexisting anemia.

Laboratory investing: falling hematocrit, reduced serum sodium.

Treatment

Calculation of Sodium Deficit

0.6 × (weight in kg) × (desired sodium –actual sodium)

Use 0.5 for women. Desired range of correction is 120–125 mmol/L. Serum sodium is corrected slowly at a rate of 0.5 mEq/L/hr (or 10–12 mEq/L in 24 hrs) to a range of 120–125 mEq/L. (in order to avoid CNS myelinolysis).

Plasma Na >120 mmol/L

- Water restriction to 0.5 liter
- 0.9% saline if volume deplete
- Stop drugs/treat specific cause
- Plasm Na >110–120 mmol/L
- Water restriction <0.5 liter
- 0.9% saline IV (if not in ECF excess) 1 liter 12 hourly
- Add frusemide 20–40 mg oral if overloaded.

Plasma Na <110 mmol/L or with Neurological Signs

1.8% or 3% (3% NaCl has 514 mmol sodium/L) saline slow IV over 3–4 hr to raise plasma Na 0.5 mmol/hour. 100 mL has 51.4 mmol.

Add frusemide 20 mg IV if overloaded or CVP rises rapidly.

Hypernateremia: Na 150 mmol/L

Likely to arise if patient is given excesss of 0.9% saline solution during early post operative period, resulting in overloading of circulation withsalt and its accompanying water.

C/F: puffiness of the face is the earliest sign, pitting edema—sacral, pedal but for pitting edema to be present at least 4.5 liters of excess fluid must be there in tissue spaces.

POTASSIUM

Major intracellular cation 98% is intracellular. Total potassium content: 3,400 mEq. Majority of it being in skeletal muscles. Each day a normal adult ingests 1 mmol/kg of potassium in food; fruit, milk, honey are rich sources an amount nearly corresponding to the intake is excreted in urine.

Augmented Potassium Excreation of Trauma

Following any trauma/surgery there is a time period, varing directly with degree of tissue damage; of increased excreation of potassium from kidneys. Loss is greatest during first 24 hrs and can last for about 2–3 days. Unless the patient was severely depleted at the time of surgery hypokalemia usually does not manifest with in 48 years.

Hypokalemia

(Serum potassium < 3.5 mmol/L) gradual hypokalemia is usually seen in surgical practice.

Etiology

Result of diarrhea from ulcerative colitis, villous tumors of the colon, losses from external fistulae of the alimentary tract, prolonged gastroduodenal aspiration, if oral feeding is withheld for more than 4 days, diuretics.

C/F: Listlessness, slurred speech, muscular hypotonia, depressed reflexes, abdominal distension (due to paralytic ileus) weakness of respiratory muscles-rapid shallow gasping respirations. Reduced BP, reduced pulse rate, cardiac arrhythmias. (ECG: prolonged QT, ST depression, flattened/inverted T wave)

Replacement

Mild hypokalemia(k^2)> 2-0 <3.5 mEq/L)
- Oral supplementation—potassium chloride syrup-30 mL with 40 mmol/L
- Intravenous KCl infusion @≤10–15 mEq/hr (1 ampoule has 20 mmol of K^+)
  Severe hypokalemia (K^+ ≤ 2.0 mEq/L, paralysis or ECG changes)
- Intravenous KCl infusion ≤40 mEq/hr
- Continuous ECG monitoring
- If life threatening, 5–6 mEq bolous IV.

Hyperkalemia

Mainly iatrogenic due to excessive infusion of potassium salts, and usually associated with severe oliguria/anuria (renal failure).

C/F: Nausea, vomiting, intermittent intestinal colic, low heart rate, low BP, mental confusion, apathy. ECG changes when serum K^+>7 mmol/L (ECG peaked T wave, wide QRS, disappearance of T wave) following are the ECG changes with increasing level of hyperkalemia.

Treatment
- Calcium gluconate infusion (10% over 10 min)—a physiologic antagonist
- Insulin with dextrose solution (30 U in 1L 10% dextrose)—drives K^+ into the cell
- Sodium polystyrene sulfonate (5 gm as enema/mouth)—decrease absorption
- Dialysis.

MAGNESIUM

An important ion in maintaining the contractility of muscle and excitability of neural tissue.

Total magnesium content in a 70 kg man: 200 mEq

Plasma concentration: 1.7 – 2.2 mEq/L

Normal dietary intake: 20–25 mEq/day. Approx 8 meq is absorbed and rest excreted.

Kidneys' has a reasonable power to conserve magnesium, during deficiency renal excretion is less than 1 mEq/day.

Deficiency

Etiology
- Prolonged loss via GI secretions—intestinal fistula
- Acute pancreatitis
- Reduce intake with increased excretion – in chronic alcoholics
- Malabsorbtion

C/F: Difficult to describe the clinical features typical to magnesium deficiency alone. In majority it is combined with other ion deficiencies. Usually characterized by—

Hyperactivity tendon reflexes, muscle tremors and tetany with a possible chvostek's sign.

When tetany is not relieved by supplementation of calcium, magnesium deficiency has to be diagnosed.

Treatment
- Parenteral administration of magnesium chloride/sulfate
- 2 mEq/kg body weight may be given when renal parameters are normal
- Monitoring of heart rate, BP, respiration, ECG
- Flowed by continuous replacement of a small dose—10–20 mEq of 50% magnesium sulfate given by IM or IV injections.

Magnesium Excess

Rare to occur as long as the renal parameters are not severely affected.

Etiology

When magnesium containing antacids or laxatives are given in a patient with an impaired renal function.

In severe acidosis and sever ECF volume deficit following burns or massive trauma.

C/F: Lethargy, weakness and progressive Loss of Deep tendon reflexes. [ECG: widening of pr interval, widening of QRS, tall T waves].

CALCIUM

Mainly extracellular cation. *Normal level in plasma 9–11 mg% (3 mEq/L),* normal daily intake is around 1–3 gm. Total body calcium in 70 kg individual is 1000–1200 gm and majority of this is found in bone as phosphate or carbonate. Majority (55%) of calcium in the serum is in bound form, bound to plasma proteins. 45% of it is in the free ionized form which is active component and responsible for neuromuscular stability.

Hypocalcemia: seen in:
- Acute pancreatitis
- Acute and chronic renal failure
- Pancreatic and small intestinal fistulae
- Accidental transient/permanent hypocalcemia following surgery on the thyroid

C/F: numbness and tingling sensation in the circumoral region and the tips of fingers.

Hyperactive tendon reflexes, muscle cramps with coropedal spasm and tetany, positive Chovstek's sign.

Treatment

Intravenous calcium gluconate. Oral supplementation—100 mg/day.

Hypocalcemia

Levels >16 mg% are fatal.
- Malignancies with bony metastasis, especially in calcium lung, CA breast

- Multiple myeloma
- Hyperparathyroidism
  Mild (11.5 mg/dL): Asymptomatic.
  Moderate 11.5–13 mg/dL): lethargy, anorexia, nausea and polyutria
  Severe (>13 mg/dL): neuromypathic symptoms, muscle weakness, depression, lethargy, impaired memory, stupor, coma.

These many signs and symptoms are commonly attribute to either the cancer treatment or the cancer itself and may make it difficult to detect hypocalcemia when it first occurs.

This disorder can be severe and difficult to manage. Severe hypocalcemia is a medical emergency requiring immediate treatment.

Treatment

Oral/slow IV inorganic phosphates, corticosteroids—decrease resorption of calcium from bone and reduce intestinal absorption of vitamin D. calcitonin, large doses of IV frusemide can excrete calcium from kidney.

Fluid Administration

The fluids can be administered alone or in combination for the replacement of body fluids are:
- Whole blood and red cells concentrates
- Colloids solution either as plasma protein fraction or synthetic colloids
- Crystalloids solution
- Hypertonic solution
- Others, e.g. solution of hemoglobin and perflorocarbons

Replacement Fluids

Use to replace abnormal loses of blood, plasma or other extracellular fluids by increasing volume of vascular compartment. Principally in:
- Treatment of patient with hypovolemia
- Maintenance of normovolemia patients with ongoing fluid losses, e.g. surgical blood loss.

General Principles
- Crystalloids replacement fluids should be infused in a volume at least 3 times the volume lost in order to correct the hypovolemia

- Colloid solution should be infused inva volume equal to the blood volume deficit
- All colloid solutions (albumin, dextrin's, gelatins, hydroxyethyl starch solutions) are replacement fluids. However, they have not show to be superior to crystalloids in resuscitation except that they are needed in a lower volume as compared to crystalloids
- Plain water should not be infused IV as it will cause hemolysis due to hypotonicity.

Other routes of administrating fluids: intraosseous, oral, rectal

---

Note: One of the many problems in the resuscitation of the shocked patient is how to gain access to the circulation to provide fluids or drugs. Since the 1830s fluids have been administered intravenously. Intravenous access is not always possible in the very shocked patient. An alternative, used in the First World War, was the rectal route. This has rarely been used on a large scale since. Just before the outbreak of the Second World War a chance discovery resulted in the development of intraosseous infusions of fluid and drugs. From its discovery it was used in adults and children. For many years it seemed to be ignored in adult resuscitation, but there are now signs of renewed interest in the technique.

J Accid Emerg Med 2000; 17:136–137

Crystalloids Solutions

- Contain a similar concentration of sodium as that of plasma
- Contain the capillary membrane from the vascular compartment to the interstial compartment
- Are distributed to the whole extracellular compartment
- Usually only a quarter of volume of crystalloid infused remains in the vascular compartment, e.g. compound sodium lactate (Ringers lactate), normal saline.

Colloid Solution

larger molecular weight compared to crystalloids

- Initially tend to remain in the intravascular space
- Mimic plasma proteins thereby maintaining or raising the colloid osmotic pressure of the blood
- Provide longer duration of plasma volume expansion than crystalloid solution
- Required in smaller volume.

Maintenance fluids: Fluids use to replace normal physiological loses through the skin, lung, faces and urine.

Volume needed varies with pyrexia, increased loss, etc. these are composed mainly of water in dextrose solution may contain some electrolytes.

All maintenance fluids are crystalloids e.g. 5% dextrose, 4% dextrose in sodium chloride 0.18%.

Crystalloid Solution

Normal Saline (Sodium Chloride 0.9%)

Indications: Replacement of blood volume and other extracellular fluid lost

Precaution: Caution in situation when local edema may aggravate pathology may precipitate volume overload

Contraindications: Do not use patient with establishes renal failure

Side effect: Tissue edema can develop with a large dose

Dosage: At least 3 time the volume of blood lost
NaCl 0.9%, Na 154 mmol/L, 4.5 gm sodium and 154 mmol/L of chloride.

Balance Salt Solutions

Ringers lactate, Hartmann's solution.

Indications: Replacement of blood volume and other extracellular fluid losses

Precautions: Caution in situations when local edema may aggravate pathology, may precipitate volume overload

Contraindications: Do not use in patient with established renal failure

Side effect: Tissue edema can develop with a large dose

Dosage: At least 3 times the volume of blood lost.

Ringer's Lactate (Compound Sodium Lactate)

Each 100 mL has: lactic acid—0.24 mL = 0.32 gm sodium lactate; NaCl—0.6 gm; KCl—0.04 gm; CaCl—0.027 gm

Na—131 mmol/L; K—5 mmol/L:Ca—2 mmol/L ; Cl—111 mmol/L; HCO_3—29 mmol/L

Isolyte M

Each 100 mL has dextrose anhyhdrous—5 mg, KCl—0.15 gm potassium phosphate—0.13 gm

Sodium acetate—0.28 gm, NaCl—0.091 gm, sodium metabisulfite—0.21 gm.

Na—39 mEql/L; K^+—35 mEq/L; Acetate—21 mEq/L; PO_4—15 mEq/L

Bisulphite: 2 mEq/L:Cl^- due to HCL: 11 mEq/L.

Dextrose and Electrolyte Solution

Example 4.3 % dextrose in sodium chloride 0.18% 2.5% dextrose in sodium chloride 0.45%

Indications: Generally to be used as maintenance fluids, but if necessary those containing higher concentrations of sodium can be used as maintenance fluids.

Each 100 mL has dextrose—5 gm: NaCl—0.9 gm

Na^+—154 mmol/L. Cl^-—154 mmol/L.

Amidst this mild controversy, it is worthy to note that 5% dextrose is not a crystalloid but *merely water rendered isotonic* by the edition of glucose. When infused 5% dextrose equilibrates not only with interstitial space but with much larger intercellular space making it quite useless as a resuscitation. On the other had, 5% dextrose is the ideal fluid for correction of cellular dehydration (Table 44.6).

Colloid solutions:

Plasma derived: Plasma, albumin, fresh frozen plasma

Table 44.6: Effect of adding 1 liter

Solution	Change in ECF	Change in ICF
D5%	333 mL	667 mL
2/3 and 1/3	555 mL	444 mL
½ normal saline	667 mL	333 mL
Normal saline	1000 mL	0 mL
Ringer's lactate	990 mL	100 mL

Albumin – 5% with 50 mg/mL of albumin.
20% with 200 mg/mL of albumin
25% with 250 mg/mL of albumin.

Indications

Replacement fluid: 5% albumin Treatment in hypo-protinemic patients: 20% albumin

Precautions

Administration of 20% albumin may cause acute expansion of intravascular volume with risk of pulmonary edema.

Not to be used for IV nutrition-expensive and poor source of essential amino acids.

No compatibility testing needed.

Synthetic Colloidal Solutions

- *Gelatins*: Hemaccel, gelofusine
- *Indications*: replacement of blood volume
- *Precautions*: can precipitate CCF
- *Cotraindications*: in established renal failure
- *Side effects*: Minor/rarely major allergic reactions due to histamine release. Transient increase in bleeding time may occur.

Hydroxyethyl Starch (Hetastarch or HES)

Available as a 6% solution of hydroxyethyl starch in 0.9% saline and a 10% hypertonic infusion.

Replacement of Blood Volume

Precautions: Coagulation defect can occur.

Can precipitate volume overload and cause heart failure.

Table 44.7: Advantages and disadvantages of crystalloids and colloids		
	Advantages	*Disadvantages*
Crystalloids	Low cost	Short duration
	Availability	May cause edema
		Large volumes
Colloids	Longer duration of action	No evidence that they are clinically more effective
	Lesser volume needed	Higher cost

Contraindications

- Not to be used in patients with preexisting disorders of coagulation
- Not to be used in renal failure.

Side effects—minor allergic reactions, transient increase in bleeding time, may raise serum amylase levels

Dose—Adults—up to 20 mL kg/day. Total dose not to exceed to 1500 mL. No data available for use in children.

Rate of infusion—0.33 mL/kg/min in hemorrhagic shock. In septic and burn patient lower rate of infusion is indicated.

Dextrans

These are inert glucose polymers.

Available in various molecular sizes:
- Dextran 40 and dextran 70

Dextran 40 is not used nowadays. Dextran 70 is used for small volume replacements. Available either in the saline (0.9%) or in the 5% dextrose forms.

Adverse Reactions

- Affects the coagulation system
- Large infusions (more than 20 mL/kg) can reduce factor VIII levels
- Interferes with the blood cross-matching
- Anaphylactic reactions (1:2000 infusions)
- Serious reaction (1:6000 infusions)

Colloid (vs) Crystalloid—the better one

Systematic reviews of available comparison of colloid vs. crystalloid suggest increased mortality (4%) associated with colloid use. Other reviews suggest that crystalloid may be superior in multiple trauma patients. Colloids are not shown to be superior to crystalloids in resuscitation except that they are needed in a lower volume as compared to crystalloids (Table 44.7).

A Routine Maintenance IV Fluid Regime

The normal daily requirement for water and electrolytes must met. In healthy adult, administration of 2000–3000 mL of water daily to produce a urine volume of 1000–1500 mL/day. Aim is to maintain urine output at rate of 0.5–1 mL/kg/hr (Table 44.8).

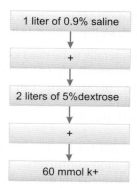

Dextrose supplementation of carbohydrate in the form of dextrose (100–150 g/day or 400–600 kcal/day) is required to minimize protein catabolism and prevent ketosis.

Postoperative Fluid Regimen

Water and electrolyte composition in surgical patients.

Surgical patients require replacement of intra-/ extravascular losses secondary to wound or burn edema, ascites and gastrointestinal secretions.

Table 44.8: Normal 24 hours requirements		
Intravenous fluid	*Additive*	*Duration*
500 mL 0.9% NaCl	20 mmol KCl	4 hours
500 mL 5% dextrose	–	4 hours
500 mL 5% dextrose	20 mmol KCl	4 hours
500 mL 0.9% NaCl	–	4 hours
500 mL 5% dextrose	20 mmol KCl	4 hours
500 mL 5% dextrose	–	4 hours

Wound, burn edema, and ascetic fluid- protein rich, contain electrolytes in concentrations similar to plasma.

Substantial loss of gastrointestinal fluids require more accurate replacement of electrolytes (potassium, magnesium and phosphate). Small losses are to be replaced by isotonic saline only.

Replacement of Fluid Losses During Surgical Procedures

For procedure involving
- Minimal trauma—4 mL/kg/hr
- Moderate trauma—6 mL/kg/hr
- Extreme trauma—8 mL/kg/hr.

First 24 Hours

- There is an increased secretion of aldosterone and anti-diuretic fluid
- Conservation of sodium and water occurs hence 2 liters of 5% dextrose is sufficient. (operative blood loss is to be considered and replaced, fluid loss to be estimated and replaced).

During the Second and Subsequent 24 Hours

2 liters of 5% dextrose and 1 liter of isotonic saline per 24 hours taking into account
- Insensible losses max of 900–1000 mL/day
- 1 liter to replace urine volume 5% dextrose

Any GI losses are to be replaced by isotonic salt solutions.

Additional replacement of distributional and sequestration losses of extra cellular fluid should be done by isotonic saline.

On the 3rd postoperative day and thereafter 40–60 mmol of potassium is added per 24 hr. with isotonic 4.3% dextrose and 0.18% isotonic saline.

Clinical Evaluation of Salt and Water Depletion

Mild (< 2 liters in adult)
- Thirst
- Concentrated urine

Moderate (2–3 liters in adult)
- As above plus:
- Dizziness, weakness
- Oliguria (<400 mL/day)
- Postural hypotension > 200 mm Hg systolic
- Low JVP.

Severe (>3 liters in adult)

As above plus

Confusion, stupor, systolic BP <10 mm Hg, Tachycardia (not in elderly), low pulse volume, cold extremities, poor capillary return, reduced skin turgor (doughy).

Replacement of Volume Deficit

Mild: 0.9% saline 1 liter IV 6–12 hourly.

Moderate
- 0.9% saline 1 liter IV over 2–4 hours
- 0.9% saline 1–2 liters IV 6–8 hourly.

Severe
- Gelatin/starch/plasma protein solution 0.5 liter over 1–3 hours
- 0.9% saline 2 liters IV over 4–6 hours
- 0.9% saline 1 liter 6 hourly until replaced.

Surgical Nutrition

45

INTRODUCTION

Nutrition in its basic sense refers to the intake of nourishment especially the fluids and the type of diet a patient need to survive, Following oral and maxilla facial surgery procedures nutrient needs are increased in order to facilitate healing. For oral and maxillofacial surgery, this may be particularly challenging for several reasons. The presence of surgical incisions around the mouth and postoperative swelling may make it more difficult to chew and swallow normally. Surgery in mouth jaw such as fracture reduction, dental implants, biopsies, oncology surgical procedure, orthognathic surgery or similar procedure may require inclusion of carbonated beverages, drinking clear fluids or Ryles tube feeding. Earlier orthognathic or jaw fracture patients had their jaw immobilized to promote healing. Of course now with the advent of rigid fixation this can be avoided to a certain extent, For those who require IMF should be advised liquid diet till IMF are released.

- Dietary requirements can be altered by the stress of injury and surgery, which will have a profound effect on the postsurgical recovery and repair of oral and maxillofacial surgery patient
- Maintenance of good nutrition is essential for both the comprehensive management and prevention of disease. Many a debilitating complications can be prevented by attention to their nutritional status.

Importance of Satisfactory Nutritional Status

- Significant correlation between preoperative malnutrition and postoperative morbidity Early and late postoperative complications
- Wound dehiscences, immune responses, infections or sepsis and other processes of recovering period
- Risk to patient's life in addition to increase in hospital stay time and costs.

Goals of nutrition therapy
Provide energy and protein sufficient to meet estimated nutrient needs and aid in wound healing
Provide adequate fluids to maintain optimal patient hydration
Provide nutrient intake in a practical, tolerable and efficacious form
Maintain an acceptable quality of life

Nutritional support team
- Head and neck surgeon
- Nutritionist
- Nurse
- Dietician
- Pharmacist.

Causes of nutritional imbalance
- Decreased nutrient intake
- Increased nutrient losses
- Increased nutritional requirements
- Increased or inefficient energy metabolism

- Post tumor nutrient substrate competition
- Deranged nutrient substrate metabolism
- No adaptation to starvation in sepsis.

Medical conditions that could predispose to malnutrition
- Liver disease
- Renal failure
- Inflammatory bowel disease
- Neoplastic disease, chemotherapy
- AIDS.

Effects of nutritional imbalance
Delayed gastric emptying
Prolonged ileus
Poor wound healing manifests as wound dehiscence
Delayed callus formation
Disordered coagulation
Decreased enzyme synthesis
Impaired oxidative metabolism of drugs by liver
Immunological depression which increases susceptibility to infection
Altered taste
Dysphagia
Decreased tolerance to radiotherapy and chemotherapy
Mental apathy

Indications for nutritional support
Maxillofacial trauma
Multiple trauma
Burns
Malignant diseases
Anorexia

Nutrients—
   6 basic nutrients required:
- Carbohydrates, fats, proteins, minerals and vitamins

Caloric value of nutrients—
- Carbohydrates   4 cal/g
- Proteins   4 cal/g
- Fat   9 cal/g

Factors associated with operative risk—
- Research is being done to predict surgical patients at risk for sepsis or death
- Prognostic nutrition index (PNI) has been developed which identifies patients who would suffer from complication, sepsis or mortality
- A positive correlation between anergy and risk of sepsis and death has been established
- Low serum albumin levels correlated with both anergy and increased risk of sepsis and mortality
- Anergy is associated with malnutrition, sepsis, and shock in hospital patients.

Nutritional Assessment

Body weight

$$\% \text{ weight loss} = \frac{\text{usual weight} - \text{present weight}}{\text{usual weight}}$$
$$> 25\% \text{ weight loss} = \text{severe}$$
$$> 33\% \text{ weight loss} = \text{fatal}$$

Physical examination
- Oral—cheliosis, glossitis, mucosal atrophy
- Abdomen—liver enlargement abdominal mass
- Extremities—muscle size and strength edema
- Integument—skin texture rash, hair quality nail deformities.

Anthropometric measurements
- Used to assess the fat and protein stores by comparing to normal values for that age and gender
- Tricep skin fold measurement, determined with calipers, is used to evaluate body fat
- Upper arm circumference is used to evaluate protein stored in skeletal muscle.

Laboratory evaluation serum albumin
- Normal   3. 5 – 4. 5 g/dL
- Moderate malnutrtion   2. 5 – 3. 5 g/dL
- Severe malnutrition   < 2. 5 g/dL

Total lymphocyte count
- Normal   1500 – 2000/mm^3
- Moderate malnutrition   1000 – 1500/mm^3
- Severe malnutrition   < 1000/mm

Creatinine height index
Used to estimate degree of protein loss
CHI = 24 hr urine creatinine excretion normal creatinine excretion for that height

Other plasma proteins transferrin
- Normal   200 mg/dL
- Mild malnutrition   < 175 mg/dL
- Severe malnutrition   < 147 mg/dL
- Retinol binding protein   < 40 g/dL
- Thyroxine binding protein   < 200 g/dL

Immunologic testing
- Skin testing that evaluates cell mediated immunity
- Anergy
- Normal daily requirements

Protein requirements
Protein balance: The body alters protein stores to compensate for changes in activity and levels of physical stress.

Daily protein requirements
Adult male: 0.8 g/kg weight/day
Children: 2–2.5 g/kg weight/day
Acute illness: 1.5 g/kg weight/day
Severely stressed patients: 2–3 g/kg weight/day

Nitrogen balance studies
- Positive nitrogen balance signifies that more nitrogen is being taken in than excreted
- Negative nitrogen balance indicates losses exceed intake and catabolic state prevails
- 1g of nitrogen = 6.25 g of protein
- Calculation of nitrogen balance

$$\text{N balance} = \frac{\text{Protein intake(g)} - (24 \text{ h urea})}{6.25}$$

- Calorie : Nitrogen ratio
The energy required for protein synthesis is expressed by a ratio of $\frac{150-200}{1}$

This means that ideal diets should have 150–200 nonprotein calories per gram of nitrogen.

This ratio increases when the body is stressed. It can be high as 400:1 in uremic patients.

Caloric requirements
- The daily requirement for calories varies with the activity level of the individual.
  - Under normal circumstances the average healthy adult requires about 2500 cal/day.
  - Basal resting level: 1500 cal/day
  - Heavy exercise: 4000–5000 cal/day
- Surgical patients have greater caloric needs than nonstressed patients. At rest these patients require 4000–5000 cal/day
- The daily caloric requirement may be determined by a variety of methods
- The patient's body weight may be used to estimate the daily caloric requirement
- Adult: 21–30 cal/kg weight/day
- A more accurate method to ascertain the daily caloric requirement involves determining the basal energy expenditure. The Harris-Benedict equation may be used to estimate this value
- Basal energy expenditure for
  Men = 13.7(weight) + 5(height) – 5(age) + 666
  Women = 10(weight) + 1.8(height) – 5(age) + 655

Recent trends
Determining the rate of muscle breakdown (urinary creatinine excretion and 3-methyl histidine excretion):
Body potassium and nitrogen assessment is used to measure the absolute size of body cell mass
^{14}C Leucine assessment measures protein synthesis rate

Hospital diets for surgical patients
Hospital diets are available in various consistencies, compositions and caloric contents
A balanced diet contains • Carbohydrate: 50–70% • Fats: 20–30% • Protein: 10–20%

NUTRITION AND MAXILLOFACIAL CANCER

- Malnutrition is commonly encountered in cancer patients
- The etiology is multifactorial: ranging from diminished dietary intake to metabolic changes induced by systemic inflammatory responses
- Cancer patients often suffer from a substantial loss in weight and energy as a result of changes in appetite and metabolism. It is a known fact that appetite in cancer patients is adversely affected as a direct consequence of the disease and/or its treatments. Cancer patients are therefore vulnerable to malnutrition and may be predisposed to a poor health and quality of life
- There are many causes of malnourishment, including pain, depression and the side effects of chemotherapy or radiation treatment. The simplest and most obvious cause is insufficient dietary intake, usually caused by loss of appetite. Loss of appetite is very common among cancer patients, whether caused by emotional depression or difficulty to chew. One cause that is sometimes overlooked is problems with the swallowing mechanism. This is extremely common in head and neck cancers
- Patients suffering from cancer of head and neck are at risk of significant nutritional depletion due to several factors. These patients have a lifestyle in which excessive alcohol consumption; smoking and poor dietary habits are notable features. The location of the tumor often leads to significant odynophagia and dysphagia resulting in a reduced dietary intake. Extensive cancers in the head and neck area may lead to anorexia secondary to chronic pain, anxiety and chemical mediators
- Malnutrition results in devastating quality-of-life, economic, and survival issues. The malnourished cancer patient responds poorly to therapeutic interventions, such as chemotherapy, radiotherapy and surgery, with increased morbidity and mortality compared with well-nourished patients

- Nutritional assessment of such patents is therefore a must to identify malnourished patients and thus be able to provide them with adequate and appropriate nutritional supplementation for better quality of life and overall success of the treatment
- The ultimate goal of nutritional assessment should be to identify patients who have a pre-existing malnutrition, or are at risk of developing malnutrition during therapy, and would benefit from nutritional intervention. The administration of adequate nutritional support before cancer therapy has been shown to significantly decrease the incidence of therapy related complications
- Because both the timing and method of administration of nutritional support are critical management should be coordinated through a multidisciplinary nutritional support team to maximize appropriate patient care
- Information should be obtained regarding the specific type and stage of the patient's tumor, the anticipated method and magnitude of oncologic therapy and the estimated extent and duration of metabolic stress and nutritional disability
- The nutritional assessment must begin before the initiation of oncologic therapy and continue throughout the course of treatment, with frequent reassessment to prevent complications
- In addition to the metabolic nutritional deficiencies that accompany malignant neoplasms in general, the patient with a head and neck tumor may also suffer from distortion of normal anatomic nutritional pathways; poor nutrient intake due to dysphagia, odynophagia or anorexia and other deficiencies associated with a history of smoking and alcohol use. Also, oncologic treatment, consisting of surgery, radiation therapy, and chemotherapy will serve to increase metabolic demand while further impairing adequate oral nutritional intake.

Following minor surgical procedures, daily caloric requirements in healthy active adults increase from 25% to 30%, while requirements following major surgeries increase from 50% to 60%; therefore the potential for nutritional deficiencies is compounded during the period of convalescence.

- It is essential that underlying causes or the nutritional problems that occur or are likely to occur are understood by the physician and the dietician so that a rational and effective nutritional support program may be developed for the individual patient
- The nutritional problem in head and neck cancer patients does not only arise from decreased intake but is further complicated due to presence of cachexia
- Cancer cachexia is a complex syndrome that includes host tissue wasting, anorexia, asthenia, and abnormal host intermediary metabolism. It is present in approximately 50% of cancer patients during treatment and nearly 100% of treated cancer patients at death. Cachexia has a detrimental impact on cancer therapy. The central problem of cancer cachexia is that energy balance is not maintained, and the host has a relative hypophagia which results in host tissue wasting. The tumor by its nature and obligate growth can continue to consume glucose, amino acids, and lipids at the expense of the host. This produces abnormal host intermediary metabolism including elevated glucose production and recycling, decreased muscle protein synthesis, and increased muscle and fat breakdown. The exact mechanisms of cancer cachexia have been only partially elucidated. The identification of signal molecules like cachectin which mediate these changes may be on the horizon
- Nutritional support can reverse some of the derangements seen with cachexia, and there is evidence that functional lean body mass or body cell mass can be restored in some (but not all) patients. However, nutritional support has improved operative mortality and morbidity in cachectic cancer patients undergoing major

surgical procedures. Optimum host nutritional support appears to be dependent on high insulin concentrations. Insulin and exercise may be methods to preserve host lean tissue and feed the host rather than the tumor.

Altered composition diets (Table 45.1)
- There are many types of diets and their compositions are changed to help manage various disease processes
- Diabetic diet
- Sodium restricted diet
- Protein controlled and potassium restricted diets
- Fat modified diet
- High fiber and low fiber diets

FEEDING METHODS ENTERAL NUTRITION

- There are multiple indications for the use of enteral feedings
- Forced enteral feedings may be indicated following mandibular or maxillofacial trauma preferred over the parenteral route
- Postoperative enteral nutritional support is safer and less expensive than parenteral nutrition and has the added benefit of preserving gut functionality

Advantages
Decreased infection
Decreased metabolic/ catheter related complications
It directly provides gut mucosa with the substrate essential for maintaining gut epithelial integrity
Maintains normal intestinal immune function
Avoids gut atrophy and amino acid transport defects
Decreased septic morbidity and increased survival rate following enteral administration.

Enteral Nutrition in Trauma Patients
- Conventional management deferred nutritional support in trauma patients till about 5 days following trauma after which time, the failure to tolerate an oral diet was considered an indication to institute TPN

	Table 45.1: Altered consistency diets			
Consistency	Purpose	Use	Adequacy	Comments
Clear liquid	Short term (1–2 days) Supplies fluid and some energy (600 kcal/d) in a form that requires minimal digestion	Initial feed after surgery. IV feed to relieve thirst and hydrate	Falls short of nutrients. If this diet is to continue beyond 3–5 days, nutritional supplementation on needed	Does not meet required dietary allowances except vitamin C Usually provides 10 g protein and 300 cal
Full liquid	Supply fluid and meet energy and nutrients more adequately	Transition between clear and solid diet after surgery. Useful for patients who are unable to chew after head and neck surgery	Inadequate in niacin, folacin, iron. Adequacy can be improved by high protein, high calorie supplements/ multivitamins supplements	More complete than former. Protein 76 g Fat 91g Carbohydrartes 312 g Calories 2300
Soft diet	Food which can be swallowed with little or no chewing	Acutely ill patients with difficulty in chewing/swallowing. Too ill to tolerate usual diet. Head and neck surgery patients	Adequate in nutrients	Protein 100 g Fat 60 g Carbohydrates 290 g Calories 2080 kcal Available in pureed/ blended form

- However recent clinical trials have suggested that an early enteral nutrition is associated with less septic complication than intravenous alimentation
- Traumatic injuries result in relative immunosuppression, manifested by neutrophil dysfunction, decreased lymphocyte reactivity and decreased antibody activity
- Enteral formulas have hence been modified to enhance the patient's immune system. One such formula uses arginine, n-3 fatty acid and nucleotide which has improved the nitrogen balance and has resulted in reduced rise in acute phase reactants.

Routes of Enteral Administeration

- When enteral administration of nutritional support is indicated, the most appropriate route of administration must be chosen

- Factors to be considered are:
  - Anticipated duration of nutritional supplementation
  - Patient's risk of aspiration
- Trauma patients who are likely to require nutritional support for more than 4 weeks are best served with a permanent gastrostomy or jejunostomy feeding tube
- When the nutrition supplementation is <4 weeks, nasoenteric feeding tube is used (Table 45.2)
- Tube feeding methods position of the tip should be radiographically documented prior to feeding
- With hyperosmolar formulas, feedings are started with a dilute, 1/4 strength solution. Then concentration is gradually increased every 2–3 days
- Initial rate of feeding should be 1/2 of the final rate to permit the GI tract to accommodate

Table 45.2: Nasoenteric feeding tubes

Type of tube	Clinical uses	Problems
Nasogastric	• Short-term usage (few weeks) • Placement can be intermittent • Normal gastric emptying required • Bolus feeds/continuous drip	• Irritation of nasopharynx (bleeding may occur) • Aspiration pneumonia
Nasoduodenal/nasojejunal	• Short-term usage • Used when gastric emptying is impaired	• Passing tube through pylorus • Tubes stiffen with time

Table 45.3: Types of enteral feeding formula

Formula	Indications	Tube of Choice	Comment
Blenderized	Normal digestion and absorption required Used with gastrostomy tubes	Large bore (12–18 bore)	Lowest cost 2 L daily Bolous feed
Polymeric	Normal digestion and absorption required	Small bore (8–10) bore	>2 L needed Bolous/pump feed
Monomeric	Transitional feeding from parenteral to enteral	Small bore (5–6) bore	Higher cost Pump feed 3 L/day
Disease related	Stress, trauma, hepatic or renal failure	Small bore (5–6n bore)	Highest cost Pump feed >2 L/day
Modular	Specific metabolic abnormalities	Varies, depending on viscosity	Bolous/pump feed

to the osmotic load. The diet is advanced by first increasing the volume and then the concentration (Table 45.3)

- Tube feedings may be administered by 3 basic methods:
  - Continuous drip
  - Bolus feeding
  - Timed feeding
- The continuous drip technique is the most preferred method

Complications of nasoenteric feeding tube

- Tube placement
  - Traumatic insertion
  - Hemorrhage
  - Pulmonary intubation
  - Aspiration pneumonia
  - Pneumothorax
  - Inadvertent placement in trachea/esophagus

- Tube maintenance
  - Patient discomfort
  - Otitis media
  - Pharyngitis
  - Rupture of esophegal varices
  - Nasal erosion/necrosis
  - Esophagitis
  - Diarrhea
  - Dehydration
  - Hypernatremia/azotemia.

Parenteral Nutrition

- The development of parenteral nutritional support in the late 1960s revolutionized care of the surgical patients, particularly those with permanent inability to obtain adequate enteral nourishment

- In general parenteral nutrition should be employed only when the gastrointestinal tract cannot be utilized
- In itself maxillofacial trauma is rarely an indication for parenteral nutrition
- Parenteral nutrition is of two types:
  - Total parenteral nutrition (TPN)
  - Peripheral parenteral nutrition (PPN)

Composition of parenteral nutrition formulas
Carbohydrate—50% and 10% dextrose in water
Lipid—20% and 10% emulsions via a piggyback in central/peripheral line
Essential vitamins and trace elements
Vitamin K—5–10 mg/week
Amino acids
Electrolytes
Regular insulin
Iron is not routinely added as it increases invading organism virulence

Total Parenteral Nutrition

- TPN provides total caloric and protein requirements but requires administration into a central vein due to its high osmolarity
- May be administered via short-term/long-term central venous access
- Hospitalized trauma patients receive TPN via catheters introduced percutaneously
- Catheter tips positioned in the SVC
- Central venous access via the IJV/ subclavian vein
- Peripherally introduced central catheters provides access via cephalic/ basilic veins.

Modification of TPN
Protein intake in renal failure patients should be restricted. Restricted amount of potassium, magnesium and phosphorus in TPN formulas. Metabolic acidosis countered by addition of acetate in formula
TPN solutions rich in BCAA and poor in AAA should be administered to patients with hepatic failure.

Peripheral Parenteral Nutrition

- PPN administered through peripheral intravenous line with osmolarity maintained below 900 mOsm/L to avoid phlebitis
- With low osmolarity solutions large volume of infusions are required to supplement them with protein and nonprotein calories
- Hence PPN is administered as partial parenteral nutrition (not supplying all macronutrients)
- Used along with TPN
- PPN administered no more than 7–10 days before TPN administration.

Administration of Parenteral Nutrition

- Confirm central line placement radiographically before infusing alimentation
- The starting infusion rate should be 50–100 mL/h. Rate is slowly increased in 25 mL/h increments everyday. Final rate and volume infused determined by the amount of calorie required.

Recent trends
Sepsis and multiorgan failure remain a major source of morbidity and mortality in critically ill trauma pts. To improve this clinical outcome, administration of amino acids rich in BCAA may improve the nitrogen balance in septic pts and reduce muscle protein catabolism and provides rapid repletion of visceral and muscle protein
Administration of gut specific fuels (glutamine) in parenteral solutions prevents postoperative gut mucosal atrophy and improves immune function
Addition of fatty acids also has a positive effect on the colon, preventing TPN associated colon atrophy

- Patient should be carefully monitored
- Hyperglycemia may occur after parenteral administration.
  Preoperative patients on TPN should have the rate reduced to 1/3–1/2 the usual rate during GA and surgery to prevent stress hyperglycemia.

Monitoring Patient on TPN

Daily
- Body weight
- Fluid balance
- CBC, urea and electrolytes
- Blood glucose
- Urine and plasma osmolality
- Acid base status
- Electrolyte and H_2 analysis

Week
- Serum Ca, Mg, PO_4
- Plasma patterns
- LFT
- Clotting studies

10 days
- Serum B_{12}, folate, iron, lactate and triglycerides
- Trace elements

Complications of TPN

- Technical complications
  - Air embolus
  - Arterial laceration
  - Arteriovenous fistula
  - Brachial plexus injury
  - Cardiac perforation
  - Catheter embolism
  - Catheter malposition
  - Hemothorax
  - Pneumothorax
  - Subclavian vein thrombosis
  - Thoracic duct injury
  - Thromboembolism
  - Venous laceration.
- Infectious
  - Catheter based bacteremia
  - Catheter colonization
  - Exit site infection/colonization.
- Metabolic
  - Azotemia
  - Essential fatty acid deficiency
  - Fluid overload
  - Hyperchloremic metabolic acidosis

- Hypercalcemia
- Hyperglycemia
- Hyperkalemia
- Hypermagnesemia
- Hypernatremia
- Hyperphosphatemia
- Hypocalcemia
- Hypokalemia
- Hypomagnesemia
- Hyponatremia
- Hypophosphatemia
- Intrinsic liver disease
- Metabolic bone disease
- Trace element deficiency
- Ventilatory failure
- Vitamin deficiency.

POSTOPERATIVE NUTRITION REQUIREMENTS

Infections
- If the patient is septic and dehydrated, hospitalization may be required to replace body fluids and electrolytes
- Infection increases nutrient requirement for protein, pyridoxine and pantothenic acid
- Fever increases the BMR and basal water requirements because of hyperventilation, sweating
- Liquids are easily tolerated than solids
- A soft regular diet may be resumed once the infection subsides
- Use of antibiotics may cause diarrohea which increases nutritional requirements.

Resection of a cyst/benign tumor
- A liquid diet is recommended for 2–3 days
- A commercial dietary supplement/blended diet may be used
- Diet may be advanced from liquid to soft consistency in 2–7 days, depending on the size of the wound.

Bone grafting
Two surgical wounds to repair—
- Adequate amount of proteins, calories, ascorbic acid, vitamin A and D and calcium required.

Resection of malignant leisons
Cancer increases the energy requirements of the patient while at the same time causing anorexia and dysgeusia, resulting in weight loss and severe malnutrition
Nutritional needs of the patient are influenced by the cancer as well as the treatment itself
Cancer and surgery increase the requirements of proteins and calories
Sufficient amounts of vitamin A and C and zinc are also required for wound healing
Nutritional care must be individualized for each patient
A liquid/ blended diet or a commercial supplement is used initially, then a soft diet can be eaten.

- Patient will usually be on a liquid diet during the entire postsurgical period due to immobilization of the jaw.

Jaw immobilization—
- Nutrition in the liquid form

- Full liquid foods/commercial liquid supplement/blended diet
- Liquid vitamin and mineral supplements to be given. The most complete liquid vitamin is MVI 12

Diabetic patients—
- In addition to nutritional concerns, it is essential to prevent hypo/hyperglycemia
- When the patient is expected to omit a meal for surgery, the insulin dosage and the type needs to be adjusted and a carbohydrate source is supplied as intravenous glucose in the morning of the surgery
- Regular insulin, every 6 hours is recommended before, during and after surgery. Dosage is usually reduced because total calories provided will be less then usual
- Glucose is given intravenously to supply 50 g of carbohydrate every 6 hr (200 g /24 hr), during surgery and when the patient is still unable to digest food (500 mL of 10% glucose)
- When the patient is able to eat, a full liquid diet, blended or soft diet can be taken according to usual caloric intake of the patient. Usual kind and amount of insulin can be reinstituted
- Those on oral hypoglycemic drugs or controlled diet only, may require a similar regimen of insulin and intravenous glucose during surgery.

Power-driven Instruments Useful in Maxillofacial Surgery

46

INTRODUCTION

Maxillofacial surgery has been redefined by the presence of many powered instruments, technological tools that in many ways have revolutionized the delicacy, precision and accuracy of the various operations performed with the use of electrosurgical instruments.

Power-driven instruments like rotary and high speed stryker precision cutting instruements, micromotor of different speed, special surgical saw, implant precision micromotor, clinical surgical micromotor and coagulation instruments, electrosurgery laser, harmonic scalpel, etc.

ELECTROSURGERY

- Electrosurgery is the application of a high-frequency electric current to biological tissue as a means to cut, coagulate, desiccate, or fulgurate tissue
- Its benefits include the ability to make precise cuts with limited blood loss. Electrosurgical devices are frequently used during surgical operations helping to prevent blood loss in hospital operating rooms or in outpatient procedures
- Electrosurgery is often incorrectly termed electrocautery, which is a separate technique
- Electrocautery is a closed circuit DC device in which current is passed through an exposed wire offering resistance to the current. The resistance causes some of the electric energy

to be dissipated as heat, increasing the temperature of the wire, which then heats tissue. In true electrocautery, no current passes through the patient
- In electrosurgical procedures, the tissue is heated by an electric current. Although electrical devices may be used for the cauterization of tissue in some applications, electrosurgery is usually used to refer to a quite different method than electrocautery. The latter uses heat conduction from a probe heated by a direct current whereas electrosurgery uses alternating current to directly heat the tissue itself.

Principles of Electrosurgery

- Electrosurgery uses high frequency electro-magnetic waves to produce a localized heating of tissues leading to localized tissue destruction
- The ability to pass high frequency current through the human body without causing excess damage makes electrosurgery possible.

Tissue Heating by Electric Current

- When voltage is applied across the material it produces electric field, which exerts force on charged particles. A flow of free charge carriers—electrons and ions—is called electric current. In metals and semiconductors the charge carriers are primarily electrons, whereas in liquids the charge is carried predominantly by ions. Electrical conduction in biological tissues is primarily due to the conductivity of the interstitial fluids and thus is predominantly ionic. Transition between the electronic and ionic conduction is governed by electrochemical processes at the electrode–electrolyte interface

- Electric current of a constant polarity is referred to as direct current (DC). A current of alternating polarity is referred to as alternating current (AC). Its frequency is measured in cycles/second or Hertz (Hz)
- Current flowing through a resistor causes the generation of Joule heating. In other words, the resistance of the tissue converts the electric energy of the voltage source into heat (thermal energy), which causes the tissue temperature to rise.

Electrical stimulation of neural and muscle cells

- Neural and muscle cells are electrically-excitable, i.e. they can be stimulated by electric current. In human patients such stimulation may cause acute pain, muscle spasms, and even cardiac arrest. Sensitivity of the nerve and muscle cells to electric field is due to the voltage-gated ion channels present in their cell membranes
- To minimize the effects of muscle and neural stimulation, electrosurgical equipment typically operates in the radio frequency (RF) range of 100 kHz to 5 MHz
- Operation at higher frequencies also helps minimizing the amount of hydrogen and oxygen generated by electrolysis of water. This is especially important consideration for applications in liquid medium in closed compartments, where generation of gas bubbles may interfere with the procedure. For example, bubbles produced during an operation inside an eye, may obscure a field of view.

Monopolar Circuits (Figs 46.1)

- The components of monopolar circuit consist of four primary parts: The electrosurgical generator, the active electrode, the patient and the return electrode

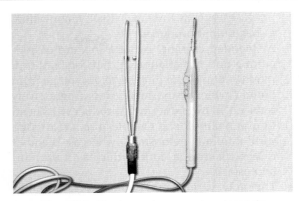

Fig. 46.1: Bipolar and monopolar electrode

- If the patient is not connected either to negative terminal or to ground, no current would flow, as there would be no way to complete the circuit
- In fact, the term monopolar circuit is incorrect, as there are in fact two poles—the active and return electrodes
- However, monopolar electrosurgery is distinguished from bipolar electrosurgery, in which both electrodes are under the surgeon's direct control.

Bipolar Circuits (Fig. 46.1)

- In this system, the active and return electrodes are in the same surgical instrument
- This allows heating of only a discrete amount of tissue.

Tissue Effects Change as the Waveform Modifies

- Electrosurgical generators are able to produce a variety of electrical waveforms. As waveforms change, so will the corresponding tissue effects. Using a constant waveform, like "cut," the surgeon is able to vaporize or cut tissue. This waveform produces heat very rapidly
- Using an intermittent waveform, like "coagulation," causes the generator to modify the waveform so that the duty cycle (on time) is reduced. This interrupted waveform will

produce less heat. Instead of tissue vaporization, a coagulum is produced

- A "blended current" is not a mixture of both cutting and coagulation current but rather a modification of the duty cycle. As you go from Blend 1 to Blend 3 the duty cycle is progressively reduced. A lower duty cycle produces less heat. Consequently, Blend 1 is able to vaporize tissue with minimal hemostasis whereas Blend 3 is less effective at cutting but has maximum hemostasis

- The only variable that determines whether one waveform vaporizes tissue and another produces a coagulum is the rate at which heat is produced. High heat produced rapidly causes vaporization. Low heat produced more slowly creates a coagulum. Any one of the five waveforms can accomplish both tasks by modifying the variables that impact tissue effect.

Electrosurgical Tissue Effects

Electrosurgical Cutting

Electrosurgical cutting divides tissue with electric sparks that focus intense heat at the surgical site. By sparking to tissue, the surgeon produces maximum current concentration. To create this spark the surgeon should hold the electrode slightly away from the tissue. This will produce the greatest amount of heat over a very short period of time, which results in vaporization of tissue.

Electrosurgical Fulguration

Electrosurgical fulguration (sparking with the coagulation waveform) coagulates and chars the tissue over a wide area. Because the duty cycle (on time) is only about 6%, less heat is produced. The result is the creation of a coagulum rather than cellular vaporization. In order to overcome the high impedance of air, the coagulation waveform has significantly higher voltage than the cutting current. Use of high voltage coagulation current has implications during minimally invasive surgery.

Electrosurgical Desiccation

- Electrosurgical desiccation occurs when the electrode is in direct contact with the tissue. Desiccation is achieved most efficiently with the "cutting" current. By touching the tissue with the electrode, the current concentration is reduced. Less heat is generated and no cutting action occurs. The cells dry out and form a coagulum rather than vaporize and explode

- Surgeons routinely "cut" with the coagulation current. Likewise, you can coagulate with the cutting current by holding the electrode in direct contact with tissue. It may be necessary to adjust power settings and electrode size to achieve the desired surgical effect. The benefit of coagulating with the cutting current is that you will be using far less voltage. Likewise, cutting with the cut current will also accomplish the task with less voltage. This is an important consideration during minimally invasive procedures.

Variables impacting tissue effect
Waveform
Power setting
Size of electrode
Time
Manipulation of electrode
Type of tissue
Eschar

Size of the electrode: The smaller the electrode, the higher the current concentration. Consequently, the same tissue effect can be achieved with a smaller electrode, even though the power setting is reduced.

Time: At any given setting, the longer the generator is activated, the more heat is produced. And the greater the heat, the farther it will travel to adjacent tissue.

Manipulation of the electrode: This can determine whether vaporization or coagulation occurs. This

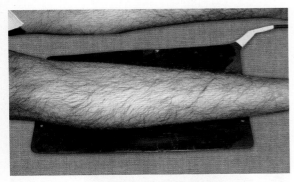

Fig. 46.2: Ground plate

is a function of current density and the resultant heat produced while sparking to tissue versus holding the electrode in direct contact with tissue (Fig. 46.2).

Type of tissue: Tissues vary widely in resistance.

Eschar: Eschar is relatively high in resistance to current. Keeping electrodes clean and free of eschar will enhance performance by maintaining lower resistance within the surgical circuit.

Grounded Electrosurgical Systems

- Electrosurgical technology has changed dramatically since its introduction in the 1920s. Generators operate by taking alternating current and increasing its frequency from 50 or 60 cycles/second to over 200,000 cycles/second
- Originally, generators used grounded current from a wall outlet. It was assumed that, once the current entered the patient's body, it would return to ground through the patient return electrode. But electricity will always seek the path of least resistance
- When there are many conductive objects touching the patient and leading to ground, the current will select as its pathway to ground the most conductive object—which may not be the patient return electrode. Current concentration at this point may lead to an alternate site burn

- A phenomenon called current division, the current may split (or divide) and follow more than one path to ground. The circuit to ground is completed whether it travels the intended electrosurgical circuit to the patient return electrode or to an alternate ground referenced site
- Many times patients are exposed to the risk of alternate site burns because (i) current follows the easiest, most conductive path; (ii) any grounded object, not just the generator, can complete the circuit; (iii) the surgical environment offers many alternative routes to ground; (iv) if the resistance of the alternate path is low enough and the current flowing to ground in that path is sufficiently concentrated, an unintended burn may be produced at the alternate grounding site.

Isolated Electrosurgical Systems

- Eelectrosurgery was revolutionized by isolated generator technology. The isolated generator isolates the therapeutic current from ground by referencing it within the generator circuitry
- In other words, in an isolated electrosurgical system, the circuit is completed not by the ground but by the generator. Even though grounded objects remain in the operating room, electrosurgical current from isolated generators will not recognize grounded objects as pathways to complete the circuit. Isolated electrosurgical energy recognizes the patient return electrode as the preferred pathway back to the generator
- By removing ground as a reference for the current, the isolated generator eliminates many of the hazards inherent in grounded systems, most importantly current division and alternate site burns
- If the circuit to the patient return electrode is broken, an isolated generator will deactivate the system because the current cannot return to its source (Fig. 46.3)

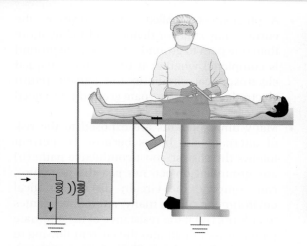

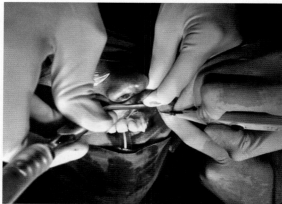

Fig. 46.4: Electrosurgery for incision

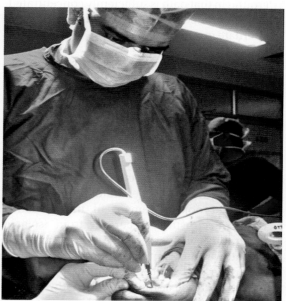

Fig. 46.3: Surgeon using electrosurgery

- Generators with isolated circuits mitigate the hazard of alternate site burns but do not protect the patient from return electrode burns, such as the one shown at right
- Historically, patient return electrode burns have accounted for 70% of the injuries reported during the use of electrosurgery. Patient return electrodes are not "inactive" or "passive". The

only difference between the "active" electrode and the patient return electrode is their size and relative conductivity. The quality of the conductivity and contact area at the pad/ patient interface must be maintained to prevent a return electrode site injury.

Patient Return Electrodes

The function of the patient return electrode is to remove current from the patient safely. A return electrode burn occurs when the heat produced, over time, is not safely dissipated by the size or conductivity of the patient return electrode (Fig. 46.4).

$$\text{Burn} = \frac{\text{Current} \times \text{Time}}{\text{Area}}$$

Ideal Return: Electrode Contact With Current Dispersion

- The ideal patient return electrode safely collects current delivered to the patient during electrosurgery and carries that current away. To eliminate the risk of current concentration, the pad should present a large low impedance contact area to the patient. Placement should be on conductive tissue that is close to the operative site
- Again, the only difference between the "active" electrode and the patient return electrode is

their relative size and conductivity. Concentrate the electrons at the active electrode and high heat is produced. Disperse this same current over a comparatively large patient return electrode and little heat is produced.

Dangerous Return: Electrode Contact with Current Concentration

If the surface area contact between the patient and the return electrode is reduced, or if the impedance of that contact is increased, a dangerous condition can develop. In the case of reduced contact area, the current flow is concentrated in a smaller area. As the current concentration increases, the temperature at the return electrode increases. If the temperature at the return electrode site increases enough, a patient burn may result. Surface area impedance can be compromised by: excessive hair, adipose tissue, bony prominences, fluid invasion, adhesive failure, scar tissue, and many other variables (Table 46.1).

Patient Return Electrode Monitoring Technology

- Return electrode monitoring contact quality monitoring was developed to protect patients from burns due to inadequate contact of the return electrode
- Pad site burns are caused by decreased contact area at the return electrode site
- Return electrode monitoring equipped generators actively monitor the amount of impedance at the patient/pad interface because there is a direct relationship between this impedance and the contact area. The system is designed to

Table 46.1: Assess pad site location	
Choose	*Well vascularized muscle mass*
Avoid	Vascular insufficiency Irregular body contours Bony prominences
Consider	Incision site/prep area Patient position Other equipment on patient

deactivate the generator before an injury can occur, if it detects a dangerously high level of impedance at the patient/pad interface
- Such an electrode can be identified by its "split" appearance—that is, it has two separate areas—and a special plug with a center pin.

Argon-enhanced Electrosurgery

Argon Flow

Argon-enhanced electrosurgery incorporates a stream of argon gas to improve the surgical effectiveness of the electrosurgical current.

Properties of Argon Gas

Argon gas is inert and noncombustible, making it a safe medium through which to pass electrosurgical current. Electrosurgical current easily ionizes argon gas, making it more conductive than air. This highly conductive stream of ionized gas provides the electrical current an efficient pathway.

- Inert
- Noncombustible
- Easily ionized by RF energy
- Creates bridge between electrode and tissue
- Heavier than air
- Displaces nitrogen and oxygen

Argon-enhanced Coagulation and Cut

There are many advantages to argon-enhanced electrosurgical cutting and coagulation.

- Decreased smoke, odor
- Noncontact in coagulation mode
- Decreased blood loss, rebleeding
- Decreased tissue damage
- Flexible eschar.

BASICS OF LASERS AND ITS EFFECTS ON TISSUES

Introduction

- Laser is an acronym, which stands for Light Amplification by Stimulated Emission of Radiation

- The image of the laser has changed significantly over the past several years. With dentistry in the high-tech era, no instrument is more representative of the term high-tech than the laser. Dental procedures performed today with the laser are so effective that they should set a new standard of care.

Laser Physics

- The concept of stimulated emission of light was first proposed (1917) by Albert Einstein. He described three processes:
  - Absorption
  - Spontaneous emission
  - Stimulated emission.
- Einstein considered the model of a basic atom to describe the production of laser. An atom consists of centrally placed nucleus, which contains positively charged particles known as protons, around which the negatively charged particles, i.e. electrons are revolving

  When an atom is struck by a photon, there is an energy transfer causing increase in energy of the atom. This process is termed as *absorption*. The photon then ceases to exist, and an electron within the atom pumps to a higher energy level. This atom is thus pumped up to an excited state from the ground state
- In the excited state, the atom is unstable and will soon spontaneously decay back to the ground state, releasing the stored energy in the form of an emitted photon. This process is called *spontaneous emission*
- If an atom in the excited state is struck by a photon of identical energy as the photon to be emitted, the emission could be stimulated to occur earlier than would occur spontaneously. This stimulated interaction causes two photons that are identical in frequency and wavelength to leave the atom. This is a process of *stimulated emission.*

Laser Design

All lasers have similar fundamental elements:

Lasing medium:
- Which may be solid, a liquid/gas
- Maiman's laser used a solid medium—ruby crystal.
- As a rule, the lasing medium gives its name to the laser, for example:
  - Ruby laser (solid)
  - Nd :YAG (solid)
  - Dye laser (liquid)
  - CO_2 (gas) and Argon (gas)
  - Semiconductor lasers

Energy source: The atoms or molecules of the lasing medium need to be excited so that protons of laser light are emitted. The energy for this may be provided by an electric discharge, high powered xenon-flash lamps or even another laser.

Optical resonator/housing tube: Is an arrangement of mirrors which both amplify the effect of the laser and ensure that when the light does emerge from the laser, it possesses the unique.

Laser Light Delivery

Light can be delivered by a number of different mechanisms. Several years ago, a hand held laser meant holding a larger, several hundred pound laser usually the size of a desk, above a patient. Although the idea was comical at the time, it is becoming more feasible as laser technology is producing smaller and lighter weight lasers. In the more future it is probable that hand held lasers will be used routinely.

Articulated Arms

Laser light can be delivered by articulated arms, which are very simple but elegant devices. Mirrors are placed at 45° angles to tubes carrying the laser light. The tubes can rotate about the normal axis of the mirrors. This results in a tremendous amount of flexibility in the arm and in delivery of the laser light. This is typically used with CO_2 laser. The arm does have some disadvantages that include the arm counter weight and the limited ability to move in a straight line.

Optical Fiber

- Laser light can be delivered by an optical fiber, which is frequently used with near infrared and visible lasers. The light is trapped in the glass and propagates down through the fiber in a process called total internal reflection
- Optical fibers can be very small. They can be either tenths of microns or greater than hundreds of microns in diameter.

Advantages

They provide easy access and transmit high intensities of light with almost no loss.

Disadvantages

- The beam is no longer collimated and coherent when emitted from the fiber, which limits the focal spot size
- The light is no longer coherent.

Mode of Delivery of Laser

Once the laser is produced, its output power may be delivered in the following modes:

Continuous Wave

When laser machine is set in a continuous wave mode the amplitude of the output beam is expressed in terms of watts. In this mode the laser emits radiation continuously at a constant power levels of 10–100 W. As for example CO_2 laser.

Chopped

The output of a continuous wave can be interrupted by a shutter that "chops" the beam into trains of short pulses. The speed of the shutter is 100–500 ms.

Gated

The term superpulsed is used to describe the output of a gated high peak power laser with a short pulse duration, typically between hundreds of microseconds (1 ms = 1 × 10^{-6} sec.). The pulse produced during superpulsing can have a repitition rate of 50–250 pulses per second that permits the laser output to appear almost continuous during use.

Pulsed

Lasers can be gated or pulsed electronically. This type of gating permits the duration of the pulses to be compressed producing a corresponding increase in peak power, that is much higher than in commonly available continuous wave mode.

Super Pulsed

The duration of pulse is one hundredth of microseconds.

Ultra Pulsed

This mode produces an output pulse of high peak power that is maintained for a longer time and delivers more energy in each pulse than in the superpulsed mode. The duration of the ultra pulse is slightly less.

Q-scotched

Even shorter and more intense pulse can be obtained with this mode. Several hundreds of millijoules of energy can be squeezed into nano second pulses.

Flash-lamp Pulsing

In these systems, a flash–lamp is used to pump the lasing medium, usually for solid state lasers.

Focusing

- Lasers can be used in either a focussed mode or in a defocused mode
- A *focussed mode* is when the laser beam hits the tissue at its focal points or smallest diameter. This diameter is dependent on the size of lens used. This mode can also be referred as cutting mode. For example, while performing biopsies
- The other method is the *defocused mode*. In which the mode is moved away from the total plane. This beam size that hits the tissue has a greater diameter, thus causing a wider area of tissue to be vaporized. However, laser intensity/power density is reduced. This method is also known as ablation mode. For example, in Frenectomies; in removal of inflammatory papillary hyperplasias

- In contact mode, the fiber handpiece is placed in contact to the tissue whereas in the non-contact, the handpiece is placed away from the target tissue.

Contact and Noncontact modes

In contact mode, the fiber tip is placed in contact with the tissue. The charred tissue formed on the fiber tip or on the tissue outline and increases the absorption of laser energy and resultant tissue effects. Char can be eliminated with a water spray and then slightly more energy will be required to provide time efficient results. Advantage is that there is control feed back for the operator.

Noncontact Mode

Fiber tip is placed away from the target tissue. In the noncontact mode the clinician operates with visual control with the aid of an aiming beam or by observing the tissue effect being created.

LASER TYPES

- Based on wavelength
  - Soft lasers
  - Hard lasers

Soft lasers

Soft lasers are lower power lasers; with a wave length around 632 mm. For example, He-Ne, diode.

These are employed to relieve pain and promote healing, e.g. in aphthous ulcers.

Hard lasers

Lasers with well known laser systems for possible surgical application are called as hard lasers, e.g. CO_2, Nd: YAG, Argon, Er:YAG, etc.
- Based on the lasing medium
  Lasers can be classified according to the state of the active medium, i.e.
  - Solid: Nd-YAG, diode
  - Liquid: Dye
  - Gas: CO_2, Argon, Er-YAG
- Based on the potential danger posed to the exposed skin and to the unaccomodated eye.

CO₂ Lasers

- The CO_2 laser first developed by Patel et al. in 1964 is a gas laser and has a wavelength of 10,600 nm or 10.6 µ deep in the infrared range of the electromagnetic spectrum
- CO_2 lasers have an affinity for wet tissues regardless of tissue color
- The laser energy weakens rapidly in most tissues because it is absorbed by water. Because of the water absorption, the CO_2 laser generates a lot of heat, which readily carbonizes tissues. Since this carbonized or charred layer acts as a biological dressing, it should not be removed
- They are highly absorbed in oral mucosa, which is more than 90% water. High absorption in small volume results although their penetration depth is only about 0.2–0.3 nm. There is no scattering, reflection, or transmission in oral mucosa. Hence, what you see is what you get
- CO_2 lasers reflect off mirrors, allowing access to difficult areas. Unfortunately, they also reflect off dental instruments, making accidental reflection to nontarget tissue a concern
- CO_2 lasers can not be delivered fiber optically advances in articulated arms and hollow wave guide technologies, now provide easy access to all areas of the mout
- Regardless of the delivery method used, all CO_2 lasers work in a noncontact mode
- Of all the lasers for oral use, CO_2 is the fastest in removing tissue
- As CO_2 lasers are invisible, an aiming helium – neon (He–Ne) beam must be used in conjunction with this laser.

Nd: YAG Laser

- Crystals of ytrium–aluminum–garnet are doped with neodymium. Nd-YAG laser, has wavelength of 1,064 nm (0.1064 µ) placing it in the near infrared range of the magnetic spectrum
- It is not well absorbed by water but is attracted to pigmented tissue, e.g. hemoglobin and melanin. Therefore various degrees of optical

scattering and penetration to the tissue, minimal absorption and no reflection
- Nd: YAG lasers work either by a contact or noncontact mode. When working on tissue, however, the contact mode in highly recommended
- The Nd-YAG laser is delivered fiber optically and many sizes of contact fibers are available
- Carbonized tissue remnants often build up on the tip of the contact fiber, creating a 'hot tip'. This increased temperature enhances the effect of the Nd-YAG laser, and it is not necessary to rinse the build up away
- Special tips, the coated sapphire tip, can be used to limit lateral thermal damage
- A helium-neon-aiming beam is generally used with Nd-YAG wavelength
- Penetration depth is $\sim$ 2–4 m, and can be varied by upto 0.5–4 mm in oral tissues by various methods
- A black enhancer can be used to speed the action
- The Nd-YAG beam is readily absorbed by amalgam, Ti and nonprecious metals, requiring careful operation in the presence of these dental materials.

Uses
- Soft tissue removal
- Hemostasis
- Coagulation

Argon Lasers
- Argon lasers are those lasers in the blue-green visible spectrum (thus, they can be seen)
- They operate at 488 nm (blue) or 514.5 nm (green), or 496 nm (blue/green). Argon is easily delivered fiber optically
- Argon lasers have an affinity for darker colored tissues and also a high affinity for hemoglobin, making them excellent coagulators. Thus argon lasers focused on bleeding vessels stop the hemorrhage. It is not absorbed well by hard tissue, and no particular care is needed to protect the teeth during surgery

- In oral tissues there is no reflection, some absorption and some scattering and transmission – travel fiberoptically is unaffected by H_2O
- Argon lasers work both in the contact and non contact mode
- Like, Nd-YAG lasers, at low powers argon lasers suffer from 'dragability' and need sweeping motion to avoid tissue from accumulating on the tip
- Enhances are not needed with Argon lasers.
- Argon lasers also have the ability to cure composite resin, a feature shared by none of the other lasers
- Argon is highly absorbed by Hb, strongly absorbed by melanin and poorly absorbed by H_2O
- The blue wavelength of 488 nm is used mainly for composite curing, while the green wavelength of 510 nm is mainly for soft tissue procedures and coagulation.

Erbium-YAG laser
- It is a promising laser system because the emission wave length coincides with the main absorption peak of water, resulting in good absorption in all biological tissues including enamel and dentin. This is the 1st Laser to be cleared by the FDA on May 7, 1997 for use in preparing human cavities
- Have a wavelength of 2.94 mm
- A number of researchers have demonstrated the Er-YAG lasers ability to cut, or ablate, dental hard tissue effectively and efficiently. The Er-YAG laser is absorbed by water and hydroxyapatite, which particularly accounts for its efficiency in cutting enamel and dentin
- A variety of restorative materials, such as Zn phosphate, Zn carboxylate, glass ionomer cements and silver amalgam can be effectively removed by the Er-YAG cases
- Pulpal response to cavity preparation with an Er-YAG laser was minimal, reversible and comparable with pulpal response created by a high-speed drill

- Er-YAG can also be used for bone ablation and has indications in soft tissue surfaces where no coagulation effect is desired, such as removal of hyperplastic gingival tissue, periodontal surgery and abrasion of large benign lesions of the oral mucosa and skin.

Ho-YAG Laser [Holmium YAG Lasers]

- Is thallium and holomium doped, chromium sensitized YAG crystal
- Has a wavelength of 2,100 nm
- Delivered through a fiber optic carrier
- A He-Ne laser is used as an aiming light
- Dragability is less compared to Nd-YAG and argon lasers
- Like Nd-YAG, can be used in both the contact and non-contact modes and are pulsed lasers.
- Ho-YAG laser has an affinity for white tissue and has ability to pass through water and acts as a good coagulator.

LASER–TISSUE INTERACTION (FIG. 46.5)

Reflection

- Reflected light bounces off the tissue surface and is directed outward
- Because the energy dissipates so effectively after reflection, there is little danger of damage to other parts of the mouth
- It also limits the amount of energy that enters the tissue.

Scattering

- It occurs when the light energy bounces from molecule to molecule within the tissue
- It distributes the energy over a larger volume of tissue, dissipating the thermal effects.

Absorption

Occurs after a characteristic amount of scattering and is responsible for the thermal effects within the tissue.

Transmission

- Light can also travel beyond a given tissue boundary. This is known as transmission

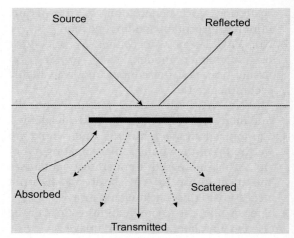

Fig. 46.5: When laser strikes a tissue surface, it can be reflected, scattered, absorbed, or transmitted

- It irradiates the surrounding tissue and must be quantified
- The distance the energy transmits into the tissue is called penetration depth
- Coagulation where as depth is the deepest level where alterations in the tissue will occur because of the laser's energy
- For example CO_2, Nd-YAG and argon have similar coagulation depths but different penetration depths.

Lasers and Soft Tissues

- The absorption of laser light by different elements of tissue is extremely wavelength dependent
- H_2O, a major constituent of soft tissue strongly absorbs wavelengths of 2 nm/above and therefore these penetrate little in soft tissues, the greater part of which is made up of H_2O.

Lasers and Hard Tissues

Many researchers felt that lasers were obvious replacement for the dental drill, as

- Lasers are 'noncontact' and their use produces much less vibration than conventional drills
- They are much quieter than drills, usually producing only a muted 'popping sound', which is generally well-tolerated
- They can sterilize as they cut

- They can also be used to seal tissues at the periphery of the cut. Therefore, cut dentinal tubules were sealed rather than left-open as pathways for microorganisms, reducing the possibility of postoperative hypersensitivity.

Thermal Effects

- The best known laser effect in dentistry is the thermal vaporization of tissue by absorbing laser light, i.e. the laser energy is converted into thermal energy or heat that destroys the tissues
- When the high peak-power of a pulsed – laser is greater, a super-heated gas called the 'plasma' may form, which can absorb the incoming laser beam, allowing less energy to reach the surface. This hot plasma, can then quickly conduct heat to the tissues surfaces and causes ablation and severe heating, which can lead to tissue damage. Flowing water down the fiber and onto the tissue has been used in an attempt to control this plasma.

LASER HAZARDS AND LASER SAFETY

The subject of dental laser safety is broad in scope, including not only an awareness of the potential risks and hazards related to how lasers are used, but also recognition of existing standards of care and a thorough understanding of safety control measures (Table 46.2).

Laser Hazard Class According to ANSI and OSHA Standards:

Class I: Low powered lasers that are safe to view

Class IIa: Low powered visible lasers that are hazardous only when viewed directly for longer than 1000 sec

Class IIb: Low powered visible lasers that are hazardous when viewed for longer than 0.25 sec

Class IIIa: Medium powered lasers or systems that are normally not hazardous if viewed for less than 0.25 sec without magnifying optics

Class IIIb : Medium powered lasers (0.5w max) that can be hazardous if viewed directly

Class IV : High powered lasers (>0.5W) that produce ocular, skin and fire hazards.

The types of hazards grouped as follows:
Ocular injury
Tissue damage
Respiratory hazards
Fire and explosion
Electrical shock

Ocular Injury

- Direct emission
- Reflection

Potential injury to the eye can occur either by direct emission from the laser or by reflection from a specular (mirror like) surface or high polished, convex curvatured instruments. Damage can manifest as injury to sclera, cornea, retina and aqueous humor and also as cataract formation. The use of carbonized and nonreflective instruments has been recommended.

Tissue Hazards

- Laser induced damage to skin and other non target tissues can result from the:
  - Thermal interaction of radiant energy with tissue proteins. Temperature elevation of 21°C above normal body temp (37°C) can produce cell destruction
  - Tissue damage can also occur due to cumulative effects of radiant exposure.

Table 46.2: Flammable objects used in surgery		
Solids	*Liquids*	*Gases*
Clothing	Ethanol	Oxygen
Paper products	Acetone	Nitrous oxide
Plastics	Methylmethacrylate	General anesthetics
Waxes and resins	Solvents	Aromatic vapors

Respiratory

- Another class of hazards involves the potential inhalation of airborne biohazardous materials that may be released as a result of the surgical application of lasers. Toxic gases and chemical used in lasers are also responsible to some extent
- During ablation or incision of oral soft tissue, cellular products are vaporized due to the rapid heating of the liquid component in the tissue.

Fire and Explosion

- Flammable solids, liquids and gases used within the clinical setting can be easily ignited if exposed to the laser beam. The use of flame-resistant materials and other precautions therefore is recommended.

Electrical Hazards

These can be:
- Electrical shock hazards
- Electrical fire or explosion hazards.

HARMONIC SCALPEL

Harmonic scalpel use and comparison with electrosurgery described recently in maxillo-facial surgery for pectoralis major myocutaneous flapdissection less operative time, and less blood loss,drainage volume with less operative time [Deos Hazarica]. Its use also done in parotidectomy, oncosurgery. The harmonic scalpel cuts and coagulates simultaneously using a mechanical vibration. Current studies also showed less incidence of nerve injury. less damage to tissues and less lymph leakage. It is also known as ultracision.

Instruments and Postexposure Prophylaxis

47

INTRODUCTION

Surgeons have access to a variety of surgical instruments that are designed to help them in treatment of abnormalities.The instruments for oral and Maxillofacial surgical use are varied and many. Most of the time an instrument is picked up the task for which it is specifically used should be adhered to. This chapter deals with the instruments that are required to perform routine ORAL AND MAXILLO-FACIAL; surgical procedures, since it is a must that one shoud have a fundamental knowledge of them and their application.

Classification of Instruments

- General surgical instruments (Common for all kind of surgeries)
- Procedure specific instruments of oral and maxillofacial surgery.

General Surgical Instruments

On the basis of type of procedure can be categorized as:

- Instruments for keeping the sterile instruments
- Instruments to transfer sterile instruments
- Instruments for preparing surgical field
- Instruments to hold towels and drapes in position
- Instruments to incise tissue

- Instruments for elevating mucoperiosteum
- Instruments for controlling hemorrhage
- Instruments to grasp tissue
- Instruments for retracting soft tissue
- Instruments for removing bone
- Instruments for holding bone
- Instruments for providing suction
- Instruments for irrigation
- Instruments to remove soft tissue from bony defects
- Instruments for draining an abscess
- Instruments for maintaining drainage
- Instruments for grafting skin/bone
- Instruments for suturing mucosa
- Instrument tray systems.

Instruments for Keeping the Sterile Instruments

Surgical Trays/Boxes (Figs 47.1 and 47.2)

- Can be solid/perforated, stainless steel/ aluminium with/without lock, small/medium/ large
- Autoclavable, heat and acid resistant, improves storage, sterilization and selection of instruments.

Surgical Containers/Drums (Fig. 47.3)

Perforated, with lock made up of aluminium, can be small/medium/large.

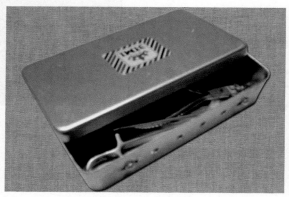

Fig. 47.1: Surgical box

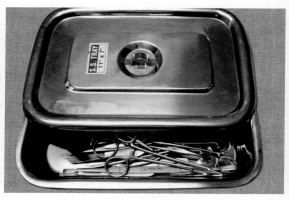

Fig. 47.2: Surgical tray

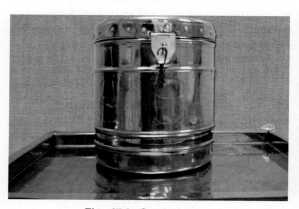

Fig. 47.3: Surgical drum

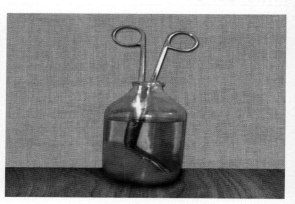

Fig. 47.4: Chittle's forceps

INSTRUMENTS TO TRANSFER STERILE INSTRUMENTS

Chittle's Forceps (Fig. 47.4)
- These are heave long forceps used to transfer sterile instruments from one sterile area to another
- These forceps are usually right angled with heavy jaws so that instruments can be moved from one area to another without dropping them.
- It is stored in a container that is filled with a bactericidal solution like Savlon. The solution must be changed every day.

INSTRUMENTS FOR PREPARING SURGICAL FIELD

Swab Holder (Fig. 47.5)
- An instrument with long blades expanded at ends forming an oblong tip
- Blades have central fenestrations and transverse serrations.

Steel Bowl
- A simple stainless steel bowl to keep betadine gauze piece.

INSTRUMENTS TO HOLD TOWELS AND DRAPES IN POSITION

Towel Clamps (Figs 47.6 and 47.7)

- Towel clamps are mainly used for fastening sterile towels and drapes placed on the patient's head and chest, as well as for securing the surgical suction tube and the tube connected to the handpiece with the sterile drape covering the patient's chest.
- They are of two types
  - The pinchter type
  - The forceps type/beckhaus towel clip.

INSTRUMENTS TO INCISE TISSUE

Scalpel (Handle and Blade) (Figs 47.8 to 47.10)

Handle

The most commonly used handle in oral surgery is the Bard–Parker no. 3. Its tip may receive different types of blades.

Blade

- Blades are disposable and are of three different types (nos. 11, 12 and 15)

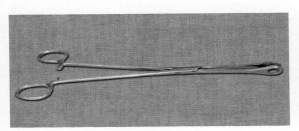

Fig. 47.5: Swab holder

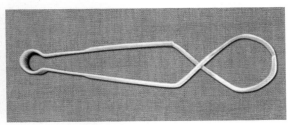

Fig. 47.6: Towel clip—pinchter type

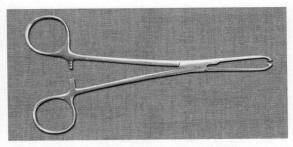

Fig. 47.7: Towel clip—forceps type

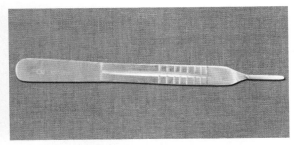

Fig. 47.8: Scalpel handle

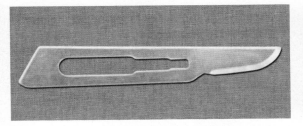

Fig. 47.9: Scalpel blade no 15

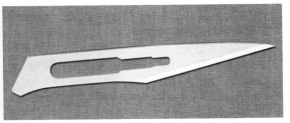

Fig. 47.10: Scalpel blade no 11

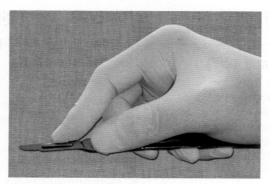

Fig. 47.11: Surgeons method of holding scalpel

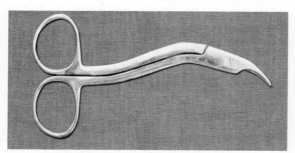

Fig. 47.12: Suture cutting scissors

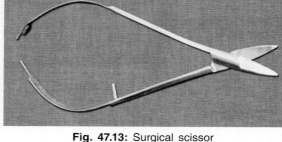

Fig. 47.13: Surgical scissor

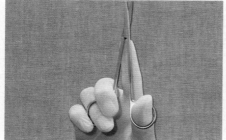

Fig. 47.14: Method of holding scissor while in use

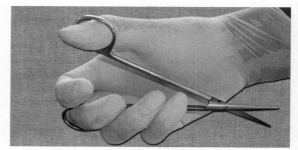

Fig. 47.15: Safe holding the scissor after use

- The most common type of blade is no. 15, which is used for flaps and incisions on edentulous alveolar ridges
- Blade no. 12 is indicated for incisions in the gingival sulcus and incisions posterior to the teeth, especially in the maxillary tuberosity area
- Blade no. 11 is used for small incisions, such as those used for incising abscesses
- The scalpel blade is placed on the handle with the help of a needle holder, or hemostat, with which it slides into the slotted receiver with the beveled end parallel to that of the handle
- The scalpel is held in a pen grasp and its cutting edge faces the surface of the skin or mucosa that is to be incised (Fig. 47.11).

Scissors (Fig. 47.12 to 47.15)

- Various types of scissors are used in oral surgery, depending on the surgical procedure. They belong to the following categories— suture scissors and soft tissue scissors

- The most commonly used scissors for cutting sutures have sharp cutting edges, while Goldman–Fox, Lagrange (which have slightly upward curved blades), and Metzenbaum are used for soft tissue. Lagrange scissors are narrow scissors with sharp blades and are mainly used for removing excess gingival tissue, while the Metzenbaum are blunt-nosed scissors and are suitable for dissecting and undermining the mucosa from the underlying soft tissues
- Scissors are held the same way as needle holders.

INSTRUMENTS FOR ELEVATING MUCOPERIOSTEUM

Periosteal Strippers (Fig. 47.16)

- A straight instrument with a handle and a blade with sharp working tip
- Comes in various shapes and sizes of handle and blade
- Curve, angle and blade width combine to elevate periosteum in quicker and easier fashion

- Light in weight
- Used in "push" stroke.

Periosteal Elevator (Figs 47.17 and 47.18)

- This instrument has many different types of end
- The most commonly used periosteal elevator in intraoral surgery is the no. 9 Molt, which has two different ends—a pointed end, used for elevating the interdental papillae of the gingiva, and a broad end, which facilitates elevating the mucoperiosteum from the bone
- The Freer elevator is used for reflecting the gingiva surrounding the tooth before extraction. This instrument is considered suitable, compared to standard elevators, because it is easy to use and has thin anatomic ends
- The elevator may also be used for holding the flap after reflecting, facilitating manipulations during the surgical procedure. The Seldin elevator is considered most suitable for this purpose.

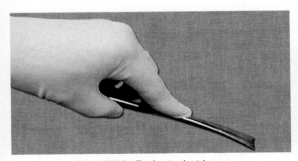

Fig. 47.16: Periosteal stripper

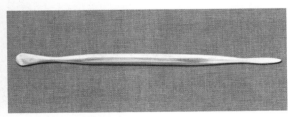

Fig. 47.17: Molt's no. 9 periosteal elevator

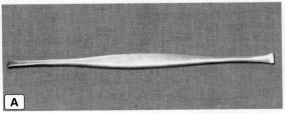

A

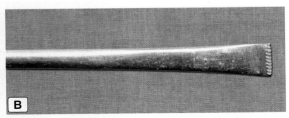

B

Figs 47.18A and B: Howarth's elevator

INSTRUMENTS FOR CONTROLLING HEMORRHAGE

Hemostats (Fig. 47.19 to 47.24)

- The hemostats used in oral surgery are either straight or curved. The most commonly used hemostat is the curved mosquito type or micro-Halsted hemostat, which has relatively small and narrow beaks so that they may grasp the vessel and stop bleeding
- Hemostats may also be used for firmly holding soft tissue, facilitating manipulations for its removal.

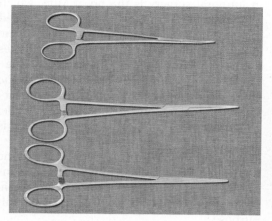

Fig. 47.19: Artery forceps mosquito, curved, and straight

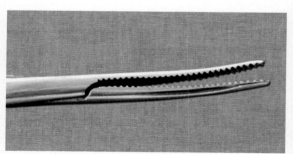

Fig. 47.20: Straight artery forceps

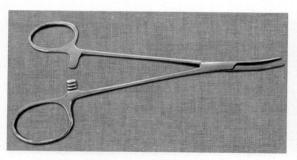

Fig. 47.21: Curved artery forceps

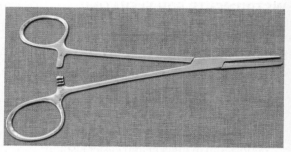

Fig. 47.22: Curved artery forceps blade near view

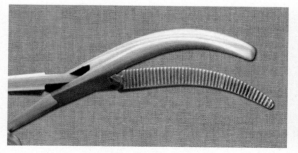

Fig. 47.23: Curved artery forceps blade notice the horizontal striations

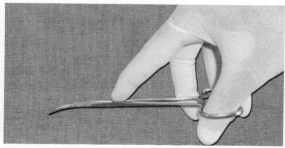

Fig. 47.24: Method of holding artery forceps when in use

Instruments to Grasp Tissue

- Skin hook
- Adson tissue holding forceps
- Allis tissue holding forceps
- Babcock's tissue holding forceps
- Vein hook
- Nerve hook.

Skin Hook (Fig. 47.25)

- A thin long instrument with a delicate pointed curved tip, which engages tissue
- Types

- Single prong – Gillies
  – Kilner
- Double prong

Uses
- To hold and retract skin edges during cutting, dissection and suturing
- To retract small amount of soft tissues
- Surgical anatomic forceps (Fig. 47.26)
- Surgical forceps are used for suturing the wound, firmly grasping the tissues while the needle is passed (Figs 47.27 and 47.28)

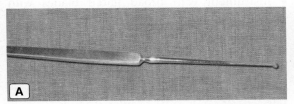
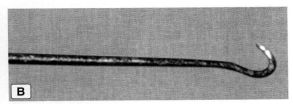

Figs 47.25A and B: Skin hook

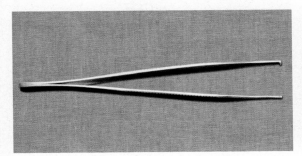

Fig. 47.26: Surgical anatomy toothed forceps

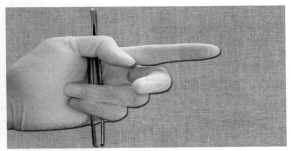

Fig. 47.27: Safe hold of forceps when not in use

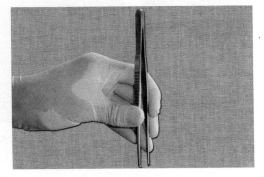

Fig. 47.28: Method of using forceps

- There are two types of forceps—the long standard surgical forceps, used in posterior areas, and the small, narrow Adson forceps, used in anterior areas
- The beak of the forceps has a wedge-shaped projection or tooth on one side, and a receptor on the other, which fit into each other when the handles are locked. This mechanism allows the forceps to grasp the soft tissues found between the beaks very tightly
- Anatomic forceps do not have a wedge-shaped projection, but parallel grooves. This type of forceps is used to aid in the suturing of the wound, as well as grasping small instruments, etc. during the surgical procedure.

Allis Tissue Forceps (Fig. 47.29 to 47.31)

- A forceps with locking handle, blades have delicate teeth
- Handle longer than beaks
- Should never be used to hold the skin directly
- Held in the same way as needle holder.

Uses

- To hold and retract tissues (generally for tissues that will be excised)
- To provide tension during tissue dissection.

Babcock's Tissue Forceps (Fig. 47.32)

- Instrument with broad flared blades with fenestrations and without teeth

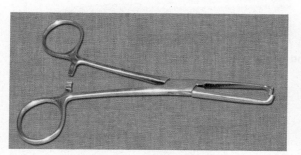

Fig. 47.29: Allis tissue forceps

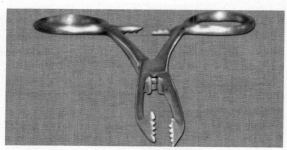

Fig. 47.30: Allis tissue forceps blade near view

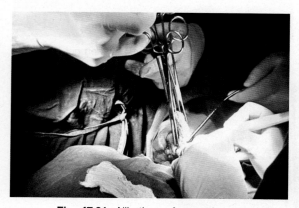

Fig. 47.31: Allis tissue forceps in use

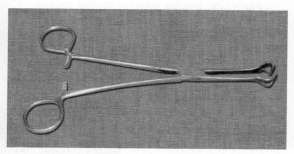

Fig. 47.32: Babcock's tissue forceps

- Handle with lock
- More delicate and less traumatic than Allis
- Used to hold enlarged lymph nodes or any glandular tissue.

Vein Hook (Desmarre's) (Fig. 47.33)

- A small instrument with broad curved blade (concave from inside) with smooth edge, which encircles the vessel
- Used to retract vessels during dissection (especially for major vessels during neck dissection).

Nerve Hook (Dandy's) (Fig. 47.34)

- A small instrument with a broad curve at the tip, tip is relatively blunt
- Used in neurectomy procedures for nerve identification and in nerve repositioning procedures.

Instruments for Retracting Soft Tissue (Fig. 47.35 to 47.40)

Retractors

- Retractors are used to retract the cheeks and mucoperiosteal flap during the surgical procedure. The most commonly used retractors are Farabeuf, Kocher–Langenbeck, and Minnesota retractors
- Tongue retractors may be used to retract the tongue medially away from the surgical field, facilitating manipulations.

Langenback retractor

- Has a long handle and a L shaped blade (Fig. 47.35)
- Available in different sizes of handle and blade (width and length)
- Can be single/double ended.
- Common types are (Fig. 47.36):
  - Standard (edge of the blade points towards handle)

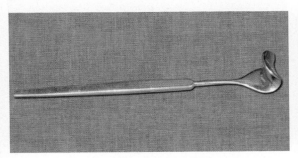

Fig. 47.33: Vein hook

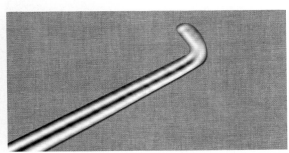

Fig. 47.34: Nerve hook

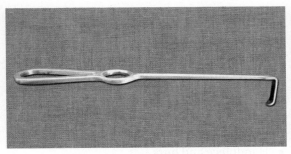

Fig. 47.35: Langenback retractor

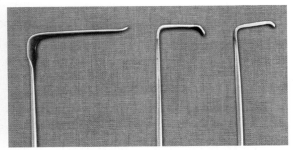

Fig. 47.36: Note different edge (both standard and reverse instruments)

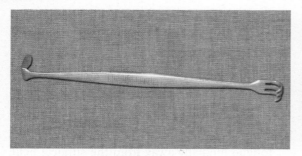

Fig. 47.37: Cats paw

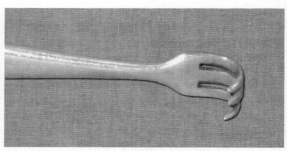

Fig. 47.38: Cats paw edge view

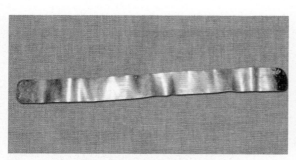

Fig. 47.39: Copper malleable retractors

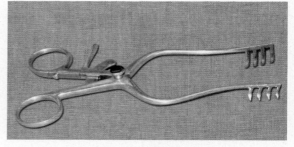

Fig. 47.40: Self retaining retractor

– Reverse (edge of the blade points away from the handle), edge of the blade can take support to retract tissues.

Uses
- To retract incised edges
- To retract soft tissue mass
- To allow visualization of deeper tissues.

Cats paw (Figs 47.37 and 47.38)
- Resembles cat's paw
- On one side of the instrument blade has prongs which are curved at the tip, on other side there is right angle retractor
- May have 3/4/5 prongs
- Used for retracting small amount of soft tissues
- Care should be taken not to apply excessive force.

Copper Malleable (Fig. 47.39)
- A universal kind of retractor made of copper, can be molded into any shape according to the need

- Only disadvantage is lack of firm retraction as given by others.

Self retaining retractors (Weitlaner) (Fig. 47.40)
- An instrument with long curved blades
- Blades have multiple prongs
- Ends can be blunt or sharp
- Have rake tips
- Ratchet to hold tissue apart.

Instruments for Removing Bone (Figs 47.41 to 47.47)

- Rongeur forceps
- Bone cutter
- Chisel and mallet
- Osteotome
- Bone gouge
- Giglis wire saw
- Handpiece and burs
- Surgical saw
- Bone file
- Smith spreader.

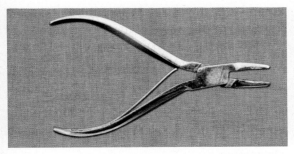

Fig. 47.41: Bone Rongeur

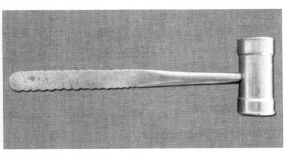

Fig. 47.42: Mallet

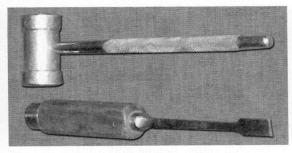

Fig. 47.43: Mallet and chisel

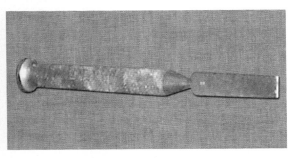

Fig. 47.44: Osteotome

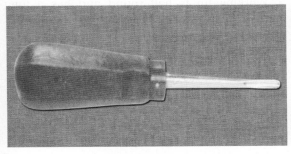

Fig. 47.45: Bone gouge

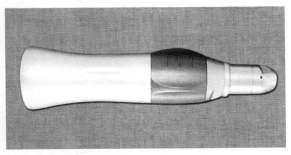

Fig. 47.46: Surgical hand piece

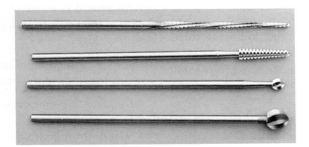

Fig. 47.47: Bone burs

Rongeur Forceps (Fig. 47.41)

- This instrument is used during intraoral surgery as well as afterwards, to remove bone and sharp bone spicules. The ends and sides of the sharp blades become narrow, so that when the handles are pressed, they cut the bone found in between without exerting particular pressure. There is a spring between the handles, which restores the handles to their original position every time pressure is applied for cutting bone
- The most practical rongeur in oral surgery is the Luer–Friedmann, because its blades are both end-cutting and side-cutting.

Uses

- To nibble sharp bony margins following extraction of teeth or surgical procedures
- To peel of thinned out bone present over cystic or tumorous pathologies
- To trim sharp bony edges during alveoloplasty procedures
- It is a delicate instrument, should not be used to remove a large amounts of bone in single bite.

Other modifications

- Luer
- Beyer.

Bone Cutter

Similar to Rongeur forceps as far as working principle is concerned, but more sturdy than Rongeur, shape of the blade is different and have a side cutting action only.

Uses

- To cut sharp bony margins following extractions or surgical procedures
- To cut sharp ridge projections during alveoloplasty procedures.

Chisel and Mallet

- Mallets are instruments with heavy-weighted ends

- The surfaces of the ends are made of lead or of plastic so that some of the shock is absorbed when the mallet strikes the chisel
- The chisels used in oral surgery have different shapes and sizes. Their cutting edges are concave, monobeveled or bibeveled. The bibevel chisel is used for sectioning multi-rooted teeth.

Osteotome

- Similar to chisel but the edges of working tip is bibeveled
- It splits bone rather than cutting or chipping it.

Uses

- Various osteotomy procedures
- Removal/recontouring of bone.

Bone Gouge

- It has a round handle and a blade that has sharp working tip that is concave on inner side.
- Working tip is half round and has a long working area.

Uses

- To make a window in anterior border of maxillary sinus (in Caldwell Luc)
- To remove cancellous bone graft material/ irregular pieces of bone.

Giglis Wire Saw

- It has three components

Wire saw: It is made by twisting a few pieces of wire together so that it acquires a sharp barbed cutting edge.

Handles: At the end of the wire there is a ring to which the hook of the handles can be fitted.

Introducer: When moved to and fro along its long axis, it cuts the bone.

Used in mandiblectomy and maxillectomy procedures.

Surgical Unit and Handpiece

The surgical unit includes the following:

- Surgical micromotor: This is a simple machine with quite satisfactory cutting ability
- Technologically advanced machines, which function with nitrous dioxide or electricity and have a much greater cutting ability than the aforementioned micromotor
- The surgical handpiece is attached to the above unit, includes many types, and is manufactured to suit the needs of oral surgery. Its advantages are as follows:
  - It functions at high speeds and has great cutting ability.
  - It does not emit air into the surgical field.
  - It may be sterilized in the autoclave.
  - The handpiece may receive various cutting instruments.

Bone Burs (Fig. 47.47)

- Burs are rotary instruments that cut the bone made up of stainless steel/carbide and available in different shapes and length
- Sharp carbide burs remove cortical bone efficiently, burs such as No.557/No. 703 fissure bur or No. 8 round bur are used.

Uses

- To aid in bone removal or splitting the tooth during surgical removal of tooth
- To round of sharp margins after extractions/minor surgical procedures and during alveoloplasty
- To make bony window for access to cystic cavities
- To release bony ankylosis
- To perform osteotomy cuts
- To perform resection of maxilla/mandible.

Surgical Saw (Fig. 47.48 to 47.52)

- It gives ease of cutting bone with precision because of different shape/movements of saw
- Unit consists of:
  - Regulator, foot control and cable.
  - Hand piece
    - Electric powered
    - Pneumatic powered (uses compressed air at 90–110 psi pressure)
  - Saw

- In handpieces speed of 10,000—1 lac cpm can be achieved
- Different kinds of saws available for various type of osteotomy
- Sagittal saw moves side to side (5–6° arc), used for wedge/transverse osteotomy
- Oscillating saw oscillates (5–6° arc), used for curved/straight osteotomy
- Reciprocating saw: Moves to and fro (2.4 mm), used for short/long osteotomy.

Bone File (Miller Colbourn) (Fig. 47.53)

- It is used for final smoothening of bony margins before suturing
- It has one long curved working end and another short oval
- Working end has horizontal serrations
- It is used unidirectionally using a "pull" stroke (push stroke causes burnishing and crushing of bone).

Modification: "Miller" bone file

Smith Spreader (Fig. 47.54)

- It has 3 blades that are separated by spring action when the handles are compressed
- Used to separate bony fragments after completion of the osteotomy cuts (in OMFS used to check separation of fragments during downward fracture of maxilla/SSO procedure).

Instruments for Holding Bone

- Crocodile bone holding forceps
- Kochers toothed heavy artery forcep
- Forcep type of towel clip.

Crocodile Bone Holding Foreps

- Named so because of appearance of beaks side ways
- Have long handles as compared to beaks
- Beaks have toothed margin to allow a good grip on the bone
- Has a catch to stabilize the instrument in required position
- Used to hold the bony fragments during manipulation (fracture reduction and fixation/osteotomy/resection procedures)

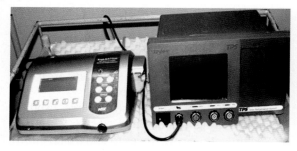

Fig. 47.48: Stryker's set

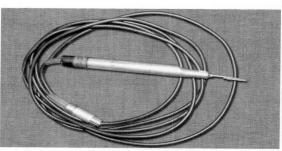

Fig. 47.49: Strikers' handpiece with connecting cable

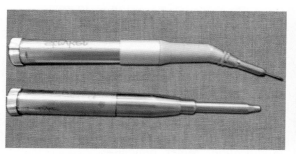

Fig. 47.50: Strikers' handpiece

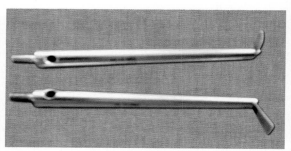

Fig. 47.51: Surgical saw

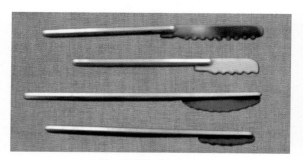

Fig. 47.52: Saw tips

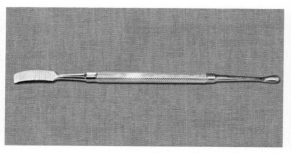

Fig. 47.53: Bone file (bone rasp)

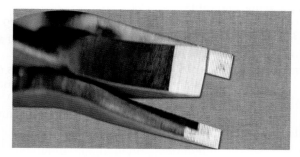

Fig. 47.54: Smith spreader

- When it comes without catch in the handle, called as Sequestrum holding forcep, used to hold sequestrum.

Kochers Toothed Heavy Artery Forceps

Similar to a long heavy artery forcep but it has toothed tips.

Uses
- Specially designed to hold the coronoid process during coronidectomy procedures
- Can be used like other bone holding forceps for stabilization of bony fragments.

Forceps Type of Towel Clip

Can be used for holding the bone piece but not for bigger ones.

Instruments for Providing Suction

Surgical Suction (Fig. 47.55)

- There are a variety of designs and sizes of surgical suctions that are used for removing blood, saliva, and saline solution from the surgical field. Certain types of surgical suctions are designed so that they have several orifices, preventing injury to soft tissues (greatest danger for sublingual mucosa) during the surgical procedure
- The standard surgical suction has a main orifice for suctioning and only one smaller orifice on the handle, for the reasons mentioned above
- This orifice is usually covered when rapid suctioning of blood and saline solution from the surgical field is required.

Instruments for Irrigation

Irrigation Instruments

- Irrigating the surgical field with saline solution during bone removal is necessary and a plastic syringe or a special irrigation system with a steady stream of saline solution may be used for this purpose
- In the first case, the syringe used is large, with a blunt needle that is angled (facilitating irrigation especially in posterior areas) with its end cut off so that it does not damage soft tissues
- In the second case, the special irrigation system is directly connected to the bottle of saline solution, with a small tube. A knob stops the flow of solution.

Instruments to Remove Soft Tissue from Bony Defects

Periapical Curettes (Fig. 47.56)

- These are angled double-ended, spoon-shaped instruments. The most commonly such used instrument is the periapical curette, whose shape facilitates its entry into bone defects and extraction sockets
- The main use of this instrument is the removal of granulation tissue, small cysts, bone chips, foreign bodies, etc.

Volkmann's Bone Scoop

Similar to curette but concavity of the working edge is more pronounced.

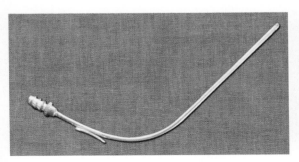

Fig. 47.55: Metal suction tip

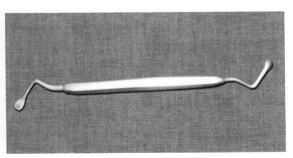

Fig. 47.56: Periapical curettes

Uses
- To collect the contents from sinus tract/fistula/ chronic abscess cavity
- To scrape bony cavities due to cystic/ tumorous/osteomyelic lesions
- To scoop out cancellous bone for grafting procedures
- To introduce graft material or antiseptic powder into the surgical area.

Instruments for Draining an Abscess
- Listers sinus forceps
- Wide bore plastic syringes.

Listers Sinus Forceps (Figs 47.57 and 47.58)
- It has long narrow blades which are serrated transversely for only ½ an inch at the tip
- Tip is rounded and bulbous.
- Instrument does not have a catch.

Uses
- To open an abscess by Hilton's method (Fig. 47.59)
- To dissect out sinus/fistulous tract in soft tissues.

Wide Bore Plastic Syringe
Commonly an 18 gauge needle is used with large plastic syringe to aspirate pus (Fig. 47.60).

Instruments for Grafting Tissues
- Skin graft set
- Instruments for bone grafting.

Skin Graft Set
This contains following instruments:
- Humpy's knife with carbon steel blade used to slice a thin layer of skin (Fig. 47.61)
- Wooden plank, used to stretch skin during harvesting and to keep graft over it for manipulation
- Spreader, used to stretch the harvested graft over wooden plank (Fig. 47.62).

Instruments for Bone Grafting
Bone trephine (Fig. 47.63 and 47.64)
- Specially designed instrument used to obtain small diameter trephines of bone for grafting/ histomorphic purposes
- Has 3 parts
  - Barrel with stands.
  - Piston (working tip has saw)
  - Stylet.

Instruments for Suturing Mucosa
- Needle holder
- Suture needles
- Tissue holding forceps
- Suture cutting scissors
- Binocular loupes with light source.

Needle Holders (Figs 47.65 and 47.66)
- Needle holders are used for suturing the wound. The Mayo-Hegar and Mathieu needle holders are considered suitable for this purpose

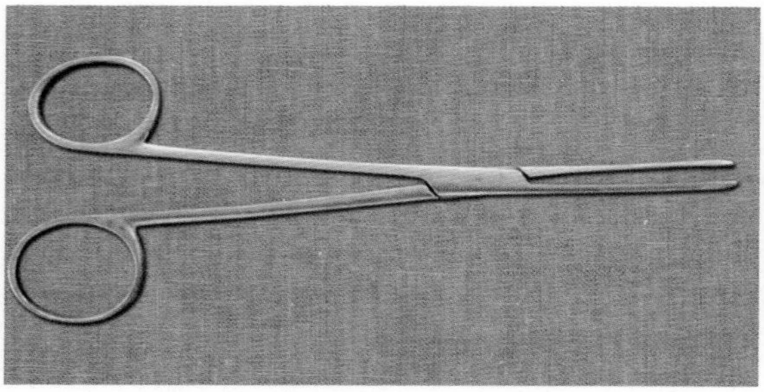

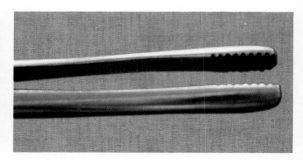

Fig. 47.57: Lister sinus forcep—no locking mechanism

Fig. 47.58: Note that only tip has serration

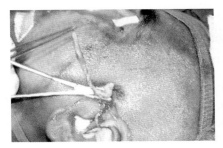

Fig. 47.59: Hiltons method use of listers sinus forceps

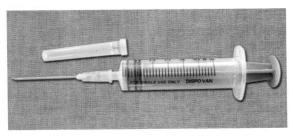

Fig. 47.60: 18 gauge needle with 5 mL syringe

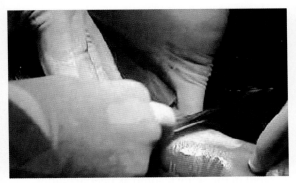

Fig. 47.61: Humpy's knife in use for harvesting

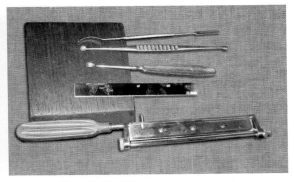

Fig. 47.62: Skin flap harvesting set

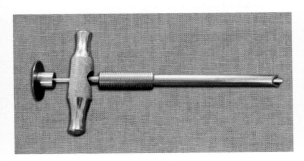

Fig. 47.63: Bone trephine

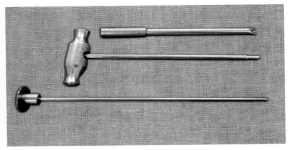

Fig. 47.64: Bone trephine disassembled

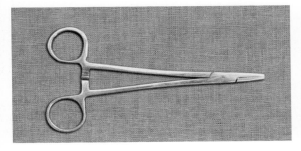

Fig. 47.65: Needle holder

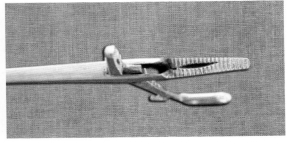

Fig. 47.66: Needle holder—note the vertical groove

- The first type looks similar to a hemostat and is preferred mainly for intraoral placement of sutures
- The hemostat and needle holder have the following differences:
  - The short beaks of the hemostat are thinner and longer compared to those of the needle holder
  - On the needle holder, the internal surface of the short beaks is grooved and cross-hatched, permitting a firm and stable grasp of the needle while the short beaks of the hemostat have parallel grooves which are perpendicular to the long axis of the instrument
  - The needle holder can release the needle with simple pressure, because of the gap in the last step of the locking handle, whereas the hemostat requires a special maneuver, because it does not have that gap in the last step of the locking handle
- The correct way to hold the needle holder is to place the thumb in one ring of the handle and the ring finger in the other. The rest of the fingers are curved around the outside of the rings, while the fingertip of the index finger is placed on the hinge or a little further up, for better control of the instrument.

Suture Needles

Surgical needles have 3 parts:
- Eye – closed (traumatic)
  - Swaged (atraumatic)
- Body/shaft/needle grasping area
  - Cross sectionally:
    - Round
    - Oval
    - Triangular
    - Trapezoidal
  - Longitudinally:
    - Straight
  - Half curved
  - Curved (1/4,1/2,3/8,5/8)
  - Compound curved

- Tip (from extreme tip to max cross section of body)
  - Cutting
  - Round (tapered).

Cutting Needles

- Have at least 2 opposite cutting edges
- Triangular in cross section
- Can be conventional/reverse cutting
- Ideal for suturing keratinized tissue (skin/mucosa).

Round Needles

Used for suturing soft and non keratinized tissues (muscle/fascia/neural sheath).

Suture Cutting Scissors (Fig. 47.67)

Dean's
- They have long delicate handles and a short blade with cutting edge and striations
- Can be—straight/curved, angulated/non angulated
- Held in the same fashion as needle holder.

Binocular Loupes with Light Source (Figs 47.68 and 47.69)

- This system is comprised of binocular loupes, which may be adapted to eyeglass frames or a headband, ensuring good vision of the surgical field
- This system also has a light source that projects intense light into difficult areas of the surgical field (e.g., posterior teeth), where vision by means of standard lighting is not satisfactory.

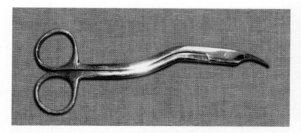

Fig. 47.67: Deans suture cutting scissors

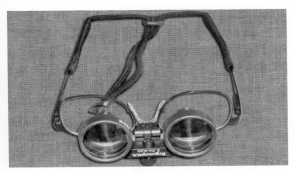

Fig. 47.68: Surgical loops

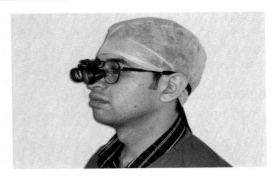

Fig. 47.69: Surgeon with surgical loops

PROCEDURE SPECIFIC INSTRUMENTS OF ORAL AND ORAL AND MAXILLOFACIAL SURGERY

- Diagnostic instruments
- For opening the mouth/keeping the mouth open
- Soft tissue retractors
- Exodontia
- Trauma and orthognathic surgery
- Cleft lip, palate and rhinoplasty.

DIAGNOSTIC INSTRUMENTS

- Mouth mirror
- Explorer/probes
- Tweezers
- Nasal speculum
- Punch biopsy forceps
- Calipers.

Mouth Mirror

- A small circular reflecting mirror
- Can be plane/concave/convex or magniying/non-magnifying
- Handle may be round/octagonal or made up of plastic/stainless steel
- Mirror holding unit can be fixed or removable from handle
- Comes in various sizes of mirror/handle
- Used for visualisation (direct/indirect) and for retracting tongue/cheek.

Explorer/Probes

- A slender stainless steel instrument, single/double ended with a fine flexible sharp working tip
- Working tip may be circular or angulated at an angle to the shank
- Used for exploring sockets/cavity.

Tweezers (Meriam)

- A long forcep with angulated blades
- Serrations on inner side of blade and on the handle
- Can be of self locking variety (specially for introducing medication).

Uses
- To catch loose tooth/bone/suture/wire pieces
- To hold and place cotton ball/gauge piece/medications.

Nasal Speculum (Killien)

- An instrument for examining nasal cavity
- Has 2 semicircular blades (with blunt edge) which flares at their distal end
- Two curved handles with spring.

Punch Biopsy Forceps

- Has got a long arm at the end of which there is a small blade with sharp margins
- Two handles, straight and oval with spring action

- Blade remains open in normal position and on activation of instrument gets fitted inside the groove of the arm and cuts the small pieces of tissue present in between

Calipers (Castroviejo) (Fig. 47.70)

- An instrument with two adjustable legs, a key and a curved scale
- Used for measurement purposes (specially for TMJ Ankylosis, orthognathic, distraction and grafting cases).

FOR OPENING THE MOUTH/ KEEPING THE MOUTH OPEN (FIG. 47.71 TO 47.73)

- Mouth gag
- Mouth prop.

Mouth Gag

An instrument for opening the mouth forcibly.

Heisters (Fig. 47.71)

Has two serrated blades that are applied between upper and lower posterior teeth and separated by turning a key.

Fergusson and Doyen's (Fig. 47.72)

Handle has a catch to fix the instrument at required opening.

Uses

- To force the mouth open when there is trismus due to infection/muscle spasm/hemarthosis of TMJ
- To give post op active jaw physiotherapy after surgery for TMJ ankylosis/SMF
- When using these instruments care must be taken to prevent luxation of teeth/TMJ.

Mouth Prop (Fig. 47.73)

- Used to keep the mouth open during any surgical procedure
- Consists of rubber blocks having concave surface on either side to fit in between upper and lower teeth
- Usually there are 3 or 4 blocks of varying vertical height arranged in ascending order and connected by a chain
- Block is placed more to posterior of mouth.

SOFT TISSUE RETRACTORS

- Tongue retractors
- Cheek retractors
- Soft tissue flap retractors.

Tongue Retractors

- Mouth mirror
- Tongue depressor

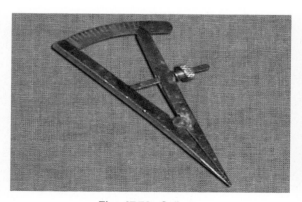

Fig. 47.70: Calipers

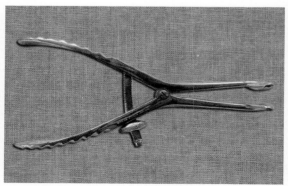

Fig. 47.71: Mouth gag—Heisters

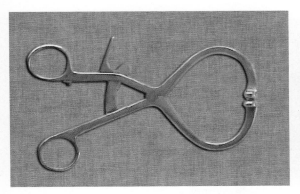

Fig. 47.72: Mouth gag—Fergusson and doyen's

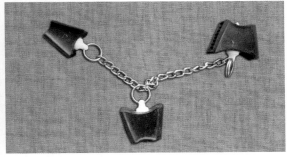

Fig. 47.73: Mouth prop

- A L shaped instrument with broad smooth blade
- Used for depressing/retracting during examination/surgical procedures
- Weiders retractor
  - A broad heart shaped retractor, serrated on one side to engage and retract the tongue firmly
- Tongue forceps
  - Swab holder variety (Young's)
    - Similar to swab holder but no fenestrations on the blade and serrations are more coarser
    - May cause damage to tongue
- Towel clip variety
  - Similar to forcep variety of towel clip but tip of the blades are not sharp
  - Better than previous variety.

Uses

- To hold and retract the tongue during tongue surgery
- To prevent tongue fall and airway obstruction in unconscious patient.

Cheek Retractors (Figs 47.74 to 47.76)

- Mouth mirror
- Tongue depressor
- Middeldorpf retractor

- Kilner's retractor (Fig. 47.74)
  - A broad curved bladed retractor may be single/double ended used to retract and hold the cheek during surgical procedures
- Photo cheek retractor (Fig. 47.75)
  - A self retaining retractor made up of autoclavable polycarbonate plastic
  - Easy to place, comes in different sizes for child and adult
  - Useful for photography and oral surgical procedures
- Austins retractor (Fig. 47.76)
  - A right angled retractor with one concave surface and a curved small tip at end
  - Used for retracting cheek and mucoperiosteal flap
- Minnesota retractor
  - A broad angulated, offset designed retractor used for retracting cheek and mucoperiosteal flap.

Soft Tissue Flap Retractors

- Woodson periosteal elevator
- No.9 Molts periosteal elevator
- Howarth periosteal elevator
- Austins retractor
- Minnesota retractor
- Seldin retractor
  - Similar to periosteal elevator but broader and leading edge is dull

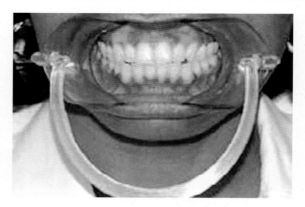

Fig. 47.74: Kilner's retractor

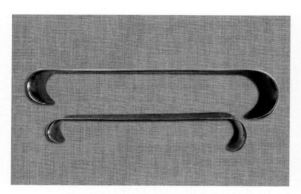

Fig. 47.75: Photo cheek retractor

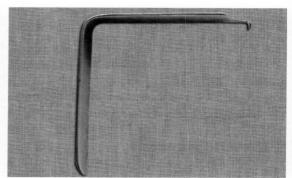

Fig. 47.76: Austin's retractor

– Provides broader retraction and increased visualization
– Used for retracting (not elevating) soft tissue flap

INSTRUMENTS FOR EXODONTIA

• Local anesthetic instruments
• Periosteal elevators
• Dental elevators
• Dental forceps.

Local Anesthetic Instruments

• Needles
• Syringes
• Cartridges containing anesthetic solution

Needles

• Has 5/3 parts
• Size of the needle
• Diameter of lumen 20–25 gauge
• Length 0.5–4 inches
• Made up of stainless steel/iridoplatinum
• Disposable needles with plastic hub ensures sterility and sharpness for each patient and saves time and work.

Syringes
Parts

• Thumb ring
• Swivel finger bar (for flexible control of syringe)
• Spool finger grip (for positive grip for aspiration)

- Spring lock (centers and holds cartridge in syringe)
- Harpoon on piston rod
- Open side (for loading and unloading)
- Chrome plated barrel
- Syringe adaptor.

Classification of Syringes

According to form
- Cartridge type
- Noncartridge type.

According to nozzle
- Luer lock
- Friction lock.

According to material
- Glass
- Metal
- Plastic.

According to size—3/5/10 cc/mL

Cartridge type syringes
- Small syringes into which a hermetically sealed cartridge (cont anesthetic solution) can be fitted
- Advantages—ensures sterility and uniformity of concentration of anesthetic solution and saves time
- Disadvantages—leakage during injection, cartridge breakage and surface deposits
- Types
  - Conventional aspirating
  - Self aspirating
  - Disposable aspirating
  - Jet injectors (syrijet)
  - Periodontal ligament injectors.

Conventional aspirating syringe
- Most commonly used syringes in dental office
- It is a side loading metal cartridge syringe which accepts hermatically sealed 1.8 mL glass cartridge.

Self aspirating syringe: This syringe relies on elasticity of rubber diaphragm of the anesthetic cartridge to produce negative pressure for aspiration.

Disposable aspirating syringe: Composed of a sterile disposable needle syringe barrel combination and a reusable plastic, barbed piston section.

Jet injectors (Syrijet): Spring loaded instrument accepting 1.8 mL cartridge, used to produce infiltration/topical anesthesia.

Periodontal ligament injector: Developed for intra-ligamentary injection, uses standard cartridge and equipped with pistol grip mechanism to express solution under high pressure

Periosteal Elevators

- Moons probe
  - A thin flat instrument with small working tip at right angle to handle
  - Tip is narrow and sharp
  - Used to separate mucoperiosteum around the tooth prior to extraction
- Woodson periosteal elevator
- Molt No.9 periosteal elevator
- Howarth elevator.

Dental Elevators

An instrument having blade that engages tooth/root and elevates them from the socket, also expands the alveolar bone

Indications
- To luxate the teeth prior to forcep application
- To remove root remnants/interradicular bone
- To remove teeth which cannot be engaged by forcep beaks (impacted/malposed/badly carious teeth).

Components
- *Handle:* Usually large in size to facilitate a good grip, may be at a line or at right angle to shank (cross bar/T – bar)
- *Shank :* Should be strong enough to withstand and transmit forces
- *Blade :* Its working tip transmits forces to tooth/root/bone, can vary in size and shape.

Classification: According to their working principle:
Lever principle—
- Straight elevator
- Crane pick elevator

Wheel and axel—
- Potts elevator
- Winter elevator
- Cryers
- Winter cryers

Wedge principle—
- Apexo elevators
- Apical elevators

According to their form:
Straight—
- Straight elevator
- Coupland elevator

Angular—
- Hockey stick
- Warwick James
- Miller elevator

Cross bar—
- Potts elevator
- Winter elevators
- Cryer
- Winter cryer

According to their function:
Tooth elevators—
- Straight
- Coupland
- Miller
- Potts
- Warwick james
- Winter elevators

Root elevators—
- Cryers
- Winter cryers
- Crane pick
- Apexo elevators

Apical elevators—
- Root tip pick.

Straight Elevator (London Hospital Pattern/ Coleman) (Figs 47.77 and 47.78)
- Having a straight blade with one convex surface and another flat serrated working surface
- Handle may be serrated
- Most commonly used elevator to luxate teeth.

Coupland Retractor (Gouge)
- Having a straight blade with one convex surface and another concave working surface
- Used to elevate teeth (smaller one for unerupted tooth whereas larger one for widely spaced teeth).

Miller Elevator
- Slight curve at end of shank which allows blade to be inserted into soft maxillary bone between distal root of second molar and crown of third molar
- Used specially for impacted third molar.

Potts Elevator
- A variant of Miller elevator which is smaller and weaker and has a cross bar
- Use, same as that of Miller.

Hockey Stick Elevator
- A variant of London hospital pattern straight elevator which has blade at an angulation to shank
- Used for maxillary molars.

Warwick James Elevator
- Similar to hockey stick elevator but smaller and more delicate
- No serrations on blade
- Used for maxillary molars.

Winter Elevators (Cross Bar/T Bar) (Fig. 47.79)
- Handle is at right angle to shank
- Working tip is at an angle to the shank
- Blade has two surfaces, one convex and another flat working surface
- Used for mandibular molars.

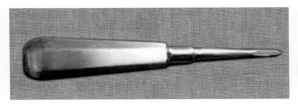

Fig. 47.77: Straight elevator

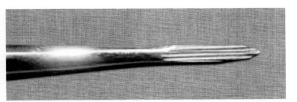

Fig. 47.78: Elevator blade close view

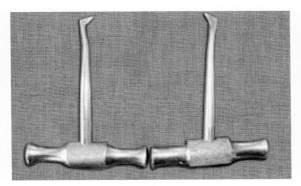

Fig. 47.79: Winters cross bar elevators

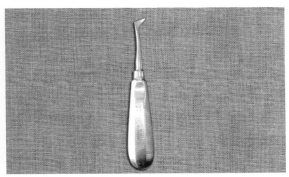

Fig. 47.80: Cryers elevators

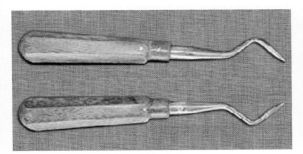

Fig. 47.81: Apexo elevators

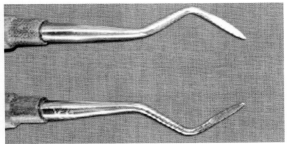

Fig. 47.82: Apexo elevators tip close view

Cryer Elevator (Fig. 47.80)

- A elevator with a triangular blade
- Working tip is angulated
- Has two surfaces one convex and another flat working surface
- Used for extraction of root stumps of mandibular molars (when one root is moved out and another left behind).

Crane Pick Elevator

- A variant of straight elevator with angulated sharp blade (in vertical direction)

- Used as a lever to elevate a broken root from tooth socket
- Usually necessary to drill a hole into the root into which the tip of blade is inserted and using buccal plate as a fulcrum, tooth is elevated.

Apexo (Wedge) Elevator (Figs 47.81 and 47.82)

- Having a biangulated sharp working tip
- Working surface is grooved
- Used to elevate root pieces by wedging in between root and bone surface.

Root Tip Pick

- A delicate instrument with sharp, pointed angulated working tip
- Used to tease small root tips from their sockets.

Rules for Using Elevators

- Never use the adjacent teeth/buccal/lingual plate as fulcrum
- Always use finger guard to protect the soft tissues incase elevator slips
- Support the shank with index finger to control forces
- Always elevate from mesial and buccal side.

Possible Complications of Elevators

- If used without caution it may damage/extract adjacent tooth fracture alveolar process/maxilla/mandible
- Slip and perforate soft tissues/vessels/nerves
- Penetrate/force a root or third molar into maxillary antrum
- Force apical 1/3 of third molar root into mandibular canal/submandibular/pterygomandibular space.

Dental Forceps

- Instruments designed to deliver the tooth from socket
- Parts—handle, hinge and beaks.

Handle

- Usually of adequate size so that can deliver sufficient pressure and leverage
- Have a serrated surface to allow a positive grip and prevent slippage
- Usually straight but may be curved on occasion
- Handles are held in two ways
- Maxillary forceps are held with palm underneth the forceps
- Mandibular forceps are held with the palm on top of forceps.

Hinge

- Connects handle to the beak and transfers and concentrates forces to the beaks
- Two kinds of forceps according to hinge

- American—hinge and handles in horizontal direction
- English—hinge and handles in vertical direction (with hand held in vertical direction).

Beaks

- Designed to adapt closely to tooth root at CEJ (not crown), thus there are different kind of beaks for single/two/three rooted teeth
- Width of beak may vary, narrow for incisors and broader for molars
- Usually angled so that can be placed parallel to long axis of tooth with handle in a comfortable position
- For maxillary forcep—beaks parallel to handle
- For mandibular forcep—beaks perpendicular to handle
- Have serrations on inner aspect to allow a better grip.

Maxillary Anterior Forceps

Maxillary Universal Forceps (No.150)

- Straight when viewed from above and slightly curved when viewed from side
- Beaks curve to meet at the tip
- Its modification – No.150A in which parallel beaks that do not touch each other are useful for maxillary premolar teeth.

Straight maxillary forceps (No.1) (Figs 47.83 and 47.84)

- Used for maxillary incisors and canines (more comfortable than No.150)
- Beaks are found on the same level as the handles, and the beaks are concave and not pointed.

Maxillary Posterior Forceps (Figs 47.85 to 47.89)

No. 53 forceps (L and R)

- Have two unidentical beaks—one rounded with inner concave surface for palatal root and other with pointed design to fit into the buccal bifurcation
- Have offset design to reach posterior aspect of mouth and remain in comfortable position.

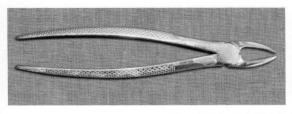

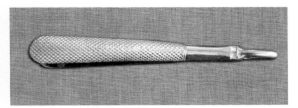

Fig. 47.83 and 47.84: Maxillary straight forceps

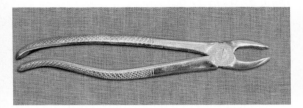

Fig. 47.85: Maxillary posterior forceps

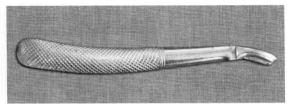

Fig. 47.86: Maxillary posterior forceps

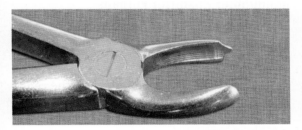

Fig. 47.87: Maxillary posterior forceps tip

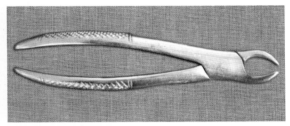

Fig. 47.88: Upper cowhorns

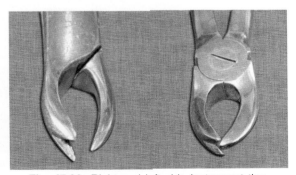

Fig. 47.89: Right and left side instrument tips

No. 88 Forceps (Upper Cowhorns) (Fig. 47.88)

- Have unidentical beaks, one of which
- Has a single pointed tip and the other has bifid pointed tip
- Single pointed tip engages the buccal furcation and other engages the palatal root
- Used when there is extensive destruction of crown but roots are not separated
- They may crush large amounts of alveolar bone.

No. 210 S Forceps (Fig. 47.90)

- Broad smooth beaks (not pointed) that offset from handle
- Useful for maxillary second and third molar that have single conical root.

Maxillary Root Forceps (Figs 47.91 to 47.92)

(No. 286 forceps)

- Offset molar forceps with very narrow beaks
- Used primarily for broken maxillary molar roots (can be used for narrow premolars).

Maxillary Primary Tooth Forceps (No.150 S)

Smaller version of No.150 forceps used as a universal primary tooth forceps.

Mandibular Anterior Forceps

Mandibular Universal Forceps (NO. 151) (Figs 47.93 to 47.94)

- Handle similar to No. 150 forceps but beaks are pointed inferiorly
- Beaks are smooth, relatively narrow and meet only at the tip
- Its modification – No. 151. A forceps in which parallel beaks that donot touch each other are useful for mandibular premolar teeth.

Mandibular Posterior Forceps

No. 17 Forceps

- Straight handled and beaks are set obliquely downward
- Beaks have bilateral pointed tips in the centre to adapt into bifurcation of molar teeth.

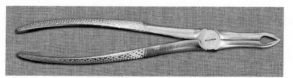

Fig. 47.90: No. 210 S forceps

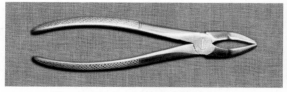

Fig. 47.91: Bayonet shaped forceps

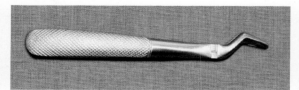

Fig. 47.92: Bayonet shaped forceps

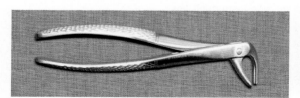

Fig. 47.93: Mandibular anterior forceps

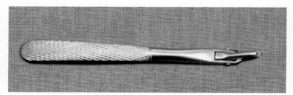

Fig. 47.94: Mandibular molar forceps

No. 222 Forceps

- Similar in design to No. 17 forceps but beaks are shorter and do not have pointed tips
- Useful for molar teeth which have fused, conical shaped roots and erupting third molars.

No. 23 Forceps (Lower Cowhorn) (Figs 47.95 to 47.96)

- Have identical short, heavy, round pointed beaks which do not meet
- Forceps grip the tooth at the furcation (tooth is elevated by squeezing the handles)
- Used to remove grossly carious mandibular molars with extensive destruction of crown.

Mandibular Primary Tooth Forceps (No. 151 S)

Smaller version of No. 151 forceps and used as a universal forcep for mandibular primary teeth.

American Pattern Forceps (Figs 47.97 and 47.98)

- American-style forceps differ from the afore-mentioned forceps in that their hinges have a vertical direction.

- Their use is limited, because large amounts of force can be generated during extraction with this type of forceps, so that if the bone is not elastic, there is increased risk of fracture of the alveolar bone.

Mandibular Root Forceps (Fig. 47.99)

- Have identical slender beaks that are closed
- Beaks are longer to take a deep grip on root stump
- Used for root stumps of all mandibular teeth

INSTRUMENTS FOR TRAUMA AND ORTHOGNATHIC SURGERY

- Wiring set
- Retractors
- Strippers
- Bone holding forceps
- Bone hook/ elevators
- Bone awl
- Chisel/osteotome
- Bone forceps for manipulation
- Bone plating instruments.

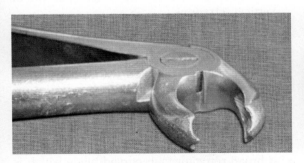

Fig. 47.95: Mandibular molar forceps

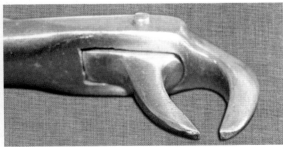

Fig. 47.96: Mandibular cowhorns forceps

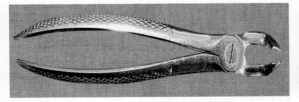

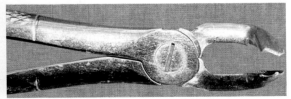

Figs 47.97 and 47.98: American pattern molar forcep

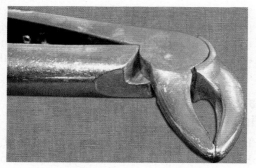

Fig. 47.99: Mandibular root forceps

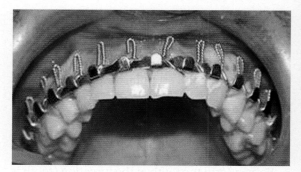

Fig. 47.100: Erich arch bar *in situ*

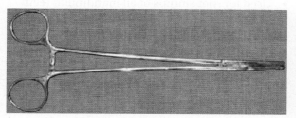

Fig. 47.101: Wire twister forceps type

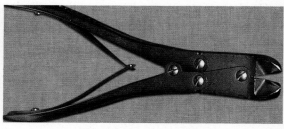

Fig. 47.102: Wire cutter

Wiring Set

Arch Bar (Erich) (Fig. 47.100)

- A prefabricated thin stainless steel strip that has hooks incorporated on it
- Malleable and can be adapted to contour of arch and fixed to teeth by wires

Uses

- To stabilize dentoalveolar fixation
- To stabilize mandibular/maxillary fracture
- To provide means of IMF
- Other prefabricated arch bars, Winter, Niro, Jelenko.

Wire

Usually a 26 gauge wire spool is used.

Uses

- To stabilize dentoalveolar fractures
- To perform IMF
- To splint the arch bar to teeth
- Fixation of fractures by trans osseous wiring
- Indirect fixation of fractures by suspension wiring.

Wire Holder/Twister (Fig. 47.101)

Two types:
- Forceps type—similar to needle holder except that it has heavy broad tip which is devoid of vertical serrations
- Pencil type.

Wire Cutter (Fig. 47.102)

It may be a simple/TC coated/with spring action/heavy duty.

Retractors (Figs 47.103 to 47.106)

Chin Retractor (Fig. 47.103)

- A broad retractor with curved blade which is bifurcated at the end having three small blades
- Used during chin surgery to provide anterior labial tissue retraction.

Channel Retractor (Fig. 47.104)

- A right angle retractor with a small angulated tip
- Used to reflect anterior/lateral soft tissues during mandibular lower border surgeries.

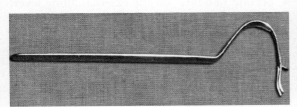

Fig. 47.103: Chin retractor

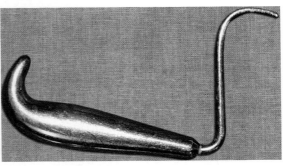

Fig. 47.104: Channel retractor

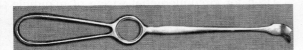

Fig. 47.105: Obwegessor ramus retractor

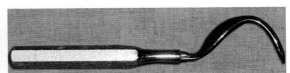

Fig. 47.106: Orbital floor retractor

Rayne Mandibular Connector

A flat retractor with angulated tip.

Obwegessor Ramus Retractor (Fig. 47.105)

- Similar to langanbacks retractor except that the edge of retracting blade is forked forming a V shaped notch (to engage anterior border of ramus)
- Used to retract soft tissues along anterior border of ramus during saggital split/ramus osteotomy/coronidectomy procedures.

Condyle retractors

- Special retractor that have an appearance similar to tongue depressor but are narrower
- Tip of blade has C shape hook that is slipped under condylar head to retract and protect medial soft tissue.

Orbital Floor Retractor (Rowe) (Fig. 47.106)

- A retractor with spoon shaped curved blades
- Used to retract globe during surgery in lateral/infra orbital/medial wall of the orbit.

Strippers

Mandibular Border Stripper

- Its working edge resembles one side of Howarth's elevator
- Used to elevate mucoperiosteum from lower border of mandible.

Ramus Stripper

- Blade is angulated for easy access to anterior border of ramus and coronoid process
- Blade is furcated at working end (the notch of the blade ensures stability of instrument).
- Used during angle surgeries, ramus osteotomy (SSO) and coronoidectomy.

Bone Holding Forceps

- Crocodile bone holding forceps
- Kochers bone holding forceps
- Forcep type of towel clip
- Harrison mandble holding forceps
- Rowes modified Harrisons mandible holding forceps
  - (Beaks having sharp tips to hold bone firmly and provided with a key).

Bone Hook/Elevators

Poswillow Zygoma (Malar) Hook

A harp curved hook with a broad handle used to elevate fractured zygoma through percutaneous approach.

Stacey Zygomatic Hook

It is also use to elevate fractured bone.

Bristows Zygomatic Elevator

- Has a flat blade on its working end for insertion medially to zygomatic arch and body
- One handle for grasping
- Indicated for reducing ZMC fracture, arch fracture thru Gillies temporal aproach
- Needs skull as a fulcrum therefore should be used with care.

Rowes Zygomatic Elevator (Figs 47.107 and 47.108)

- Has a flat border on its working end for insertion medially to zygomatic arch and body

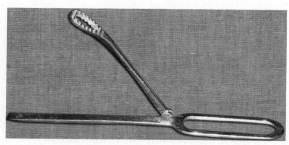

Fig. 47.107: Rowes modified Bristows elevator

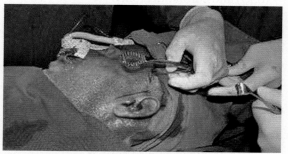

Fig. 47.108: Rowes modified Bristows elevator in use

- Two handles for grasping
- One handle is in direct line with working end (used for stabilization)
- Second handle is on the external lifting lever, its length is almost equal to that of working blade (used for activation)
- Indication is same as that for Bristos elevator but it is more safe and effective.

Bone AWL

- An instrument with thin long arm with a key at the end of arm
- Working tip is sharp and pointed
- Used for circumferential wiring of mandible and zygoma.

Chisel/Osteotome

Nasal Wall Guarded Osteotome

- Has a flat thin blade with sharp edge, which is having a small guard at corner
- Used to separate nasal floor from lateral nasal wall in maxillary osteotomy.

Nasal Rasp

- Has a flat thin blade with sharp edge, and a slit that engages anterior nasal spine
- Used to separate nasal septum and vomer from nasal floor in maxillary osteotomy.

Tessier Pterygoid Plate Osteotome

These are curved osteotomes used to separate maxilla from pterygoid plates.

Bone Forceps for Manipulation/Disimpaction (Figs 47.109 to 47.112)

Rowes Maxillary Disimpaction Forcep (Fig. 47.109)

- Consists of a straight unpadded blade and a curved padded blade
- Unpadded blade is passed up in nostril and padded one enters the mouth and grips the maxilla
- Operator should stand behind the patient and grasp each forceps for manipulation.

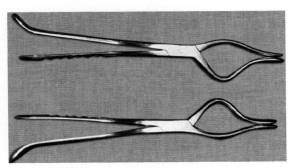

Fig. 47.109: Rowes maxillary disimpaction forceps

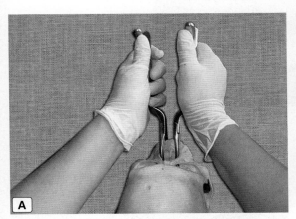

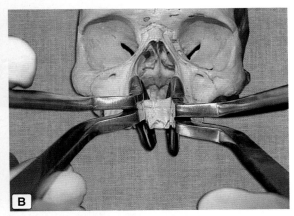

Figs 47.110A and B: Method of using disimpaction forcep

Uses
- To disimpact maxilla in fresh Le Fort I fracture and malunited fracture (Fig. 47.110)
- To check free movements of maxilla after Le Fort I osteotomy

Hayton William Maxillary Forceps (Fig. 47.111)
- Has to widely divergent curved beaks that engage the maxilla behind the tuberosity
- Usually used in conjuction with Rowes disimpaction forceps to mobilize the maxilla (Fig. 47.112).

Tessier Maxillary Mobilizer

An instrument with curved beaks, used to mobilize maxilla (by forward traction) after its disimpaction by Rowes maxillary disimpaction forcep.

Walsham's Nasal Wall Forceps
- Used to manipulate the fractured nasal fragments
- Has a unpadded and padded blade that are curved
- The unpadded blade is passed in the nostrils and the nasal bone and the associated fragment of the frontal process of maxilla are secured between the padded blade externally and unpadded internally, the fragments are then manipulated in their correct position.

Ash nasal septum forceps (Fig. 47.113)
- Used to align the nasal septum and reduce the fracture of nasal bone
- Has to identical straight blades that are close
- Blades are passed on either side of nasal septum and vomer and perpendicular plate of ethmoid are ironed out.

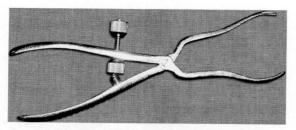

Fig. 47.111: Hayton William maxillary forceps

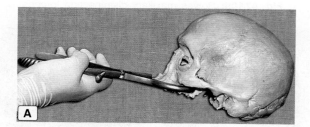

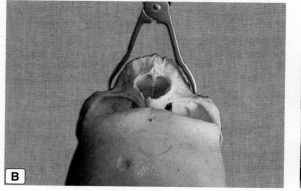

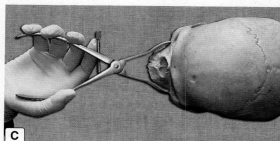

Figs 47.112A to C: Method of using Hayton William maxillary forceps

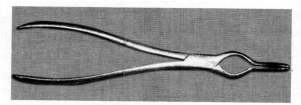

Fig. 47.113: Ash nasal septum forceps

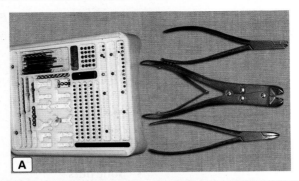

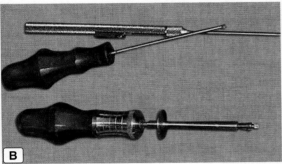
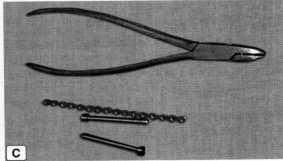

Figs 47.114A to C: Bone plating kit with plates, drivers, and screws

Bone Plating Instruments (Fig. 47.114)

Drill bits
- Made up of stainless steel/titanium
- Available in 1/1.5/2 mm diameter.

Drill guide: Transbuccal device.

Miniplates (Noncompression)
- Made up of stainless steel/Ti
- Available in various sizes and form
- Thicknes—0.9 mm
- Width—6 mm
- Diameter of hole—1.5/2/2.5 mm
- Bevel of hole—at 30°
- Length—2/3/4/5/6 holes with or without gap
- Various forms—orbital/chin/nose/L/I/T shaped
- High elasticity of the material tolerates deformation in all 3 planes so that exact adaptation is possible.

Plate bending forceps: This plier allows the plates to be adapted over margins and surfaces (by virtue of special indentation in the plate).

Modeling lever: Similar to plate bending forceps in action but it has got holding pins inside the beaks.

Plate holding forceps: Used to hold the plate during drilling and screw placement.

Mini screws (Monocortical)
- It is self tapping cortical screws
- Length—5–15 mm
- Screw thread diameter—1.5/2/2.5 mm
- Thread core diameter—0.4 mm lesser than that of thread diameter
- Diameter of screw head—2.8 mm
- One turn of the screw corresponds to 1 mm penetration into the bone
- Screw gauge
- Depth gauge.

Screw holding forceps: It has got spring action, used to hold the screw

Screw driver: Two kinds:
- Ordinary
- Self holding (it can hold as well as drive the screw).

INSTRUMENTS FOR CLEFT SURGERY (FIGS 47.115 TO 47.121)

For Palatoplasty

- Jaboma elevator
- Flat plastic elevator

For Rhinoplasty

- Septal holding forceps
- Aufreez retractor
- Kilner's ala retractor

Sets of Necessary Instruments

For practical reasons, sterilized and packaged full sets of instruments for the most common surgical procedures must always be available. These sets include:

Set for Simple Tooth Extraction

- Local anesthesia syringe, needle and ampule.
- Periosteal elevator
- Retractor or mouth mirror
- Extraction forceps
-        (depending on the tooth to be removed)
- Surgical or anatomic forceps
- Elevators
- Sterile gauze
- Periapical curette
- Suction tip
- Towel clamp
- Needle holder.

Set for Surgical Tooth Extraction/Impaction

- Local anesthesia syringe, needle, and ampule
- Scalpel and blade
- Periosteal elevators
- Elevators
- Bone chisel
- Mallet
- Rongeur forceps
- Bone file
- Periapical curette
- Bone burs
- Hemostat
- Retractors
- Needle holder
- Surgical forceps and anatomic forceps
- Scissors
- Towel clamps
- Disposable plastic syringe
- Suction tip
- Straight handpiece
- Bowl for saline solution
- Sutures
- Sterile gauze.

Set of Instruments for Surgical Biopsy (Bone and Soft Tissue)

- Local anesthesia syringe, needle, and ampule
- Scalpel and blade

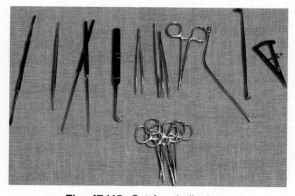

Fig. 47.115: Set for cheiloplasty

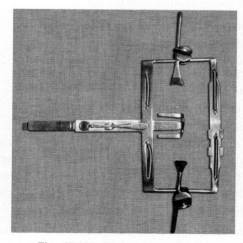

Fig. 47.116: Dingman mouth gag

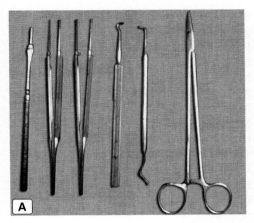
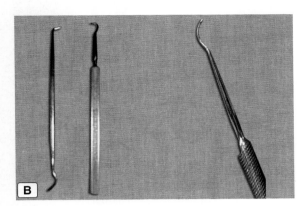

Fig. 47.117: Palatoplasty set

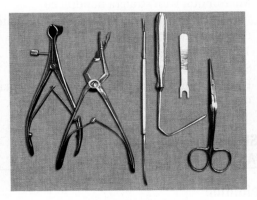

Fig. 47.118: Rhinoplasty set

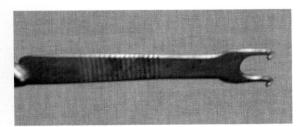

Fig. 47.119: Nasal septum holder

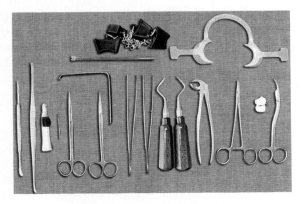

Fig. 47.120: Set for impaction

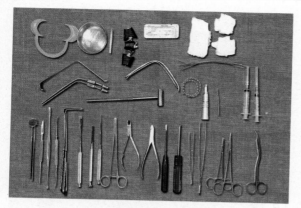

Fig. 47.121: Trauma set

- Periosteal elevator
- Scissors
- Surgical forceps and anatomic forceps
- Periapical curette
- Needle holder
- Hemostats
- Rongeur forceps
- Towel clamps
- Suction tip
- Sutures
- Sterile gauze
- Retractors.

Set of Instruments for Incision and Drainage of Abscess

- Local anesthesia syringe, needle, and ampule
- Scalpel and blade
- Hemostats
- Surgical and anatomic forceps
- Scissors
- Needle holder
- Suction tip
- Towel clamps
- Sutures
- Sterilized Penrose rubber drain 1/4 in
- Sterile gauze.

Trauma Kit Tray (Fig. 47.121)

- 2% lignocaine injection with 1:200000 adrenaline

- 2 mL and 5 mL disposable syringes with 26 gauge needle.
- Photo cheek retractor
- Mouth prop
- Mouth mirror and probe
- Adson's toothed and non-toothed forceps
- No.3 Bard Parker handle with no. 15 blade
- Moltz no. 9 periosteal elevator
- Howarth's periosteal elevator
- Tongue depressor
- Langenback retractors
- Lower border channel retractor
- Chisel
- Mallet
- Osteotome
- Metal suction tips no. 2-4
- Micromotor with straight handpiece
- 2.0 mm titanium mini plates, locking plates, three dimensional plates
- Titanium plating kit
- Suture material: 4-0 vicryl
- Dean's Suture cutting scissors and Mayo Hegard needle holder.

USE OF DRAINS IN ORAL AND MAXILLOFACIAL SURGERY

Definition

Drain is defined as a channel by which surplus liquid is drained or gradually carried off.

It is an appliance or piece of material that acts as a channel for escape of fluid.

Drains inserted after surgery help the wound to heal faster and assist in preventing infection.

Rationale

Two types of drains are:
- Prophylactic drains
- Therapeutic drains.

Prophylactic Drains

A drain placed at the end of an operative procedure to prevent accumulation of fluids.

Thought to aid in the detection of fuild accumulation or leakage specially from anastomosed breakdown.

Therapeutic Drains

A drain placed to evacuate an existing collection of pus or to promote escape of fluids already accumulated.

These drains are placed surgically or under radiological guidance.

Mechanism

Two mechanisms are:
- Open drains
- Closed drains

Open Drains

These drain freely to the exterior and not into the reservoir.

There is a risk of bacteria and other organisms ascending along the drain into the cavity being drained.

Open drains such as penrose or corrugated drain can be useful in certain situations. They are softer than tube drains, more comfortable for the patient and less likely to get blocked.

Closed Drains

Allow fluid to drain externally into a sealed container and offer a number of advantages over open drains.

Lower risk of infections when compared with open drains. Protect patient's skin by keeping fluid away from it, easier to care for and provide an accurate assessment of fluid drainage.

Principle

The simplest and most effective method of drainage is to bring the cavity to be drained to the surface. But this is not always possible, alternatively an artificial drain is passed down to the cavity to be drained.

Advantages

- Drainage of the collected fluids removes the nidus for the infection
- It monitors the future development of the complications like hemorrhage or leakage from the suture line
- Removes the separating fluid from the cavity, so that raw surfaces can collapse and come into contact which will enhance the rapid healing.

Disadvantages

- Forms a portal of entry for the bacteria
- Delays the healing
- Can break down suture lines
- Initiates the tissue reaction
- Gets sealed within 6 hours.

Sites of Drain Placement

Area	Preferable drain
Subcutaneous	Gauze wicks, corrugated sheet, glove drain, soft tube drain
Subfascial	Tube drain
Intramuscular	Tube drain
Cysts	Closed tube drain
Abscess	Corrugated rubber drain

Drain Placement

The drain used should be:
- Soft, so as not to erode the surrounding tissues
- Smooth, so as not to permit fibrin to cling to it
- Preferably radiopaque
- Of a material that will not disintegrate and leave foreign bodies in the wound
- Brought out through a separate stab wound and fixed properly
- Nonirritant
- The stab wound that gives access to the drainage cavity should be large enough to permit free drainage

- Drain must be placed in the dependent position
- Proper daliy dressing of the drainage site should be done to prevent infection
- When prosthesis is present, closed tube system should be used to prevent infection
- Should not damage the nerve or blood vessel
- Inner end should not be placed near the suture lines.

TYPES OF DRAINS

Cotton Gauze

Acts as a drain by capillary action. Once it becomes saturated, acts as a plug rather than a drain. So should be changed twice daily or every 24 hours.

Uses

To pack a cavity to prevent its closure and to allow healing from floor or to control diffuse oozing.

Advantages

Acts as a temporary drainage.

Disadvantages

- Soaked rapidly
- Sealed within 6 hours by fibrin network
- When soaked it acts as a moist channel for the penetration of bacteria
- When a soaked gauze is removed, it is often followed by a gush of accumulated fluid from the cavity
- When a pack is left in contact with the raw surfaces, it damages the raw surfaces as it becomes adherent to it.

Wicks

Formed from threads of ligatures or suture material twisted together or bound loosely.

Disadvantages

- Becomes soaked by fluid
- Can adhere to the surface
- Requires frequent change as it becomes ineffective due to soaked fluid

- When made of folded gauze, it swells when it becomes soaked which will obstruct the tract.

Glove Rubber Drain

A strip of glove rubber made of latex is used to drain the superficial dead space. However it is a poor drain and gets blocked easily, but it is least irritant.

Uses

- To drain dead space after removal of large subcutaneous lipoma, sebaceous cyst
- After thyroidectomy.

Disadvantages

Drains only deeper tissue since its surface sticks to the raw area.

Red Rubber Corrugated Drain (Fig. 47.122 to 47.126)

Made up of red rubber available in the form of unsterile sheets, from which the strips required length and breadth are cut and sterilized by autoclaving.

Advantages

- Drainage of fluid occurs along the grooves of the drain so less chances of blockage
- Used only when there is minimal amount of discharge.

Disadvantages

- If used for a prolonged period and removed at a time, then the track will heal from superficial and deep aspects and the middle part of the track remains infected which leads to sinus formation or pocket formation
- Might be sucked into the wound if not fixed properly to the surface.

Uses

- Drainage of large abscess cavity
- Drainage of subcutaneous tissue after removal of multiple enlarged nodes in neck, etc.

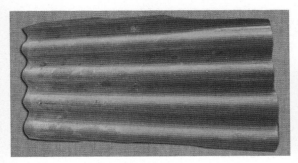

Fig. 47.122: Rubber drain

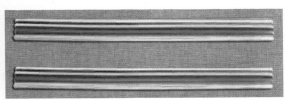

Fig. 47.123: Transparent disposable drain (pre sterilized)

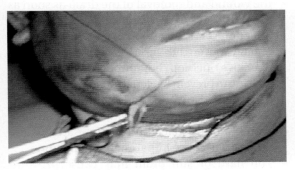

Fig. 47.124: Drain placement

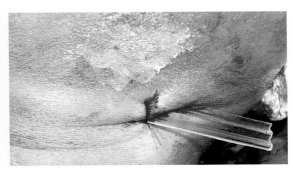

Fig. 47.125: Drain *in situ*

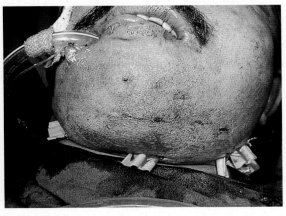

Fig. 47.126: Multiple drain *in situ* in case of Ludwig's angina

Tube Drain

When the fluid enters the tube, it can be guided into a collecting apparatus.

Advantages

Forms the closed drainage system so that the raw surface cannot be contaminated due to entry of bacteria.

Disadvantages

- Drains only in the direction of gravity
- Cannot drain viscous fluid
- If tube is too thin, the force of capillarity tends to retard the free flow of fluid through it
- When continuous negative suction is applied to a tube drain, the tissue is drawn into the inner hole
- Drains the fluid only when the tube is larger, so fluid can be replaced by the air.

Catheters

(Red rubber catheter, malecot catheter and Foley catheter).

Use is similar to that of sheet drain but are used particularly when the amount of drainage is high.

Advantages

Can be directly connected to the apparatus, so the contamination of the wound with the drainage is less.

Disadvantages

Inner end of a catheter can be blocked, by draining material obstructing the drainage.

Uses

To drain large abscess cavity.

Yeates Drain

Formed of parallel tubes of plastic material.

Disadvantages

Very little fluid passes through the tubes they are filled and it tends to track alongside the drain.

Penrose Drain

Hollow tube of latex rubber with thin wall and can be made by cutting the finger stall of surgical glove. Its tip is cut so that both the ends are open.

Uses

- As a cigarette drain
- As a simple drain.

Cigarette Drain

Penrose drain that has gauze within it is called a cigarette drain. In these drains the ooze exists along and not through the gauze. The rubber acts as a conduit *Advantages* and *uses* are same as penrose drain.

Disadvantages

- Secretions cannot be collected in bags, so cannot be measured
- More chances of infection
- Skin irritation and excoriation may occur due to seepage of irritant effluent.

Shirley Drain

Drain is incorporated with a side tube guarded by a bacterial filter so that the sterile air can be drawn down to the tip of the drain. When a suction is

applied to this drain, the air leak prevents tissues being sucked into the drain holes and blocking them.

T-Tube

T-shaped with body and two flanges made up of polyvinyl chloride. Available presterilized by gamma rays or ethylene oxide.

Precautions

- Acts as a two way conduits. Careful dressing of the wound and removal of the drain as soon as the purpose is over to reduce the likelihood of infection
- Should never be brought out through the operative incision but through separate stab incision to prevent bacterial ingress and infection of the operative wound and to prevent its closure
- Should be fixed properly with skin stitches
- Should not be placed through an area where fibrosis will cause impairment of function
- Too hard or stiff drain may cause pressure necrosis of the surrounding tissues especially one near a large blood vessel, tendon or nerve.

Sump Suction

Commercially available but can also be made by inserting one plastic tube within the other. The outer tube projects for 2–3 cm outside the wound. The inner tube is longer and connected to the suction. Number of holes are made on the lower part of the outer tube, and the inner tube has a single side hole, made close to its end.

Mechanism of Action

A continuous current of air, activated by the suction, passes down through the outer tube and up through the inner tube. Any fluid collecting in the outer tube is immediately sucked away. No suction occurs at the openings in the outer tube, so that the surrounding tissues are not drawn against it.

Uses

Used to accomplish drainage against the force of gravity. For irrigation, irrigating fluid flows through the airvent while intermittent suction continues.

Advantages

- Prevents skin damage from irritating secretions
- Permits accurate measurement of the volume of drainage fluid
- No vacuum plugging of the drain during continuous low pressure suction.

Disadvantages

- Lack of pliability so drain is uncomfortable to the patient
- Erosion of surrounding tissues may occur.

Plastic Tube Drains

Two Types

- Silastic tube connected to closed gravity drainage or to a suction apparatus
- Polyvinyl chloride tube attached to a suction apparatus or negative suction bottle, or closed gravity drainage.

Advantages

- Fluid is collected without soiling the surrounding skin
- Accurate measurement of fluid possible.

Uses

- Negative suction tube drain (redivac drain)
  - Drainage of wound to prevent hematoma
  - After lymph node resection in neck
- Plastic Tube without suction.

Redivac Drain (Fig. 47.127)

Principle

Active suction is applied in a continuous manner. Does not allow secretions to collect inside and indirectly also maintains patency of the drainage tube and does not allow secretions to dry and occlude the drain site.

Advantages

- Less irritating to the tissues
- Less likely to cause infection as it is a closed system
- Effective under large skin flaps, e.g. after radical neck dissection

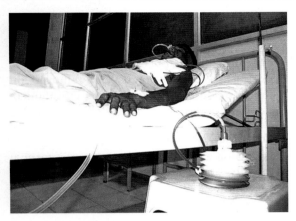

Fig. 47.127: Activated drain in place

- Closed suction drainage decreases the incidence of infection occurring secondary to contamination of the drain itself and is mandatory in the presence of a foreign body.

Equipment

- Negative suction bottle either single or three
- K-60/61 suction tube usually from latex rubber, polyvinyl chloride and silastic
- IV set.

Other types of suction drainage (pleurevac device) is used a chest drain following thoracotomy, etc

Usually 15–20 cm of H_2O effective negative suction is applied. The effectiveness of active negative suction can be judged by observing Murphy's chamber. When this chamber is ballooned, negativity is lost. On such an event the suction bottle should be charged by suction apparatus after emptying or a new negative suction bottle may be used.

Removal of drain should be done as soon as the discharge diminishes, usually after 48–72 hours.

Removal of Drain

- The prophylactically placed drain should be removed as soon as drainage has subsided
- The therapeutically placed drain is kept in position until the drainage subsides, then it is removed gradually, a 3–4 cm of drain is withdrawn each day and refixed to allow

closure of the drainage tract from its depth thus preventing pocketing
- Tube drains are removed when drainage output is minimal or ceased
- Corrugated drains are usually removed on the third day or when there is cessation of discharge.

Nasogastric Tubes (Fig. 47.128)

- Following abdominal surgery gastrointestinal motility is reduced for a variable period of time
- Gastrointestinal secretions accumulate in stoma and proximal small bowel
- May result in:
  - Postoperative distension and vomiting
  - Aspiration pneumonia
- Little clinical evidence is available to support the routine use of nasogastric tubes
- May increase the risk of pulmonary complications
- Of proven value for gastrointestinal decompression in intestinal obstruction
- Tubes are usually left on free drainage
- Can be also aspirated may be every 4 hours
- Can be removed when volume of nasogastric aspirate is reduced.

Urinary Catheters (Fig. 47.129)

- A urinary catheter is a form of drain
- Commonly used to:
  - Alleviate or prevent urinary retention
  - Monitor urine output
- Can be inserted transurethrally or suprapubically

- Catheters vary by:
  - The material from which they are made (latex, plastic, silastic, teflon-coated)
  - The length of the catheter (38 cm 'male' or '22 cm 'female')
  - The diameter of the catheter (10 Fr to 24 Fr)
  - The number of channels (two or three)
  - The size of the balloon (5 mL to 30 mL)
  - The shape of the tip.
- Special catheters exist such as:
  - Gibbon catheters
  - Nelaton catheters
  - Tiemann catheters
  - Malecot catheters.

Complications

- Paraphimosis
- Blockage
- By-passing
- Infection
- Failure of balloon to deflate
- Urethral strictures.

Do's and Don'ts of Urinary Catheters

- Choose an appropriate sized catheter
- Insert using an aseptic technique
- Never insert using force
- Do not inflate the balloon until urine has been seen coming from the catheter
- Record the residual volume
- Do not use a catheter introducer unless you have been trained in its use

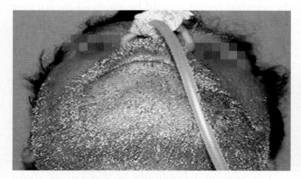

Fig. 47.128: Nasogastric tube in place

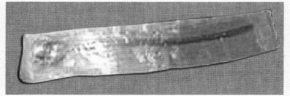

Fig. 47.129: Foley's catheter

- If difficulty is encountered inserting a urinary catheter consider a suprapubic
- Remove at the earliest possibility.

Needle Stick Injury

The needle stick injury is defined as a penetrating injury wound from a needle (or other sharp objects like scalpel, broken glass vial, etc.) that may result in exposure to blood or other body fluids.

POSTEXPOSURE PROPHYLAXIS (PEP) FOLLOWING NEEDLE STICK INJURY

Postexposure prophylaxis (PEP) is just what the name suggests; prophylaxis (preventative) medications given after an HIV or suspected HIV exposure in hopes of decreasing the likelihood of HIV infection from the exposure. The PEP medication combinations used depends on the degree of exposure and the HIV status of the source of the exposure. But before any medications are prescribed, it has to be determined if PEP is indicated and appropriate.

Exposure Reporting

First step in managing exposure is to ensure reporting. It should be accurate and prompt. Usually there is under reporting of exposure to blood by health workers.

After reporting of exposure arrangement should be made for follow up care of exposed. Confidentiality of exposed worker must be protected. Proper pre-test and post-test counseling should be offered to HCW.

Management of Exposure Site

This should be treated as medical emergency and treatment should begin at the earliest possibly , preferably within 2 hours. Exposure site should be decontaminated as soon as possible. Puncture and other cutaneous injuries should be washed with soap and water. Do not try to squeeze the blood out because it can push the blood and inoculums towards systemic circulation. Mucosal exposures involving mouth and nose should be flushed with water. Following an ocular exposure, eyes should be irrigated with clean water, saline or sterile irrigants designed for this purpose.

Clinical Evaluation Assessment of Exposure and Source Patient

Detail assessment of exposure incident and thorough evaluation of source patient should be carried out. If source patient's status with respect to HIV is not known, the relevant test should be carried out with all protocols after pre-test and post-test counselimg. Rapid testing should be confirmed by ELISA as soon as possible. If results are not immediately available or results are awaited and exposure has occurred, the best strategy is to begin prophylaxis immediately and either discontinue or modify regimen when results of test are available. In case source patients is known to be HIV infected then all information about the patient which include time since patient is infected. CD4 counts, viral load assays and detailed history aboutand current antiretroviral therapy should be obtained.

If source patient's serological status is unknown and cannot be learned, detailed epidemiological assessment of exposure should be made and expert consultation should be taken.

Selecting Chemoprophylaxis Regimen

A number of retroviral agents have been used for postexposure prophylaxis. CDC guidelines recommend a "basic" two drug regimens, the preferred regimen are as follows:

- Zidovudine plus lamivudine
- Tenofovir plus lamivudine
- Tenofovir plus emtriciatabine.

Other alternative "basic" two drug regimes recommended are:

- Stavudine plus lamivudine
- Didanosine plus lamivudine.

For exposure ascertained with an increased risk for exposure, i.e. from large bore hollow needle exposure, deep puncture wounds, exposure to needle that had been in artery or vein and exposure to blood from source patients who have symptomatic HIV infection , AIDS , the primary HIV infection or known high viral dose loads CDC recommends a three drug "expanded" regimen. The recommended three drug "expanded" regimen consists of a two drug "basic" regimen plus one of the following agents.

- Lopinavir + ritonavir(preferred)
- Indinavir + ritonavir (Avoid in pregnancy)
- Atazanavir + ritonavir (must be boosted, if tenofovir used in basic regimen)
- Saquinavir + ritonavir
- Nelfinavir
- Efavirenz (teratogenic ; avoid in pregnancy)

A variety of other regimens have been used, particularly in settings in which the source patient for an exposure has extensive antiretroviral experience and in instances in which antiretroviral resistance is known or highly suspected. In those cases prophylaxis should be initiated under expert consultation.

There are certain drugs which are not generally recommended for PEP. These are; nevirapine, abacavir, delaviridine and zalcitabine.

When is PEP Indicated?

Clinically following scenarios warrant PEP.

Two-drug PEP Recommended

- Exposure to asymptomatic HIV+ person by solid needle stick or superficial injury that break the skin
- A mucous membrane exposure to a large volume of HIV infected blood that's source is asymptomatic (consider for a lesser volume, a few drops)
- A mucous membrane exposure to a small volume of HIV infected blood that's source is symptomatic.

Three-drug PEP Recommended

- Exposure to asymptomatic HIV+ person via deep puncture from a large bore hollow needle
- A puncture from a needle with visible blood on the needle
- A puncture from a needle used in a patient's vein or artery.

Three or More Drug PEP Recommended

- Any needle stick exposure from any type needle used on a symptomatic HIV+ person
- A mucous membrane exposure to a large volume of HIV infected blood whose source is symptomatic.

Two-drug PEP under Certain Circumstances

- Needle stick with any type needle and any degree of exposure if the source has an unknown HIV status but has HIV risk factors
- Needle stick with any type needle and any degree of exposure if the source has an unknown HIV status and unknown risk factors but a setting in which exposure to HIV+ persons is likely
- A mucous membrane exposure to any volume of blood whose source has an unknown HIV status but has HIV risk factors
- A mucous membrane exposure to any volume of blood whose source has an unknown HIV status but is in a setting where HIV exposure is likely, no PEP warranted
- Any needle stick injury involving a known HIV negative source
- A mucous membrane exposure to any volume of HIV negative blood.

Best Medication Combination

PEP regimens are chosen depending on the type of exposure. Typically regimens are prescribed for a 4 week period. PEP should be started within hours of the potential exposure not days. The sooner the PEP is begun the better.

Preferred Two-drug Regimen

- Option 1—retrovir (zidovudine, AZT)+ epivir (lamivudine) twice daily. Combivir (retrovir + epivir) twice daily is typically substituted for ease of administration. This twice a day regimen is a bit harder to take but is recommended in pregnancy.
- Option 2—truvada (tenofovir + emtricitabine) taken once daily. This one drug regimen is easier to take but does have the risk of liver toxicity.

Preferred Three-drug Expanded Regimen

- Basic two drug regimen option 1 or 2 above with the addition of Kaletra (lopinavir + ritonavir) twice daily.
  HIV Medication Fact Sheets

Concerns Associated with PEP

While the benefits of PEP have been documented, there are some concerns as well. It's these concerns that cause practitioners to consider the need for PEP thoroughly before prescribing it. PEP is not without risk and should only be given in those people that absolutely need it.

Adherence issues and the problem of resistance: It's no secret that HIV medications have some unpleasant side effects. Because of these side effects the people who have been exposed find it difficult to take their PEP regimen as prescribed and/or complete the 4 week course. Both of these barriers result in poor adherence. And as in the case of HIV+ people on medication, poor adherence leads to viral resistance and poor control of HIV. That could make the difference between the PEP being successful or not.

PEP is a viable option for occupational exposures to HIV. While it is not without it's downfalls, it is effective in reducing the risk of HIV infection from a needle stick. But, without addressing the problem of needle sticks, more people are going to become infected by this route, health care cost will continue to rise and the epidemic will continue to grow.

Adherence to Prophylaxis Regimen

All strategies should be undertaken to increase and or to ensure complete adherence. This includes counseling of individual on seriousness of exposure , effectiveness of PEP regimen , need for 100% adherence and regular follow up for management of toxicities if encountered.

Duration of postexposure prophylaxis regimen the optimal course of treatment is 4 weeks.

Follow-up

Serological tests for HIV for exposed person should be done at base line, 6 weeks, 3 months and 6 months with proper pre-test and post-test counseling. Person receiving prophylaxis should follow up with the clinician at least once in a week. He should be advised to refrain from donating blood , semen or organs/tissues and abstain from sexual intercourse. In case sexual intercourse is undertaken by exposed person a latex condom to be used consistently. In addition , women health care personnel should not breast–feed their infants during the follow up period.

Questions and Answers

1. **What is the most commonly used blood group system?**
   ABO system.

2. **How many types of blood group present?**
   Totally 21 types, some of them are Landstein system, rhesus system, kell system, kidd system, duff system, ketheram system, MNS system, lewis system, P-system, etc.

3. **Which are the antibodies commonly found in the serum?**
   Anti A and anti B antibodies (iso agglutatinin).

4. **Which is the most common benign tumor of parotid gland?**
   Pleomorphic adenoma.

5. **Name the other terminology for pleomorphic adenoma.**
   Mixed tumor, enclavoma, branchioma, endothelioma, enchondroma.

6. **Which salivary tumor is radioresistant?**
   Pleomorphic adenoma.

7. **What is the other name for oxyphilic adenoma?**
   Acidophilic adenoma.

8. **Which parts are affected in Sjögren's syndrome?**
   Affected sites are:
   - Kerratoconjunctivitis sicca (eye)
   - Rheumatoid arthritis (joint)
   - Xerostomia (mouth).

9 **What investigation you do in Sjögren's syndrome?**
   ESR—normally raised,
   Unstimulated saliva level, tear production-rose Bengal dye test.

10. **What is the radiographic picture of Sjögren's syndrome?**
    In sialography it shows cherry blossom, branchless fruit laden tree.

11. **What are the other names for adenoid cystic carcinoma?**
    Cylindroma, adenocystic carcinoma, adenocystic basal cell carcinoma, baseloid mixed tumor.

12. **Name a salivary gland tumor commonly seen in children.**
    Mucoepidermoid carcinoma.

13. **Which giant cell is responsible for root resorption?**
    Osteoclast.

14. **What is the other name for osteitis deformans?**
    Pagets diseases.

15. **What is phlebolith ?**
    Thrombi calcified in vein.

16. **How primordial cyst is formed?**
    It develops through the cystic degeneration and liquefaction of stellate reticulum in an enamel organ before any calcified enamel formed.

17. **What is Kutner's tumor?**
    It is benign chronic sclerosing sialdenitis usually occur in submandibular gland is regarded as salivary gland neoplasm first described in 1896 by Dr H. Kutners. Few cases are also reported in parotid and lacrimal gland.

18. **What are the types of dentigerous cyst?**
    Lateral dentigerous cyst, circumferential dentigerous cyst, para dental dentigerous cyst, central dentigerous cyst. Central type is most common.

19. **What are the complications of dentigerous cyst?**

Formation of ameloblastoma from lining epithelium epidermoid carcinoma, mucoepidermoid carcinoma, basically malignant salivary gland tumor (mucous-secreting cells).

20. **What is residual cyst?**

It is a periapical cyst that remains after or develops after extraction.

21. **What are the treatment options for growth deformities of TMJ?**

Treatment option includes—
Ankylosis release with or without graft.
Growth center transplants, functional appliances, serial lengthening procedures during growth, osteotomies and camouflages after cessation of growth.
Choice of treatment depends on patient's age, joint function and severity of deformity. In general early treatment of growth abnormalities is advocated to prevent further deformities; active physiotherapy is followed closely: costochondral grafts are still the most supported treatment for growth restriction.

22. **What do you understand by synostosis?**

Early closure of cranial sutures like in Apert's syndrome.

23. **What type of jaw movements are involved in opening of mouth?**

Hinge followed by translation.

24. **Posterior belly of digastric is supplied by which nerve?**

Facial nerve.

25. **At what level tracheal bifurcation lies?**

Sternal angle.

26. **What do you call point of bifurcation of trachea and at what level it lies?**

Carina, i.e. angle of Louis. At the level of T_4 vertebrae.

27. **Embryologically lip is derived from which process?**

Maxillary, mandibular, lateral nasal, and medial nasal processes.

28. **What is pheochromocytoma? What is its significance?**

It is tumor of adrenal medulla, and is an absolute contraindication for use of local anesthesia with adrenaline; because of hypertensive effect.

29. **What is glossopyrosis?**

It is used to define a burning tongue.

30. **Why staging of malignancy are done?**

It is done to determine prognosis.

31. **What do you understand by lucid interval in extradural hemorrhage?**

A lucid interval is a temporary improvement in a patient's condition after a traumatic brain injury, after which the condition deteriorates. A lucid interval is especially indicative of an extradural hematoma. An estimated 20 to 50% of patients with extradural hematoma experience such a lucid interval. The time taken to form such a big hematoma as to cause sufficient rise in intracranial pressure to cause unconsciousness following injury is the period known as lucid-interval and this taken by hemorrhage to be big enough to cause cerebral compression.

32. **A patient reports with elevated Bence-Jones protein and multiple radiolucent lesions of mandible and skull, what is your probable diagnosis?**

Multiple myeloma.

33. **What is antidote for heparin?**

Protamine sulfate

34. **Where nasal antrostomy after Caldwell-Luc operation is created?**

Inferior meatus.

35. **What do you understand by saltatory conduction?**

    Saltatory conduction (from the Latin *saltare*, to hop or leap) is the propagation of action potentials along myelinated axons from one node of Ranvier to the next node, increasing the conduction velocity of action potentials without needing to increase the diameter of an axon.

36. **What is encephalation?**

    It is irrigation of salivary duct after surgical procedure on duct.

37. **Premature synostosis with syndactyle is seen in which condition?**

    Apert's syndrome.

38. **What does characteristic feature you see in skull radiograph of Apert's syndrome?**

    Metal beaten or copper beaten apprence.

39. **What do you call increase in number of platelet and decrease in there number?**

    Thrombocytosis and thrombocytopenia respectively.

40. **What is the screening test for hemophilia?**

    PTT—Partial thromboplastin time.

41. **Describe flail chest.**

    A flail chest is a life-threatening medical condition that occurs when a segment of the chest wall bones breaks under extreme stress and becomes detached from the rest of the chest wall.

42. **What is Coleman's sign? Where it is seen?**

    Sublingual echhymosis seen in case of mandibular fracture.

43. **What is Chevosteck's sign and Trousseau's sign?**

    Chovosteck's sign: When the facial nerve is tapped at the angle of the jaw (i.e. masseter muscle), the facial muscles on the same side of the face will contract momentarily (typically a twitch of the nose or lips) because of hypocalcemia (i.e. from hypoparathyroidism, pseudohypoparathyroidism, hypovitaminosis D) with resultant hyperexcitability of nerves.

    Trousseau's sign: A sphygmomanometer is placed on the arm and inflated to greater than systolic blood pressure and left in place for at least 2 minutes, a positive response is carpal spasm of the ipsilateral arm. Relaxation takes 5–10 seconds after pressure is released.

44. **For a costochondral graft which rib is taken and why?**

    5th or 6th rib because it has got maximum amount of cartilage.

45. **Which side rib is taken and why?**

    Right side rib is taken as there no important organ on that side at this level.

46. **A 50-year-patient reports with epiphora, what are the reasons?**

    Irritation and inflammation, aging (a spontaneous process), infection (i.e. dacryocystitis), rhinitis, and in neonates or infants, failure of the nasolacrimal duct to open.

47. **What is the mode of inheritance in neurofibromatosis?**

    Autosomal dominant.

48. **What is the lymphatic drainage of tongue?**

    Tip of the tongue to submental nodes, ant 2/3rd in sublingual and post 1/3rd in deep cervical.

49. **What are the complications associated with nasal fracture?**

    Septal deviation
    Contour irregularities,
    Breathing difficulty, and
    Septal hematoma.

50. **What are complications associated with naso-orbital ethmoidal fracture?**

Telecanthesis
Septal devation
Unsightly scar
Enopthalmos
Diplopia
Nasolacrimal obstruction
Sinusitis
Ocular injury
CSF leak, etc.

51. **What factors are considered for ventilation in ICU or after a major trauma?**

Hypoventilation—flail chest, diaphramatic injury, spinal injury
GCS score less than or equal to 9. Metabolic-hypoxia, hypercapnea, hypothermia, apnea

52. **Tell me something about CT scan and its units.**

Difference in tissue density detected by passage of a thin collimated beam of X-rays is the basis of CT scan. Density of the tissue is expressed in Hounsfield units. Bone is having a +1000 and air is having -1000 HU's. Helical and spiral CT scans are supplementary to conventional scanning. Contrast can be used to enhance certain tissue and thereby increasing the accuracy of diagnosis.

53. **What slice machine is used normally?**

It may be 16 slice or 64 slice.

54. **What do you mean by Tesla?**

Tesla (unit) (symbol T), SI derived unit of magnetic flux density (or magnetic inductivity), named after Nikola Tesla.

55. **What is MRI?**

In MRI hydrogen nuclei behaves like small spinning magnetic field this is the principle. The character of T1 and T2 images vary depending on the tissue characteristics. The major role of MRI is in intracranial, spinal and musculoskeletal imaging.

56. **What is the rate of recovery of axon in nerve injury?**

1 mm/day.

57. **What is Wallerian degeneration?**

The part of nerve distal to the point of injury undergoes secondary or wallerian degeneration.

58. **Which is the most commonly used nerve for grafting?**

Most commonly used nerve is Sural nerve; others are Saphinous nerve, superficial branch of radial nerve, intercostals nerve. Radial nerve has better prognosis, primarily because it is a motor nerve as well as the muscle innervated by it are not involved in fine movements.

59. **What are pupillary reflexes?**

Pupillary reflexes are light reflex, near reflex and pshychosensory reflex.

Light reflex: direct reflex –contraction of pupil if light enter directly to eye.

Consensual reflex: pupil contracts if light enters in opposite eye.

Pathways: retina → optic nerve → optic tract → nucleus in midbrain → short ciliary nerve → sphincter papillae.

60. **What is the importance of pupillary reflexes?**

These are used to evaluate the severity of head injuries.

61. **What are the causes of CSF rhinorrhea and how it is diagnosed?**

Common cause of CSF rhinorrhea is fracture of cribriform plate. Its clinical history include leakage of clear watery fluid from nose, which cannot be sniffed back.

62. **What are the confirmatory tests for CSF?**

Handkerchief test: no stiffening of handkerchief with CSF.

Halo sign (target sign)

Glucose concentration: glucose level of > 30 mg% is confirmatory.

Beta 2 transferrin on electrophoresis: specific for CSF.

63. **Give example of colloids.**

Dextran 70 (molecular wight 70000 dalton), Dextran 40 (molecular wight 40000 dalton)

64. **Give examples of crystalloids.**

Ringer lactate, Hartmans solution is crystalloid of choice for restoration of blood with osmolarity of 273 mOs/L.

65. **Can you infuse blood in the same drip of dextrose 5%?**

Blood cannot be given by same drip because there is Rouleoux formation.

66. **What are the disadvantages of colloids?**

Anaphylactic reaction, interference with blood grouping, interference with platelet function, can block renal tubules.

67. **What are the complications of blood transfusion?**

Hemolytic reactions—

Symptoms: fever with chills and rigor Nausea, vomiting, chest pain.

In anesthetized patients—tachycardia, hypotension, blood oozing from surgical sites,

Hemoglobinuria

Allergic reaction

Febrile reaction

Infections

Metabolic reaction—hyperkalemia

Hypocalcemia

Acid base abnormalities

Coagulation abnormalities

Thrombocytopenia

Hypothermia

Immunosuppression.

68. **What is massive blood transfusion?**

More than patient's blood volume in less than 24 hr or greater than 10% blood volume in less than 10 minutes.

69. **What are the complications of massive blood transfusion?**

Hyperkalemia, hypocalcemia, hypothermia, metabolic alkalosis and dilutional coagulopathies.

70. **What are the different indicative colors of cylinders for various gases?**

Oxygen—black with white shoulder

Nitrous oxide—blue

Carbondioxide—gray

Air—gray body with blue and white shoulder

Cyclopropane—orange.

71. **What is CVP?**

Central venous pressure—ideal vein is right internal juglar vein because it is valveless.

Indication: fluid management in shock, TPN, aspiratory air embolous.

Normal CVP is 3–10 cm of water.

CVP is increased in the following condition-fluid overloading, congestive cardiac failure, pulmonary emboli and hemothorax.

72. **What is capnography?**

It is of respiratory monitor. Which continuously measures end tidal CO_2 gas movement it uses infrared sensor for this. The mere presence of a carbondioxide waveform indicates breathing is occurring. It is most useful indicator of adequacy of ventilation than the pulse oximeter, because of its instantaneous measurement of gas exchange. Often capnography is more complicated than pulse oximetery in its interpretation of data.

Use: confirmation if correct intubation

Intraoperative displacement of tube

Diagnosis of malignant hyperthermia

For detection of obstructive disconnection

Indicator cardiac output.

73. **Give some examples of muscle relaxants.**

They can be depolarizing or nondepolarizing blocking

Depolarizing block—succinylcholine, decamethonium

Nondepolarizing competitive blocking

Benzylisoquinoline, d-tubocurain, metocurin, doxacurium.

74. **Name some long-acting local anesthesia agent?**

Bupivacain,tetracain, dibucaine (longest duration) agents with high protein binding like bupivacaine have prolonged action.

75. **What is malignant hypertyhermia? Tell clinical features and treatment.**

It is an autosomal dominant inherited disease characterized by uncontrolled skeletal muscle hypermetabolism, due to abnormality of ryanodine receptor, which is a calcium releasing channel of sarcoplasmic reticulum. Its etiology also said to be multi factorial. Causative agents: succinylchloine-most common, halothane, isofurane, enfurane, lignocaine

Clinical freature: hyperthermia, increase end tidal CO_2, hypoxia, hypertension, cardiac arrhythmia, severe metabolic acidosis.

Treatment: General—stop all anesthesia, hyperventilate with 100% O_2, control temperature correct acidosis, correct electrolyte.

Specific: Dantrolene 2 mg/kg to maximum of 10 mg/kg.

76. **What is propofol?**

It is an induction agent of choice for day care anesthesia (but painful on injection given with xylocain not recommended in childrens below 3 years , causes hypotension and myocardial depression. It is agent of choice for total IV anesthesia and in malignant hyperthermia) specially for a young adult for 3rd molar extraction under GA and if he wishes to attend to duty after 6 hr.

77. **Which muscle moves condyle downward and forward?**

Lateral pterygoid.

78. **What is the use of Walsham's forceps?**

Reduction of nasal septum.

79. **Which structure is known as peripheral heart?**

Lateral pterygoid muscle with pterygoid plexus.

80. **When there is an increased prothrombin time in a patient, what does it indicate?**

The prothrombin time can be prolonged as a result of deficiencies in vitamin K, which can be caused by warfarin, malabsorption, or lack of intestinal colonization by bacteria (such as in newborns). In addition, poor factor VII synthesis (due to liver disease) or increased consumption (in disseminated intravascular coagulation) may prolong the PT.

81. **What is Battle's sign?**

Fracture of middle cranial fossa presenting as echymosis behind the ear in mastoid region.

82. **What is the occlusion you see in a patient with bilateral subcondylar fracture?**

Anterior openbite.

83. **Which is a target cell for HIV?**

CD4 cells.

84. **Where is Risdons wiring indicated?**

For symphysis fracture.

85. **Suppose if you transfuse one unit of fresh Blood how much of hemoglobin can it increase?**

1 gm%.

86. **What is Eburnation, where it is seen?**

Eburnation describes a degenerative process of bone commonly found in patients with osteoarthritis or non-union of fractures.

87. **What are the sign of stage III and plane II in general anesthesia?**

Surgical Plane from the cessation of REM to the onset of paresis of the intercostal muscle.

88. **What is Gorlin's sign?**

Gorlin sign is the ability to touch the tip of the nose with the tongue and touch the elbow with the tongue. Approximately ten percent of the general population can perform this act, whereas five times as many people with Ehlers Danlos.

89. **How do you test the function of facial nerve?**
Voluntary facial movements, such as wrinkling the brow, showing teeth, frowning, closing the eyes tightly, pursing the lips and puffing out the cheeks, all test the facial nerve. There should be no noticeable asymmetry. Taste can be tested on the anterior 2/3 of the tongue.

90. **What is the best radiographic view for TMJ?**
Trans pharyngeal, trans orbital and trans cranial.

91. **Which salivary gland malignancy presents with perineural invasion?**
Adenoid cystic carcinoma.

92. **What is the nerve supply to stylopharengeous muscle?**
Glossopharyngeal nerve.

93. **How do you assess growth in children?**
Cervical vertebrae ossification seen in cephalogram.

94. **What is Eagles syndrome?**
Ossification of styloid ligament.

95. **What is sensory supply of TMJ?**
Auriculotemporal and masseteric branches of cranial nerve V.

96. **What is Bowen's diseases?**
Squamous cell carcinoma *in situ*.

97. **Name a syndrome where micrognathia is a feature?**
Pierre Robin syndrome.

98. **What is Heberdin's node? Where it is seen?**
They are hard or bony swellings that can develop in the distal interphalangeal joints (DIP) (the joints closest to the end of the fingers and toes). They are a sign of osteoarthritis and are caused by formation of osteophytes (calcific spurs) of the articular (joint) cartilage in response to repeated trauma at the joint.

99. **What are Osler's nodes?**
Tender, raised, pea-sized, red or purple lesions that erupts on the palms, soles and especially the pads of the figure and toes; they're a rare but reliable sign of infective endocarditis and pathognomonic of subacute form.

100. **What are the screening tests done for renal functions?**
Serum creatinine, serum urea and uric acid level.

101. **What is potato tumor of neck?**
A firm nodular mass in the neck, usually a carotid body tumor (chemodectoma)

102. **Middle nasal concha is part of which bone?**
Ethymoid bone.

103. **What type of giant cells seen in Hodgkin's diseases?**
Reed–Sternbergs cells (owl eye nucleus).

104. **What is Ackerman's tumor?**
Verrucous carcinoma of larynx.

105. **What do you mean by Frankfort horizontal plane?**
A craniometric surface determined by the inferior borders of the bony orbits and the upper margin of the auditory meatus.

106. **Which salivary gland often affected by Warthins tumor? And what other names it is known?**
Parotid gland, and it is also known as adeno-lymphoma, papillary cystadenoma lymphomatosum.

107. **Which giant cells are responsible for root resorption?**
Osteoclast.

108. **What is eruption hematoma/eruption cyst?**
It is dilatation of follicular space which contains tissue fluid and blood.

109. What condition is seen with multiple dentigerous cyst?

Basal cell nevoid syndrome, bifid rib syndrome.

110. Name the lesions where ghost cells are seen.

Calcifying odontogenic cyst, ameloblastic fibrodontoma, craniopharyngioma, complex compound odontome.

111. What is Trotter's syndrome?

Tumors of nasopharynx.

112. What are the other names for sphenopalatine neuralgia?

Periodic migranious neuralgia, cluster headache, histamine cephalgia, vidian nerve neuralgia, sludders headache.

113. What is Rubberman's syndrome?

Ehlers–Danlos syndrome.

114. What is Fanconi's anemia?

Aplastic anemia with congenital defects, bone abnormalities and microcephalous.

115. What is normal bilirubin level in plasma?

5.1–17.0 µmol/L or 0.2–0.8 mg/100 mL.

116. What is skip metastasis?

When oral cancer metastasizes to the cervical region it metastasizes predictably to certain lymph node groups. The anatomic limits of the Supra Omohyoid Neck Dissection are based on studies that have shown that oral SCC follows predictable patterns of lymphatic metastasis. Lindbergs (1972) classic study demonstrated oral cavity SCCs metastasize to submandibular triangle, the upperjugular chain, and the mid-jugular chain of lymph nodes Lymberg described "Skip" metastasize where metastatic tumor could "skip" the upper echelon of nodes, i.e. the jugulodigastric or submandibular nodes, and be found in the mid-jugular chain. These skip metastasis were rarely found in the lowerjugular chain(level iv)or in the posterior triangle of the neck (v).

Generally regional lymph nodes drains the tumor involved but sometimes lymphatic metastasis does not develop first in lymph node nearest to tumor, because of various lymph node anastomosis or due to obstruction of lymphatics by inflammation or radiation and it is called as skip metastasis.

117. What is apoptosis?

It is a form of programmed cell death, unlike necrosis apoptosis is an orderly event. Genes, such as p53, that can activate apoptosis function as tumor suppressor gene.

118. What is progeria?

Dwarfism, Hutchinson-Gilferal syndrome, premature senility, high pitched squeaking voice, beak like nose, hypoplastic mandible, normal or above normal intelligence.

119. What are characteristics of basal cell carcinoma?

It does not occur in oral cavity because of difference in surface epithelium and it does not metastasize.

120. What do you know about lymphangioma?

It is a benign tumor of the lymphatic vessel: classified as- simple lymphangioma, cavernous lymphangioma, cellular lymphangioma, hypertrophic lymphangioma, diffuse systemic lymphangioma, cystic lymphangioma or hygroma. Lymphangioma occur at birth. In the oral cavity it can be seen in tongue and tongue lymphangioma can cause macroglossia. Over the tongue they are seen on anterior dorsal part as grey pink projection.

121. What do you call excess respiration rate?

Tachyapnea.

122. How facial vein is connected to cavernous sinus?

By superior ophthalmic vein.

123. If normal SNA is 82 degree, a patient with SNA 90 degree what does it suggest?

Maxillary protrusion.

124. What are the options for reconstruction of tongue?

The fasciocutaneous radial forearm flap remains the first choice for hemiglossectomy and floor of the mouth defect.

Lateral arm flap (but posterior collateral artery of fore-arm is smaller than radial artery and remains narrow until the proximal part, which reduces the options in placement of pedicle).

Free vastus lateralis muscle flap- anterolateral thigh flap is a fasciocutaneous flap based on a cutaneous perforator, in obese patient flap can be difficult to raise and identification of perforator vessel is difficult.

125. What is a harmonic scalpel?

Harmonic scalpel is a cutting instrument used during surgical procedure to simultaneously cut and coagulate tissues. Harmonic scalpel cuts, coagulates simultaneously using high frequency mechanical vibration rather than high temperature. It can cut through thicker tissues create less smoke and offers greater precision Hemostasis by coagulation of vessels with the scalpel surface itself cuts through tissues by vibration range of 55,500 Hz.

Advantages: lesser operating time, lesser postoperative drainage, minimal intraoperative blood loss.

It is a safe and efficient alternative to cold knife or electrocautery.

126. What are the complication of LeFort I Pterygomaxillary separation?

Mobilization difficulty, vascular injury commonly to descending palatine artery during pterygomaxillary separation, risk of pterygoid venous plexus bleeding.

127. Complication related to LeFort III osteotomy.

Complication can be minor or major:

Minor complication can be infraorbital nerve injury, ptosis, strabismus, partial anosmia, fracture of zygoma, infection or abscess

Major complications are: CSF leakage, respiratory distress (sometimes even requiring tracheostomy), skull base fracture leading to severe bleeding.

128. What radiograph you advice for visualizing impacted 3rd molar to see whether it has 2 or 3 roots?

An occlusal film should be taken to understand the problem in 3 dimensions. Occlusal view will provide an alternative view to periapical film of the roots of horizontal teeth especially when the presence of third root is suspected. It will also determine whether the crown faces lingually or bucally.

129. What is burns space?

A narrow interval between the deep and superficial layers of the cervical fascia above the manubrium of the sternum through which pass the anterior jugular veins.

130. In case of Ludwigs angina how will you assess respiratory obstruction which may indicate need for tracheostomy even when patient is not in distress?

Immediate blood gas analysis, clinical presentation of edema.

131. What is photodynamic therapy?

It is a new treatment that involves interaction of light and drug in the presence of oxygen which result in cell death, it is a cutting edge treatment modality used in head and neck neoplasia. The technique is based on the combination of a photosensitive drug and visible light which cause distruption of cell function and induction of cytotoxicity.

132. What are the pathognomonic features of pyogenic osteomyelitis of mandible?

Loss of sensation in the affected area, rise in pressure from edema in the inferior alveolar canal are the pathgnomonic feature of acute pyogenic osteomyelities of mandible. Following the drainage of pus as a result of sius formation the temperature falls and pain reduces. If this condition is not treated it may proceed to chronic osteomylities from this stage.

133. What are the sign of fluid excess in extracellular fluid?

Loud heart sound, elevated venous pressure, increased cardiac output, anasarca with severe increase in fluid volume, vomiting and diarrhea.

134. What is the method of maintaining fluid volume?

Crystalloids is the first line of therapy (parentral IV).

135. Why wound healing is slow in jaundice?

Reduction in number of fibroblast, reduction in formation of new fibroblast, reduction in enzyme polyhydroxylase.

136. What is piezosurgery?

Piezosurgery is a term used for a collection of ultrasonic technology device which applies electric vibrations to cut bone tissues. The technique is named after piezoelectricity, a consept founded by Italian physician Tomaso Vercellottin 1988, though the device used for ultrasonic cutting by piezoelectric effect, first described by French physicist Jean and Marie Curie in 1880. Advantage is it can be used for implant, endodontic sinus lift procedure.

137. What is acetazolamide?

It is a carbonic anhydrase inhibitor used in retrobulbar hemorrhage to decrease intra ocular pressure. It works by decreasing systemic pressure which can help control hemorrhage. It reduces production of aqueous humor so used in treatment of glaucoma.

138. What is sialosis?

It is a non inflammatory, non neoplastic bilateral enlargement of parotid also known as parotid hypertrophy. Exact etiology is unclear, occurs in various endocrine and nutritional aberrations, suggesting a metabolic basis. Sialosis also associated with alcoholism with or without cirrhosis, malnutrition obesity, or pregnancy. Also it has been described as a reaction to number of pharmacological agents including iodine, thioracil and isoproterenol.

139. What is puffed check AP view? Where it is useful?

Useful to assessing distal segment of parotid and submandibular salivary ducts.

140. Name some molecular tumor markers.

Molecular tumor markers according to their function are:
- Tumor growth marker
- Tumor suppression marker
- Immune response
- Angiogenesis, tumor invasion and metastatic potential.

141. Name molecular marker involved in tumor growth, proliferation, and apoptosis.

Epidermal growth factor receptor
Tranforming growth factor
Alpha and other regulating protein
HER-2/ne4, HER-3
HER-4
Cyclin D1
Ki-67, BCL-2
BCL-2 is an antiapoptotic protein
FAS and its ligand Fas L are important mediators of apoptosis.

142. Can you tell molecular markers involved in tumor suppression?

P27 is a cyclin dependent kinase inhibitor which negatively regulates G1 phase progression of all cycle.
P53 involved in poor prognosis in most studies.

143. Molecular markers involved in tumor angiogenesis?

Angiogenesis is the growth of new microvessels and this process depends on the motility, proliferation and tube formation of endothelial cells.
VEGF (vascular endothelial growth factor), VEGF-B, VEGF-C, VEGF-E

Studies show that high level of serum VEGF correlated with nodal metastasis and clinical stage.

144. What are molecular markers involved in tumor invasion and metastatic potential?

Matrix metalloproteinases (MMPS) and collagenases, gelatinases, strome lysins and new mmps are involved in extracellularly matrix remodeling.

MMP-2 expression was significantly correlated with nodal status and overall survival in 106 patient with advanced HNSC.

145. Name some more molecular markers.

Melanoma antigen

NY-ESO-1, MAGE-1, MAGE-3

146. What is lines of tension and Langers concept regarding skin tension?

The lines of tension are those which represent the direction of greatest tension of the skin in a given area in part; they are dependent upon the structural arrangement of the elastic fibres in the dermis.

147. Who are the contributors's for concept of skin tension line?

Karl Langer, a Vienniese professor of anatomy in 1861 studied incision and puncture wound in cadaver. Earlier Filhos in 1833 had reported this, followed by Eischricht 1837 and Voight 1857.

148. What is Castleman's disease?

Castleman's disease is a very rare disorder characterized by non-cancerous growths (tumors) that may develop in the lymph node tissue at a single site or throughout the body. It involves hyperproliferation of certain B cells that often produce Cytokines. While not officially considered a cancer, the overgrowth of lymphatic cells with this disease is similar to lymphoma.

It is named for Benjamin Castleman.

149. What are types of Castleman's disease?

They are of two types:

Unicentric Castleman's disease involves tissue growths at only a single site. It usually has few or no symptoms other than those directly associated with the physical enlargement of the lymph node. In 90% or more, removal of the enlarged node is curative, with no further complications.

Multicentric Castleman's disease (MCD) involves growths at multiple sites.

150. What are Halstead's principles?

Halstead's principles are the basic principles of surgical technique regarding tissue handling, vascular occlusion, etc. If followed, they improve soft tissue surgical success rate. The principles are:

Strict asepsis during preparation and surgery.

Good hemostasis to improve conditions for the procedure and limit infection and dead space.

Minimize tissue trauma.

Use good surgical judgment ensuring elimination of dead space and adequate removal of material.

Minimize surgery time through knowledge of anatomy and technique.

Correct use of instruments and materials used.

151. What are subtriangles located within carotid and submandibular triangle?

Beclard's triangle

Lessers triangle

Pirogoff's triangle

Pirogoff's triangle is also known as lingual hypoglossohyoid or Pinaud's triangle. It is the posterior part of Lesser's triangle.

152. What are precise anatomic boundaries of Beclard's triangle, Lessers triangle, and Pirogoff's triangle?

Beclard's triangle: Boundaries are the posterior border of the hyoglossus, the posterior belly of the digastric muscle and the greater horn of the hyoid bone.

Lesser's triangle: The space between the bellies of the digastric muscle and the hypoglossal nerve.

Pirogoff's triangle: A triangle formed by the intermediate tendon of the digastric muscle, the posterior border of the mylohyoid muscle, and the hypoglossal nerve.

153. How do you manage animal bite injuries in maxillofacial region?

Bite wounds are especially prone to infectious complications, both local and systemic. In bite wounds to the face, such complications can create more difficulties than the initial tissue damage itself for the task of restoring an esthetic appearance. Management should aim to neutralize potential for infection and provide an infection-free environment for wound healing. Wound cleansing followed by primary closure is the treatment of choice, and the use of prophylactic antibiotics may further decrease the risk of infection. Delay in presentation beyond 24 hours is not necessarily a contraindication to immediate repair, but excessive crushing of the tissues or extensive edema usually dictates a more conservative approach, such as delayed closure.

154. What are revision techniques used in managing facial scar?

Z-plasty

Z-plasty is one of the most versatile scar revision techniques available. As a transposition flap, Z-plasty allows for 2 adjacent undermined triangular flaps, constructed from the same central axis, to transpose over each other and to lie in the other's originating bed. In essence, these 2 triangular flaps are transposed from areas of relative excess into areas of relative deficiency and eventually lie at near right angles to the original central axis.

W-plasty

The primary utility of the W-plasty (also termed the running W-plasty or zig-zag plasty) is in rendering a lengthy linear scar irregular. In addition to linear scar revision, the W-plasty is useful in the closure of semicircular incisions in which the sweeping unbroken curvilinear scar is more noticeable and under greater tension and, thus, over time more likely to become depressed or pincushioned. Note that while the W-plasty makes irregular a linear scar and spares unwanted lengthening that may arise from using small multiple Z-plasties, the final result is often readily visible because the eye easily can follow the predictable zig-zag configuration. Finally, in its basic execution, this technique incorporates neither transposition nor rotation of adjacent flaps; therefore, the final scar is not elongated but only increased in the final total length.

M-plasty

Often, scar revision creates angles greater than 30° at the lateral wound margins. While a greater angle at the wound's ends maximally preserves normal surrounding tissue, revision efforts under these circumstances are more likely to create a standing cone (i.e. dog-ear) deformity. Decreasing the likelihood of a standing cone deformity ultimately leads to greater loss of healthy surrounding tissue and vice versa. A useful technique to preserve healthy tissue and lessen the chance of secondary tissue deformity is the M-plasty. The M-plasty, by creating 2 separate 30° angles instead of one, decreases the loss of surrounding healthy tissue by nearly 50%.

155. What is tissue engineering and stem cells?

It is the use of a combination of cells, engineering and materials methods, and suitable biochemical and physiochemical factors to improve or replace biological functions. While most definitions of tissue engineering cover a broad range of applications, in practice the term is closely associated with applications that repair or replace portions of or whole tissues (i.e. bone, cartilage, blood vessels, bladder, skin, etc.). Often, the tissues involved require certain mechanical and structural properties for proper functioning. The term has also been applied to efforts to perform specific biochemical functions using cells within an artificially-created support system (e.g. an artificial pancreas, or a bioartificial liver). The term regenerative medicine is often used synonymously with tissue engineering, although those involved in regenerative medicine place more emphasis on the use of stem cells to produce tissues.

A commonly applied definition of tissue engineering, as stated by Langer and Vacanti, is "an interdisciplinary field that applies the principles of engineering and life sciences toward the development of biological substitutes that restore, maintain, or improve tissue function or a whole organ." Tissue engineering has also been defined as "understanding the principles of tissue growth, and applying this to produce functional replacement tissue for clinical use." A further description goes on to say that an "underlying supposition of tissue engineering is that the employment of natural biology of the system will allow for greater success in developing therapeutic strategies aimed at the replacement, repair, maintenance, and/or enhancement of tissue function.

156. At what age can the follicles of third molars be diagnosed?

7–9 yr.

157. What are 3 basic mechanism of healing?

Matrix deposition
Epithelialization
Contraction.

158. What are the reasons for postoperative complication in 3rd molar surgery?

Increased surgical time, trauma, difficulty in removal are some factors

Type of healing of surgical wound is linked to postoperative swelling.

159. Describe type of surgical wound.

Dirty wound
Contaminated
Clean contaminated
Clean wound.

160. How do you manage infections of surgical wound in maxillofacial region?

Local care
Anesthesia
Irrigation: For a small low risk wound, a minimum of 200 ml of irrigant is necessary.
Hemostasis
Closure of the wound
Sutures
Staples
Adhesives
Antibiotics
Topical
Systemic
Dressings.

161. Why injury to lingual nerve will cause anesthesia of anterior 2/3rd of tongue? Explain.

The lingual nerve provides tactile sensory innervations to the ipsilateral aspect of the tongue, the lower lingual gingivae and the floor of the mouth. It also provides the taste sensation in the anterior two-thirds of the tongue via the chorda tympani branch of the facial nerve and secretomotor innervation to the submandibular ganglion via preganglionic parasympathetic fibers.

162. What are determining factors for surgical difficulty of 3rd molar?

Difficulty in surgical extraction is associated with:

Depth (depth is deep occlusal level: level C),

Ramus relationship/space available (ramus relationship/space available is no space: class 3),

Width of root (the width of the middle root is thicker than that of the neck and the roots do not separate, incomplete roots excluded: bulbous).

163. What is normal cardiac output? What are the factors regulating cardiac output?

Normal cardiac output is 5 L/min for a human male and 4.5 L/min for a female. It is determined by the stroke volume and the heart rate.

164. Tell briefly about the development of palate.

Development of palate

The development of the secondary palate commences in the sixth week of human embryological development. It is characterised by the formation of two palatal shelves on the maxillary prominences, the elevation of these shelves to a horizontal position, and then a process of palatal fusion between the horizontal shelves. The shelves will also fuse anteriorly upon the primary palate, with the incisive foramen being the landmark between the primary palate and secondary palate. This forms what is known as the roof of the mouth, or the hard palate. The formation and development of the secondary palate occurs through signaling molecules BMP-2, FGF-8 among others.

Formation of palatal shelves

The formation of the vertical palatal shelves occurs during week 7 of embryological development, on the maxillary processes of the head of embryo, lateral to the developing tongue.

Palatal shelf elevation

The elevation of the palatal shelves from a vertical position to a horizontal one occurs during week 8 of embryological development. It is unknown as to what exactly is the direct cause of this movement is, but a number of possibilities have been identified as follows:
Muscular contraction;
Hydrostatic forces exerted by glycosaminoglycans and hyaluronin;
Mesenchymal reorganization;
Mesenchyme cell contraction;
Epithelial reorganization
Movement of the developing tongue

Suggested mechanisms for palatal fusion
Fusion between the two palatal shelves occurs during week 9 of embryonic development. In this time, the elevated palatal shelves join together to form one continuous structure, with the medial edge epithelium (the shelf surfaces which are closest to each other) disappearing.

The specific mechanism by which the medial edge epithelium disappears has been differed over by academics. The three most distinguished theories related to the explanation of palatal fusion are as follows:
Epithelial apoptosis;
Epithelial-to-mesenchymal transformation.

165. Define shock. Classify different types of shock and discuss its pathogenesis.

The state in which profound and wide spread reduction of effective perfusion leads first to reversible, and then, if prolonged, to irreversible cellular injury.

Types of shock—
Hypovolemic
Cardiogenic
Distributive or vasogenic
Extracardiac obstructive

Pathophysiology
Shocks of all form involve common cellular metabolic processes that typically end in cell injury, organ failure and death. The pathogenesis of shock involves multiple interrelated factors including
cellular ischemia,
circulating or local inflammatory mediators, and
free radical injury.

166. Why TMJ ankylosis occurs particularly in less than 10 yr of age?

In the first 2-3 yr condyle is very thin, vascular, thin cortical shell, abundant marrow and a short neck.

Marrow is highly osteogenic with self imposed immobilization especially in younger age and rapid fusion occurs.

Other factors may be: ongoing high periosteal activity

High metabolic rate.

Prolonged fixation (IMF).

Hemarthrosis.

Articular damage with loss of disk.

Disk may be lost due to infection, traumatic distraction or through displacement.

Infection destroys cartilage.

167. Define wound contraction.

It is defined as the decrease in the area of wound by the drawing together of the margins, independent of the phenomenon of re-epithelialization.

168. What is wound regeneration, wound healing and tissue repair?

A wound is defined as any anatomic or functional interruptions in the continuity of a tissue that is accompanied by cellular damage and death.

Wound healing encompasses two distinct categories of tissue restoration, regeneration and repair.

Regeneration yields a healed tissue that is structurally and functionally indistinguishable from the original tissue.

In contrast repair process achieves structural integrity through generation of a fibrous connective tissue scar.

169. What do you understand by hypertrophic scars?

Hypertrophic scarring and keloid formation represents series of derangements in orofacial healing defined as an abnormal accumulation of extracellular matrix. In the formation and remodelling of normal cutaneous scar, matrix production and degradation ordinarily balance each other and catabolism leads to matrix accumulation. The cause of this disequilibrium is not clearly understood. Scars showing largest deposition of matrix is called as keloids. Keloid scars differs from hypertrophic scars only in the relative amount of matrix produced. So

the largest deposits that are larger than anticipate are termed hypertrophic.

170. Tell me something about diabetes and wound healing.

Diabetic patients are predisposed to diversity of systemic disorders, including peripheral vascular disease, neuropathy, infection and impaired healing vascular changes, impaired blood flow, neurologic abnormalities in diabetic patients are closely related. Infection plays a major role. Several factors contributing to reduction in healing in diabetes

Reduced hypermic response to injury

A defect in inflammatory response

Impaired migration of neutrophils and macrophages

171. What are the factors affecting wound repair?

Infection

Hypoxia

Radiation

Age—younger age heals efficiently, than elderly, because aged patient show overall deterioration in general health or nutrition, perfusion and environment.

172. What are growth factors and their role in wound healing?

By definition growth factors are signaling peptides that exert various actions through specific cell surface receptors.

Biologic activity, chemical structure, molecular mechanism and target receptors of some growth factors referred to as biologic response modifiers are key regulatory roles in the process of wound healing.

The growth factors that appear to contribute to wound healing include—

Platelet derived growth factor

Transforming growth factor

Epidermal growth factor

Basic fibroblast growth factor

Insulin like growth factor

Tumour necrosis factor

173. Which fascial space infection you think is life threatening?

Lateral pharyngeal space infection.

174. What is the blood supply of a nerve?

Major supply is from 'Vasa Nervorum' contained within the epineurium. The axon which transmits electrical impulse is the functional unit of the nerve and is covered by a layer of connective tissue, the endoneurium and in turn they are surrounded by perineurium. Nerve may contain few or many fascicles. The intrabony portion of Facial nerve contain one fascicle: where as I.D nerve may have as many as 18 to 21 fascicles. The more epineurium contained in a nerve diameter the better is the ability of the nerve to withstand prolonged retraction forces during surgery and–resist injury.

175. Describe the extracranial course of facial nerve.

The posterior auricular nerve, nerve to the posterior belly of the digastric and the nerve to the stylohyoid muscle are given off upon the facial nerve's exit from the stylomastoid foramen.

The remaining fibers enter the substance of the parotid gland and divide to form the temporal, zygomatic, buccal, mandibular, and cervical branches to innervate the muscles of facial expression.

176. What are the situations when facial nerve is at risk for injury?

Orthognathic surgery
Facial trauma, laceration, fractures
TMJ surgery, arthrocentesis
Arthroscopy
Parotid surgery.

177. What is facial nerve function index devised by Peckitt and Fields?

It is a method of measuring asymmetric facial movement, also helps for monitoring progress of returning facial nerve function after surgery.

178. Which preservative is used for catgut packing?

Isopropyl alcohol.

179. What is the pharmacological mangment for keloid?

Intralesional injection of triamcinolone acetonide (an intermediate acting cortico steroid).

Since all hypertrophic scar undergo some degree of spontaneous regression, they are not treated in early phases. If the scar is still hypertrophic after 6 months surgical excision and primary closure of wound is indicated.

180. How do you classify surgical wounds?

Class I—Clean wound
Class II—Clean contaminated wound
Class III—Contaminated wound
Class IV—Dirty wound.

181. If a maxillofacial trauma patient after RTA seen in casualty after 30% loss of blood, what is your management?

30% loss of blood volume is a moderate grade of hypovolemia and can be managed adequately by IV fluids only. Cardiac stimulant, dopamine or vasopressor required in severe hypovolemia i.e. more than 40% loss.

182. What are grades of hypovolemic shock?

Mild < 20% blood loss
Cool extremeties
Diaphoresis
Anxiety
Increase capillary refill time.
Moderate 20%–40%
Same condition in addition
Tachycardia
Tachypnoea
Decreased urine output
Severe (more than 40% loss)
Same in addition they will have
Decreased blood pressure
Marked tachycardia
Hypodynamic instability

Mental status deterioration

With continued blood loss, hemoglobin <10.8 g/dL blood transfusion should be initiated.

183. What is the best guideline in case of severe trauma for quick replacement of fluids?

Urine output is a quantitative and relatively reliable indicator of organ perfusion.

184. How much of hemoglobin %concentration increases by one unit of fresh blood?

1.0 gm% whole blood of one unit will rise the hemoglobin by 1 gm% in an average size adult.

185. What do you understand by massive blood transfusion?

Transfusion greater than patients total blood volume in 24 hr or as of more than half the patients estimated blood volume over a few hours.

186. What are the complications of massive transfusion?

Hypothermia

Volume overload

Dilutional thrombocytopenia

Oxygen affinity changes

Hyperkalemia

Hypocalcemia

Hypomagnesemia

Acid/base disturbance

ARDS (acute respiratory distress syndrome)

Coagulation factor depletion.

187. What is Wolfe's graft?

Full thickness graft [includes all epidermis and dermis].

188. What is Thiersch's graft ?

Partial thickness graft [includes all epidermis and part of dermis].

189. Tell me something about split skin graft.

A rich vascular supply is essential for support of split thickness graft. It does not survive when placed directly over bone, cartilage or tendon. It is best applied over a muscle.

190. What is a port-wine stain?

It is a vascular malformation, present at birth, grows along with the child, does not regress.

191. What is strawberry hemangioma?

It is a type of capillary hemangioma.

Appears at 1–3 wk of birth.

Grows with the child up to 1 yr, the ceases to grow.

By 9 yr 90% shows complete involution.

192. A 45-year-old man presents with Progressive cervical lymph node enlargement since 4 months. What diagnostic test you would advise?

Harrison describes that in case of lymphadenopathy if the patients history and physical findings are informative of malignancy, then a prompt lymph node biopsy (excisional) should be done. FNAC is not of much use as it does not provide enough tissue to reach a diagnosis.

193. Most common organ injured in blunt abdominal trauma.

Spleen is the most common organ injured in blunt abdominal trauma. Followed by spleen are liver and kidney. Extreme blunt force to upper abdomen may fractures the pancreas, which is subjected to injury because of its position overlying rigid vertebral column. Most common abdominal organ to rupture following blunt trauma is spleen.

194. A 25-year-old man presented in casualty with fracture of 4th to 10th rib with respiratory distress after RTA. What would be your diagnosis?

Flail chest and PaO_2 of less than 60%.

195. Describe flail chest symptoms and treatment.

Result of multiple rib fracture, creating an unstable fragment of chest wall. This fragment moves paradoxically during respiration. The problem that occurs with a flailches is a contused lung paradoxical movement of the chest wall fragment, pain on respiration, assymetrical and uncoordinated movement of the thorax result in poor ventilation.

Management: First stage: Stabilization of loose segment with an external splint. Splinting decrease vital capacity but increased ventilation efficiency.

Seocnd stage: Pain relief via intercostals nerve blocks. Allows the patient to breathe deeply and cough.

Third/final stage: Volume cycled respirator with endotracheal intubation to provide intermittent mandatory ventilation (IMV).

196. Which LA agent is having vasoconstrictor action?

Cocaine.

197. What are commonly used modes of Ventilation?

Controlled mechanical ventilation (CMV).
Assisted/Controlled mechanical ventilation (A/C).
Pressure support ventilation (PSV).
Synchronized intermittent mandatory ventilation (SIMV) with or without PSV.
Continuous positive airway pressure (CPAP).

198. What is trigeminocardiac reflex?

The oculocardiac reflex, also known as Aschner phenomenon, Aschner reflex, or Aschner-Dagnini reflex, is a decrease in pulse rate associated with traction applied to extraocular muscles and/or compression of the eyeball.

199. What is parotid sialocele? How do you manage?

Sialoceles are known complications of penetrating trauma to the parotid gland. A sialocele typically presents a few days after trauma or surgery as a cystic mass in the area. However, isolated injury of the parotid duct without facial nerve injury is rare, and almost all reported cases have occurred in adults following an assault with a knife, bottle, or firearm. Failure to detect and repair a ductal injury can result in a salivary fistula, sialocele,

facial abscess, or atrophy of the involved parotid gland.

Surgical modalities usually involve an operation with possible facial nerve injury, with the risk of a general anesthetic, and with prolonged hospitalization to be considered. Among non-surgical modalities radiation and laissez-faire are of questionable efficacy.

200. What is paralytic lagophthalmos?

Inability to close the eyelid seen in facial nerve palsy is known as paralytic lagophthalmos. Corrected by gold implant, tarsorrhaphy.

201. What is Heyton Williams wiring?

Figure of eight wiring.

202. What is primary intraosseous carcinoma?

It is the squamous cell carcinoma arising with in the jaw and has no initial connection with oral mucosa and develops from the residues of odontogenic epithelium.

203. How you classify primary intraosseous carcinoma?

Type I: PIOC exodontogenic cyst
Type IIA: Malignant ameloblastoma
Type IIB: Ameloblastic carcinoma arising *de novo* exameloblastoma or exodontoganic cyst
Type III: PIOC arising *de novo*
Keratinizing type
Non keratinizing type
Type IV: Intraosseous mucoepidermoid carcinoma.

204. What is adjuvant chemotherapy?

Adjuvant chemotherapy is administration of chemo therapic agents after definitive treatment with radiation or chemotherapy in a effort to reduce locoregional and systemic recurrence.

205. What is the rationale behind chemoradio-therapy and concurrent therapy?

rational for combining chemotherapy and radiotherapy concomitantly in the treatment of head and neck cancer exist chemotherapy can sensitize the tumor to radiotherapy by inhibiting tumor repopulation, preferentially killing hypoxic cell, sterilizing micro metastatic diseases outside the radiation field and decreasing the tumor mass. Which lead to improve blood supply and reoxygenation.

206. What is normal factor VIII level in blood?
0.5–1.5 IU per ml.

207. What is Erbs point?
It is a point located on lateral surface of neck where a confluence of nerve is seen.

208. What is normal CD4 count?
CD4 are those cells which express CD4 category of antigen on their surface, helper T-cell are a type of cd4 cell. Its normal count is 590–1120 cells/cubic mm.
If it is less than 100:
Evaluate the patient for severe opportunistic diseases.
If white count is expected to decrease then delay the elective surgical procedure till white count increases.

209. What is optical coherence tomography?
Optical coherence tomography was first used by Huang et al. in 1991, it is a non invasive interferometric tomographic method of imaging that allows millimeter penetration with micrometer scale with axial and lateral resolution, this time resolve technique extensively used in ophthalmology now has been used in head and neck for hemangioma skin lesion, nasopharynx and orophayrnx lesion and tried to detect areas of inflammation, dysplasia and cancer.

210. How you will classify neck dissection?
It can be comprehensive neck dissection or selective neck dissection,
Comprehensive: radical neck dissection, extended neck dissection, modified neck dissection type I, II and III.
Selective neck dissection: supraomohyoid neck dissection, jugular neck dissection, central compartment neck dissection, posterolateral neck dissection.

211. Explain elective and therapeutic neck dissection.
If a neck dissection is carried out when there is no evidence of neck diseases it is termed as elective.
If a neck dissection is undertaken for metastatic diseases in the neck it is called a therapeutic neck dissection.

212. What is Kole's procedure?
It is done for correction of anterior open bite. A standard subapical osteotomy is performed after which a portion is removed of the lower border is as in a genioplasty and wedged into the space produced btween the dentoalveolar segment, this newly formed chin is then reshaped and wound closed in layers.

213. What is brown tumor?
Brown tumor is an uncommon sequel of hyperparathyroidism. The lesion localizes in areas of intense bone resorption, and the bone defect becomes filled with fibroblastic tissue that can deform the bone and stimulate a neoplastic process. These tumors have a brown or yellow hue.

214. How many lymph nodes present in the body?
800.

214. How many lymph nodes are there in head and neck region?
300.

216. What is collar-stud abscess?
Cervical lymphadenitis seen in tuberculosis.

217. Examples of simple fractures in mandible.
Fracture of condyle.

218. Commonest cause of death in fracture of jaw.
Airway obstruction.

219. Is seqesterum more radiopaque or radiolucent then surrounding bone. And why?
It is more radio opaque as there is no blood supply to it, i.e. it is avascular.

220. What is involucrum?
It is a sheath of new bone formed around new bone.

221. Which component of radiation is used in radiotherapy?
Gamma radiation.

222. Uses of radioactive materials in diagnosis?
They are use in radioassays and to study tissue metabolism.

223. What is parotid plexus?
Facial nerve forms a plexus of nerves within the gland and divides the gland arbitrarily into two lobes (not a true division) is known as parotid plexus.

224. What is carotid plexus?
It is a plexus of nerve surrounding the internal carotid artery, or a autonomic plexus that is formed around external carotid and its branch.

225. Where exactly external carotid artery ligation done?
External carotid artery is ligated after it gives superior thyroid artery. It is ligated here because:
1. It makes certain that we are ligating external carotid artery as there is no branch of internal carotid in neck.
2. Most important factor is to avoid transfer of emboli from site of formation (ligation site) to internal carotid system.

226. How will you differentiate between Cushing;'s syndrome from Cushing's disease?
Cushing's syndrome refers to hypercortisolemia and its associated signs and symptoms due to any cause.
Cushing's disease refers to hypercortisolemia due to ACTH overproduction by a pituitory adenoma.

227. What are tumor markers?
Tumors include enzymes, harmones gene loci, and oncofetal antigens that are associated with particular tumors. The markers reflect the presence of the tumor or the quantity of tumor.

228. Define carcinogegesis.
Carcinogenesis is the alteration of normal cells into malignant cells. It is generally a multistage evolution of genetic and epigenetic alterations that causes cells to escape the normal growth constraints of the host.

229. What do you know about oncogenes?
Oncogenes in humans have the capacity to transform normal cells into malignant ones. These genes acquire or mutated during life make the patient susceptible to cancer by altering or impairing several processes.

230. What is field cancerization?
Slaughter and colleages first proposed concept of field cancerisation in 1953 as the preconditioning of an are of epithelium to cancer growth by a carcinogenic agent this definition was in response to a significant proportion of oral squamous carcinoma occurred multifocally and that tumor tended to be located within a patch of histologically abnormal cells.

231. What is metachronous tumor?
Patients diagnosed with a head and neck cancers are predisposed to the development of a second tumor within aerodigestive tract. The detection of second primary lesion more than 6 months after the initial diagnosis is referred to as metachronous tumor.

232. What is delphian node?
It is a pretracheal lymph node which may become involved by advanced tumors of the glottis with subglottic spread.

233. Skull base fracture what are clinical signs you look for?
Otorrhea, rhinorrhea, raccoon eye, and Battles sign (ecchymosis behind the ear).

234. What is seed and soil theory?

Several types of tumors metastasize in an organ specific pattern depedance of the seed or cancer cells on the soil (the secondary organ) that is once cells have reached secondary organ, their growth efficiency in that organ is based on the compatibility of the cancer cells "biology" with its new microenvironment.

235. What are contraindication for tracheal intubation (oral and nasal)?

1. Tracheal fracture
2. Coagulopathy
3. CSF rhinorrhea
4. Nasal occlusion, nasal fracture.

236. What is the main content of hemaccel?

Degraded gelatin.

237. Which is the best vein for parenteral nutrition?

Subclavian vein. The preferred site for central vein infusion is superior vena cava and preferred access sites are subclavien, jugular, femoral vein.

238. How do you assess shock clinically?

Urine output.

239. What is Mohs surgery?

It is indicated for tumors of eyelid or nose. Where minimal amount of skin tissue is removed in this micrographically controlled Surgery clinically apparent tumor is removed by curettage or excision the surgeon then removes thin layer of tissue usually 1 mm in thickness. Its advantage is highest cure rate for primary Basal cell carcinoma but the disadvantage is time consuming and additional anesthesia.

240. What is chemodectoma?

That is also known as carotid body tumor or potato tumor, arises from chemoreceptor cells on the medial side of carotid bulb Histologocally it is a non chromaffin paraganglioma which has a association with "pheochromocytoma" present most commonly in 5th decade approximately 10% have family history Patient often presents with a long history of several years of a slowly enlarging painless lump at the carotid bifurcation, the mass is often rubbery, pusatile and is mobile from side to side but not up and down A bruit may also be present. These tumors rarely metastasize and their ovrerall rate of growth is slow and need for surgical removal must be considered carefully as complication of surgery are potentially serious.

241. What are the structures preserved in functional neck dissection?

Sternocleidomas oid muscle and Internal jugular vein.

242. What are structures preserved in radical neck dissection?

Vagus nerve

243. What is classical radical neck dissection?

This involves the removal of:

a. Cervical lymphatics and lymph nodes
b. Internal jugular vein
c. Accessary nerve
d. Submandibular gland
e. Sternomastoid muscle.

244. Where branchial cyst is seen?

Branchial cysts are characteristically seen anterior and deep to upper third of sternocleidomastoid muscle and are remnants of branchial apparatus present in fetal life.

245. What is vicryl?

It is a copolymer of glycolide and lactide a synthetic absorbable suture material which completely absorbs by hydrolysis slower than catgut causes less of a reaction on implantation. Its tensile streanth lasts for approximately 3–4 weeks and is indicated for soft tissue approximation.

246. What are biological principles behind osseointegration in implantology?
1. The main principle is implant stability and load consideration .
2. The formation of direct bone implant contact is the prerequisite before loading could be commenced and bone healing is one of the several important factors.
3. Absence of mobility which is the main clinical manifestation of a successful implant.

247. What are the main determination of implant stability?
The main determination of implant stability are:
1. Mechanical property of bone tissue at the implant site which is determined by the composition bone at the implant site and is influenced by stage of healing since soft trabecular bone is transformed to dense cortical bone near the implant surface.
2. Second factor is influenced by surgical technique, the design of implant, and the osseointegration process. Successful healing results in bone formation that reinforces the interface zone and forms bridges with a direct contact between implant surface and the surrounding bone.

248. Name some lateral neck mass as a differential diagnosis.
Neoplastic—Metastatic upper jugular and jugulodigastric oral cavitry oropharynx and laryngeal primaries.
Lower jugular hypopharynx and thyroid primaries, submandibular gland nasal paranasal sinuses and facial skin primaries
Carotid body tumor
Non-Hodgkin's lymphoma
Hodgekin's lymphoma
Hemangioma
Schwannoma
Salivary gland tumor

Congenital/developmental-branchial cyst Sialadenopathy, lymphangioma,
Inflammatory—Bacterial adenitis, viraladenitis, sialadenitis, scrofula (tuberculosis).

249. Patient aged 45 reports with lymphadenopathy. What are the clinical assessments?
Clinical examination by careful palpation of different levels palpable nodes are described by location size, tenderness, temperature. compressibility,texture fluctuation induration whether it is freely mobile in horizontal verticalor, or is fixed to underlying tissue or whether there are changes in overlying skin. Trans-illumination may aid in determining whether the lesion is fluid filled.
If in the midline the swelling should be evaluated while patient is swallowing.
Swelling which moves while swallowing (rise and fall) are likely thyroglossal duct cysts. Swelling that are pulsatile with palpable thrill or bruit on auscultation may be indicative of a vascular lesion.

250. What are oncogenes and how they are related to cancer?
Oncogene is a gene that has the potential to cause cancer, they are often mutated or expressed at highloads. Anoncogene is a gene found in chromosome of tumor cells whose action is associated with initial and continuing conversion of normal cells into cancer cells. Most normal cells undergo programmed form of death (apoptosis) Activated oncogenes cause those cells that ought to die to survive and proliferate instead. Oncogenes require an additional step such as mutation in another gene or environmental factors such as viral infection to cause cancer.

251. What is proto–oncogene?
A proto-oncogene is a normal gene that can become an oncogene due to mutations or increased expression. The resultant protein may be termed as oncogene by a relatively small modification of its original function.

252. What are lymph node?

Lymph nodes are smallnnround organs that are part of the bodys lymphatic system, found throughout the body and are connected to one another by lymph vessels A clear fluid called lymph flows through lymph vessels and lymph nodes. Lymph nodes are important parts of bodys immune system. They contain B lymphocutes, T lymphocytes and other types of immune system cells. Lymph nodes are also important in helping to determine whether cancer cells have developed the ability to spread to other parts of body.

253. What is a sentinel lymph node?

A sentinel lymph node is defined as the first lymph node to which cancer cells are most likely to spread from a primary tumor. Sometime there can be more than one sentinel lymph node.

254. What is a sentinel lymph node biopsy?

Sentinel lymph node biopsy technique involves injection of radio labeld tracer around the periphery of the tumor, allowing tracer to drain via the lymphatic system to the first echelon of nodes. The sentinel node are then delineated using gamma probe followed by surgical removal of the node(s) in a manner that is oncologically safe. These nodes are then examined by frozen section if micro-metastasis are identified the patient recieves a SND. If negative SLNB result suggests that malignancy has not developed the ability to spread to lymph nodes. This information helps the surgeon to stage the cancer and plan treatment .

255. What is Kuffners osteotomy?

Kuffner's os teotomy is another name to Lefort III osteotomy.

256. What is McEwans triangle?

McEwans triangle is formed by posterior border of mandible, posterior belly of digastrics and the tympanic plates.

257. How much is the hydrostatic pressure within a radicular cyst?

Hydrostatic pressure is around 70 cm H_2O.

258. How do you decide intubation in trauma patient?

When there is respiratory distress and GCS less than 9 due to head injury.

259. Which cervical vertebra has no body and spine?

Atlas.

260. Name hypothesis related to trigeminal neuralgia.

1. Blood vessel—usually artery compressing the Trigeminal nerve root.
2. Bioresonance hypothesis—states that when vibration frequency of a structure surrounding trigeminal nerve becomes to its natural frequency the resonance of the Tri. nerve occurs. This bioresonance can damage tri. nerve fibers and lead to the abnormal transmission of the impulse which may finally result in facial pain.
3. The ignition hypothesis—This is based on recent advances in the understanding of abnormal electrical behavior in injured sensory neurons. Neuralgia results from specific abnormality of tri.afferent neurons in the trigeminal root or ganglion. The injury renders axons hyperexcitable. This hyprexcitable afferents in turn give rise to pain paroxysm.

261. What are biomechanics of mandible with regards to osteosynthesis?

Mainly 2 basic functionally adequate types of fixation which are semirigid load bearing and load sharing (a) superior portion designed as the tention zone (b) inferior portion designed as compression zone

262. What is hunting bow concept?

Mandible is similar to hunting bow in shape; strongest in symphysis (midline) and weakest at both ends (condyle)

263. **What are advantages of Champy's principle?**
    1. Plate placement sites are easily accessible intraorally.
    2. Small miniplates are required for fixation.
    3. Technique uses natural functional forces, thus, minimizing surgical exposure.

264. **How lymphatics originates?**
    They originate as lymph capillaries.

265. **What is prelaryngeal node?**
    Prelaryngeal node lies on cricothyroid membrane and drain subglottic region of larynx and pyriform sinuses also known as Delphian node.

266. **What order lymph nodes examined?**
    – Upper horizontal chain
    – External jugular chain
    – Internal jugular chain, spinal accessory,
    – Transeverse cervical chain
    – Anterior jugular chain
    – Juxta visceral chain.

267. **What are 3 lymph tissues?**
    a. Diffuse lymph tissues—no capsule present found in all organs.
    b. Lymphatic nodes—no capsule found singly or in clusters.
    c. Lymphatic organ—Capsule present, found in lymph node, thymus, spleen.

268. **What are methods of assessment of airway?**
    a. Mallampatti classification.
    b. Wilsons scoring system.
    c. Mentohyoid, thyromental and sternomental distance.
    d. Mouthopening less than 4 cm suggestsdifficulty in intubation.
    e. Reduced TMJ movements.

269. **What is primary goal of early treatment of trauma patient?**
    To provide sufficient tissue oxygenation to avoid lethal organ failure and secondary CNS damage.

270. **How do you perform airway with cervical spine injury?**
    Looking for foreign bodies, noisy breathing is a good indicator of airway obstruction.

271. **What are the indication for a definitive airway?**
    Obstruction definitive:
    – Inadequate breathing oxygen saturation less than 90%
    – Inadequate circulation systolic BP less than 75 despite adequate fluid

272. **Which sign necessitate urgent intubation?**
    Strider.

273. **Other than airway, what else ensures ventilation?**
    a. Adequate gas exchange is mandatory
    b. Artificial Ventilation

274. **What is hypogeusia?**
    Diminished taste.

275. **What is odynophagia?**
    Painful swallowing.

276. **What is the goal of IMRT? (intencity modulated radiotherapy)**
    a. It is a novel technique for unknown primary SCCHN.
    b. Reduces local failure by improved target volume, localization, dose escalation, etc.
    c. Reduces toxicity by improved dose distribution especially to parotid region.

277. **What is the origin of nasolacrimal duct?**
    It originates few millimeters posterior to the medial canthal tendon and courses from lacrimal sac inferiorly and posteriorly before becoming enclosed in the bony canal and draining through the valve of Hasner into inferior meatus of nose.

278. **Mention signs of skull-base fracture.**
    a. Battle sign
    b. CSF leakage
    c. Panda face
    d. Hemotympanum.

279. **What are indications for intubation in head injury?**

a. Deppressed level of consciousness

b. Cannot maintain airway

c. Need for hyperventilation

d. Extensive maxillofacial fracture.

280. What is the normal intracranial pressure?
Normal intracranial pressure varies from 8 to 12 mm Hg.

281. Name the longest cranial nerve which is injured in head injury.
Abducent nerve.

282. Mention 2 important alarming finding in head injury.
a. Bradycardia
b. Pupillary dilatation.

283. Mention 2 causes of death due to head injury.
a. Raised intracranial pressure
b. Injury to vital organ.

284. Blood-brain barrier is formed by which process?
Astrocyte food process.

285. Which is the most extensively distributed cranial nerve?
Vagus nerve.

286. What is the dangerous zone of scalp?
Fourth layer or loose subcutaneous tissue containing Emissary vein allowing free movement of layer 1 to 3 and 4th layer to spread infection through emissary vien to intracranially.

287. What is the clinical finding in acute increase in intracranial pressure?
Reaspiratory irregularity.

288. In head injury, what do you mean contusion? Explain.
Contusions are areas of brain injury Intracranial Hematoma showing areas of mixed density in CT image signs of which include severe headache dizziness, vomiting, increase size of one pupilor sudden weakness in an arm or leg. The person may seem restlessagitated or irritable lasting for several hours to weeks depending on the seriousness of injury diagnosis made through CT scan or MRI.

289. What are the guidelines for advising CT scan for head injury patients?
a. GCS <13 at any point of time
b. GCS 13 or 14 at 2 hr
c. Focal neurological deficit
d. Siezures.

290. What is boering therapy ?
Educating the patient about the nature of their problem especially TMJ about limiting eccentric jaw movement, eliminating any pathologic habits instructing about habitually perform nonclenching techniques for TMJ dysfunction syndrome cases.

Index

Page numbers followed by '*f*' and '*t*' indicate figures and tables, respectively.